Master Techniques in Blepharoplasty and Periorbital Rejuvenation

Guy G. Massry • Mark R. Murphy
Babak Azizzadeh
Editors

Master Techniques in Blepharoplasty and Periorbital Rejuvenation

Foreword by Allen Putterman, MD and Norman Pastorek, MD

Springer

Editors
Guy G. Massry, MD
Director
Ophthalmic Plastic Surgery
Spaulding Drive Cosmetic Surgery and Dermatology
Beverly Hills, California, USA
gmassry@aol.com

Mark R. Murphy, MD
Director
Palm Beach Facial Plastic Surgery
Palm Beach Gardens, Florida, USA
mrm9002@gmail.com

Babak Azizzadeh, MD
Center for Advanced Facial Plastic Surgery
Assistant Clinical Professor of Surgery
Department of Facial Plastic and Reconstructive Surgery
David Geffen School of Medicine at UCLA
Beverly Hills, California, USA
md@facialplastics.info

ISBN 978-1-4614-0066-0 ISBN 978-1-4614-0067-7 (eBook)
DOI 10.1007/978-1-4614-0067-7
Springer New York Dordrecht Heidelberg London

Library of Congress Control Number: 2011933599

© Springer Science+Business Media, LLC 2011
All rights reserved. This work may not be translated or copied in whole or in part without the written permission of the publisher (Springer Science+Business Media, LLC, 233 Spring Street, New York, NY 10013, USA), except for brief excerpts in connection with reviews or scholarly analysis. Use in connection with any form of information storage and retrieval, electronic adaptation, computer software, or by similar or dissimilar methodology now known or hereafter developed is forbidden.
The use in this publication of trade names, trademarks, service marks, and similar terms, even if they are not identified as such, is not to be taken as an expression of opinion as to whether or not they are subject to proprietary rights.
While the advice and information in this book are believed to be true and accurate at the date of going to press, neither the authors nor the editors nor the publisher can accept any legal responsibility for any errors or omissions that may be made. The publisher makes no warranty, express or implied, with respect to the material contained herein.

Printed on acid-free paper

Springer is part of Springer Science+Business Media (www.springer.com)

Foreword

In *Master Techniques in Blepharoplasty and Periorbital Rejuvenation*, the latest textbook on this specialized area of aesthetic facial surgery, Drs. Massry, Azizzadeh, and Murphy have skillfully combined the talent of various leaders in their fields to create a comprehensive and well-detailed reference. Other texts have described the many considerations and techniques of extended cosmetic blepharoplasty but this book is unique. It provides the most updated and comprehensive information on the discipline. The editors have reached out of the realm of their specific subspecialties and engaged in a multidisciplinary approach by adding the expertise of oculoplastic, facial plastic, and plastic surgeons, in addition to contributions from dermatologists. A textbook on the shared experience of authorities in these fields is a tremendous contribution, has been sorely lacking in the literature, and will add significantly to our approach to and performance of surgery.

I have been privileged to observe the evolution of blepharoplasty through a long career in oculoplastic surgery. During my initial introduction to this subject, there were short chapters on upper and lower blepharoplasty in several textbooks that dealt with all other aspects of oculoplastic surgery or general plastic surgery. The usual description of upper blepharoplasty was to excise large amounts of skin and fat with direct closure of the wound. Lower eyelid blepharoplasty was performed externally with excision of as much fat as could be prolapsed, in addition to significant skin excision. The elevation of the eyebrow was usually accomplished by a direct excision of an ellipse of skin above the brow. It took some time before the complications of lagophthalmos, lower lid retraction and ectropion, hollowing of the lower lid, lowering of the eyebrow, and significant eyebrow scars were noted as problems. With time, we learned to be more conservative in the excision of eyelid skin and fat, to reconstruct upper eyelid creases, to address the lower lid from a transconjunctival approach, to reposition fat, and to horizontally tighten the lower eyelid. We also learned to lift the forehead with small skin incisions in the hairline and with the use of endoscopic-guided technology. Finally, midface lifting and laser resurfacing the eyelid and periorbital areas were added to our armamentarium. This textbook "masterfully" covers all these topics and their evolution in a concise and clear way.

In this text Dr. Massry and colleagues have added chapters on the beautiful eye, the prominent globe, and wound modulation after surgery. These topics are not routinely covered in most standard texts, and are ones which provide information critical to our contemporary understanding of patient evaluation and surgery. In addition, the editors have included sections on brow lifting, blepharoplasty, midface lifting, neuromodulation, volume preservation/replacement with fat and fillers, the management of festoons, and laser incisional surgery and skin resurfacing. The book is truly comprehensive; and like the title of the first chapter, it is an "evolution" in the field. I commend Drs. Massry, Azizzadeh, and Murphy as they are master editors in creating this fine textbook.

Chicago, IL — Allen M. Putterman, MD

Foreword

This textbook, *Master Techniques in Blepharoplasty and Periorbital Rejuvenation*, is an anthology of great significance in the advancement of the art and science of aesthetic surgery and in the treatment of the eyelids and periorbita. Much has been written about this area of the face, as it is imperative that the initial recommendations and treatment options be accurate in planning, and exceedingly as perfect in execution. The textbook promotes this supposition. It is well known that no secondary surgery of the face is more difficult than that involving the eyelids. It is not hard to appreciate why in prose, poetry, and song, the eyes more than any other facial feature have been recognized through the ages as the portal of the soul, and a true reflection of our humanity. It is little wonder then, that so many medical and surgical disciplines, such as facial plastic surgery, plastic surgery, oculoplastic surgery, and dermatology, intersect at aesthetic eyelid and periorbital care.

Drs. Guy Massry, Babak Azizzadeh, and Mark Murphy have brought together in this book the brightest and most forward thinking physicians and surgeons whose interest, experience, expertise, and intellectual focus is on beautification and restoration of the aging eye and periorbita. Herein, these experts have given us a view of what is new, innovative, and progressive in aesthetic treatment of the eyelids and periorbital region. They also have looked back to remind us of the essential truths discovered by the masters who have gone before into surgical care of this precious facial real estate. This textbook is truly worthy of its title.

New York, NY — Norman Pastorek, MD

Preface

Aesthetic eyelid surgery is perhaps the most complex and controversial area of facial aesthetic rejuvenation. Surgical outcomes determine patient appearance, function, psychology, and – most importantly – vision. There is truly no room for error as surgical results cannot be hidden and complications may render significant consequence. Fortunately, the history of eyelid surgery and its contemporary practice is founded on the contributions of expert physicians and surgeons who have molded the field into a unique and specialized discipline. We have been acutely aware of this concept and have been privileged to bring it to the forefront in *Master Techniques in Blepharoplasty and Periorbital Rejuvenation.*

This text follows on the footsteps of its predecessors *Master Techniques in Facial Rejuvenation* (2006) and *Master Techniques in Rhinoplasty* (2011). What differentiates this particular book from others in its field is that to bring justice to the understanding, planning, and performance of eyelid and periorbital surgery requires the perspective of the varied specialties which contribute to the constant evolution of the field. We have been blessed with this perspective as the influence of leaders in oculoplastic, facial plastic, and plastic surgery and dermatology have been molded into the development of this text. We are proud to have been involved in this project and hope it helps guide other as it has ourselves.

We have also been fortunate to have been surrounded with a unique and dedicated core of individuals at Springer who have made our job much easier than it could have been. We are deeply indebted to all who have contributed. We are especially appreciative of the tireless efforts of Catherine Paduani, Barbara Lopez-Lucio (developmental editors), and Sara Krause (illustrator), without whom this project would not have been completed. Their dedication, long hours, and unwavering commitment have been unparalleled and cannot be emphasized with words alone.

Finally, nothing in life comes easy or without a price. This textbook has been a labor of love, an education, and an honor for us to be involved in. It has also been a very time-consuming and all-encompassing project. It would not be here today if not for the support, patience, and constant motivation of our friends, family, and loved ones who make our life endeavors worthwhile. We are fortunate to have them at our sides and thank them all for bringing such value and meaning to our lives.

Guy G. Massry, MD
Mark R. Murphy, MD
Babak Azizzadeh, MD

Contents

Contributors

Richard L. Anderson, MD, FACS Medical Director, Center for Facial Appearances, Salt Lake City, UT, USA

Babak Azizzadeh, MD Center for Advanced Facial Plastic Surgery, Assistant Clinical Professor of Surgery, Department of Facial Plastic and Reconstructive Surgery, David Geffen School of Medicine at UCLA, Beverly Hills, CA, USA

Sterling S. Baker, MD Assistant Clinical Professor, Department of Ophthalmology and Dermatology, University of Oklahoma College of Medicine, Oklahoma City, OK, USA

Adjunct Clinical Professor, Department of Dermatology, University of Oklahoma College of Medicine, Oklahoma City, OK, USA

Geeta Belsare, MD Instructor, Department of Ophthalmology, Loyola University Medical Center, Stritch School of Medicine, Maywood, IL, USA

Adam G. Buchanan, MD Assistant Chief, Department of Ophthalmology, Madigan Army Medical Center, Tacoma, WA, USA

Craig N. Czyz, DO, FACOS Chair, Section Head, and Clinical Faculty, Department of Ophthalmology, Section of Oculofacial Plastic and Reconstructive Surgery, Ohio University, OhioHealth Doctors Hospital, Columbus, OH, USA

Raymond S. Douglas, MD, PhD Associate Professor, Department of Ophthalmology and Visual Sciences, University of Michigan, Ann Arbor, MI, USA

Jill A. Foster, MD, FACS Associate Clinical Professor, Director, Division of Oculofacial Plastic and Reconstructive Surgery, Department of Ophthalmology, Ohio State University, Columbus, OH, USA

Dan Georgescu, MD, PhD Clinical Assistant Professor, Wilmer Eye Institute, Johns Hopkins Medical Center, Baltimore, MD, USA

Mark J. Glasgold, MD Clinical Associate Professor of Surgery, Department of Surgery, UMDNJ-Robert Wood Johnson Medical School, Highland Park, NJ, USA

Robert A. Glasgold, MD Clinical Assistant Professor of Surgery, Department of Surgery, UMDNJ-Robert Wood Johnson Medical School, Highland Park, NJ, USA

Robert A. Goldberg, MD Professor, Department of Ophthalmology and Oribitofacial Surgery, Jules Stein Eye Institute at UCLA, Los Angeles, CA, USA

Gregory J. Griepentrog, MD Clinical Instructor, Department of Ophthalmology and Visual Sciences, University of Wisconsin-Madison, Madison, WI, USA

Douglas G. Hamilton, MD Private Practice, Dermatologist and Assistant Clinical Professor, David Geffen School of Medicine at UCLA, Beverly Hills, CA, USA

Morris E. Hartstein, MD, FACS Clinical Associate Professor, Department of Ophthalmology and Division of Plastic Surgery, St. Louis University School of Medicine, St. Louis, MO, USA

Director, Oculoplastic Surgery, Department of Ophthalmology, Assaf Harofeh Medical Center, Beer Yaacov, Israel

Jonathan A. Hoenig, MD Assistant Professor, Jules Stein Eye Institute, UCLA Medical Center, Private Practice, Beverly Hills, California, USA

Paul K. Holden, MD, MS Holden Facial Plastic Surgery, Scottsdale, AZ, USA

John B. Holds, MD, FACS Clinical Professor, Departments of Ophthalmology and Otolaryngology Head and Neck Surgery, St. Louis University School of Medicine, Director, Ophthalmic Plastic and Cosmetic Surgery, Inc., Des Peres, MO, USA

Amina Husain, MD Oculoplastic Fellow, Department of Ophthalmology, Duke Eye Center, Durham, NC, USA

Amir M. Karam, MD Director of Facial Plastic Surgery, Carmel Valley Facial Plastic Surgery, San Diego, CA, USA

Don O. Kikkawa, MD Professor of Clinical Ophthalmology and Chief of Division of Ophthalmic Plastic and Reconstructive Surgery, Department of Ophthalmology, Shiley Eye Center, University of California, La Jolla, San Diego, CA, USA

Bobby S. Korn, MD Assistant Professor of Clinical Ophthalmology, Department of Ophthalmology, Shiley Eye Center, University of California, La Jolla, San Diego, CA, USA

Jonathan S. Kulbersh, MD Fellow in Facial Plastic Surgery, Spaulding Drive Cosmetic Surgery and Dermatology, Beverly Hills, CA, USA

Samuel M. Lam, MD, FACS Director, Willow Bend Wellness Center, Plano, TX, USA

Vincent B. Lam, MD Department of Ophthalmology, Drexel University College of Medicine, Columbus, OH, USA

Kimberly J. Lee, MD Assistant Clinical Professor, Department of Surgery, Division of Head and Neck Surgery, University of California, Los Angeles, CA, USA

Attending Surgery, Department of Facial Plastic and Reconstructive Surgery, Cedars-Sinai Medical Center, Los Angeles, CA, USA

Seongmu Lee, MD Department of Ophthalmology, David Geffen School of Medicine at UCLA, Los Angeles, CA, USA

Mark J. Lucarelli, MD, FACS Professor, Director, Oculofacial and Orbital Surgery, Department of Ophthalmology and Visual Sciences, University of Wisconsin-Madison, Madison, WI, USA

Ronald Mancini, MD Assistant Professor, Department of Ophthalmology, UT Southwestern Medical Center, Dallas, TX, USA

Corey S. Maas, MD, FACS The Maas Clinic, Associate Clinical Professor, University of California-San Francisco, San Francisco, CA, USA

Guy G. Massry, MD Director, Ophthalmic Plastic Surgery, Spaulding Drive Cosmetic Surgery and Dermatology, Beverly Hills, CA, USA

John D. McCann, MD, PhD Medical Director, Center for Facial Appearances, Salt Lake City, UT, USA

Asa D. Morton, MD, BA Director of Oculoplastic and Facial Reconstruction, Eye Care of San Diego, San Diego, CA, USA

Mark R. Murphy, MD Director, Palm Beach Facial Plastic Surgery, Palm Beach Gardens, FL, USA

Paul S. Nassif, MD Spaulding Drive Cosmetic Surgery and Dermatology, Assistant Clinical Professor, Department of Otolarlaryngology–Head and Neck Surgery, University of Southern California School of Medicine, Beverly Hills, California, USA

Kartik D. Nettar, MD The Maas Clinic, San Francisco, CA, USA

Joe Niamtu III, DMD Cosmetic Facial Surgeon, Private Practice, Midlothian, VA, USA

Sang-Rog Oh, MD Clinical Fellow in Oculofacial and Reconstructive Surgery, Department of Ophthalmology, Shiley Eye Center, University of California, La Jolla, San Diego, CA, USA

Stephen W. Perkins, MD Meridian Plastic Surgeons, Indianapolis, IN, USA

Ayelet Priel, MD Clinical Fellow in Oculofacial and Reconstructive Surgery, Department of Ophthalmology, Shiley Eye Center, University of California, San Diego, La Jolla, CA, USA

Allen M. Putterman, MD Professor, Department of Ophthalmology and Visual Sciences, Illinois Eye and Ear Infirmary, University of Illinois at Chicago, Chicago, IL, USA

Nicholas A. Ramey, MD Resident, Department of Ophthalmology, Duke Eye Center, Durham, NC, USA

Oscar M. Ramirez, MD, FACS Director, Sanctuary Plastic Surgery, Boca Raton, FL, USA

Usha P. Reddy, MD Fellow in Oculoplastic and Reconstructive Surgery, Department of Ophthalmology, Duke University Medical Center, Durham, NC, USA

Kiran Sajja, MD Clinical Assistant Professor, Department of Ophthalmology and Visual Sciences, Havener Eye Institute, The Ohio State University, Columbus, OH, USA

Adam J. Scheiner, MD Oculoplastic Surgeon, Tampa Eye Clinic, Tampa, FL, USA

Christian L. Stallworth, MD Assistant Professor, Department of Otolaryngology–Head and Neck Surgery, University of Texas Health Science Center at San Antonio, San Antonia, TX, USA

Mehryar Taban, MD Associate Diplomate, Department of Ophthalmology and Orbitofacial Surgery, Jules Stein Eye Institute, David Geffen School of Medicine at UCLA, Los Angeles, CA, USA

Kevin S. Tan, MD Resident Physician, Department of Ophthalmology, Shiley Eye Center, University of California, La Jolla, San Diego, CA, USA

Jeremiah P. Tao, MD, FACS Assitant Professor, Director, Oculoplastic Surgery, Department of Ophthalmology, University of California, Irvine, CA, USA

Betina Wachter, MD Clinical Instructor, Oculoplastic Surgery, Department of Ophthalmology, University of California, Irvine, CA, USA

Tom D. Wang, MD Professor and Chief, Division of Facial Plastic and Reconstructive Surgery, Department of Otolaryngology–Head and Neck Surgery, Oregon Health and Science University, Portland, OR, USA

Daniel J. Woodward, MD Pediatric Cardiac Anesthesiologist, Department of Anesthesiology, Oregon Health and Sciences University, Portland, OR, USA

Julie A. Woodward, MD Associate Professor, Chief Division of Oculofacial Surgery, Department of Ophthalmology, Duke University, Durham, NC, USA

Steven Yoon, MD Clinical Instructor, Oculoplastic Surgery, Department of Ophthalmology, University of California, Irvine, CA, USA

Kenneth C.Y. Yu, MD Department of Otolaryngology-Head and Neck Surgery, Wilford Hall Medical Center, Lackland Air Force Base, TX, USA

Part I

General Considerations

1 Periorbital Aesthetic Surgery: The Evolution of a Multidisciplinary Surgical Subspecialty

Jonathan S. Kulbersh, Guy G. Massry, and Babak Azizzadeh

Key Points

- Aesthetic eyelid and periorbital surgery is a multidisciplinary field of cosmetic surgery.
- Ophthalmologists, oculoplastic surgeons, otolaryngologists, facial plastic surgeons, plastic surgeons, and dermatologists have contributed to the evolution of the field.
- Early surgical procedures focused on excisional or "subtractive" techniques.
- Our current understanding of periorbital and facial aging is that volume loss is one of the major factors leading to involutional changes.
- Modern surgery has led to a paradigm shift of tissue preservation and augmentation, associated with less aggressive tissue excision, to prevent further volume depletion.
- Endoscopic surgical technology has become an essential part of forehead, eyebrow, and midface surgery.
- Neuromodulators and fillers are widely used for less invasive cosmetic improvement of the periorbital area.

1.1 Introduction

The ancient Greek word *aisthetikos* describes a passion for that which is beautiful. It is this passion that has driven the evolution of aesthetic and reconstructive periorbital surgery. The treatment of "relaxed skin of the upper eyelid" was first described by Aulus Cornelius Celsus, a Roman encyclopedic, in his textbook *De re Medica* in 25–30 AD [1] (Fig. 1.1). Here, we have the beginnings of the numerous and varied contributions to the evolution of periocular surgery. Over the last 2,000 years, there have been great advances in the field, and it has been due to continued contributions from physicians, scientists, and scholars from a variety of disciplines. In the current age of medical subspecialization, there are many different physicians/surgeons with overlapping expertise in the treatment of the aging eyelids and surrounding regions. The evolution of how we approach and provide surgical options in this area could not be possible without the contributions of ophthalmologists, oculoplastic surgeons, facial plastic surgeons, otolaryngologists, plastic surgeons, and dermatologists. Their combined contributions have been a synergistic and collaborative movement that has resulted in a better comprehension of the appropriate techniques in periorbital aesthetic surgery. More importantly, this evolution has led to fewer surgical complications, better patient care, and improved surgical outcomes. In this chapter, we will highlight the varied contributions to the art and science of blepharoplasty and periorbital rejuvenation, and how these multidisciplinary contributions have allowed the field to evolve.

G.G. Massry (✉)
Director, Ophthalmic Plastic Surgery, Spaulding Drive Cosmetic Surgery and Dermatology, Beverly Hills, CA, USA
e-mail: gmassry@aol.com

1.2 Blepharoplasty

Blepharoplasty is derived from the Greek words *blepharon*, meaning eyelid, and *plastos*, meaning formed. It is one of the oldest described treatments of the aging face [2]. The first recorded surgical treatment of the eyelid was by a Spanish surgeon, Albucasis, a pioneer in the creation of surgical instrumentation, including cautery [3]. He described a crescent shaped partial thickness excision of upper eyelid skin using cautery in 1000 AD. About the same time in Baghdad, Ali Ibn Isa – who researched and described many ophthalmologic pathologic processes including the etiology of epiphoria and Vogt–Koyanagi–Harada syndrome (VKH) – described using two wooden bars to pinch excess upper eyelid skin for 10 days [4]. This led to tissue necrosis, and the subsequent removal of the resultant skin without a scar. Excess skin of the upper lids did not appear in the literature until Beers, a Viennese ophthalmic pioneer described it in 1792 [5]. The first illustration of the condition was published 25 years later in a subsequent edition of the text *Lehre der Augenkrankheiten* [6]. In 1818, a German ophthalmologist, Von Graefe, was the first to term blepharoplastik

G.G. Massry et al. (eds.), *Master Techniques in Blepharoplasty and Periorbital Rejuvenation*,
DOI 10.1007/978-1-4614-0067-7_1, © Springer Science+Business Media, LLC 2011

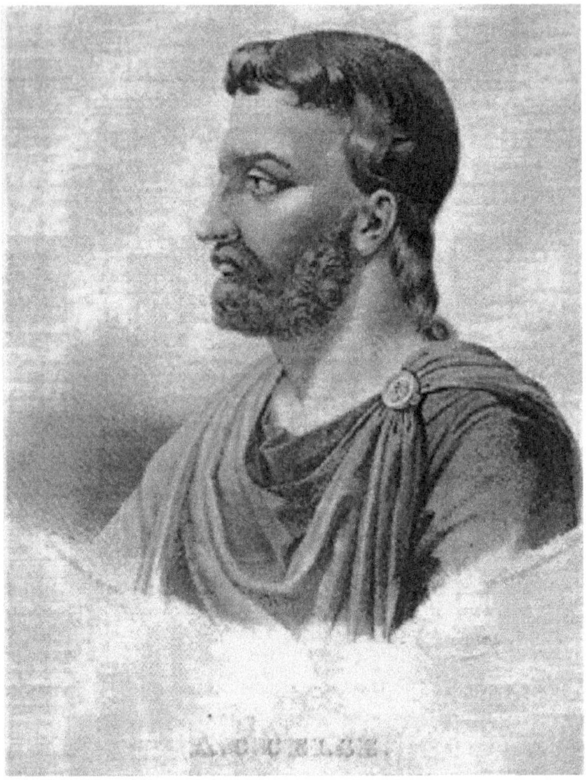

Fig. 1.1 Aulus Cornelius Celsus was the first to describe treatment of relaxed skin of the upper skin in 25–30 AD

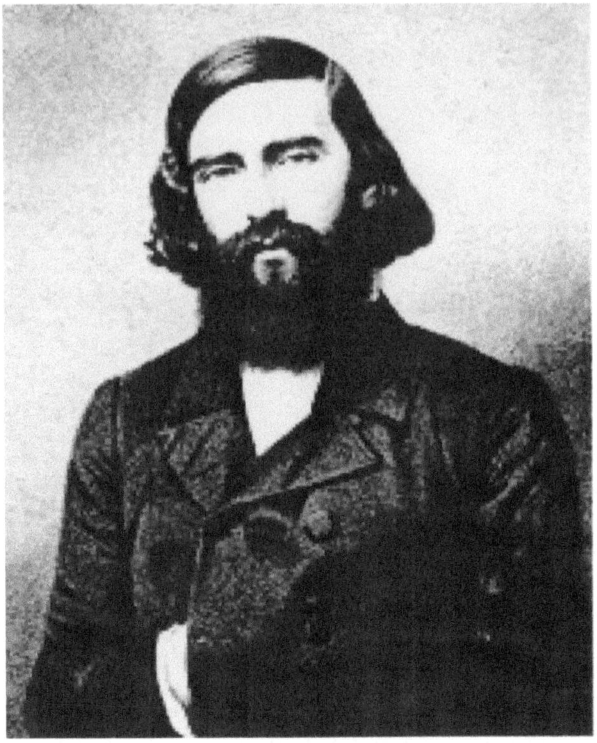

Fig. 1.2 Von Graefe is credited with coining the term blepharoplastik for excision of excess upper lid skin related to carcinoma

(blepharoplasty) for removal of excess skin of the upper lid for the treatment of eyelid carcinoma [7] (Fig. 1.2). The term has remained over the last 150 years.

In the first half of the nineteenth century, a number of Von Graefe's contemporaries, including Mackenzie, Alibert, Graf, and Dupuytren, were also performing similar upper lid skin excisions [8–11]. In 1844, Sichel was the first to describe herniated fat in the upper lid, and later in the century Fuchs described the reformation of the eyelid crease [12, 13].

In the early 1900, plastic surgeons began to focus on aesthetic eyelid surgery. In 1907, Conrad Miller, one of the modern day founders of plastic surgery, published the first textbook on cosmetic surgery, *Cosmetic Surgery: The Correction of Featural Imperfections* [14]. He included the first photographs of upper and lower blepharoplasty incisions. In his following textbook in 1924, he illustrated blepharoplasty incisions [15]. In 1911, Frederick Kolle, another early contributor to modern plastic surgery, elaborated on the value of preoperative markings for blepharoplasty skin excision [16]. In a series of publications in the 1920, Albert Bettman added to our understanding of blepharoplasty by detailing surgical techniques to reduce wound scarring (minimal tension, apposition of wound edges, timely removal of sutures) [17–19]. Interestingly, these early observations are still considered dogma today.

In the 1920, Julian Bourguet, a French surgeon, was the first to describe removal of herniated orbital fat from the upper lids, transconjuctival fat excision from the lower lids, and the importance of taking pre- and postoperative photographs [20–22]. Susan Noel, one of the first influential female aesthetic surgeons, included numerous pre- and postoperative photographs of cosmetic eyelid surgery in her 1926 textbook *La Chirurgie Esthetique: Son Role social* [23]. She emphasized the importance of reviewing photographs with patients and is credited for highlighting the importance of the psychological issues related to cosmetic surgery. Even in the infancy of cosmetic surgery, Noel had the foresight and wisdom to identify that photo-documentation and patient psychology were basic tenets for successful surgical outcome.

Modern blepharoplasty techniques have focused on excision of variable amounts of skin, muscle, and fat. Costaneres first elaborated these techniques in a 1951 paper that also included a detailed anatomical description of the orbital fat compartments [24]. Costaneres also recognized the significance of the orbicularis muscle, including its excision, when necessary, as part of the scope of cosmetic eyelid surgery. In the 1950 and 1960, Sayoc, Pang, and Knou Boo-Chai published on Asian upper lid blepharoplasty, including the formation of a double eyelid crease [25–27]. In 1970,

Sheen emphasized the role of the levator aponeurosis in eyelid crease formation (supra-tarsal fixation) [28, 29]. Dryden and Liebsohn then described levator advancement for simultaneous ptosis repair during blepharoplasty [30]. During this time, Smith, Patrelli, and Lisman elaborated on the surgical correction of lacrimal gland prolapse by suture repositioning for correction of temporal lid fullness [31, 32]. Over the next 20 years, the idealized goal for upper lid blepharoplasty was a high and deep lid fold. This was due in part to the contributions by Flowers and Siegel [33–35]. Today a high crease and deep fold in the upper lid have fallen out of favor. In 2002, Fagien reviewed current concepts of a fuller, more youthful appearing upper lid [36].

Increased interest in lower lid blepharoplasty surgery has primarily focused on preventing lower eyelid malposition and volume depletion, both inherent to the excisional surgery first described by Costaneras. The role of lower eyelid laxity as a predisposing factor for postsurgical eyelid malposition was first described by Edgerton in the 1970 [37]. Webster et al., Tenzel, and Kantzen et al. described lower lid horizontal shortening or canthal suspension techniques, which reduced the incidence of this aesthetic and functional complication [38–40]. Anderson and Gordy's "tarsal strip" procedure [41] is noteworthy in that it has remained a mainstay in canthal suspension surgery until today. A number of less disruptive (more aesthetic) canthal suspension techniques have also been described to prevent eyelid malposition after lower lid blepharoplasty [42–46]. Fagien elaborated on the limitations of the lateral tarsal strip, including asymmetry, globe lid disjunction, canthal dystopia, and long-term shortening of the horizontal palpebral aperture. He advocated a lateral retinacular suspension (suture canthopexy) for reinforcement of the lateral canthus to enhance or maintain vertical lower eyelid position [47]. Shorr and colleagues described combined cheek lift, lateral canthal suspension, and posterior eyelid spacer grafting with hard palate mucosa, for correction of post-blepharoplasty cicatricial lower eyelid retraction [48–50]. His work demonstrated a means of raising the lower lid without skin grafting in appropriate patients. It also emphasized the need to assess and address when necessary, deficiencies in the anterior, middle, and posterior lamella of the lower lid to attain better outcomes.

The incidence of lower lid malposition has significantly decreased with the repopularization of the transconjunctival lower lid blepharoplasty by Tomlinson and Hovey in 1975 [51]. In 1989, Baylis and colleagues further elaborated and refined the technique [52]. In 1991, Kamer and Mikaelian described a simple skin pinch excision as an adjunct to transconjunctival lower blepharoplasty surgery to address excess skin [53].

Fat preservation and repositioning in lower lid blepharoplasty was first described by Loeb and later modified by Hamra and Goldberg in an effort to prevent postoperative orbital skeletonization (hollowing) and improve the tear trough deformity (nasojugal groove) [54–56]. Volume augmentation/preservation with fat has been a paradigm shift away from traditional excisional blepharoplasty. Sydney Coleman pioneered the technique of fat grafting in the periorbital area to restore volume deficiencies [57]. Massry recently presented results of combined fat repositioning and grafting for effacement of the tear trough and orbitomalar groove [45]. In addition to modifications in lower lid blepharoplasty surgical techniques, and an awareness of the importance of volume restoration, creating a smooth contour between the lower lids and cheek requires modification of the midface (discussed later) [58].

1.3 Forehead Lift

In contemporary times, there is a clear understanding of the relationship of the forehead and brows to the eyelids. Historically, however, this relationship has been generally overlooked. In 1919, Passott was one of the first to describe excising multiple skin ellipses from the face for lifting of the brow, midface, and neck [59] (Fig. 1.3). Lexer also recognized the aesthetic importance of the brow. He performed early brow lifts by excising an ellipse of skin from the forehead [60]

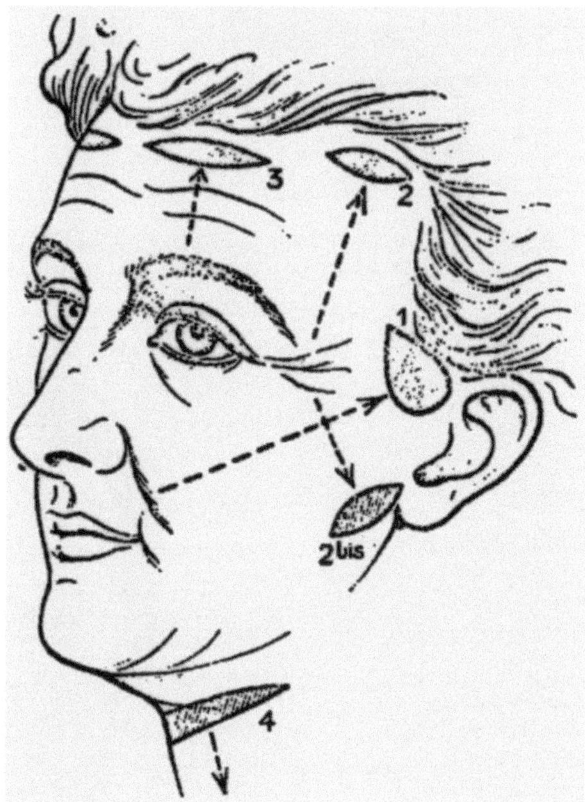

Fig. 1.3 Early elevation of the brows through elliptical excisions. (Adapted from Passot [59])

(Fig. 1.4). In 1929, the coronal browlift technique was described by Hunt in New York [61] (Fig. 1.5). Shortly afterwards, Claoue dissected the forehead in an attempt to get a better lift of the brow, and Fomon published an article describing subcutaneous dissection before transection of the pericranium [62, 63]. Passot also described the use of a supraciliary brow incision for the correction of brow ptosis, and Vinas clarified the relationship of the coronal incision and the change to a patient's hairline [60, 64]. In the 1960 and 1970, he described using a pretrichial incision for high foreheads and coronal incisions for patients with average forehead height. He was revolutionary in advocating release of fibrous attachments in the glabellar and supraorbital regions.

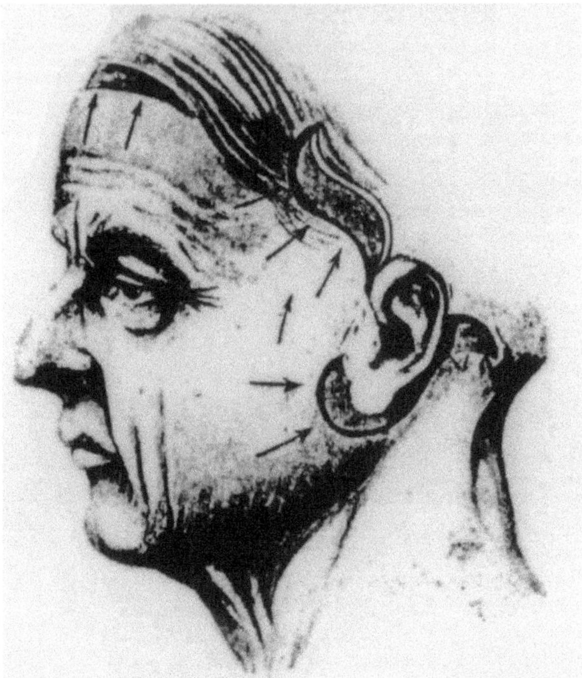

Fig. 1.4 Early approaches for browlifting included a direct excision of ellipse of skin from the forehead. (Adapted from Lexner [60])

Modern browlifting has gradually changed since George Brennan repopularized the bi-coronal lift in 1980 [65]. In 1991, Flowers stressed the true importance of the brow position in regards to periorbital rejuvenation [66]. He advocated that lifting a ptotic brow in select cases would result in a better aesthetic outcome than excision of tissue from the upper lid. Internal fixation of the brow was first described by McCord and Doxanas in 1990. This procedure, termed "Browpexy," was described to address mild temporal brow ptosis [67]. It is performed at the time of blepharoplasty, through the same eyelid crease incision, and is minimally invasive. Anderson and others have reported on modifications of the initial description to improve outcome [68–70].

In 1992, Isse was the first plastic surgeon to describe the use of an endoscope for brow rejuvenation [71]. Many modifications of the "endoscopic brow lift" have been described since its introduction. Ramirez was integral in modifying the technique and defining surgical landmarks with the aid of the endoscope [72]. Different planes of dissection have been advocated and remain controversial [73]. In addition, various methods of brow fixation have been described, including the use of bolsters, v–y scalp closure, externalized or buried permanent/resorbable devices anchored to calvarium, and drilled tunnels in calvarial cortex [74–86]. There is general agreement that temporal fixation is best achieved by securing the superficial to deep temporal fascia with suture. Otherwise, cost, operative time, and potential complications such as allopecia, scarring, and palpation of, or pain, from the anchoring device have dictated surgeon preference. While no single suspension mechanism has proved superior, most surgeons agree that the optimal elevation of the brow complex requires complete release of the arcus marginalis and all the attachments of the brow depressors [87, 88].

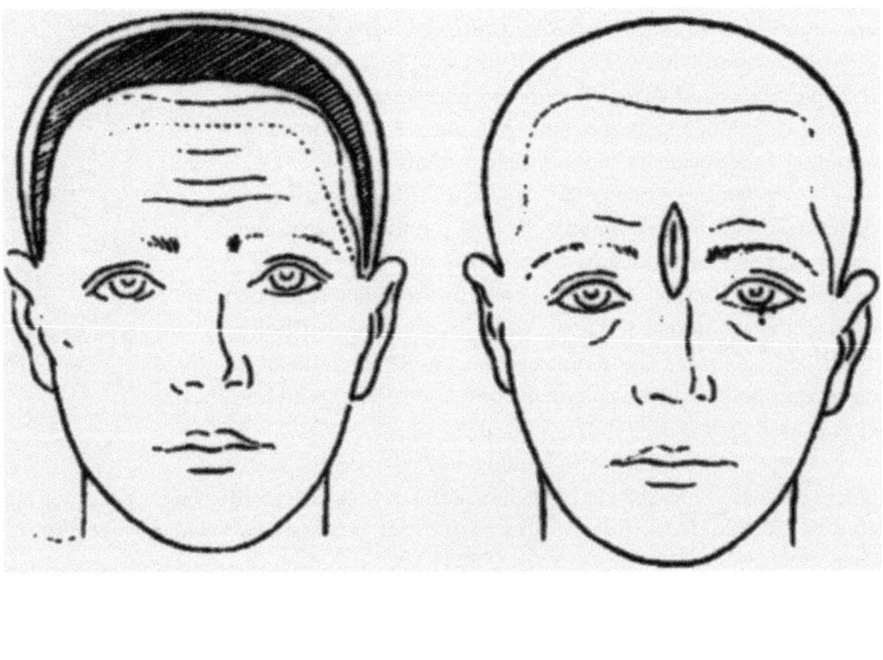

Fig. 1.5 Incisions for early browlift in the pretrichial and hair bearing regions. (Adapted from Hunt [61])

The use of neuromodulators to enhance the position of the brow in a nonsurgical manner has been a very recent phenomenon. In 1997, Blitzer et al. reported on a collaborative study of 162 patients for the treatment of forehead and periocular rhytids with botulinum toxin-A (BTX). They demonstrated a predictable, reproducible, and consistent decrease in dynamic rhytid formation in the glabellar and forehead [89]. In 1998, Frankel and Kamer reported reproducible medial brow elevation using BTX injections into the glabellar depressors – the procerus, and corrugator muscles [90]. Ahn and Maas evaluated injecting BTX to the lateral brow depressors (temporal aspect of the orbital orbicularis oculi muscle) to produce lateral brow elevation [91]. Huang et al. reported reproducible "chemical browlift" over the entire course of the brow by injecting BTX in medial and lateral depressors of the brow [92]. Today, neuromodulators are used as adjunctive treatments in the rejuvenation of the brow and offer a conservative option for patients with limited brow ptosis.

1.4 Midface

In comparison to surgical rejuvenation of the eyelid and brow, the midface has only gained the interest of aesthetic surgeons over the past two decades. There are a number of aging changes that contribute to midface aging, including: laxity of the suspending ligaments of the eyelid and cheek, descent of the malar fat pad, loss of the malar prominence, and generalized soft tissue and bony volume loss. These changes can lead to contour irregularities of the lower lid, cheek, and their associated interface, which manifest as an orbitomalar and nasojugal depression (tear trough), irregular malar contour, and deepening of the nasolabial fold.

The major advances in midface rejuvenation have been the deep plane/composite facelift, the endoscopic midface lift, and volume restoration. The works of Skoog, Mitz, and Peyronie in the 1970 defined the superficial musculoaponeurotic system (SMAS) and demonstrated that surgical repositioning of the SMAS improves lower facial rejuvenation [93, 94]. The deep plane facelift which utilizes a sub-SMAS dissection was first described in 1990 by Hamra as a more reliable method to elevate the midface [95]. In 1992, Hamra described the composite facelift, which went one step further by elevating the orbicularis oculi muscle with the SMAS as a single flap in the facelift procedure, in order to enhance midface and lower lid appearance [96]. Kamer and others further popularized and validated the deep plane technique [97, 98]. The deep plane rhytidectomy remains a mainstay in contemporary rhytidectomy surgery.

Subperiosteal midface rejuvenation sprouted from the work of Tessier, a craniofacial pioneer, who had vast experience with this technique. During this work, he discovered that lifting the temporal region, lateral canthus, and midface with dissection to the level of the maxilla would reverse the changes of aging midface [99]. In 1988, Psillakis and colleagues published results on facial rejuvenation via subperiosteal midface dissection, reporting a 6.7% incidence of injury to the facial nerve [100]. In 1989, Tessier and Krastinova-Lolov described their midface lift technique (mask lift) which elevated the midface with a combination of intraoral and coronal incisions, and a subperiosteal dissection of the malar eminence, zygomatic arch, and orbital margin [101, 102]. Open midface lift methods were further modified in the 1990 by Ortiz-Monasterio, Tapia et al., and De la Plaza et al. in order to protect the fascial nerve. Ortiz-Monasterio and Tapia et al. used multiple interconnected subperiosteal pockets below both layers of the temporalis facia to protect the facial nerve [103, 104]. De la Plaza et al. stayed supraperiosteal anterior to zygomatic arch to protect the facial nerve [105]. The early midface lifts had a relatively high rate of facial nerve injury and were mostly "open" techniques utilizing wide coronal and temporal incisions.

The endoscopic assisted subperiosteal midface lift is currently the preferred method for surgical midface lifting. Endoscopic midface rejuvenation followed in the footsteps of the endoscopic browlift techniques. Isse, in 1994, described using an endoscope for surgical manipulation of the midface and brow complex [77]. Fuente del Campo was the first to report that the endoscopic technique was less traumatic than "open" procedures, and that it led to less postoperative edema and a speedier recovery [106]. Burnett el al. described an endoscopic dissection from temporal and subciliary incisions. With the assistance of the endoscope and retrograde dissection, they described a decreased incidence of frontal nerve branch injury [107]. In the late 1990, Paul and McCord et al. popularized the transblepharoplasty approach to midface rejuvenation [108, 109]. Their techniques aggressively excised skin and required a lateral canthotomy. Many of the contemporary techniques for endoscopic midface rejuvenation have been modified and elaborated on by Ramirez over the last decade [110–113].

Recently, volume restoration has taken a more prominent role in midface rejuvenation. In 1893, Neuber first reported using autologous fat to help correct facial scars [114]. Modern day liposuction, developed by Italian surgeons in the 1970, continued to modify the techniques used today for autologous fat grafting [115]. Illouz was the first to demonstrate that the fat removed during liposuction could survive and be transferred to fill depressions [116]. In 2001, Ramirez described a hybrid technique of midface rejuvenation utilizing autologous fat grafting, rotation of the Bichat's fat pad, and an endoscopic midface lift [111]. Coleman wrote the first dedicated textbook on autologous fat grafting in 2004 [117]. He was able to show facial volume enhancement through injecting small aliquots of autologous fat in different facial soft tissue planes. Glasgold and Lam have also been central in the paradigm shift of periocular and midface rejuvenation with the use of autologous fat grafting [118, 119]. Autologous fat grafting is now an integral part of the rejuvenation of the periocular region.

Synthetic fillers have also gained attention for facial rejuvenation; beginning in the 1970, when bovine collagen was first introduced [120]. Initially, fillers such as collagen, hyaluronic acid gel, and calcium hydroxylapatite were utilized for nasolabial effacement. However, more recently, the use of fillers for lower eyelid and midface volume rejuvenation has become widely accepted. In 2004, Goldberg et al. reported a series of patients who obtained excellent results with the use of hyaluronic acid gel filler in the tear trough region [121]. Poly-L-lactic acid (PLLA, Sculptra, Sanofi-Aventix, Bridgewater, NJ), a collagen stimulator was introduced to the North American market for use of human immunodeficiency virus (HIV) related lipoatrophy in 2004. Although, the product was initially approved for HIV-related lipoatrophy, it has been successfully used in midface and lower facial rejuvenation to reverse age-related lipoatrophy [122].

Beginning in the 1970, Spadafora et al., Hinder, and Gonzalez Uloa introduced the use of alloplastic facial implants for volume restoration of the face [123–125]. In the 1980, Binder described the use of alloplastic midface implants as an independent method to restore volume secondary to soft tissue atrophy [126]. Terrino further advocated the use of midface implantation in the 1990 to enhance facial aesthetics [127]. In the periorbital area, alloplastic implants have been used to augment the orbital rim, fill the tear trough, and mask a prominent globe [128–130].

1.5 Conclusion

Contemporary periorbital aesthetic surgery has evolved with the contributions of surgeons from a variety of subspecialties. Ophthalmologists have been integral in the early descriptions of eyelid surgery. Plastic surgeons, facial plastic surgeons, oculoplastic surgeons, and dermatologists have since added immense insight, intellect, and technique to the field. Each contribution has served as a building block for the next. This has significantly improved our ability to evaluate the periocular region, has fueled a wealth of growth and development in our understanding of the procedures we perform, and has laid the foundation for improved outcomes to both surgical and nonsurgical rejuvenation of this area of the face. None of this could have been accomplished without the cumulative contributions of each of the specialties previously mentioned.

References

1. Arrington G. A history of ophthalmology. MD Publications: New York; 1959.
2. Adamson P, Moran M. Historical trends in surgery for the aging face. Plast Surg. 1993;9:133–42.
3. Wolfort FG, Colon F, Wolfort S, et al. The history of blepharoplasty. In: Wolfort FG, Kanroe WR, editors. Aesthetic blepharoplasty. Boston: Little Brown; 1995. p. 1–16.
4. Wood C. The Tadhkirat of Ali ibn Isa of Baghdad (transl). Chicago: Northwestern University; 1936. p. 98, 115, 118–119.
5. Beer GJ. Lehre der Augenkrankheiten. Vienna, C.F. Wappler; 1792.
6. Beer GJ. Lehre von den Augenkrankheiten als Leitfaden Zuseinen Offentlechen Vorlesungen Entworsen. Vol. 11. Vienna, Lamesina: Heubner & Volke, 1817. p. 109–11.
7. Von Graefe CF. De Rhinoplastice. Berlin: Dietrich Reimer; 1818. p. 13.
8. Mackenzie W. Practical treatise of the diseases of the eye. London: Longman; 1830. p. 170–1.
9. Albert JL. Monographie des Dermatoses ou Precis Theorique et Practique des Maladies de la Peau; 1832. p. 795.
10. Graf D. Oertliche erbliche Erschlaffung der haut. Wochensche Gesamte Heilkd; 1836. p. 225–227.
11. Dupuytren G, editor. De l'oedeme chronique des tumeurs enkystees des paupieres. In Locons Orales de Clinique Chirurgicale. Paris: Germer-Bailliere; 1839. p. 377–8.
12. Sichel J. Aphorismes pratiques sur divers points d'ophthalmologie (Practical aphorisms on various points of ophthalomogy). Ann Ocul (Paris). 1844;12:185.
13. Fuchs E. Textbook of ophthalmology. New York: D Appleton; 1982.
14. Miller CC. Cosmetic surgery: the correction of featural imperfections. Chicago: Oak; 1908. p. 40–2.
15. Miller CC. Cosmetic surgery. In: Cosmetic surgery: the correction of featural imperfections. Philadelphia: FA Davis; 1924. p. 30–2.
16. Kolle FS. Plastic and cosmetic surgery. New York: S Appleton; 1911.
17. Bettman AG. Plastic and cosmetic surgery of the face. Northwest Med. 1920;19:205.
18. Bettman AG. Plastic surgery about the eye. Ann Surg. 1928;88: 994–1006.
19. Betman AG. The minimal scar. Portland, OR: Medical Sentinel; 1926.
20. Bourguet J. Les hernies graissueses de l'orbite: Notre traitement chirurigical. Bull Acad Med. 1934;92:1270.
21. Bourguet J. Chirurgie esthetique de la face: Lex nez concaves, les rides et les "poches" sous les yeux. Arch Franco Belg Chir. 1925;28:293.
22. Bourguet J. La chirurgie esthetique de l'oeil et des paupieres. Monde Méd. 1929;39:725–31.
23. La NA. Chirurgie Esthetque: son role social. Masson et Cie: Paris; 1926.
24. Costaneras S. Blepharoplasty for herniated intraorbital fat: anatomic basis for a new approach. Plast Reconstr Surg. 1951;8:46.
25. Sayoc BT. Plastic reconstruction of the superior palpebral fold. J Ophthalmol. 1954;38:556–9.
26. Pang RG. Surgical formation of the upper lid fold. Arch Ophthalmol. 1961;65:783–4.
27. Boo-Chai K. Plastic construction of the superior palpebral fold. Plast Reconstr Surg. 1963;31:74–8.
28. Sheen JH. Supratarsal fixation in upper lid blepharoplasty. Plast Reconstr Surg. 1974;54:424–31.
29. Sheen JH. A change in the technique of supratarsal fixation in upper lid blepharoplasty. Plast Reconstr Surg. 1977;59:831–4.
30. Dryden R, Leibsohn J. The levator aponeurosis in blepharoplasty. Ophthalmology. 1978;85:718–25.
31. Smith B, Petrelli R. Surgical repair of prolapsed lacrimal glands. Arch Ophthalmol. 1978;96:113–4.
32. Smith B, Lisman R. Dacryoadenopexy as a recognized factor in upper lid blepharoplasty. Plast Reconstr Surg. 1983;71:629–32.
33. Flowers RS. Upper blepharoplasty by eyelid invagination: anchor blepharoplasty. Clin Plast Surg. 1993;20:193–207.
34. Siegel RJ. Essential anatomy of contemporary upper lid blepharoplasty. Clin Plast Surg. 1993;20:209–12.
35. Siegel RJ. Contemporary upper lid blepharoplasty. Tissue invagination. Clin Plast Surg. 1993;20:239–46.

36. Fagien S. Advanced rejuvenative upper blepharoplasty: enhancing aesthetics of the upper periorbita. Plast Reconstr Surg. 2002;110: 278–92.
37. Edgerton M. Causes and prevention of lower lid ectropion following blepharoplasty. Plast Reconstr Surg. 1972;49:367–73.
38. Webster RC, Davidson TM, Reardon EJ, Smith RC. Suspending sutures in blepharoplasty. Arch Otolaryngol. 1979;105:601–4.
39. Tenzel RR. Cosmetic blepharoplasty. In: Soll DB, editor. Management of complications in ophthalmic plastic surgery. Birmingham, AL: Aesculapiuus; 1976. p. 119–31.
40. Kantzen LB, Tenzel RR. Canthal laxity and eyelid malpositions. Adv Ophthalmol Plast Reconstr Surg. 1983;2:229–43.
41. Anderson RL, Gordy DD. The tarsal strip procedure. Arch Ophthalmol. 1979;97:2192.
42. Hamra ST. The role of the septal reset in creating a youthful eyelid-cheek complex in facial rejuvenation. Plast Reconstr Surg. 2004;113(7)2124–41; discussion 2142–4.
43. Hamra ST. The zygorbicular dissection in composite rhytidectomy: an ideal midface plane. Plast Reconstr Surg. 1998;102(5):1646–57.
44. Rizvi M, Lypka M, Gaon M, Kovacev T, Eisemann B, Eisemann MJ. Minimally invasive lateral canthopexy (MILC). J Plast Reconstr Aesthet Surg. 2010;63(9):1434–6.
45. Massry GG. Comprehensive lower eyelid rejuvenation. Facial Plast Surg. 2010;26(3):209–21.
46. Kam-Lung CK, Goldberg RA. Lateral canthal surgery. Facial Plast Surg. 2010;26(3):193–200.
47. Fagien S. Algorithm for canthoplasty: the lateral retinacular suspensions: a simplified suture canthopexy. Plast Reconstr Surg. 1999;103:2042–53.
48. Shorr M, Fallor NK. "Madame Butterfly" procedure: combined cheek and lateral canthal suspension procedure for post-blepharoplasty, rounded eye, and lower eyelid retraction. Ophthal Plast Reconstr Surg. 1985;1:229–35.
49. Shorr N. Madame Butterfly procedure with hard palate graft: management of post-blepharoplasty rounded eye and sclera show. Facial Plast Surg. 1994;10:90–118.
50. Cohen MS, Shorr N. Eyelid reconstruction with hard palate mucosal grafts. Ophthal Plast Reconstr Surg. 2000;16:223–30.
51. Tomlinson FB, Hovey LM. Transconjunctival lower lid blepharoplasty for removal of fat. Plast Reconstr Surg. 1975;56:314–8.
52. Baylis HI, Long JA, Groth MJ. Transconjunctival lower eyelid blepharoplasty. Technique and complications. Ophthalmology. 1989;96(7):1027–32.
53. Kamer F, Mikaelian AJ. Pre-excision blepharoplasty. Arch Otolaryngol Head Neck Surg. 1991;117(9):995–9.
54. Loeb R. Fat pad sliding and fat grafting for leveling lid depressions. Clin Plast Surg. 1981;8:757–76.
55. Hamra S. The role of orbital fat preservation in facial aesthetic surgery: a new concept. Clin Plast Surg. 1996;23:17–28.
56. Goldberg RA. Transconjunctival orbital fat repositioning: transposition of orbital fat pedicles into a subperiosteal pocket. Plast Reconstr Surg. 2000;105:743–58.
57. Coleman SR. Structural fat grafts: the ideal filler. Clin Plast Surg. 2001;28:111–9.
58. Hester TR, Codner MA, McCord CD, et al. Evolution of technique of the direct transblepharoplasty approach for the correction of lower lid and midfacial aging: maximizing results and minimizing complications in a 5 year experience. Plast Reconstr Surg. 2000;105:393–406.
59. Passot R. La chururgie esthetique des rides du visage. Presse Méd. 1919;27:258.
60. Lexer E. Die Gesamte Wiederherstellungs-Chirurgie, vol. 1 and 2. Leipzig: Jahann Ambrosius Barth; 1931.
61. Hunt HL. Plastic surgery of the head, face, and neck. Philadelphia: Lea & Febiger; 1926.
62. Claoue C. La ridectomie cervico-faciale par accrochage parieto-temporo-occipital et resection cutanee. Bull Acad Med (Paris). 1933;109:257–65.
63. Fomon S. Surgery of injury and plastic repair. Baltimore: Williams & Wilkins; 1939.
64. Vinas JC. Plan general de la ritidoplastia y zona tabu. In: Transactions of the 4th Brasilian congress on plastic surgery, Porto Alegre, 5–8 Oct 1965. p. 32.
65. Brennan GH. The forehead lift. Otolaryngol Clin North Am. 1980;13:209–23.
66. Flowers RS. Periorbital aesthetic surgery for men: eyelids and related structures. Clin Plast Surg. 1991;18:689–729.
67. McCord CD, Doxanas MT. Browplasty and browpexy: an adjunct to blepharoplasty. Plast Reconstr Surg. 1990;86(2):248–54.
68. Georgescu D, Anderson RL, McCann JD. Brow ptosis correction: a comparison of five techniques. Facial Plast Surg. 2010;26(3): 186–92.
69. Burroughs JR, Bearden WH, Anderson RL, McCann JD. Internal brow elevation at blepharoplasty. Arch Facial Plast Surg. 2006;8(1):36–41.
70. Walden JL, Orseck MJ, Aston SJ. Current methods for brow fixation: are they safe? Aesthet Plast Surg. 2006;30(5):541–8.
71. Isse NG. Endoscopic forehead lift. Presented at the Annual Meeting of the Los Angeles County Society of Plastic Surgeons, Los Angeles, 12 September 1992.
72. Ramirez OM. Endoscopic techniques in facial rejuvenation; an overview. Part I. Aesthet Plast Surg. 1994;18:111–47.
73. Nassif PN. Evolution in techniques for endoscopic brow lift with deep temporal fixation only and lower blepharoplasty-transconjunctival fat repositioning. Facial Plast Surg. 2007;23:27–42.
74. Matarasso A. Endoscopically assisted forehead-brow rhytidoplasty: theory and practice. Aesthet Plast Surg. 1995;9:141–7.
75. Smith DS. A simple method for forehead fixation following endoscopy. Plast Reconstr Surg. 1996;98:1117.
76. Fodor PB, Isse NG. Forehead rejuvenation. In: Endoscopically assisted aesthetic plastic surgery. St. Louis: Mosby; 1996.
77. Isse NG. Endoscopic facial rejuvenation: endoforehead, the functional lift. Aesthet Plast Surg. 1994;18:21–9.
78. Ramirez OM. Endoscopically assisted biplanar forehead lift. Plast Reconstr Surg. 1995;96:323–33.
79. Isse NG. Endoscopic forehead lift: evolution and update. Clin Plast Surg. 1995;22:661–73.
80. Morselli PG. Fixation for forehead endoscopic lifting: a simple, easy, no-cost procedure. Plast Reconstr Surg. 1996;97:1309–10.
81. Core GB, Vasconez LO, Graham III HD. Endoscopic browlift. Clin Plast Surg. 1995;22:619.
82. Ramirez OM. Endoscopic full facelift. Aesthet Plast Surg. 1994;18:363–71.
83. Pakkanen M, Salisbury AV, Ersek RA. Biodegradable positive fixation for the endoscopic brow lift. Plast Reconstr Surg. 1996;98:1087–91.
84. Lorenc ZP, Ivy E, Aston SJ. Neurosensory preservation in endoscopic forehead plasty. Aesthet Plast Surg. 1995;19:411–3.
85. Kim SK. Endoscopic forehead-scalp flap fixation with K-wire. Aesthet Plast Surg. 1996;20:217–20.
86. Gunter JP, Antrobus SD. Aesthetics of the eye-brows. Presented at Endoscopic-assisted aesthetic plastic surgery, Dallas, December 1995.
87. De La Fuente A, Samtamaria AB. Facial rejuvenation: a combined conventional and endoscopic assisted lift. Aesthet Plast Surg. 1996;20:471–9.
88. Oslin B, Core GB, Vasconez LO. The biplanar endoscopically assisted forehead lift. Clin Plast Surg. 1995;22:633–8.
89. Blitzer A, Binder WF, Aviv JE, et al. The management of hyperfunctional facial lines with botulinum toxin: a collaborative study of 210 injection sites in 162 patients. Arch Otolaryngol Head Neck Surg. 1997;123:389–92.
90. Frankel AS, Kamer FM. Chemical browlift. Arch Otolaryngol Head Neck Surg. 1998;124:321–33.
91. Ahn MS, Catten M, Maas CS. Temporal brow lift using botulinum toxin A. Plast Reconstr Surg. 2000;105:1129–35.

92. Huang W, Rogachefsky AS, Foster JA. Browlift with botulinum toxin. Dermatol Surg. 2001;26(1):55–60.
93. Skoog T. Plastic surgery: new methods and refinements. Philadelphia: Saunders; 1974.
94. Mitz V, Peyronie M. The superficial musclo-aponeurotic system (SMAS) in the parotid and cheek area. Plast Reconstr Surg. 1976;58:80–8.
95. Hamra T. The deep-plane rhytidectomy. Plast Reconstr Surg. 1990;86:53–61.
96. Hamra ST. Composite rhytidectomy. Plast Reconstr Surg. 1992;90:1–13.
97. Kamer FM. One hundred consecutive deep plane face-lifts. Arch Otolaryngol Head Neck Surg. 1996;122:17–22.
98. Bonnefon A. Deep "en bloc" facial lift. Ann Chir Plast Esthét. 1992;37(1):85–94.
99. Tessier P. Face lifting and frontal rhytidectomy. 1979:393.
100. Psillakis JM, Rumley TO, Camargos A. Subperiosteal approach as an improved concept for correction of the aging face. Plast Reconstr Surg. 1988;82:383–94.
101. Tessier P. Le lifting facial sous-perioste. Ann Chir Plast Esthét. 1989;34:193.
102. Krastinova-Lolov D. Le lifting facial sous-perioste. Ann Chir Plast Esthét. 1989;34:199–211.
103. Ortiz-Monasterio F. Aesthetic surgery of the facial skeleton: the forehead. Clin Plast Surg. 1991;18:19–27.
104. Tapia A, Ferreria B, Blanch A. Subperiostic lifting. Aesthet Plast Surg. 1991;15:155–60.
105. De la Plaza R, Valiente E, Arroyo JM. Supraperiosteal lifting of the upper two-thirds of the face. Br J Plast Surg. 1991;44:325–32.
106. Fuente del Campo A. Ritidectomia subperiostica endoscopia. Cirugia Plastica Ibero-Latino Americana. 1994;20:393.
107. Burnett CD, Rabinowitz S, Rauscher GE. Endoscopic-assisted midface lift utilizing retrograde dissection. Ann Plast Surg. 1996;36:449–52.
108. Paul MD. The periosteal hinge flap in the subperiosteal cheek-lift. Oper Tech Plast Reconstr Surg. 1997;5:145.
109. McCord D, Codner MA, Hester TR. Redraping the inferior orbicularis arc. Plast Reconstr Surg. 1998;102:2471–9.
110. Ramirez OM. The central oval of the face: tridimensional endoscopic rejuvenation. Facial Plast Surg. 2000;16:283–98.
111. Ramirez OM. Full face rejuvenation in three dimensions: "a face lifting" for the new millennium. Aesthet Plast Surg. 2001;25:152–64.
112. Ramirez OM. Three-dimensional endoscopic midface enhancement. A personal quest for the ideal cheek rejuvenation. Plast Reconstr Surg. 2002;109:329–40.
113. Ramirez OM, Volpe CR. Double ogee facial rejuvenation, Chap. 43. In: Panfilov DE, editor. Aesthetic surgery of the facial mosaic. Berlin: Springer; 2007. p. 288–99.
114. Neuber F. Fettransplantation. Verh Dtsch Ges Chir. 1893;22:66.
115. Fischer A, Fischer G. First surgical treatment for molding body's cellulite with three 5 mm incisions. Bull Int Acad Cosmet Surg. 1976;3:35.
116. Illouz YG. The fat cell "graft": a new technique to fill depressions. Plast Reconstr Surg. 1986;78(1):122–3.
117. Coleman S. Structural Fat Grafting. St Louis, MO: Quality Medical; 2004.
118. Lam SM. A new paradigm for the aging face. Facial Plast Surg Clin North Am. 2010;18:1–6.
119. Meier JD, Glasgold RA, Glasgold MJ. Autologous fat grafting long-term evidence of its efficacy in midfacial rejuvenation. Arch Facial Plast Surg. 2009;11(1):24–8.
120. Thomas JR. Advanced therapy in facial plastic and reconstructive surgery. Shelton, CT: People's Medical; 2010.
121. Goldberg RA, Fiaschetti D. Filling the periorbital hollows with hyaluronic acid gel: initial experience with 244 injections. Ophthal Plast Reconstr Surg. 2006;5(22):335–43.
122. Vleggaar D. Soft-tissue augmentation and the role of poly-L-lactic acid. Plast Reconstr Surg. 2006;118:46S–54.
123. Spadafora A, De los Rios E, Toledo Rios R. Pomulos planos (platizigion): endoprotesis de polietileno insertadas por via sub periostica de arco cigomatico (flat cheeks: polyethelene endoprostheses inserted subperiosteally along the zygomatic arch). Prensa Med Argent 1971;58(40):1946–50.
124. Hinderer UT. Malar implants for improvement of the facial appearance. Plast Reconstr Surg. 1975;56(2):157–65.
125. Gonzales-Uloa M. Building out the malar prominences as an addition to rhytidectomy. Plast Reconstr Surg. 1974;53(3):293–6.
126. Binder WJ. Submalar augmentation. An alternative to facelift surgery. Arch Otolaryngol Head Neck Surg. 1989;115(7):797–801.
127. Terrino EO. Allpoplastic facial contouring by zonal principals of skeletal anatomy. Clin Plast Surg. 1992;19(2):487–510.
128. Weinberg DA, Goldberg RA, Hoenig J, Shorr N, Baylis HI. Management of relative proptosis with a porous polyethylene orbital rim onlay implant. Ophthal Plast Reconstr Surg. 1999; 15:67–73.
129. Yaremchuk MJ. Infraorbital rim augmentation. Plast Reconstr Surg. 2001;107:1585–92; discussion 1593–5.
130. Yaremchuk MJ, Kahn DM. Periorbital skeletal augmentation to improve blepharoplasty and midfacial results. Plast Reconstr Surg. 2009;124:2151–60.

2 Surgical Anatomy of the Forehead, Eyelids, and Midface for the Aesthetic Surgeon

Kevin S. Tan, Sang-Rog Oh, Ayelet Priel, Bobby S. Korn, and Don O. Kikkawa

Key Points

- The eyes are a central feature of the face, and patients commonly present for aesthetic rejuvenation of the eyelids and surrounding areas.
- A detailed comprehension of forehead/eyebrow, eyelid and midface anatomy, and how these separate units interrelate with each other, is critical to successful aesthetic surgery of the upper face.
- Eyebrow position is maintained by a delicate balance of muscles which elevate the brow (frontalis muscle), and those that depress the brow (orbital orbicularis oculi, corrugators supercilii, procerus and depressor supracilii).
- Eyebrow lifts can be achieved surgically with variety of browlifting procedures, or chemically (along with treatment of dynamic rhytids) with selective chemodenervation.
- The eyelids are complex structures composed of multiple delicate layers. A comprehensive familiarity with their anatomy and function is essential for successful aesthetic and functional surgical outcomes.
- Involutional lower lid and midface changes lead to lower lid "bags," lid/cheek interface depressions (tear trough), and loss of malar projection. An understanding of these changes allows appropriate planning for surgical correction
- The temporal, zygomatic, and to a lesser degree, the buccal, branches of the facial nerve innervate the eyelids and periorbital region. It is important to understand the course of these nerves when performing surgery.

D.O. Kikkawa (✉)
Professor of Clinical Ophthalmology and Chief of Division of Ophthalmic Plastic and Reconstructive Surgery, Department of Ophthalmology, Shiley Eye Center, University of California, La Jolla, San Diego, CA, USA
e-mail: dkikkawa@ucsd.edu

2.1 Introduction

The expanding indications and array of procedures available to the aesthetic surgeon demand a thorough understanding and knowledge of the intricate anatomy of the face. Novel surgical approaches and evolving instrumentation offer tremendous opportunities to improve clinical and surgical skills and outcomes. An intimate appreciation of facial anatomy is critical in choosing and performing the appropriate surgical procedure. This chapter will review eyelid and periorbital facial anatomy essential to all aesthetic surgeons.

2.2 Facial Proportions

Evidence from historical texts and art dating back to the Renaissance period show that appreciation of ideal facial proportions has persisted for ages. Many regard the ideal face as five eye widths wide and eight eye widths high [1]. In a study examining North American Caucasians, the horizontal proportions were defined by the width of the nose, with one nose width equaling interorbital width or one fourth of the face width [2].

More recent studies have emphasized the importance of recognizing ethnic, gender, and age-related differences in facial proportions when performing aesthetic and reconstructive surgery. One guideline of beauty is "the golden ratio" introduced by Euclid approximately three centuries before Christ. The "golden ratio" (1:1.618), sometimes called "phi," is a ratio obtained when a line is divided into two unequal segments, where the ratio of the longer segment to the whole line is equal to the ratio of the shorter segment to the longer one. This ratio is naturally observed in both nature and the human body. This "golden ratio" was used to develop a "facial golden mask" [3]. Aesthetic surgeons can use the facial golden mask to represent idealized facial structures that are reported to remain consistent regardless of race or culture. The facial golden mask can be overlaid on standard

G.G. Massry et al. (eds.), *Master Techniques in Blepharoplasty and Periorbital Rejuvenation*,
DOI 10.1007/978-1-4614-0067-7_2, © Springer Science+Business Media, LLC 2011

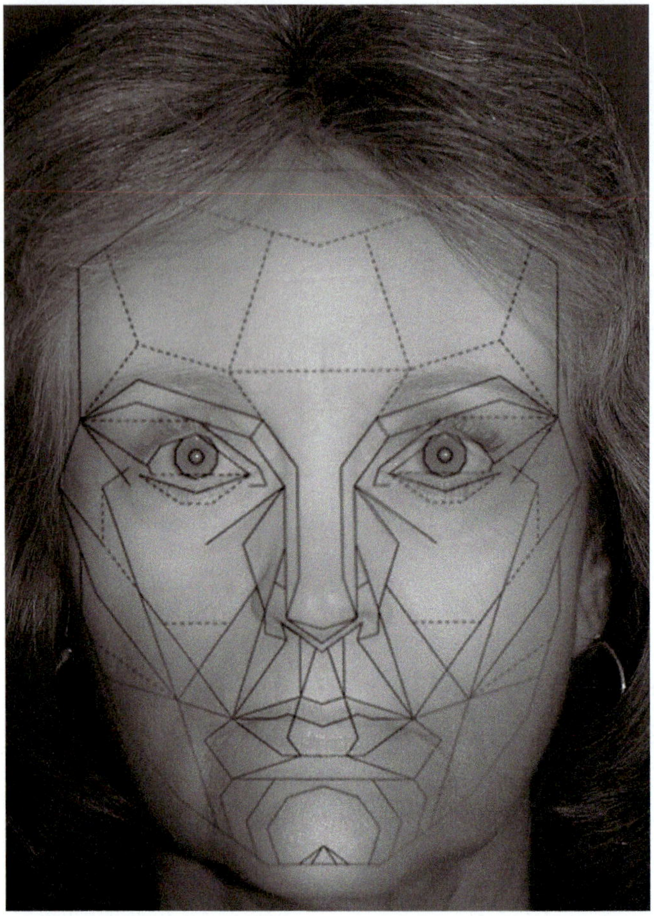

Fig. 2.1 A 55-year-old woman with the golden facial mask superimposed on a digital photograph

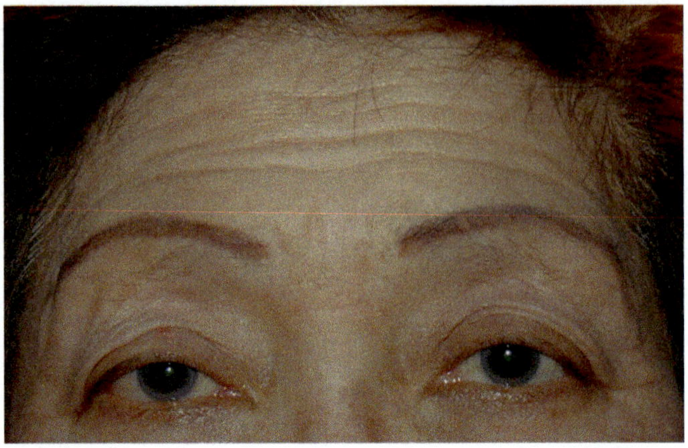

Fig. 2.2 A 76-year-old woman with visually significant bilateral upper eyelid ptosis and compensatory contraction of the frontalis muscle

photographs and used as an analytical tool to recognize the balance and arrangement of facial structures based on soft tissues in pre- and postoperative patients [4] (Fig. 2.1).

2.3 Forehead

Since the upper face forms the platform for facial recognition, beauty, and age estimation, it is a focus of many patients seeking aesthetic facial surgery. The importance of the upper facial appearance was studied with eye tracking devices to determine which facial regions on a photograph were used by observers to gauge age and tiredness. By far, the periorbital areas were the most scrutinized by observers [5].

The forehead is composed of multiple layers, including skin, connective tissue, and muscle. The skin of the forehead is the thickest of the face and contains transverse oriented septae extending from the dermis to the frontalis muscle. These are thought to play a distinct role in the transverse forehead furrows that occur with aging. The vertically oriented frontalis muscle is the main retractor of the upper face whose primary function is to raise the forehead/eyebrows. Its fibers originate from the galea aponeurotica on the scalp and it inserts on the skin of the eyebrows and nose. The galea aponeurotica divides into a superficial layer, encompassing the frontalis muscle and a deep layer, which attaches to the supraorbital margin and merges into the postorbicular fascial plane at the upper eyelid [6]. It is common to see chronic contraction of the frontalis muscle with secondary horizontal forehead rhytids in patients with visually significant upper eyelid ptosis or dermatochalasis (Fig. 2.2).

The primary depressors of the forehead and eyebrows are the procerus, corrugator supercilii, orbicularis oculi, and depressor supracilii muscles (Fig. 2.3). The procerus is a small, triangular muscle that originates from the fascia of the nasal bone and inserts into the glabellar and forehead skin, between the paired bellies of the frontalis muscle. It draws the medial angle of the eyebrow downward and is responsible for the horizontal wrinkles seen over the nasal bridge.

Superior to the procerus is the corrugator supercilii muscle, which lies at the medial one-third of the orbicularis oculi muscle. It originates from the nasal process of the frontal bone and extends obliquely over the supraorbital rim where it interdigitates with fibers from the frontalis and orbicularis muscles and inserts into the deep surface of the skin. Its action is to pull the forehead and eyebrow in an inferomedial direction. Contraction of the corrugator causes vertical "frown lines" rhytids (glabellar folds) medial to the eyebrow. Aesthetic evaluation should include testing for corrugator function to detect the presence of dynamic rhytids. Chemodenervation of the corrugator and procerus muscles with botulinum toxin injections provide temporary yet powerful treatment for dynamic rhytids in this region (Fig. 2.4). The corrugator muscle is supplied by the temporal branch of the facial nerve, and the procerus is innervated by the buccal branch of the facial nerve (cranial nerve VII).

The orbicularis oculi is divided into an orbital, preseptal, and pretarsal portions based on the anatomic structures that lie beneath (Fig. 2.3). The orbital fibers arise from the medial canthal tendon, arch along the orbital rim, and meet laterally

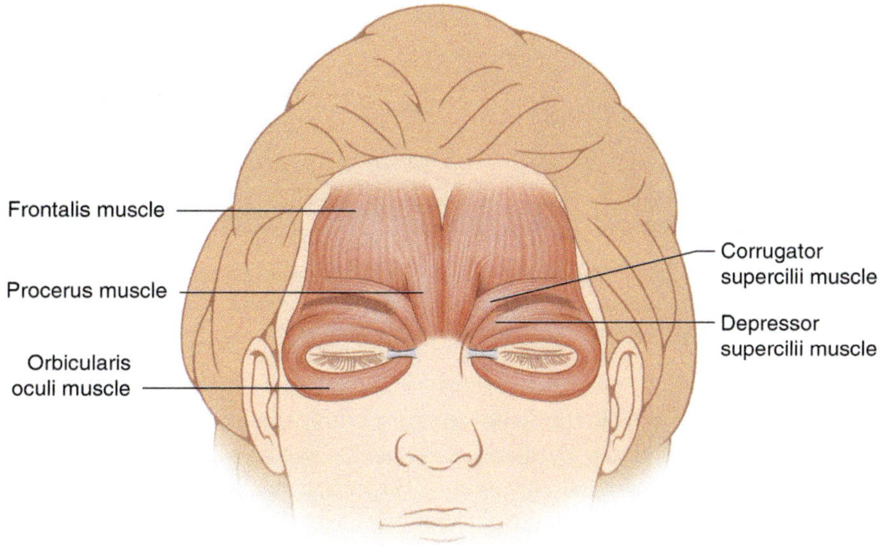

Fig. 2.3 Upper face retractors and depressors

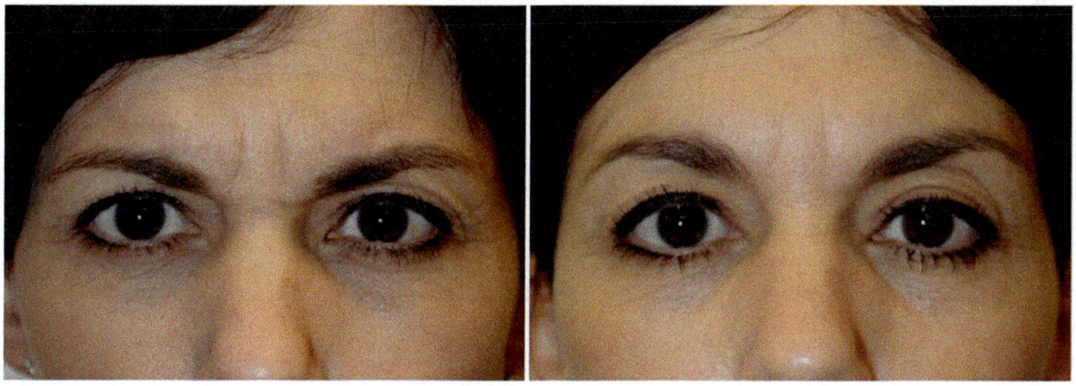

Fig. 2.4 This patient desired nonsurgical treatment for her glabellar rhytids (*left*). Four weeks after botulinum injection, she was satisfied with resolution of her rhytids (*right*). Patient still has presence of static rhytids and may benefit from soft tissue fillers

at the zygoma. The preseptal fibers overlie the orbital septum, originate at the medial canthal tendon and meet laterally to contribute to the lateral palpebral raphe. The pretarsal fibers are firmly adhered to the tarsus and travel in an elliptical path around the palpebral fissure. Medially, the pretarsal orbicularis splits into superficial and deep heads. The superficial head (along with the preseptal and orbital orbicularis) originate above and below the anterior reflection of the medial canthal tendon. The deep head arises at the posterior lacrimal crest (posterior reflection of medial canthal tendon). Laterally, the pretarsal orbicularis also forms superficial and deep heads. The deep head contributes to the lateral canthal tendon which inserts 3 mm posterior to the orbital rim at Whitnall's tubercle.

The orbicularis muscle functions as a protractor of the eyelids (blinking, squinting and forceful eyelid closure), with its orbital component an accessory depressor of the forehead. The superior fibers of the orbicularis oculi (upper eyelid) are innervated by the temporal branch of the facial nerve, while the inferior fibers (lower eyelid) are innervated by the zygomatic branch. The orbital fibers of the orbicularis muscle interdigitate superiorly with the frontalis muscle fibers, pulling the skin of the forehead and eyelid downward, while elevating the cheek toward the eye from their inferior function, resulting in dynamic "crow's feet." With aging and thinning of the overlying dermis and fascia, static rhytids develop over time.

Finally, the depressor supercilii originates on the medial orbital rim, near the lacrimal sac and inserts on the medial aspect of the bony orbit, inferior to the corrugators supracilii [7]. It is also innervated by the temporal branch of the facial nerve, and acts as an accessory depressor of the medial eyebrow.

2.4 Eyebrows

The eyebrows serve as a foundation for the eyelids. Freund and Nolan reported a study showing that, in general, men have straighter eyebrows, remaining at the level of the superior orbital rim, while women tend to have a greater arc that

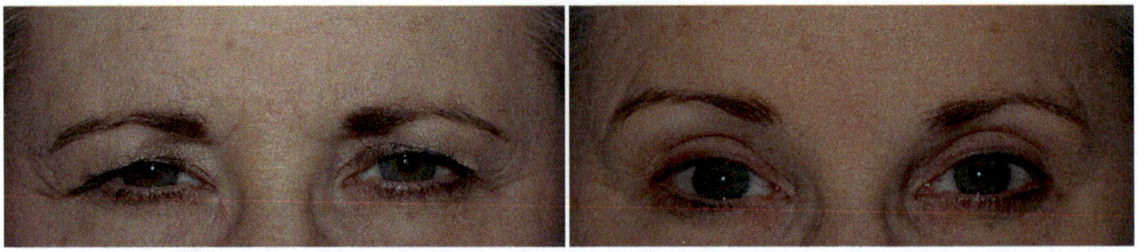

Fig. 2.5 Pre- and postoperative photographs of a 58-year-old patient after bilateral endoscopic eyebrow lift and upper eyelid blepharoplasty. Preoperatively, she had a flat brow with ptosis of the lateral tail (*left*). Postoperatively, a more youthful brow shape is achieved with the eyebrow apex located at the lateral limbus (*right*)

remains above the orbital rim, with the apex at the lateral limbus [8]. There is also a preference for a medial eyebrow below or at the supraorbital rim, with a shape that has a lateral slant in females [9]. A more contemporary assessment of favorable eyebrow shape, taking into account cultural preferences, indicates that a more lateral brow apex is preferable [10].

The orientation of eyebrow cilia is remarkably constant among individuals. Angular and lateralized cilia are much more abundant in the medial eyebrow, with decreasing degree as the eyebrow arcs laterally. The upper portion of the eyebrow contains cilia directed downward from the vertical plane, while in the lower portion they are directed upward from the vertical plane [11]. Incisions in the brow should to be beveled in the appropriate angle to preserve cilia.

With aging, the classical notion of eyebrow descent from the effects of gravity has been widely described. Recent studies, however, suggest that eyebrows can actually remain level or even elevate with age [12]. Some studies have shown a higher and more arched brow in older adults [13]. When eyebrow height in an older cohort was compared to a younger one, the older subjects had higher eyebrows and a flatter configuration, with the lateral and central regions having similar heights [12]. Lateral brow ptosis is more common due to lack of frontalis contraction in the lateral brow and also from gravitational pull from the heavy cheek and lateral facial tissues. Because of this, when rejuvenating the upper face, consideration should be given to selectively elevate the lateral brow, more than the nasal brow (Fig. 2.5).

Deep to the interdigitation of the frontalis/orbicularis muscles is a fibro-fatty layer termed the eyebrow fat pad, or retroorbicularis oculi fat pad (ROOF) (Fig. 2.6). The ROOF contributes to eyebrow volume and mobility of the lateral eyebrow and eyelid. However, in some individuals who have prominent eyebrow fullness, the ROOF can be debulked. The ROOF is continuous with the posterior orbicularis fascia in the eyelid [14].

There are variable amounts of eyebrow fat present among different ethnicities. Studies suggest that in the Asian eyelid, there is a more substantial fatty extension of the ROOF into the preseptal space, which has been denoted as "submuscular fibroadipose layer" or "preseptal fat pad" [15, 16]. The anatomic relationship of the ROOF and the eyelid must be remembered when operating on the eyelid, as the eyebrow fat can often be mistaken for preaponeurotic fat of the eyelid.

Treatment consideration – forehead and brow rejuvenation: Dynamic rhytids in the glabellar and lateral periorbital regions can be temporarily treated with chemodenervation. Surgically, eyebrow ptosis repair, either internally through a concurrent blepharoplasty incision or externally above the brow, can provide minimally invasive functional and aesthetic improvement. Finally, endoscopic or open coronal brow and forehead elevation is an excellent option for those seeking maximal yet more invasive rejuvenation.

2.5 Eyelid

2.5.1 Topography

The contour of the eyelid is highly dependent on gender, race, and age. The typical eyelid has a lateral canthus which is approximately 2 mm superior to the medial canthus. In Asians, this vertical elevation may be slightly higher, and is referred to as the "Mongoloid slant." The palpebral fissure in the adult averages 10–12 mm vertically, and 28–30 mm horizontally. In adults, about 1–2 mm of the superior cornea is covered by the upper eyelid margin and the apex of the upper lid margin is found nasal to a vertical line drawn through the center of the pupil.

The vertical palpebral fissure and position of the upper eyelid crease varies among different ethnic groups. This finding has important implications in both ptosis and upper eyelid blepharoplasty surgery. When eyelids of patients of African, Latino, and Asian ancestry were studied, all groups had a lower upper lid (relative ptosis) than Caucasian patients [17]. This was identified by measuring the margin reflex distance (MRD). This is the distance from the upper (MRD1) or lower (MRD2) lid margins to a light reflex in the center of the pupil created by shining a light at the patient's eyes. This is the best parameter of lid position (i.e., ptosis or lower lid retraction), as it is unaffected by the position of its upper or lower lid counterpart.

The upper eyelid crease (formed by attachments of the levator aponeurosis to the skin) in Caucasians is 7–8 mm above the lid margin in men and 10–12 mm in women. In Asians, the crease is lower and the upper sulcus more full. It has traditionally been thought that this occurs because the orbital septum and levator aponeurosis fuse lower on the lid, below the superior tarsal border. However, a recent study by Kakizaki et al. showed that this fusion occurred above the tarsal border [17]. In either case, the preaponeurotic fat pad (PFP) descends and prevents a higher insertion of the levator aponeurosis to the upper lid skin [18]. These variations result in an inferiorly positioned or absent upper eyelid crease in Asians.

The lower lid margin rests at the inferior limbus of the cornea, with a crease that is 2 mm below the lash line medially and 5 mm laterally. The nadir of the lower lid margin is slightly lateral to the center of the pupil.

2.5.2 Lamellae

The upper and lower eyelid layers are classically divided into the anterior, middle, and posterior lamellae. The skin and underlying orbicularis oculi muscle comprise the anterior lamella of the upper eyelid. The orbital septum forms the middle lamella, separating the true orbit from the eyelid. The posterior lamella is composed of the tarsal plate, eyelid retractors, and conjunctiva (Fig. 2.6).

Deep to the orbicularis muscle and above the tarsus is the fibrous orbital septum. The orbital septum originates from the arcus marginalis, a band of thickened periosteum at the superior orbital rim [19]. The anterior layer of the orbital septum fuses with the levator aponeurosis which forms extensions into the orbicularis muscle and skin to form the eyelid crease [20, 21]. If the septum is mistaken for the levator aponeurosis and advanced during ptosis repair, lagophthalmos and eyelid retraction may develop [22].

The upper eyelid fat is found posterior to the orbital septum and is divided into two components, the preaponeurotic fat pad (PFP) and the medial (or nasal) fat pad (Fig. 2.7). The PFP is found just anterior to the levator aponeurosis. The orbital lobe of the lacrimal gland, found laterally and posterior to the septum can be mistaken for the PFP and must be carefully identified and avoided in upper eyelid fat removal. The PFP is made up of fat encased in a thin membranous sac, the wall of which harbors small blood vessels and is innervated by terminal branches of the supraorbital nerve [23].

The nasal fat pad is surrounded by the medial horn of the levator aponeurosis and the tendon of the superior

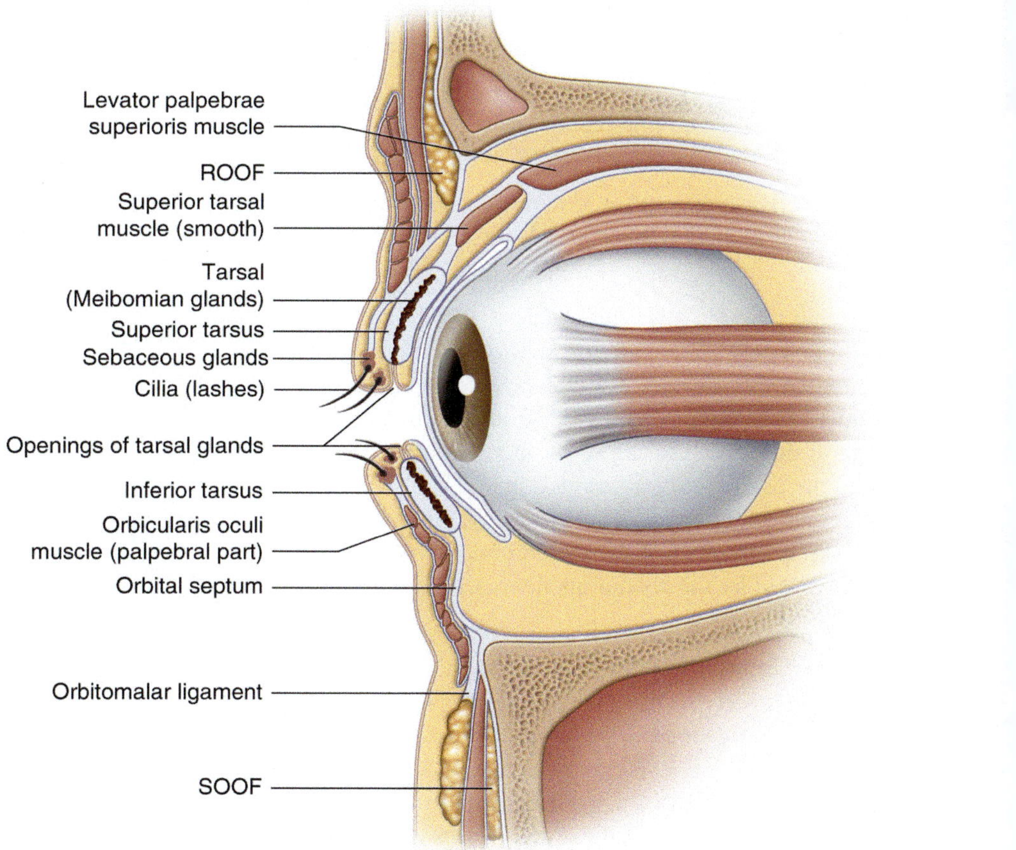

Fig. 2.6 The ROOF sits posterior to the orbital portion of the orbicularis oculi muscle

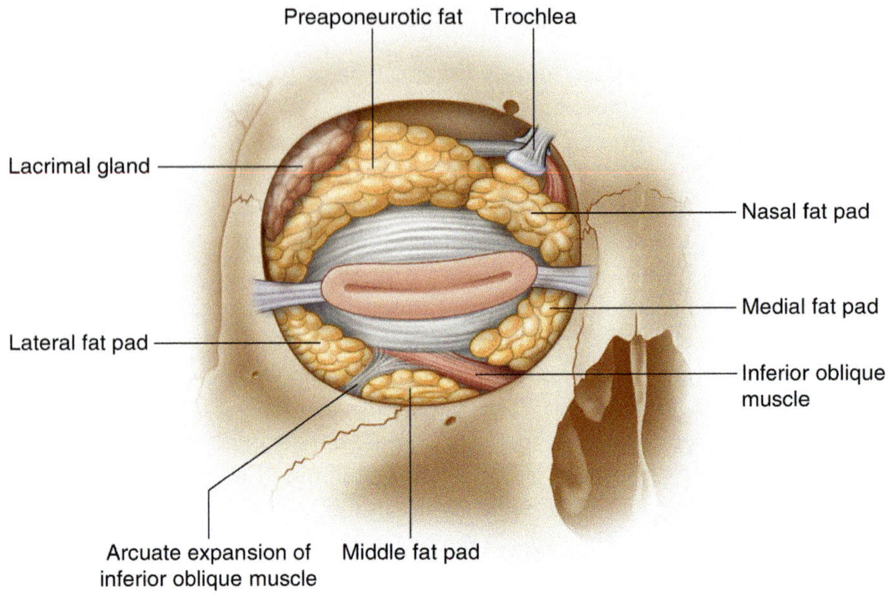

Fig. 2.7 Upper and lower eyelid fat pads

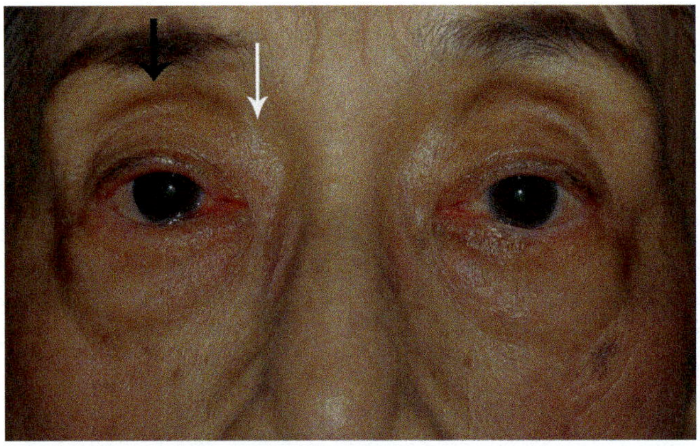

Fig. 2.8 This 72-year-old man has atrophy of the central fat pad (*black arrow*) with preservation of the nasal fat pad (*white arrow*)

oblique muscle. It is whiter than the PFP and noted to be similar in character to intraconal orbital fat [24]. The trochlea of the superior oblique muscle separates the nasal and PFP. During surgical procedures in this region, damage to this structure can result in strabismus, i.e., superior oblique palsy or Brown's syndrome [25]. During transconjunctival upper eyelid blepharoplasty, the nasal fat pad can be safely approached via the conjunctiva because it is not interrupted by the levator aponeurosis [26].

Treatment considerations – fat pad contouring in upper eyelid blepharoplasty: Korn et al. noted an abundance of adult stem cells derived from human orbital adipose tissue in the upper lid fat pads [27]. Although these cells were noted in both the nasal and PFP, there was two-fold higher staining of putative neural-crest stem cell markers in the nasal fat pad. A higher population of these cells in the nasal fat pad may explain the prominence of the nasal pad and atrophy of the PFP with aging. During fat removal in blepharoplasty, we recommend preservation of the PFP with conservative excision of the nasal fat pad if clinically indicated (Fig. 2.8).

2.5.3 Upper Eyelid Retractors

The levator palpebrae superioris (LPS) is the main retractor of the upper eyelid and arises from the orbital apex. The muscular portion is 40 mm in length with a terminal tendonous sheath that extends for about 14–20 mm, termed the levator aponeurosis (LA) [28]. The transition from muscle to tendon of the LPS is at the region of Whitnall's ligament. Whitnall's ligament, in concert with the intermuscular transverse ligament, may act to elevate the LPS like a pulley [29]. The central portion of the LA inserts onto the tarsal surface via elastic attachments. It also sends attachments to the orbicularis muscle and skin forming the eyelid crease (Fig. 2.6). With age, the LA may become attenuated or disinserted, compromising lid height, and leading to ptosis [30]. In thyroid-related orbitopathy, lid contour may change as the peak of the upper eyelid is situated laterally (temporal flare) [31] (Fig. 2.9).

Müller's muscle is an accessory retractor and is a smooth muscle that lies deep to the levator and firmly attaches to underlying conjunctiva near the superior margin of the tarsus [32]. It is innervated by the sympathetic nervous system and contraction causes approximately 2 mm of eyelid retraction. Aging causes thinning, fat deposition, and lengthening of Müller's muscle, which can be effectively resected for mild to moderate ptosis. Classically, topical phenylephrine is used as a diagnostic tool to determine if resection of Müller's

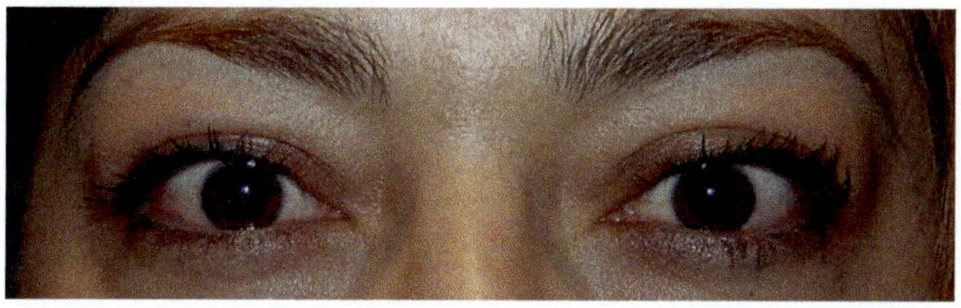

Fig. 2.9 A 47-year-old woman with thyroid related orbitopathy, exhibits lateral upper eyelid flare in both eyes

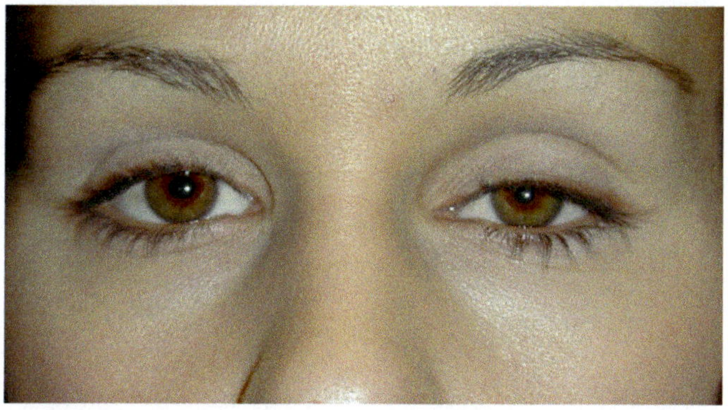

Fig. 2.10 This 26-year-old woman was initially referred for left upper eyelid ptosis. Examination revealed miosis of the left eye, with greater aniscoria in dim light. Horner's syndrome was confirmed with pharmacologic testing, and she was referred for systemic evaluation

muscle could correct the existing ptosis (see Chap. 13). There is now evidence that patients who are both positive and negative for this test may benefit from a Müllerectomy [33].

Clinical pearls: During ptosis evaluation, it is imperative to examine the pupils for anisocoria. Patients with ptosis and ipsilateral miosis must be evaluated for Horner's syndrome (Fig. 2.10). Whereas patients with ptosis and an ipsilaterally enlarged pupil, require evaluation for acute or chronic third nerve paresis.

2.5.4 Tarsus

The tarsus of the upper and lower eyelids have attachments to the periosteum of the orbital rim via the medial and lateral canthal tendons. The upper eyelid tarsal plate measures 10–12 mm vertically and tapers at the medial and lateral ends. The lower eyelid tarsal plate is 4 mm vertically and also taper at its medial and lateral ends. The tarsal plates are composed of dense connective tissue and function as rigid structural support to the eyelids. Both the medial and lateral canthal tendons secure the tarsus to their corresponding orbital rims. Medially the canthal tendon has a deep attachment to the posterior lacrimal crest and a superficial attachment to the anterior lacrimal crest. Laterally, the canthal tendon also has a deep attachment 3 mm posterior to the orbital rim of a Whitnall's tubercle. These posterior attachments are important in maintaining appropriate lid position and continuity with the globe. With age, stretching and attenuation of the canthal tendons can result in a variety of involutional eyelid malpositions (ectropion, entropion, retraction).

2.5.5 Lower Eyelid

The layered lamellae of the lower eyelid are analogous to those of the upper eyelid. The capsulopalpebral fascia (CF) and the inferior tarsal muscle make up the lower eyelid retractors. The CF and the inferior tarsal muscle are akin to the levator aponeurosis and Müller's muscle in the upper eyelid, respectively. The capsulopalpebral head originates from the fascia of the inferior rectus muscle, then envelopes the inferior oblique muscle to become the CF, inserting at the inferior tarsal border along with the orbital septum. The inferior tarsal muscle receives sympathetic innervation and is located posterior to the CF.

Until recently, it was thought that the lower eyelid retractors were a single layer consisting of the CF and inferior tarsal muscle [34]. Recent studies demonstrate that the lower lid retractors are actually made of two layers, which can be separated using either blunt or sharp dissection [35, 36]. The CF transmits forces exerted by the inferior rectus muscle on the lower lid. This intimate relationship can result in lower eyelid retraction after inferior rectus recession surgery (Fig. 2.11). The lower eyelid crease is formed by small fibers of the CF that attach to the skin-orbicularis complex just a few millimeters below the tarsus.

The position of the lower eyelid margin is highly dependent on the three-dimensional vector forces imposed by the lower eyelid retractors and the canthal ligaments. Mechanical and involutional forces from either acquired or developmental abnormalities may cause eyelid problems, such as entropion and ectropion. In lower eyelid entropion, upward forces cause internal rotation of the inferior tarsal plate, an observation seen more frequently in Asians because of more prominent adipose tissue [37]. On the other hand, Caucasians more frequently exhibit ectropion, possibly due to loss of soft tissue support and greater tendency for actinic changes in the skin. The posterior layer of the lower eyelid retractors has been shown to provide the vertical vector force of the eyelid and should be targeted during surgical correction of both eyelid ectropion and entropion [36].

The orbital septum of the lower eyelid arises as a fibrous extension of the arcus marginalis. The orbital septum fuses with the lower eyelid retractors below the tarsal plate. In Caucasians, this conjoined area begins 3–4 mm lower than it does in Asians. As a result of these anatomic differences,

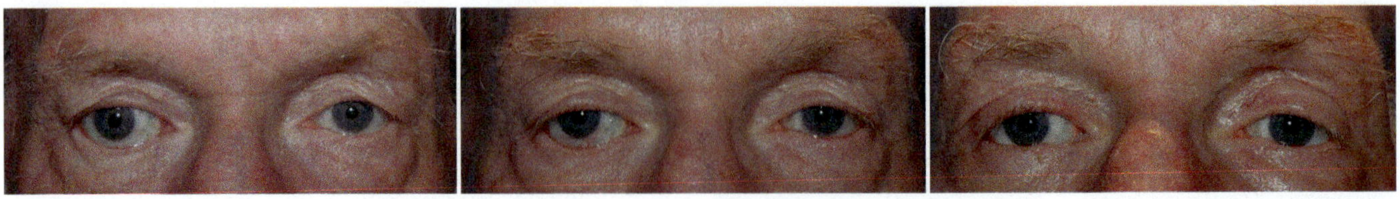

Fig. 2.11 This patient initially presented with left hypertropia and right lower eyelid retraction (*left*). After right inferior rectus recession, his right lower eyelid retraction worsened (*center*). He had right lower eyelid retraction repair with posterior lamellar grafting with hard palate mucosa (*right*). This case demonstrates the intimate relationship between the inferior rectus muscle and the lower eyelid retractors

the length of unreinforced septum is about 12.3 mm in Asians and only 9.3 mm in Caucasians. Attenuation of the inferior orbital septum thereby allows anterior and superior extension of the lower eyelid fat pads in Asians, analogous to inferior extension of the same tissue in the upper eyelid [38].

There are three clinically apparent fat pads in the lower eyelid: the medial, central, and lateral fat pads. The belly of the inferior oblique muscle divides the medial and central fat pads, while its arcuate expansion separates the central and lateral fat pads. Anatomic variations do exist where only two compartments or a non-compartmentalized single fat pad is found. A pretarsal fat pad has also been described and is located at the lateral half of the tarsal plate, just superior to the lateral fat pad [39]. This pretarsal fat can contribute to the visible bulk of the eyelid below the eyelashes.

Lockwood's ligament is the primary suspensory ligament in the lower eyelid. It can be divided into an inferior ligament (which supports the eyelid retractors), the main ligament, and an arcuate expansion. The main ligament inserts onto Whitnall's tubercle at the lateral orbital wall, approximately 11 mm below the frontozygomatic suture [40]. Lockwood's ligament acts as one of the suspensory support systems of the inferior orbit [41]. The arcuate expansion divides the central and lateral fat pads of the lower eyelid.

Clinical pearls: One of the dreaded complications after lower eyelid blepharoplasty is lower eyelid retraction. Both anterior lamellar shortening and middle or posterior lamellar cicatrices can cause retraction. Spacer grafts may be necessary for posterior lamellar shortening. If minimal anterior lamellar deficiency coexists with middle or posterior lamellar scarring, a cheek or midface lift may be simultaneously performed to recruit anterior lamellar tissue. Severe cases of anterior lamellar deficiency resulting in eyelid marginal ectropion and keratinization of the palpebral conjunctiva require a full-thickness skin graft.

2.6 Midface

Aging of the midface is associated with descent of soft tissue, demarcation of the nasojugal and nasolabial folds, deflation of the facial soft tissues, and loss of bone. These varied structural age-related midface changes make comprehensive rejuvenation challenging.

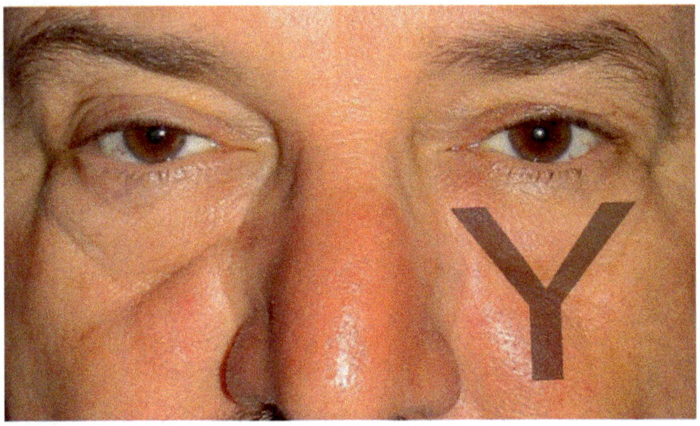

Fig. 2.12 A 61-year man with midface ptosis exhibiting an obliquely oriented "Y," formed by the palpebromalar groove superolaterally, the nasojugal groove medially, and the midcheek furrow/groove inferolaterally (*right*)

2.6.1 Topography

The term "midface" is a defined region demarcated superiorly from an imaginary line between the medial and lateral canthi, and inferiorly from an imaginary line between the inferior border of the tragal cartilage to just below the oral commissure.

In youth, the midface has a uniformly rounded fullness. With age, it tends to assume an obliquely oriented "Y," formed by the palpebromalar groove superolaterally, the nasojugal groove medially, and the midcheek furrow/groove inferolaterally [42] (Fig. 2.12). Loss of the maxillary projection (bone) below the orbit is a major contributor to laxity and descent of the medial cheek soft tissue. Some studies have advocated augmentation of the infraorbital rim with alloplastic implants to provide convexity to this region [43]. Schematically, the prominent, youthful midface can be viewed as a "base up triangle," with the cheeks forming the base. With age, midface ptosis and lower face jowls transform the triangle to a base down configuration (Fig. 2.13).

2.6.2 Soft Tissue Lamellae

The soft tissues of the face can be categorically divided into five concentric layers: (1) skin, (2) subcutaneous layer, (3) musculoaponeurotic layer, (4) loose areolar tissue, and (5) periosteum and deep fascia [44].

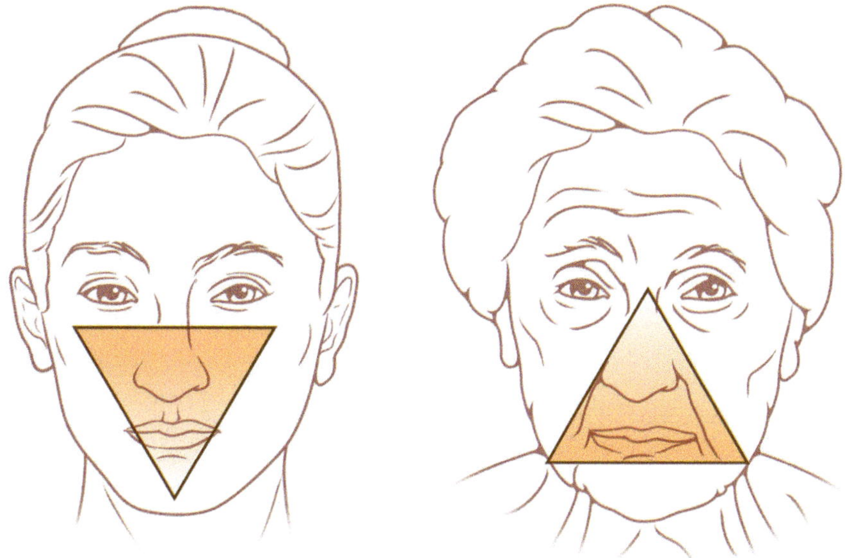

Fig. 2.13 In youth, the lower face has a base up triangle (*left*). However, with aging changes, the lower face takes on a base down triangular configuration (*right*)

The musculoaponeurotic layer, termed the superficial musculoaponeurotic system (SMAS), is firmly attached to the skin by retinacular cutis fibers within the subcutaneous layer. The SMAS has only limited attachments to the underlying bony skeleton, likely contributing to its inferior descent seen with aging [45]. The SMAS spreads out in a fanlike fashion and functions to transmit and distribute the facial muscle contractions to the skin. The fibrous network of the SMAS invests the orbicularis oculi and attaches to the orbital rim via the orbitomalar ligament (OML) [46]. With age, the elastin fibers of the SMAS degenerate, leading to descent of the SMAS and development of senile facial changes, such as malar festoons, eyelid ectropion, and orbital fat prolapse [17].

The areolar layer lies posterior to the SMAS and is composed of ligaments anchoring the overlying soft tissue to the facial bones [47]. With aging, these areas without deep attachments become distended and appear as bulges on the surface. In contrast, areas firmly attached to the dermis resist this distention and result in cutaneous grooves or folds.

2.6.3 Nasojugal Groove

The nasojugal groove, also known as the "tear trough" or medial lid-cheek junction, becomes more visible with age. This region is a natural depression, extending inferolaterally from the medial canthus to the midpupillary line [48].

With age-related midface descent, atrophy of skin and soft tissue, the tear trough is accentuated as thin eyelid tissue overlies the inferior orbital rim. In addition, elongation of the area between the OML and the eyelid margin leads to prolapse of orbital fat over the inferior orbital rim. The increased visibility of this region adds to the formation of "eyelid bags" and often motivates patients to seek periorbital aesthetic surgery.

Clinical pearls: Filler injection to restore volume to the tear trough has gained popularity as a nonsurgical alternative to lower lid blepharoplasty. However, the long-term efficacy of these materials has not been well studied. In a study by Donath, an 85% average maintenance effect of augmentation was noted at 15 months [49]. One patient, at 23 months, had a 73% volume retention. Limited soft tissue movement (facial dynamics) in this area compared to other facial sites, may explain the longer retention of hyaluronic acid fillers in the tear trough as compared to other facial areas.

2.6.4 Malar Region

The malar segment is a triangular region between the lid-cheek junction and the nasolabial region. This area of the midface is formed superiorly by the OML along the inferior orbital rim, the zygomatic ligaments laterally, and a transverse line from the zygomatic ligaments through the zygomaticus muscles. The zygomaticus minor and major muscles, which appear clinically as one complex, draw the mouth superolaterally, as exemplified in smiling. Since the facial nerve courses deep to the plane of the zygomaticus major, it provides a reliable guide to dissection into the medial portion of the face.

On the deep surface of the orbicularis muscle, at the superior border of the malar region, lies a significant layer of fat overlying the periosteum, termed the suborbicularis oculi fat (SOOF). It has been shown that the SOOF is actually a continuation from the ROOF superiorly [42]. In one study, the SOOF was shown to have two distinct areas, termed the lateral and medial suborbicularis oculi fat [50]. In addition, Rohrich describes a third, distinct fat pad, the deep cheek fat, which is found medial to the medial suborbicularis oculi fat. Since there can be differential loss and preservation of the

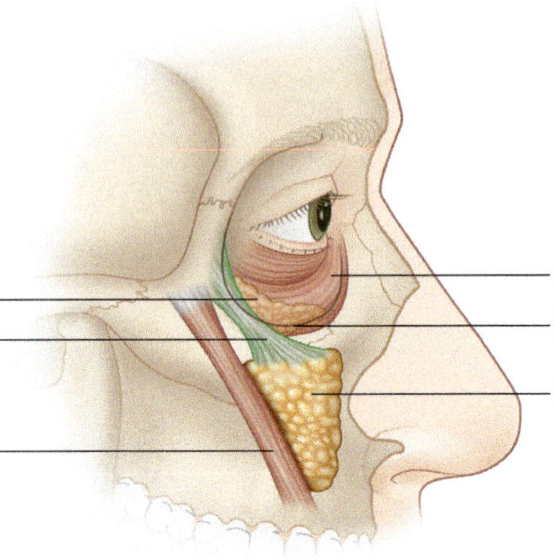

Fig. 2.14 With aging, there is laxity of the orbitomalar ligament (*green*), leading to inferior descent of the SOOF and skeletonization of the inferior orbital rim

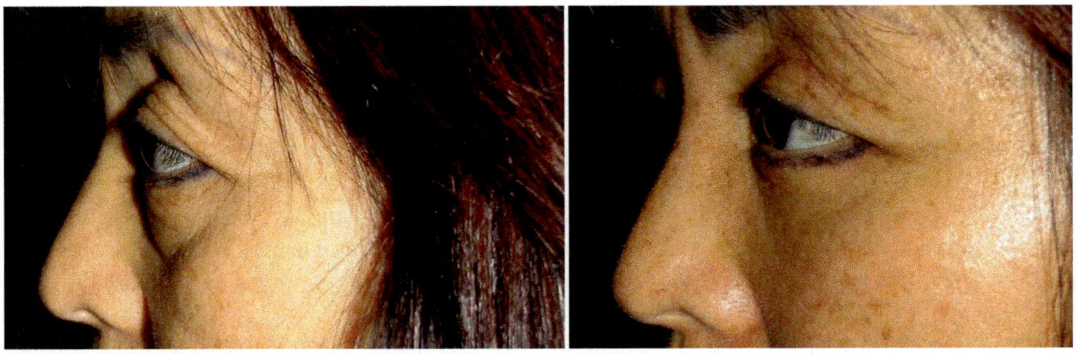

Fig. 2.15 A 56-year-old patient with superior sulcus hollowing, double convex deformity of lower eyelids, and unmasking of the inferior orbital rim (*left*). She had upper and lower eyelid blepharoplasty along with resuspension of the orbitomalar ligament and elevation of the SOOF (*right*). Note the elevation of her midface and softening of the nasojugal groove

three fat compartments, any facial rejuvenation procedure should aim to treat only the deficient regions, and targeted soft tissue augmentation is ideal for this purpose.

The SOOF has variable thickness, being most prominent in the central and lateral malar region. Medially, the SOOF engulfs the mimetic muscles and lies superficial to the periosteum. Many theorize that loss and/or ptosis of the SOOF and its adjacent deep fat compartments, in combination with the attenuation and relaxation of connective tissue, contributes to "malar bags" associated with aging [51, 52]. In severe cases, the "double convexity" deformity is noted. In this case, the prolapsed orbital fat is the superior convexity, below which is the concavity caused by the deflated skeletonized inferior orbital rim. The inferior convexity is defined by the malar mound.

The role of the SMAS, OML, and SOOF should be understood to access anatomic changes that occur in the lower eyelid. Inferior descent of the SMAS and SOOF contributes to unmasking of the inferior orbital rim (Fig. 2.14). Concurrent lengthening of the OML can result in apparent vertical elongation of the lower eyelid. In these cases, SOOF lifting and anatomic reconstitution of the OML should be considered [53].

Clinical pearls: Resuspension of the SOOF with the OML, in conjunction with lower eyelid blepharoplasty, provide powerful elevation and support for the entire midface [47] (Fig. 2.15).

2.6.5 Nasolabial Region

The nasolabial region of the midface is trapezoidal in shape, encompassing the side of the nose between the malar segment and lip, and continuing as the lower cheek beyond the oral commissure. It can be divided into two segments, an upper and lower segment. The upper segment overlies the maxilla and the levator labii superioris and levator labii superioris alaequae nasi, two mimetic muscles involved in raising the upper lip. The lower segment of the nasolabial region forms the roof of the oral cavity and is predominantly mobile. Its lateral segment, however, is directly fixed with strong

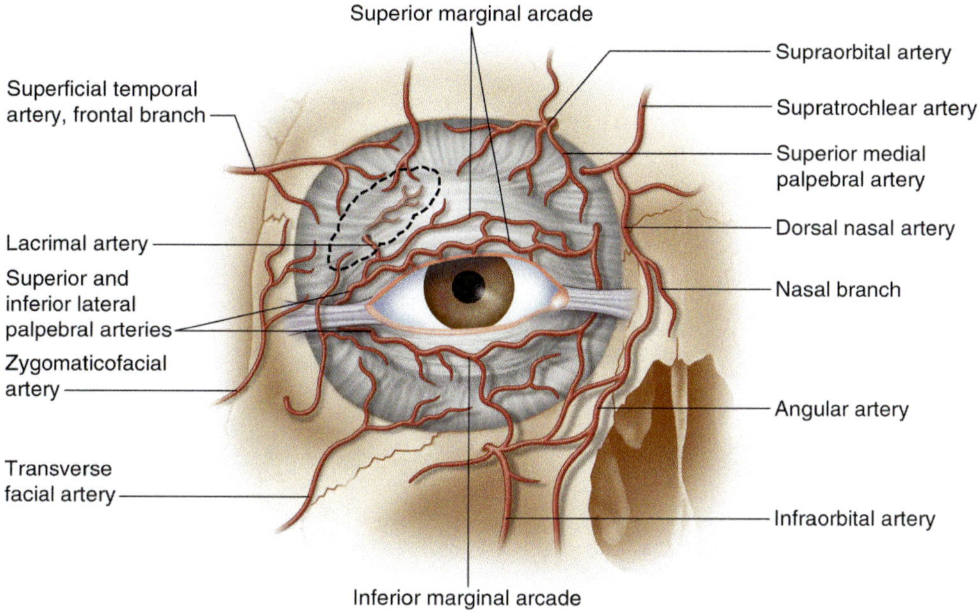

Fig. 2.16 Eyelid vasculature

ligamentous attachments to the zygoma and has additional support from the upper masseteric ligaments.

The subcutaneous layer in the nasolabial region is composed of thicker and more mobile fat termed the "malar fat pad" [54]. In older individuals, laxity of suspensory attachment of the nasolabial area by the zygomatic ligaments, leads to loss of the youthful, rounded fullness. In addition, as the lateral portion of the nasolabial region in the midface disinserts from the bony girdle beneath, hollowing of the midcheek also become prominent.

2.7 Facial Vasculature, Innervation, and Lymphatic Drainage

The internal and external carotid arteries provide the blood supply to the face. The superficial temporal artery and the terminal branch of the external carotid artery, supplies the lateral forehead and eyebrow. The medial forehead is supplied by terminal branches of the ophthalmic artery, including the supraorbital and supratrochlear arteries.

The upper eyelid is supplied by the marginal and peripheral arcades from the ophthalmic artery [55] (Fig. 2.16). Terminal branches of the ophthalmic and facial arteries provide additional vasculature to the medial eyelid. The angular artery, the terminal branch of the facial artery, lies about 6–8 mm medial to the medial canthus and 5 mm anterior to the lacrimal sac.

Clinical pearls: When grafting fat in the periorbital region, care must be taken to inject the fat while withdrawing the needle or cannula. Fat emboli injected into the arterial system anywhere in the face, can lead to end organ infarction [56].

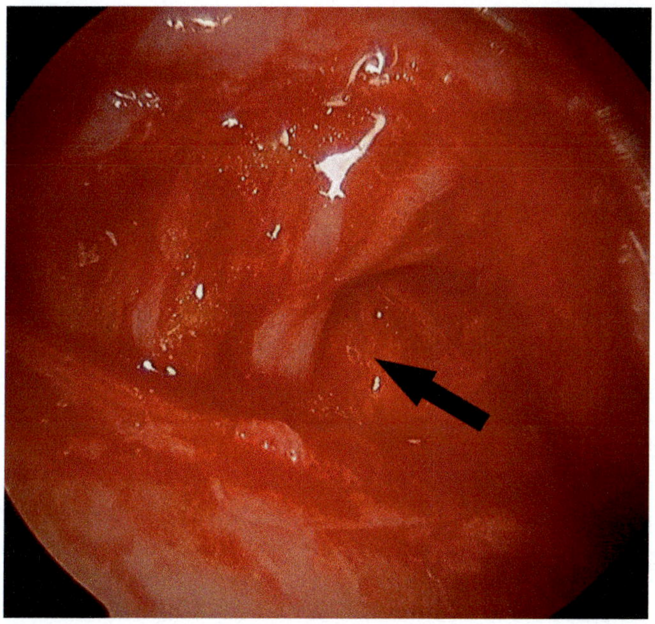

Fig. 2.17 During endoscopic browlift procedures, the supraorbital neurovascular bundle (*arrow*) must be preserved

The trigeminal nerve (cranial nerve V) provides sensation to the face. The brow receives sensory innervation from the ophthalmic division of the nerve (V1). The supratrochlear nerve conveys sensation to the bridge of the nose and medial part of the upper eyelid and forehead. The supraorbital neurovascular bundle exits the orbit through a notch or foramen in the superior orbital rim and provides sensation to the rest of the forehead and scalp. Care must be taken to preserve the supraorbital neurovascular bundle during endoscopic forehead surgery [57] (Fig. 2.17).

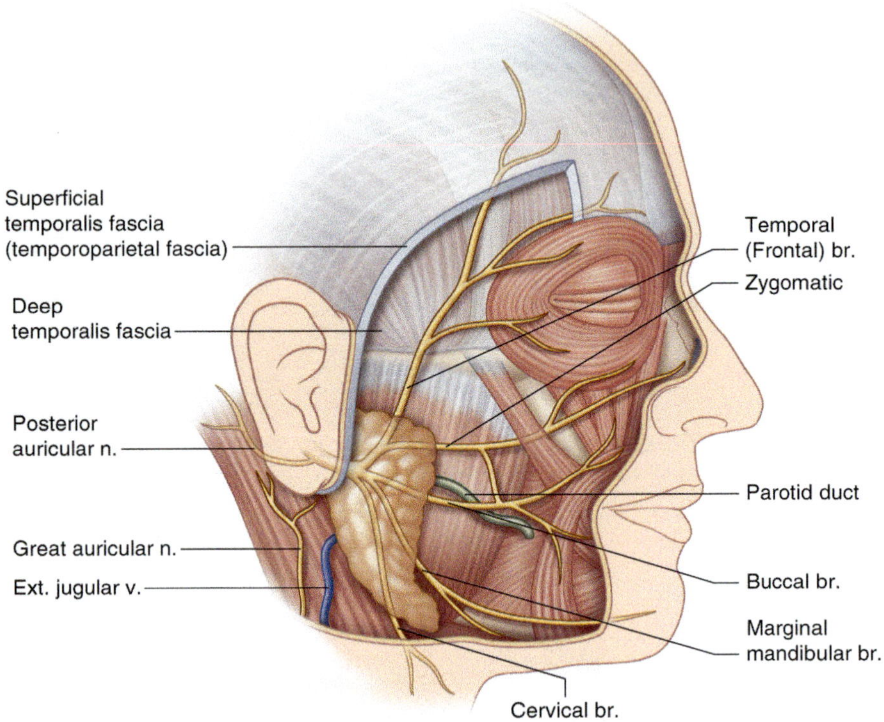

Fig. 2.18 The course of the facial nerve. In the temporal region, the facial nerve is found within the superficial temporalis fascia, and superficial to the deep temporalis fascia

Sensory innervation to the skin overlying the malar region is provided by the maxillary branch (V2) of the trigeminal nerve. It innervates the lower eyelid, cheek, side of the nose, nasal vestibule, and the skin and mucosa of the upper lip. Subperiosteal midface cheek lifts may injure the infraorbital nerve resulting in hypesthesia of the maxillary region.

Facial motor function is provided by the facial nerve (cranial nerve VII) and the oculomotor nerve (cranial nerve III – eyelid elevation) (Fig. 2.18). CNVII divides into its major trunks within the parotid gland. The superior division of CNVII innervates the upper eyelids via its temporal (frontal) branch, and the lower lids via its zygomatic and buccal branches [58]. In the temporal region, branches of the temporal nerve are found in the deep portion of the superficial temporal fascia (Fig. 2.18). During manipulation in this region, dissection must be deep to this layer (on top of the deep temporal fascia) to protect the nerve [59]. In addition to the upper eyelids (orbicularis muscle), the temporal branch also innervates the frontalis muscle, the corrugator muscle, the depressor supercilii muscle, and the anterior and superior auricular muscles.

In the lower face, the branches of the facial nerve are deep to the SMAS and become superficial medial to the masseter muscle. Because of its location, dissection during rhytidectomy must be performed superficial to the SMAS to avoid injury to the nerve.

The face has a rich lymphatic drainage system. The eyelids drain into the preauricular and submandibular lymph nodes; the midface drains to the submental and submandibular nodes; and the lateral face drains to the preauricular and retroauricular nodes. Disruption of the lymphatics during aesthetic surgical procedures can lead to prolonged lymphadenopathy and chemosis.

2.8 Conclusion

A sound anatomic approach to surgery remains the basis for all successful cosmetic and reconstructive procedures. This is especially true is regards to surgery on the eyelids and adjacent areas. The forehead/eyebrows and the upper lids, and the lower lids and midface act and function as a continuum. Understanding the clinical, surgical, and functional anatomy of how these structures interrelate is essential to attaining successful outcomes to surgery. In addition to relevant anatomic knowledge, it is imperative to be cognizant of the important changes associated with aging in order to effectively rejuvenate this area of the face. Only with mastery of these two principals can the aesthetic surgeon provide the best care for patients.

References

1. Tolleth H. Concepts for the plastic surgeon from art and sculpture. Clin Plastic Surg. 1987;14(4):585–98.
2. Farkas LG, Hreczko TA, et al. Vertical and horizontal proportions of the face in young adult North American Caucasians: revision of neoclassical canons. Plast Reconstr Surg. 1985;73:328–37.

3. Marquardt SR, Stephen R. Marquardt on the Golden Decagon and human facial beauty. Interview by Dr. Gottlieb. J Clin Orthodont. 2002;36:339–47.
4. Lee JH, Kim TG, Park GW, Kim YH. Cumulative frequency distribution in East Asian facial widths using the facial golden mask. J Craniofac Surg. 2009;20(5):1378–82.
5. Nguyen HT, Isaacowitz DM, Rubin PA. Age- and fatigue-related markers of human faces: an eye-tracking study. Ophthalmology. 2009;116(2):355–60. (The visual cues of facial aging and mood are noted by observers in periorbital areas).
6. Lemke B, Stasior OG. The anatomy of eyebrow ptosis. Arch Ophthalmol. 1982;100:981–6.
7. Cook Jr BE, Lucarelli MJ, Lemke BN. Depressor supercilii muscle: anatomy, histology, and cosmetic implications. Ophthal Plast Reconstr Surg. 2001;17(6):404–11.
8. Freund RM, Nolan III WB. Correlation between brow lift outcomes and aesthetic ideals for eyebrow height and shape in females. Plast Reconstr Surg. 1996;97:1343–8.
9. Westmore M. Facial cosmetics in conjunction with surgery. Paper presented at the Aesthetic Plastic Surgical Society Meeting, Vancouver, BC, May 1974.
10. Biller JA, Kim DW. A contemporary assessment of facial aesthetic preferences. Arch Facial Plast Surg. 2009;11(2):91–7.
11. Lemke BN, Stasior OG. Eyebrow incision making. Adv Ophthalmic Plast Reconstr Surg. 1983;2:19–23.
12. Matros E, Garcia JA, Yaremchuk MJ. Changes in eyebrow position and shape with aging. Plast Reconstr Surg. 2009;124(4): 1296–301.
13. Ramirez OM. Subperiosteal brow lifts without fixation. Plast Reconstr Surg. 2004;114:1604–5.
14. Putterman AM, Urist MJ. Surgical anatomy of the orbital septum. Ann Ophthalmol. 1974;6:290–4.
15. Meyer DR, Linberg JV, et al. Anatomy of the orbital septum and associated eyelid connective tissues. Ophthal Plast Reconstr Surg. 1991;7:104–13.
16. Seiff SR, Seiff BD. Anatomy of the Asian eyelid. Facial Plast Surg Clin North Am. 2007;15(3):309–14.
17. Kakizaki H, Leibovitch I, Selva D, et al. Orbital septum attachment on the levator aponeurosis in Asians: in vivo and cadaver study. Ophthalmology. 2009;116(10):2031–5.
18. Chen WP. Asian blepharoplasty: update on anatomy and techniques. Ophthal Plast Reconstr Surg. 1987;3(3):135–40.
19. Jordan DR, Anderson RL. Surgical anatomy of the ocular adnexa: a clinical approach. Ophthalmology Monograph 9. San Francisco: American Academy of Ophthalmology; 1996: p. 16, 17, 26.
20. Malik KJ, Lee MS, et al. Lash ptosis in congenital and acquired blepharoptosis. Arch Ophthalmol. 2007;125:1613–5.
21. Murchison AP, Sires BA, Jian-Amadi A. Margin reflex distance in different ethnic groups. Arch Facial Plast Surg. 2009;11(5):303–5.
22. Tarbet KJ, Lemke BN. Clinical anatomy of the upper face. Int Ophthalmol Clin. 1997 Summer;37(3):11–28.
23. Persichetti P, Lella FD, et al. Adipose compartments of the upper eyelid: anatomy applied to blepharoplasty. Plast Reconstr Surg. 2004;113:373–8.
24. Johnston MC, Noden DM, Hazelton RD, et al. Origins of avian ocular and periocular tissues. Exp Eye Res. 1979;29:27–43.
25. Neely KA, Ernest JT, et al. Combined superior oblique paresis and Brown's syndrome after blepharoplasty. Am J Ophthalmol. 1990;109(3):347–9.
26. Gausas RE. Advances in applied anatomy of the eyelid and orbit. Curr Opin Ophthalmol. 2004;15:422–5.
27. Korn BS, Kikkawa DO, Hicok KC. Identification and characterization of adult stem cells from human orbital adipose tissue. Ophthal Plast Reconstr Surg. 2009;25:27–32.
28. Most SP, Mobley SR, et al. Anatomy of the eyelids. Facial Plast Surg Clin North Am. 2005;13:487–92.
29. Ettl A, Priglinger S, et al. Functional anatomy of the levator palpebrae superioris muscle and its connective tissue system. Br J Ophthalmol. 1996;80:702–7.
30. Karesh JW. Diagnosis and management of acquired blepharoptosis and dermatochalasis. Facial Plast Surg. 1994;10(2):185–201.
31. Kakizaki H. Modified marginal myotomy for thyroid-related upper eyelid retraction. Eur J Plast Surg. 2008;31:9–13.
32. Kakizaki H, Zako M, et al. The levator aponeurosis consists of two layers that include smooth muscle. Ophthal Plast Reconstr Surg. 2005;21:379–82.
33. Baldwin HC, Bhagey J, et al. Open sky Müller muscle-conjunctival resection in phenylephrine test-negative blepharoptosis patients. Ophthal Plast Reconstr Surg. 2001;21:276–80.
34. Hawes MJ, Dortzbach RK. The microscopic anatomy of the lower eyelid retractors. Arch Ophthalmol. 1982;100:1313–8.
35. Kakizaki H, Zhao J, et al. The lower eyelid retractor consists of definite double layers. Ophthalmology. 2006;113:2346–50.
36. Kakizaki H, Malhotra R, et al. Lower eyelid anatomy: an update. Ann Plast Surg. 2009;63(3):344–51.
37. Carter SR, Chang J, et al. Involutional entropion and ectropion of the Asian lower eyelid. Ophthal Plast Reconstr Surg. 2000;16:45–9.
38. Kakizaki H, Jinsong Z, et al. Microscopic anatomy of the Asian lower eyelids. Ophthal Plast Reconstr Surg. 2006;22:430–3.
39. Hwang K, Joong Kim D, Chung RS. Pretarsal fat compartment in the lower eyelid. Clin Anat. 2001;14(3):179–83.
40. Lockwood CB. The anatomy of the muscles, ligaments, and fasciae of the orbit, including an account of the capsule of Tenon, the cheek ligaments of the recti, and of the suspensory ligament of the eye. J Anat Physiol. 1885;20:1–25.
41. Camirind A, Doucet J, et al. Anatomy, pathophysiology, and prevention of senile enophthalmia and associated herniated lower eyelid fat pads. Plast Reconstr Surg. 1997;100:1535–46.
42. Mendelson BC, Jacobson SR. Surgical anatomy of the midcheek: facial layers, spaces, and the midcheek segments. Clin Plast Surg. 2008;35:395–404.
43. Yaremchuk MJ, Kahn DM. Periorbital skeletal augmentation to improve blepharoplasty and midface results. Plast Reconstr Surg. 2009;124(6):2151–60.
44. Yousif NJ, Mendelson BC. Anatomy of the midface. Clin Plast Surg. 1995;22(2):227–40.
45. Haddock NT, Saadeh PB, et al. The tear trough and lid/cheek junction: anatomy and implications for surgical correction. Plast Reconstr Surg. 2009;123:1332–40.
46. Ghassemi A, Prescher A, et al. Anatomy of the SMAS revisited. Aesth Plast Surg. 2003;27:258–64.
47. Furnas DW. The retaining ligaments of the cheek. Plast Reconstr Surg. 1989;83(1):11–6.
48. Mendelson BC, Muzaffar AR, Adams WP. Surgical anatomy of the midcheek and malar mounds. Plast Reconstr Surg. 2002;110:885–96.
49. Donath AS, Glasgold RA, Meier J, Glasgold MJ. Quantitative evaluation of volume augmentation in the tear trough with a hyaluronic acid-based filler: a three-dimensional analysis. Plast Reconstr Surg. 2010;125(5):1515–22. (The authors highlight the longer than expected duration of hyaluronic acid filler augmentation in the tear trough.)
50. Rohrich RJ, Arbique GM, et al. The anatomy of suborbicularis fat: implications for periorbital rejuvenation. Plast Reconstr Surg. 2009;124(3):946–51.
51. Kikkawa DO, Lemke BN, et al. Relations of the SMAS to the orbit characterization of the orbitomalar ligament. Ophthal Plast Reconstr Surg. 1996;12(2):77–8.
52. Lucarelli MJ, Khwarg SI, et al. The anatomy of midfacial ptosis. Ophthal Plast Reconstr Surg. 2000;16(1):7–22.
53. Korn BS, Kikkawa DO, Cohen SR. Transcutaneous lower eyelid blepharoplasty with orbitomalar suspension: retrospective review of 212 consecutive cases. Plast Reconstr Surg. 2009;125(1): 315–23.

54. Owsley JQ, Fiala TG. Update: lifting the malar fat pad for correction of prominent nasolabial folds. Plast Reconstr Surg. 1997;100(3):715–22.
55. Kawai K, Imanishi N, et al. Arterial anatomic features of the upper palpebra. Plast Reconstr Surg. 2004;113:479–84.
56. Park SH, Sun HJ, Choi KS. Sudden unilateral visual loss after autologous fat injection into the nasolabial fold. Clin Ophthalmol. 2008;2(3):679–83.
57. Knize DM. Anatomic concepts for brow lift procedures. Plast Reconstr Surg. 2009;124:2118–26.
58. Davis RA, Anson BJ, et al. Surgical anatomy of the facial nerve and parotid gland based upon a study of 350 cervicofacial halves. Surg Gynecol Obstet. 1956;102:385.
59. Ramirez OM. Why I prefer the endoscopic forehead lift. Plast Reconstr Surg. 1997;100(4):1033–9; discussion 1043–46.

3 The Beautiful Eye: Perception of Beauty in the Periocular Area

Adam G. Buchanan and John B. Holds

Key Points

- The eye and periocular structures are central to the perception of facial beauty.
- Symmetry, averageness, and feature size are core concepts in facial beauty.
- Features should be evaluated in the context of patient age, ethnicity, and gender.
- Preoperative asymmetries should be photo-documented and discussed.
- A knowledge of what is perceived as beautiful is essential for surgical success.

3.1 Introduction

The eye and periocular area are not only central features of the face, but house the organ responsible for sight. As such, the eye and adjacent area are instinctively perceived as an essential feature of facial beauty. Characteristic changes in the periocular area with age signal the onset of puberty to senescence. For this reason, we all intuitively look to the eye to assess age, beauty, health, mood, level of consciousness, and intelligence. Fair or not, these judgments are wired into our psyche, and patients often wish to modify appearance to alter perception. A study of what is perceived as "beautiful" in the periocular area will help the surgeon to appropriately guide patients and assess whether their goals are realistic.

When addressing perception of the periocular region, there are several core concepts that form a foundation for beauty. These general characteristics span the borders of age, race, and ethnicity, and include facial symmetry, averageness, and feature size. While not overtly apparent to the unschooled observer, these characteristics are instinctively perceived and provide an important background for one's perception of individual features.

The presence of symmetry is one key to facial beauty. The periocular region often displays marked asymmetry, particularly in the areas of the brow, eyelid margin, eyelid skin fold, globe prominence, and cheek projection [1]. In a study of facial symmetry by Rhodes et al. [2], the photos of digitalized mirror-image faces were found to be more attractive than the unaltered asymmetric ones. The degree of asymmetry was found to inversely correlate with perceived attractiveness.

The importance of symmetry to the oculofacial surgeon cannot be overstated. All patients have a degree of facial asymmetry; however, many lack awareness of it. It is the surgeon's responsibility to photo-document these asymmetries preoperatively, and to thoroughly discuss with the patient their impact on the surgical plan and projected outcome. It should be stressed that a certain degree of asymmetry will persist postoperatively. These issues must always be discussed preoperatively and the patient must acknowledge the surgeon's concerns regarding asymmetry and the ability of surgery to address it. A failure to resolve these issues preoperatively is a common cause of postoperative patient unhappiness.

The concept of "averageness" holds that the average facial features of a particular population form the ideal [3]. This theory was evaluated by Langlois and Roggman [4], who compared the photos of individuals to the composite images of the group. Their results showed that the composites were rated as more attractive. Similarly, the Virtual Miss Germany project, performed at the University of Regensburg, morphed the faces of 22 Miss Germany finalists into one digital composite face. When compared to the face of the actual winner and all other contestants, the composite Virtual Miss Germany was selected as more attractive by all examiners.

Finally, feature size is another general characteristic that plays a role in the perception of what is beautiful. There are some anatomical features that in deviating from the mean, tend to enhance beauty [5]. The size of these "desirable" features deviates from the concept of averageness. Examples

J.B. Holds (✉)
Clinical Professor, Departments of Ophthalmology and Otolaryngology Head and Neck Surgery St. Louis University School of Medicine, Director, Ophthalmic Plastic and Cosmetic Surgery, Inc., Des Peres, MO, USA
e-mail: jholds@sbcglobal.net

G.G. Massry et al. (eds.), *Master Techniques in Blepharoplasty and Periorbital Rejuvenation*,
DOI 10.1007/978-1-4614-0067-7_3, © Springer Science+Business Media, LLC 2011

of this concept in the periocular area include increased eye width, malar prominence, and orbit size, all of which are typically perceived as more attractive.

3.2 Specific Anatomic Subunits

Skin is not only the largest organ in the body, but often the first indicator of health and beauty when observing a face. The presence of good skin tone and clarity can change the perception of an average face to an exceptional one. Skin should be uniform and smooth, without fine wrinkles or deeper rhytids. Ideally, it is free of blemishes, with no dyschromias or abrupt changes in quality, texture, or contour (Fig. 3.1).

The upper eyelids display a gently curved marginal contour, with a more acute angle medially, and a peak height displaced towards the lateral limbus. Along with the lower eyelid margin, this achieves a desirable almond shaped configuration of the palpebral fissure (Fig. 3.2). Centrally, the upper eyelid margin falls just below the limbus, with no superior scleral show [6]. The upper eyelid should have a healthy, full appearance with neither significant fat pad protrusion, nor superior sulcus hollowing (Fig. 3.3). The lashes should be long and thick, with a gentle outward curve

A well defined eyelid crease is located approximately 10 mm above the lash line, with notable variation based on sex and ethnicity. There should be a platform of visible, well fixated pretarsal skin inferior to the crease which on average measures 3–6 mm (Fig. 3.4). The eyelid crease tends to be slightly lower in males, and is often markedly lower or absent in many Asians. While beyond the scope of this chapter, a thorough discussion of patient expectations and desires pertaining to eyelid crease and skin fold configuration must be held preoperatively. This is especially true with the Asian blepharoplasty patient.

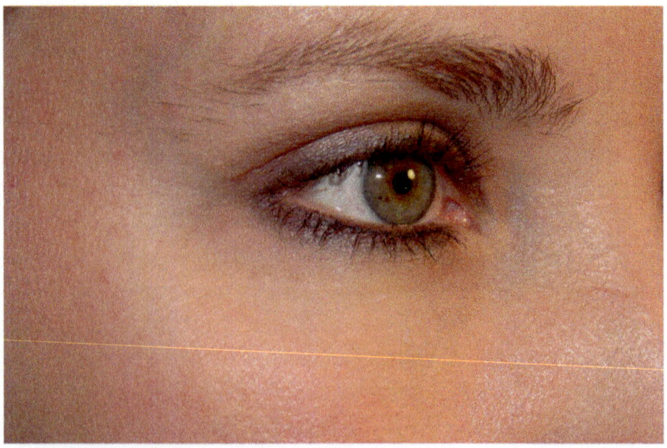

Fig. 3.1 Oblique view of the right brow and eyelids of a woman in her mid-30s. Note the smooth skin without obvious rhytids or dyschromia. There is uniform texture, quality, and contour of the skin from the brow to the lids to the midface. (Photo courtesy Guy G. Massry, MD)

The contour of the lower eyelid follows a gentle downward curve from lateral to medial, with the central margin at the level of the limbus and no inferior scleral show. Laterally, the insertion of the lower eyelid forms a lateral canthal angle that is slightly higher than the medial canthal angle (Fig. 3.5). The lateral canthal angle is fixated laterally, appropriately acute,

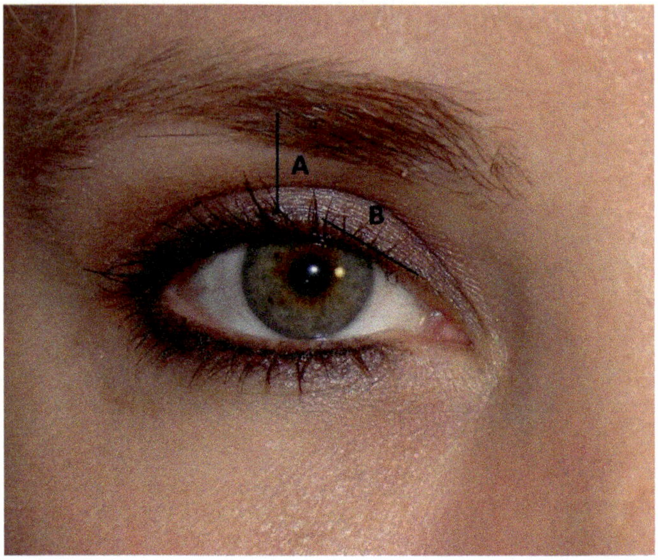

Fig. 3.2 Frontal view of the same woman as Fig. 3.1. The upper eyelid displays a regular curved marginal contour, with (**A**) an eyelid peak tending towards the lateral limbus and (**B**) a more acute angle nasally. (Photo courtesy Guy G. Massry, MD)

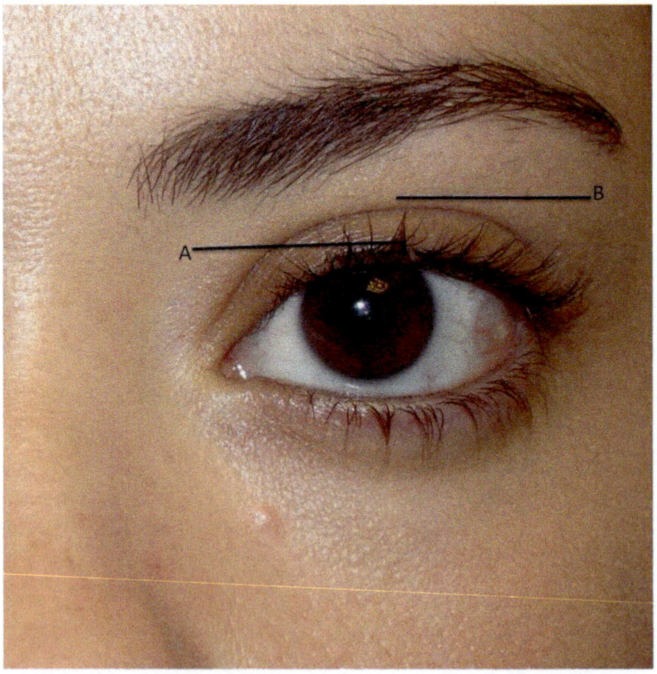

Fig. 3.3 Frontal view of another woman. (**A**) Superior lid margin falls just below the upper limbus without sclera show. (**B**) There is neither fat protrusion or sulcus hollowing. (Photos courtesy Guy G. Massry, MD)

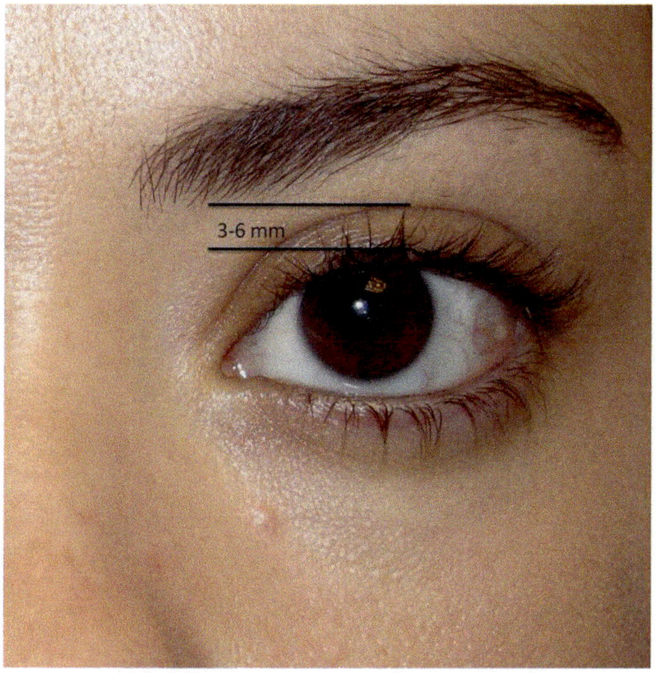

Fig. 3.4 Note smooth pretarsal skin with a visible lid platform measuring 3–6 mm. (Photo courtesy Guy G. Massry, MD)

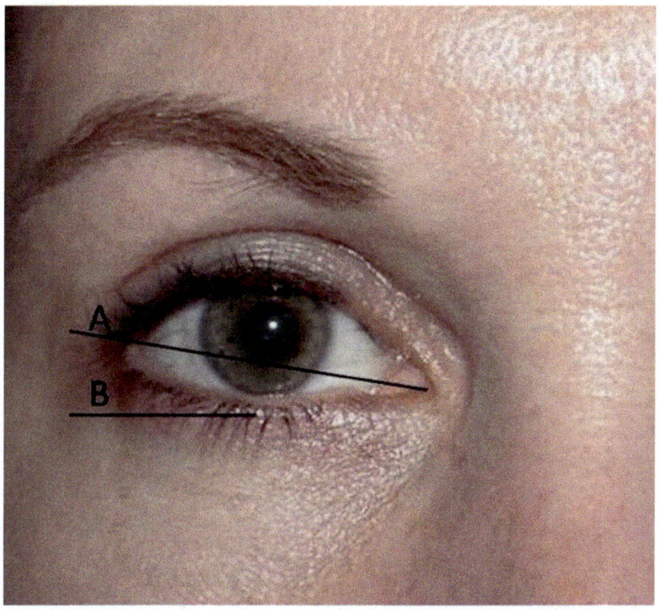

Fig. 3.5 (**A**) The lateral canthal angle is slightly higher than the medial canthal angle. (**B**) The central margin of the lower lid is at the level of the limbus with no inferior scleral show. (Photos courtesy Guy G. Massry, MD)

and sharply defined. The eyelid skin is tight with a smooth transition from thin eyelid skin to thicker cheek skin inferiorly. A subtle roll of plump pretarsal orbicularis muscle just inferior to the lashes provides a youthful look [7].

It is difficult to describe the lower eyelid without consideration of the midface. There should be a gradual

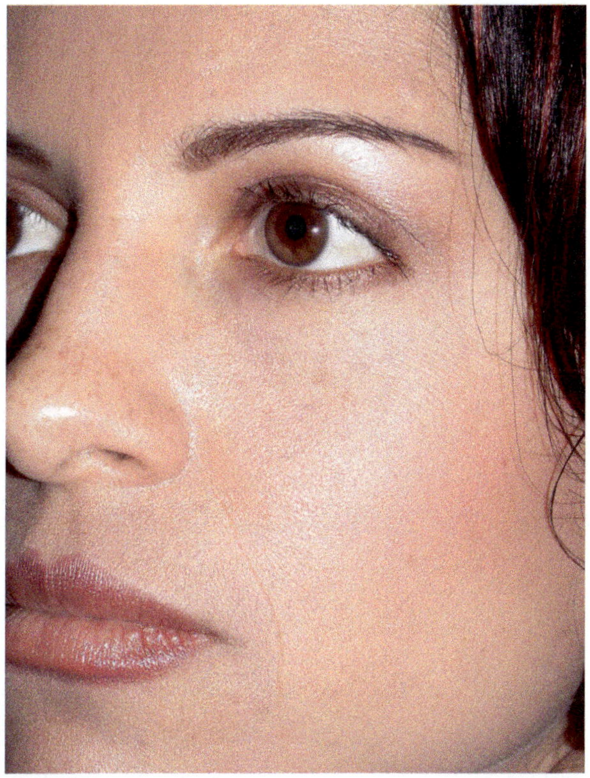

Fig. 3.6 Oblique view of a woman in her mid-30s. Note the smooth transition from the lower lid to the midface without contour irregularities. (Photo courtesy Guy G. Massry, MD)

transition of contour from eyelid to cheek (Fig. 3.6) without the double convexity that may arise from bulging fat pads and tear trough deformity (Fig. 3.7). High, prominent cheeks with a youthful fullness are aesthetically desirable.

Like the cheek, the eyebrow helps frame the eye, and is integral to its beauty. The head of the eyebrow should be positioned at the superomedial orbital rim, in a vertical line with the medial canthus and nasal ala. Its head and tail should be aligned horizontally. In the female the brow arcs gently upwards over the orbital rim, with the maximal arch in line with an imaginary line between the nasal ala and the lateral limbus. The tail of the brow should terminate in a similar line drawn between the nasal ala and the lateral canthus [7] (Fig. 3.8). In the male, the brow is flatter, of thicker hair, lies at the superior orbital rim, with a lower positioned tail. An attractive eyebrow has a gradual transition from thicker subbrow skin to thinner upper eyelid skin, and lacks prominent glabellar furrows or "frown lines."

The forehead is intimately associated with the eyebrow, and has a width approximately twice its height [8] (eyebrow to hairline – Fig. 3.8). There should be a normal hair line superiorly, with the forehead well fixated without contributing to glabellar or eyebrow ptosis. The skin of the forehead and brow is smooth without visible furrows in women. With men,

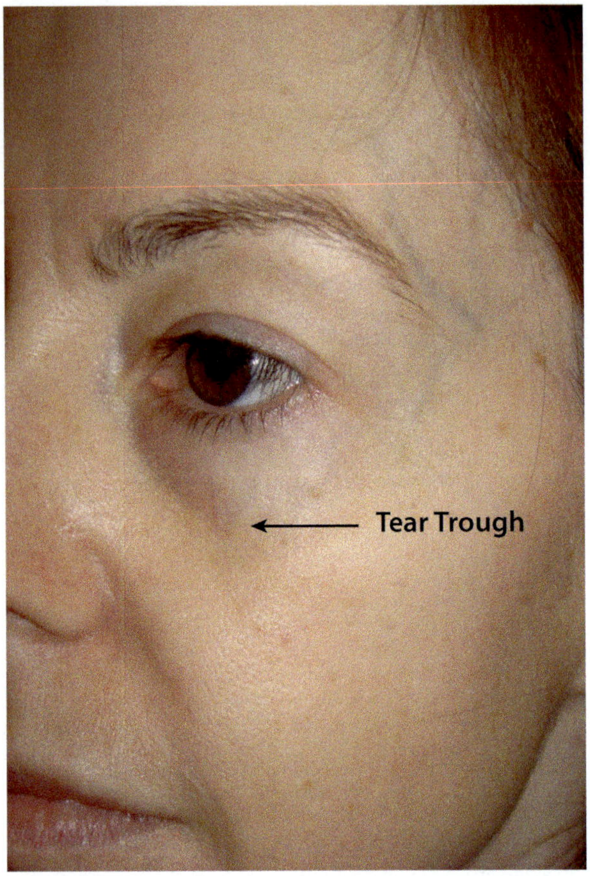

Fig. 3.7 Compare Fig. 3.6 to this woman. In this patient the lid/cheek junction demonstrates the typical double convexity formed by bulging lower lid fat, a nasojugal groove (tear trough) and descent of the midface. (Photo courtesy Guy G. Massry, MD)

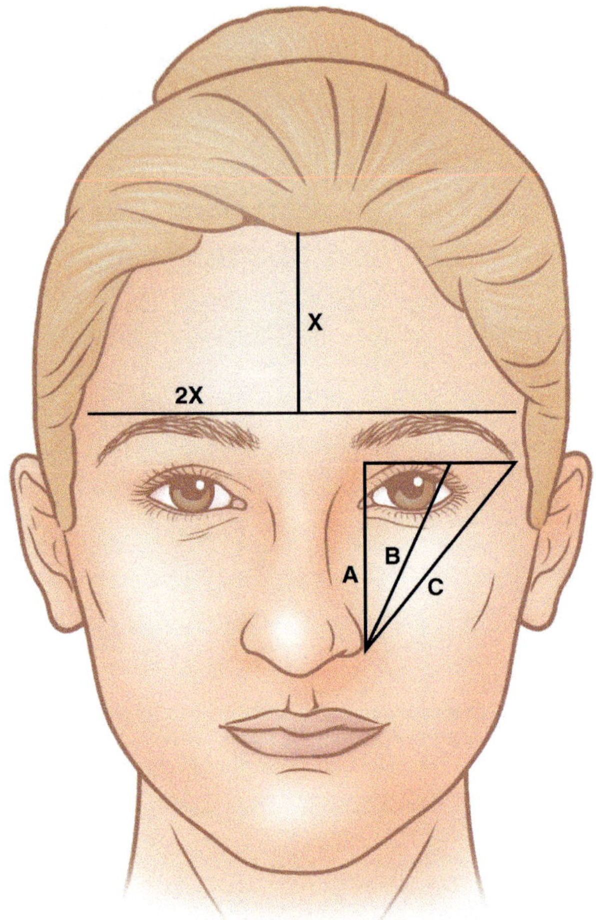

Fig. 3.8 The ideal female brow begins and ends on as horizontal plane. (**A**) Medially it is in line with the medial canthus and nasal ala. (**B**) It peaks in an imaginary line drawn from the nasal ala through the lateral limbus. (**C**) It end is a similar line from the nasal ala through the lateral canthus. The forehead is twice as wide (2×) as its vertical height (×). (Photos courtesy Guy G. Massry, MD)

some furrowing of the brow may confer a desirable rugged appearance.

While not visible or easily amenable to cosmetic surgical alteration, the bony orbit provides a foundation that affects the overall perception of beauty. Faces with a larger orbital width in the horizontal axis are perceived to be more attractive [9]. A slightly higher superior vertical height also decreases crowding of the upper eyelids, allowing increased visualization of the lid crease and pretarsal platform. In general, the intercanthal distance should approximate the width of the palpebral fissure (Fig. 3.9).

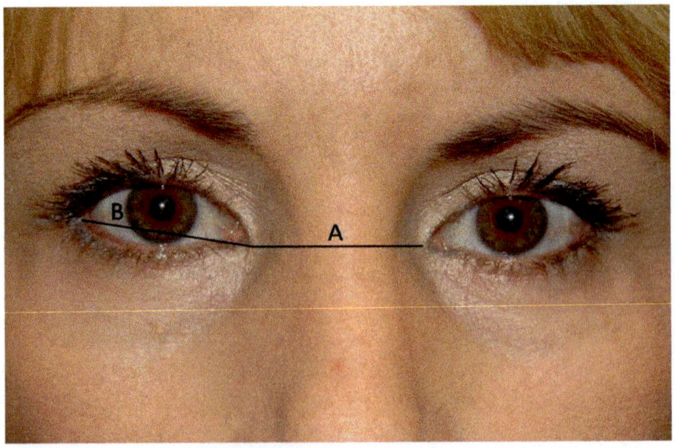

Fig. 3.9 In the ideal situation, the (**A**) intercanthal distance is equal to the (**B**) horizontal palpebral fissure distance. (Photo courtesy Guy G. Massry, MD)

3.3 Conclusion

There are a number of general characteristics and specific anatomic relationships that affect our perception of attractiveness in the periocular region. While some of these factors are amenable to medical or surgical alteration, others are not.

An understanding of what is considered beautiful can shape our approach to the evaluation and management of patients seeking rejuvenation in this critical area.

References

1. McCurdy JA. Beautiful eyes: characteristics and application to aesthetic surgery. Facial Plast Surg. 2006;22(3):204–14.
2. Rhodes G, Profitt F, Grady JM, et al. Facial symmetry and the perception of beauty. Psychon Bull Rev. 1998;5:659–69.
3. Volpe CR, Ramirez OM. The beautiful eye. Facial Plast Surg Clin North Am. 2005;13:493–504.
4. Langlois JH, Roggman LA. Attractive faces are only average. Psychol Sci. 1990;1:115–21.
5. Baudouin JY, Tiberghian G. Symmetry, averageness, and feature size in facial attractiveness of women. Acta Psychol (Amst). 2004;117(3):313–32.
6. Shorr N, Enzer YR. Considerations in aesthetic eyelid surgery. J Dermatol Surg Oncol. 1992;18(12):1081–9.
7. Wolfert FG, Gee J, Pan D, et al. Nuances of aesthetic blepharoplasty. Ann Plast Surg. 1997;38:257–62.
8. Wolfort FG, Baker T, Kanter WR. Aesthetic goals in blepharoplasty. In: Wolfort FG, Kanter WR, editors. Aesthetic blepharoplasty. Boston: Little Brown; 1995. p. 17–34.
9. Farkas LG. Anthropometry of the head and face. New York: Raven; 1994.

Critical Evaluation of the Periorbital Aesthetic Patient

4

Jeremiah P. Tao, Betina Wachter, and Steven Yoon

Key Points

- Underlying general medical, ophthalmic, dermatologic, and psychologic pathology may warrant prior attention in the periorbital aesthetic assessment.
- The periorbital face may subdivided into: (1) orbitoskeleton and globe, (2) the forehead and upper eyelid complex, and (3) the lower eyelid and midface complex.
- Orbito-skeletal changes such as midface hypoplasia can contribute to the aging or "tired" face.
- Enophthalmos may abet eyelid ptosis or pseudoptosis and also cause a superior sulcus "hollow" deformity.
- Exophthalmos may produce an undesirable "surprised" appearance and may exacerbate eyelid retraction and ocular surface disease.
- Dynamic rhytids and static rhytids should be identified and contrasted since the treatments vary.
- Brow ptosis independently causes dyscosmesis, but also increases the amount of apparent upper eyelid dermatochalasis.
- Levator function and the eyelid crease are critical in the assessment of the upper eyelid and ptosis. Race and sex variations in the crease should be recognized.
- Eyelid malposition, skin quality, laxity, orbital fat herniation, and cheek descent are important findings. Palpation and digital repositioning are helpful in surgical planning.
- The nasojugal and palpebro-malar grooves may create a midfacial double convexity that may be a key rejuvenation target.

J.P. Tao (✉)
Assitant Professor, Director, Oculoplastic Surgery,
Department of Ophthalmology, University of California,
Irvine, CA, USA
e-mail: j.tao@uci.edu

4.1 Introduction

Facial aesthetics and beauty standards vary across society, cultures, and over time. Additionally, physical beauty is highly subjective. Today, media presents a benchmark of beauty, however these are often unrealistic. Yet, the individual contemplating cosmetic surgery may have these ideals in mind. Working with these expectations may be challenging and requires an organized approach [1].

The oculofacial cosmetic patient commonly desires correction for an aging or fatigued appearance. Common complaints include "bags," "puffiness," "dark circles," "wrinkles," or looking "tired" (Fig. 4.1). Other requests include looking "natural" with particular avoidance of a "surprised" or "overdone" appearance. In general, patients seek to look like themselves, but "refreshed," "rested," or "younger."

In addition to identifying the cosmetic goals, the evaluation includes a thorough medical assessment to establish surgical candidacy. Conditions directly affecting the eyes and periocular structures, in particular, thyroid ophthalmopathy or myasthenia gravis, mandate consideration and treatment prior to considering aesthetic interventions. Additionally, prior facial surgery – cosmetic or otherwise – should be recorded. Ophthalmic disease, such as dry eyes or blepharitis, should be addressed and dermatologic issues such as keloid formation or hyperpigmentation should be identified.

A psychological assessment is also critical. Identifying unrealistic, manipulative, unstable, or even hostile patients is imperative since their response to the results may be unpredictable.

The periorbital surgeon must understand common misconceptions. For example, perfect symmetry is often equated with beauty. However, even ideal, model faces exhibit subtle asymmetry and some of the natural variations may actually correlate with attractiveness. Ultimately, balanced proportions are desirable, but perfect symmetry is generally not possible or preferred [2, 3].

Photo-documentation (pre- and postoperative) is important. Furthermore, reviewing photographs of the patient at a

G.G. Massry et al. (eds.), *Master Techniques in Blepharoplasty and Periorbital Rejuvenation*,
DOI 10.1007/978-1-4614-0067-7_4, © Springer Science+Business Media, LLC 2011

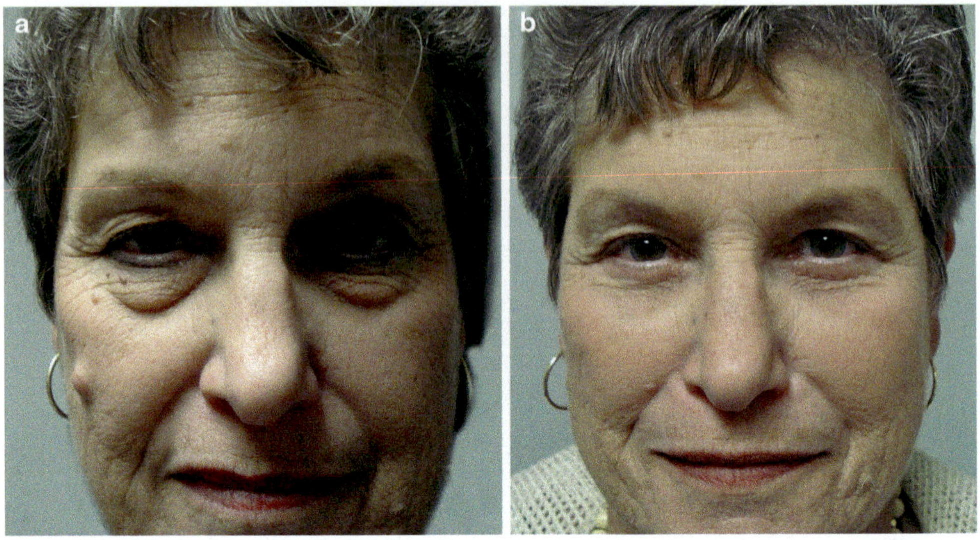

Fig. 4.1 (**a**) A fatigued appearance due to rhytids, eyelid ptosis, and orbital fat pad herniation. (**b**) Same patient after periorbital rejuvenative procedures

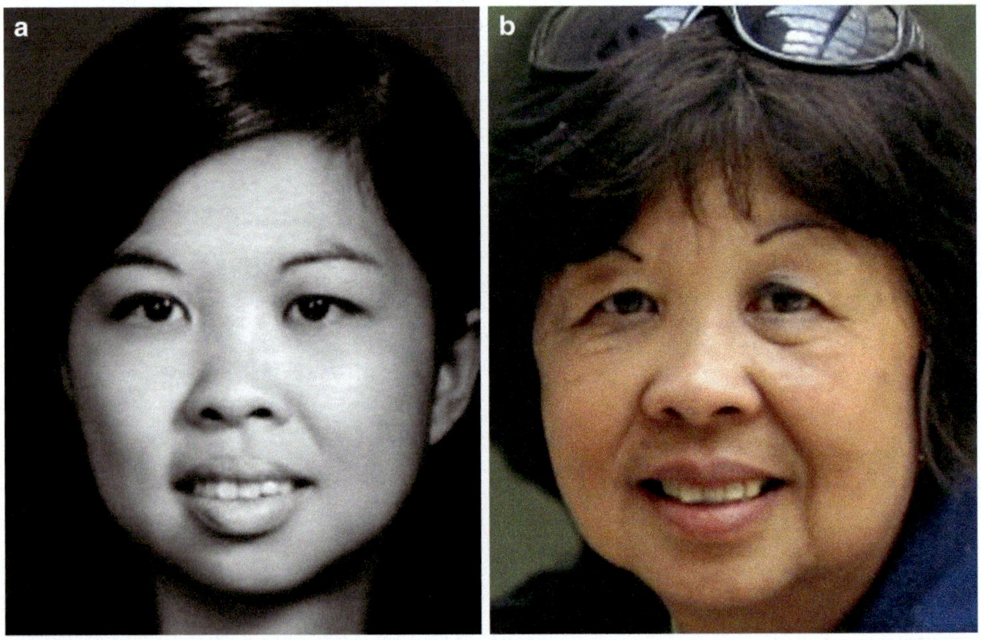

Fig. 4.2 (**a**) Age 22 and (**b**) 67. Note age-related upper eyelid redundancy, increase in tear trough and laugh lines, and descent of the midface over time

younger age may be useful to identify intervention targets (Fig. 4.2). A portable facial mirror is useful to enhance the doctor–patient aesthetic facial dialogue [4].

With patient objectives in mind, the face must be analyzed both as a single unit as well as in components. The periorbital region is particularly important since the eyes are key defining facial features, and eye contact naturally draws attention to this zone. Additionally, the periorbital anatomy and musculature are central in facial expressions, mood, and offer "tell-tale" signs of age or fatigue [5].

Ultimately, the surgeon must connect the exam findings to an array of interventions and surgical procedures. Successful outcomes can be achieved when the correct approach is combined with good technique. The periorbital face may be considered in the following units: (1) orbitoskeleton and globe, (2) the forehead and upper eyelid complex, and (3) the lower eyelid and midface complex.

4.2 Orbito-skeletal and Globe Assessment

The facial bones form the framework and base of attachments for ligaments and muscles that define the face. These deep structures contribute significantly to the external appearance.

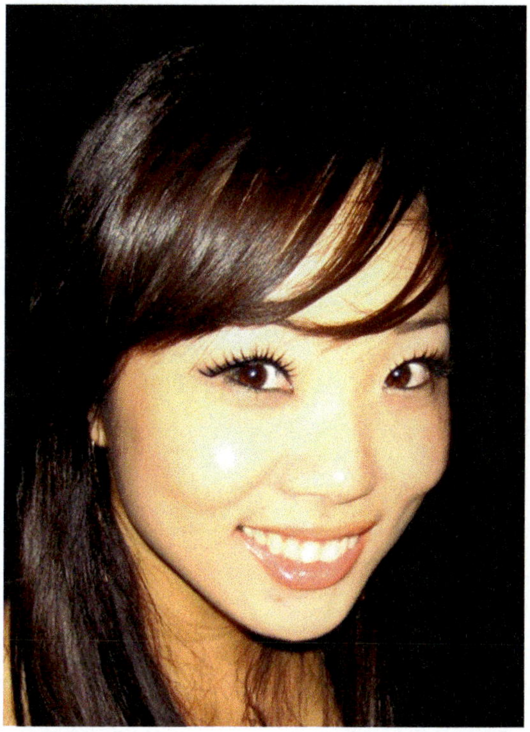

Fig. 4.3 Prominent malar eminences and cheekbones are considered youthful and beautiful

The midfacial or "cheek" bones, including the zygoma laterally and the maxilla medially, are of particular importance. A prominent malar eminence is generally considered a sign of beauty and youth, and is seen more commonly in those of Asian and African descent (Fig. 4.3). Increasing age may subtract from this feature.

Morphologic studies have demonstrated that the orbital skeletal subunit remodels over time. With increasing age, the orbit may become progressively longer vertically and the infraorbital rim may resorb [6].

While radiographic imaging is usually not necessary, visual inspection and palpation can help identify a hypoplastic or flat malar zone that can contribute to a tired or aged appearance. Individuals with midface hypoplasia, whether congenital, age-related, traumatic, or post-surgical, may benefit from facial skeletal augmentation, such as onlay implants.

The relationship of the globe to the orbitofacial skeleton is important. Enophthalmos, or a sunken eye, may produce eyelid ptosis or pseudoptosis and also cause a superior sulcus "hollow" deformity – all, which contribute to a tired or aged appearance (Fig. 4.4). Exophthalmos, or a prominent eye, may exacerbate eyelid retraction and produce a "surprised" or a "deer-in-headlights" look (Fig. 4.5). Proptosis also increases the risk of postoperative eyelid malposition [7].

Anterior globe prominence is commonly measured with the Hertel exophthalmometer, which provides the distance in millimeters to the corneal apex, from an imaginary line between the left and right lateral orbital rim, drawn in the coronal plane (Fig. 4.6). Normal readings are 15–17 mm for adults with a range from 12 to 22 mm. This distance tends to vary with race, with African-American having higher readings, due to a shallower orbit when compared with Caucasians or Asians, in general. A difference between the two eyes of greater than 2 mm is considered abnormal and further workup may be necessary.

The results of exophthalmometry can influence surgical planning. For instance, the position of lateral canthal fixation, as in lower eyelid blepharoplasty or midface lifting, must be tailored according to the degree of eye prominence. Also, higher degrees of exophthalmos may require modifications to standard blepharoplasty, such as orbicularis muscle suspension or spacer grafts [8]. Very high proptosis may in fact be an indication for further workup and potentially other procedures, such as orbital decompression (especially if the patient has thyroid-associated ophthalmopathy – see Chap. 26).

An ophthalmic examination and globe assessment are essential. The principal components include visual acuity, extraocular muscle motility, eyelid/external exam, pupil exam, visual field testing, and anterior segment exam.

The eyelids should be assessed for malposition, closure, tumors, and skin disease. Ectropion, entropion, retraction, trichiasis, blepharitis, and meibomian gland dysfunction should be identified and addressed. Lash loss or margin notching may signify malignancy. Eyelid closure and the spontaneous blink dynamics should be documented. Incomplete closure, or lagophthalmos, can cause significant corneal, conjunctival, and ocular surface pathology.

Conjunctival findings may include injection, inflammation, or neoplasms such as pinguecula or squamous neoplasia. Prior glaucoma surgery, especially the presence of a trabeculectomy conjunctival bleb, is important to note since eyelid surgery may compromise the delicate aqueous filtering conduit.

The cornea should be inspected for clarity, the overlying tear film break up time, exposure, keratitis, and sensation. Fluorescein or rose Bengal dye may be helpful in detecting superficial cornea disease or dry eye syndrome, which may be exacerbated with eyelid surgery.

Reflexive eye protective mechanisms should be checked. Some surgeons assess tear production with Schirmer's testing. The Bell's phenomenon should be evaluated by digitally elevating the upper eyelid while asking the patient to forcefully close his/her eyes. The normal finding should be an upward eye movement shifting the cornea under the upper eyelid.

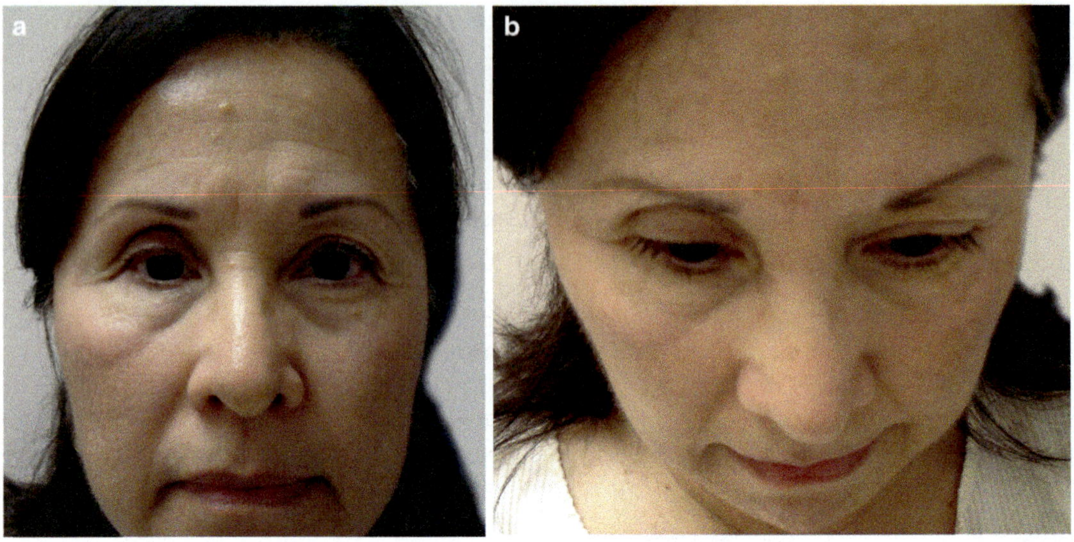

Fig. 4.4 (**a**) Pseudoptosis of the right upper eyelid and (**b**) deep superior sulcus due to enophthalmos

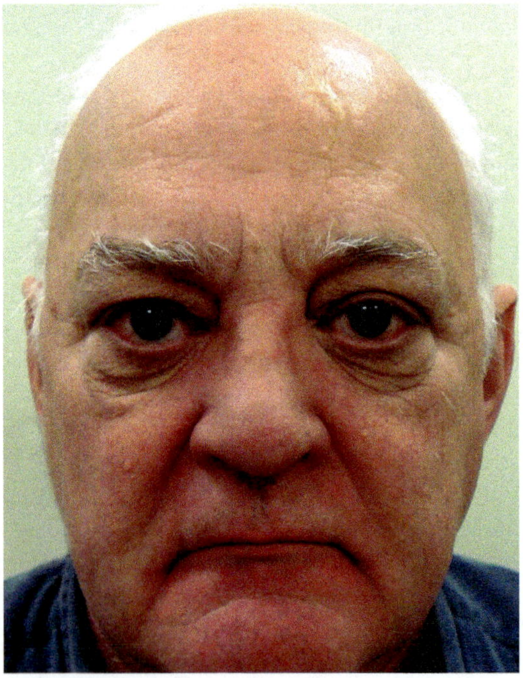

Fig. 4.5 Prominent eyes with lower eyelid retraction right greater than left

4.3 Examination of the Brow and Upper Eyelid Continuum

The forehead, brows, and upper eyelids are the major constituents of the upper face. The assessment of this zone can be subdivided into assessments of skin, rhytids, brows, and the eyelids, but it is imperative to recognize the interrelationships and continuity of these structures [9].

Beginning with a macroscopic assessment, the forehead and scalp are evaluated. The forehead shape, hairline, and hair quality (e.g., thickness) should be inspected. Mild male pattern baldness may respond favorably to pre-trichial incisions, which can lower the hairline. However, it is important to recognize that a mildly elevated hairline is not always objectionable to men. Its manipulation should be discussed before surgery to avoid patient dissatisfaction.

The skin in the periorbital region is vulnerable to aging changes, which should be noted. As the reparative and regenerative mechanisms slow, the skin becomes more fragile and thin. The effects of gravity, sun exposure, environmental factors and genetics accumulate, resulting in damaged collagen cross-linking, and the loss of elasticity and strength. Wrinkles may first appear with facial expressions, but with age and the loss of subcutaneous fat, the dynamic rhytids may become permanent with years of repetitive facial muscle contracture. However, most facial static rhytids occur independent to underlying muscle contracture and may be best treated with resurfacing techniques.

Alternatively, dynamic rhytids and furrows correlate to underlying muscle anatomy. Forehead rhytids develop secondary to facial muscle contracture: one brow elevator (frontalis) and three brow depressor muscles (corrugator supercilii, procerus, orbicularis oculi). The horizontal forehead furrows are due to the vertically oriented frontalis muscle. The vertical lines between the eyebrows, sometimes called "11s," are due to the corrugator supercilii. Horizontal nasal dorsum rhytids or "bunny lines" are due to the procerus. The orbicularis oculi muscle creates the lateral canthal "crows feet."

The assessment of dynamic rhytids may include asking the patient to frown, squint, raise the brow, or grimace, which will usually accentuate or deepen the wrinkles or lines. Dynamic rhytids may respond favorably to muscle weakening

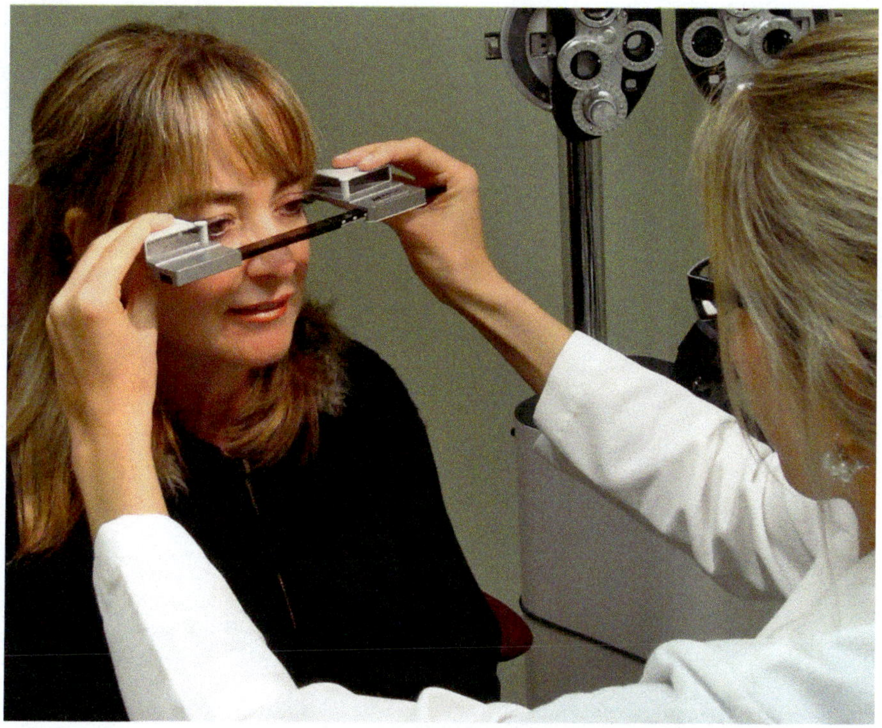

Fig. 4.6 Measurement of the degree of prominence with Hertel exophthalmometer

strategies, such as myectomy, myotomy, or chemodenervation with botulinum toxin.

The eyebrow position should be recorded. In males, the brow is typically flat and lies at the level of the supraorbital rim. In females, the brow is arched and lies above the orbital rim, with the highest point at the level of the lateral limbus or lateral canthus. Brow symmetry, or lack thereof, especially the medial and lateral extremes, is important to identify (Fig. 4.7) [10, 11]. Tattooed brows should be noted since they are often placed superior to the actual brow. Brow-elevating procedures may reposition the tattoos to an unnatural midforehead zone.

Downward gravitational pull and age-related, soft tissue laxity, and bone loss may create brow ptosis, which is diagnosed when the position of the eyebrow is below the supraorbital rim. Frontalis muscle overuse is an additional sign. Prominent horizontal forehead furrows may indicate frontalis muscle compensation (Fig. 4.8). Having patients close their eyes and gently open with the eyebrows relaxed may help identify the resting brow position [12].

The brows may directly affect the upper eyelids. Excess upper eyelid skin, or dermatochalasis, due to brow ptosis, may be especially evident laterally, where the depressor function of the orbicularis is primarily unopposed (Fig. 4.9). Digital elevation of the eyebrows to the correct anatomic position and demonstrating the effect with a mirror or photograph may help patients understand this relationship. Unrecognized brow ptosis may predispose to excessive eyelid skin excision during blepharoplasty and the complications of eyebrow depression or eyelid retraction [13].

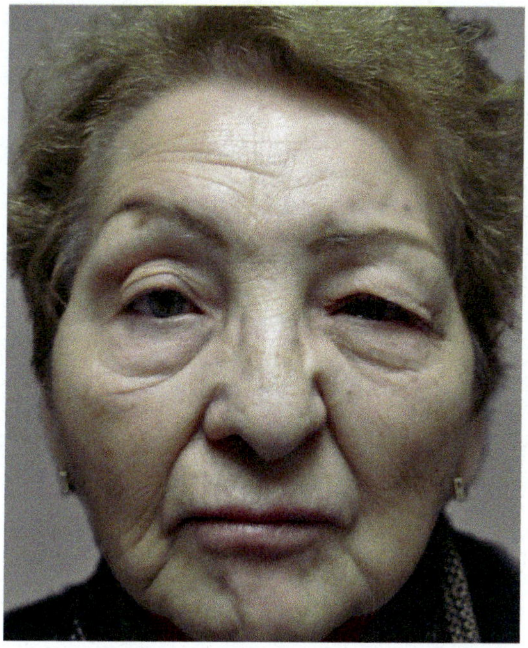

Fig. 4.7 Brow and facial asymmetry due to a facial nerve palsy

The upper eyelids, independently and profoundly impact the overall facial appearance and expression. The aging eyelid may create the false impression of fatigue or unhappiness (Fig. 4.10). Droopy, wrinkled, and hooded eyelids can diminish a prior youthful and brighter appearance (Fig. 4.11) [14].

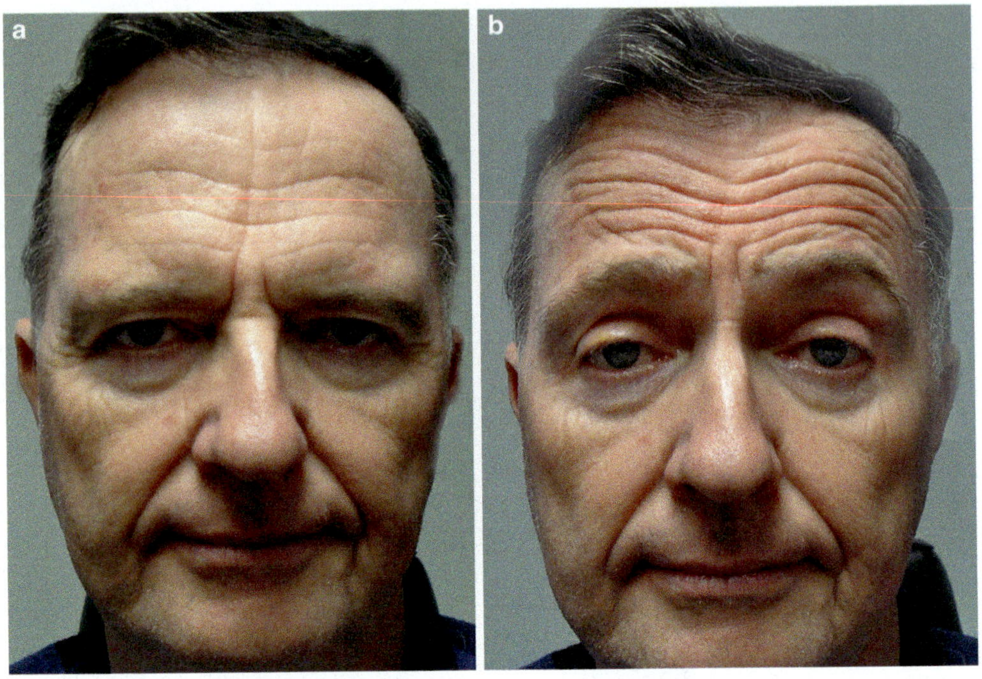

Fig. 4.8 (**a**) Brow ptosis causes excessive upper eyelids folds. (**b**) Frontalis muscle overuse with deep horizontal forehead rhytids compensates for heavy lids

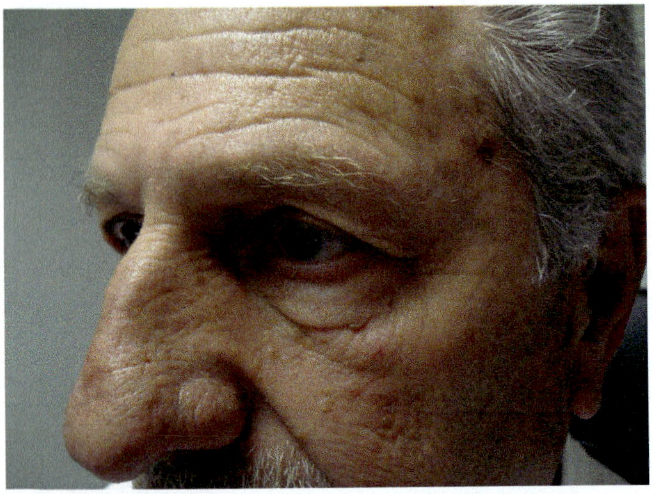

Fig. 4.9 Brow ptosis, prominent horizontal forehead furrows, and excessive upper eyelid folds laterally

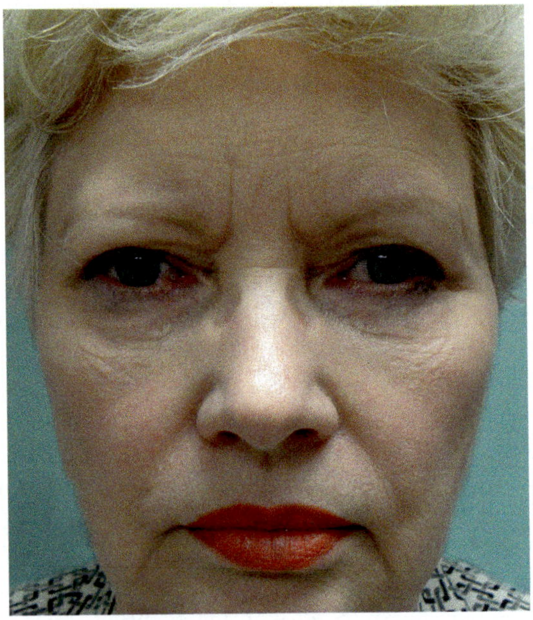

Fig. 4.10 Tired and unhappy appearance related to excess upper eyelid skin

Upper eyelid dermatochalasis is commonly caused by reduced collagen and elastic fibers in the dermis. In addition to brow ptosis, loss of integrity of the orbital septum causing fat protrusion, displacement of the orbital portion of the lacrimal gland laterally, and prominent eyebrow fat pads, all contribute to excess eyelid skin or fullness of the upper eyelid fold (Fig. 4.12) [15].

A significant landmark is the eyelid crease, which determines the position of the skin fold. The crease is formed by the fusion of fibers from the levator aponeurosis into the overlying orbicularis muscle and dermis. In non-Asians, the crease is typically 8–10 mm above the eyelid margin in females and 6–8 mm in males. The space between the margin and the crease has been referred to as the "eyeshadow space" or tarsal platform, is often desirable, and may be feminizing, especially in non-Asians (Fig. 4.13).

In the Asian eyelid, the crease may be significantly lower or even absent due to a lower inferior septal insertion and

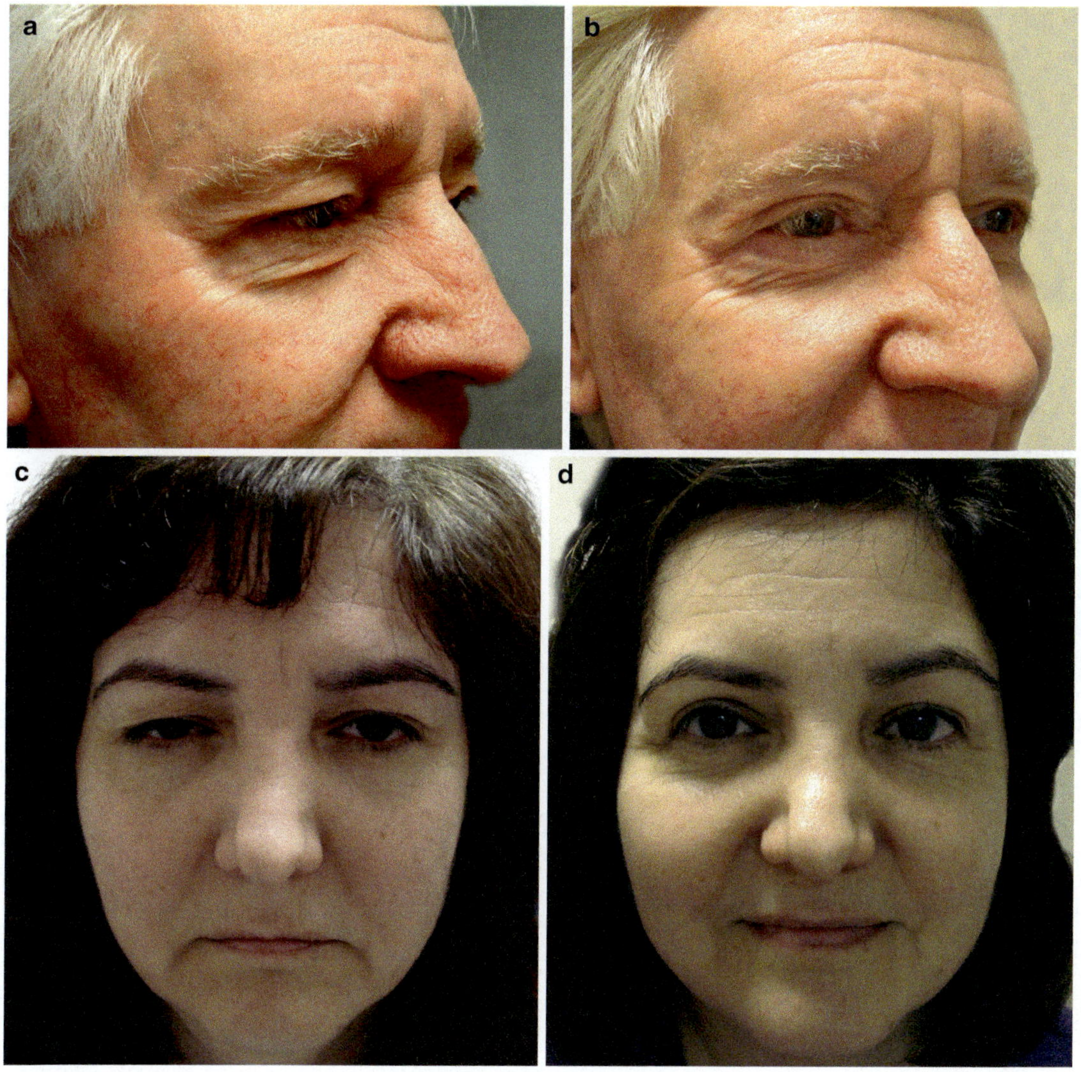

Fig. 4.11 (**a**, **b**) Preoperative and postoperative appearance after blepharoplasty and (**c**, **d**) ptosis repair

orbital fat pad obliteration of the crease-forming levator fibers. It is important to maintain the low crease configuration in the Asian eyelid since an unnaturally high crease may make obvious that the patient had surgery and overly "westernize" the appearance.

Asymmetry, elevation, or loss of the eyelid crease may signify levator aponeurosis pathology. Stretching or dehiscence of the levator aponeurosis may result in a high eyelid crease (Fig. 4.14). Volume depletion from fat atrophy or retraction of the central preaponeurotic fat pad may exacerbate the deep, hollow, upper eyelid sulcus from ptosis or enophthalmos.

Critical measurements in the assessment of upper eyelid ptosis are the vertical palpebral fissure, margin-to-reflex distance one (MRD_1), and especially levator function. Evaluation should be conducted in primary gaze, with the frontalis muscle relaxed and the brow in a fixed position.

The average vertical palpebral fissure is approximately 10 mm. The vertical excursion of the eyelid (ask the patient to look down and then up), determines the levator function. The normal range is between 12 and 18 mm. It is important to negate the effect of the frontalis muscle with a thumb or digit, when assessing the levator function. The correct procedure in treating eyelid ptosis depends critically on levator function.

The margin-to-reflex distance (MRD_1) is the space in millimeter between the central corneal light reflex and the upper eyelid margin, and typically ranges between 4 and 4.5 mm. A diminished MRD_1 typically signifies ptosis of the upper eyelid, whereas an elevated MRD_1 indicates eyelid retraction (Fig. 4.15). Upper eyelid retraction is most commonly a manifestation of thyroid-associated ophthalmopathy, but may be secondary to a host of other causes, including high myopia, buphthalmos, facial nerve palsy, or trauma.

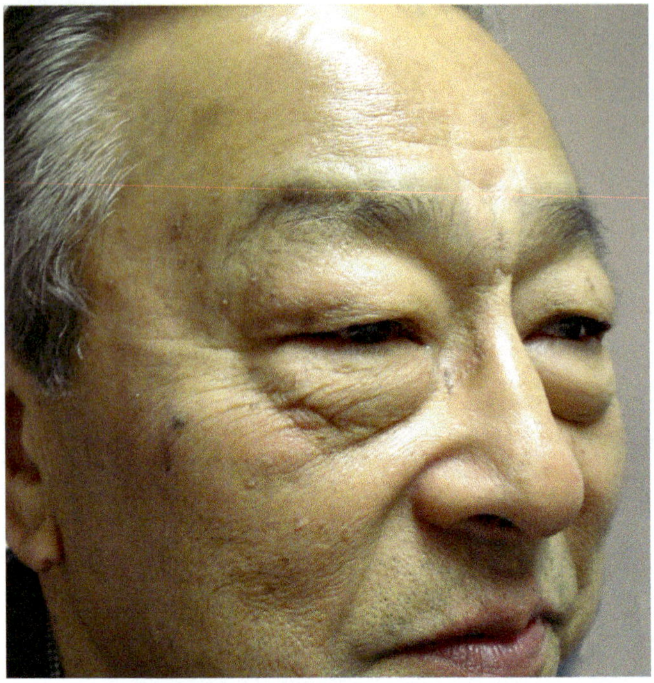

Fig. 4.12 Multifactorial nature of upper eyelid fullness (redundant skin, fat herniation, etc.)

4.4 Examination of the Lower Eyelid and Cheek Continuum

The inferior midface analysis can be subdivided to the skin, the lower eyelids, and the cheeks. These structures should be inspected independently, as well as a continuous unit [16].

The skin should be evaluated for the effects of age, sun exposure, and heritable disease. With time and loss of elasticity, the eyelids and cheeks may exhibit laxity. The presence of skin conditions, pigmentation, rhytids, and scars are also important considerations. Depending on the texture, thickness, and degree of solar damage, skin-resurfacing techniques may be indicated instead, or in conjunction with, incisional procedures (Fig. 4.16). The amount of redundant skin should also be noted to avoid excessive skin resection [17].

Orbital fat herniation, evident through the eyelids, may contribute to the aging face appearance (Fig. 4.17). Orbital septal weakening, orbicularis atrophy, and supporting ligamentous laxity, combine to incite orbital fat protrusion. Examining the patient in up-gaze position may assist in identifying problematic fat compartments [18, 19].

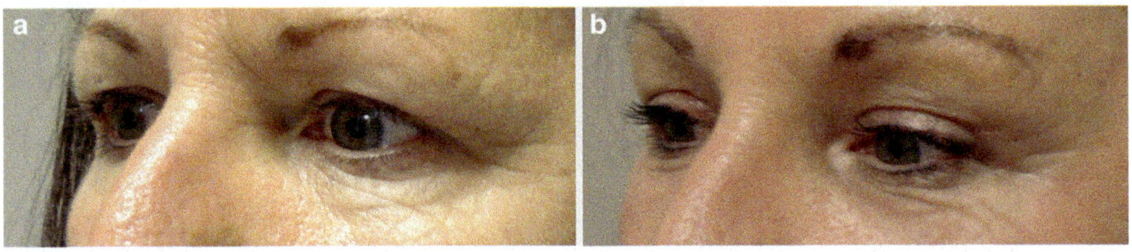

Fig. 4.13 (**a**) Eyelid crease with a minimal tarsal platform; (**b**) After brow elevation with blepharoplasty, an enlarged space between the eyelid margin and crease is achieved, giving a feminizing eyeshadow space

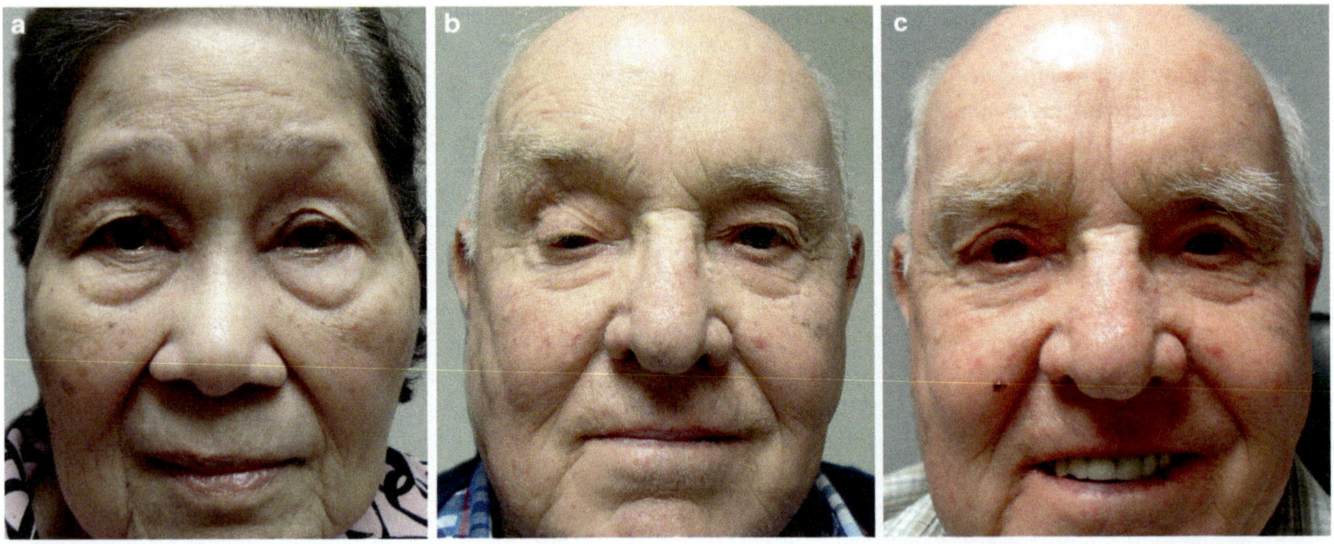

Fig. 4.14 (**a**) Dehiscence of the levator aponeurosis on the left resulting in ptosis and high eyelid crease; (**b**) right upper eyelid ptosis and compensatory right brow elevation and eyebrow asymmetry; (**c**) equalization of the brows after bilateral upper lid blepharoplasty and ptosis repair

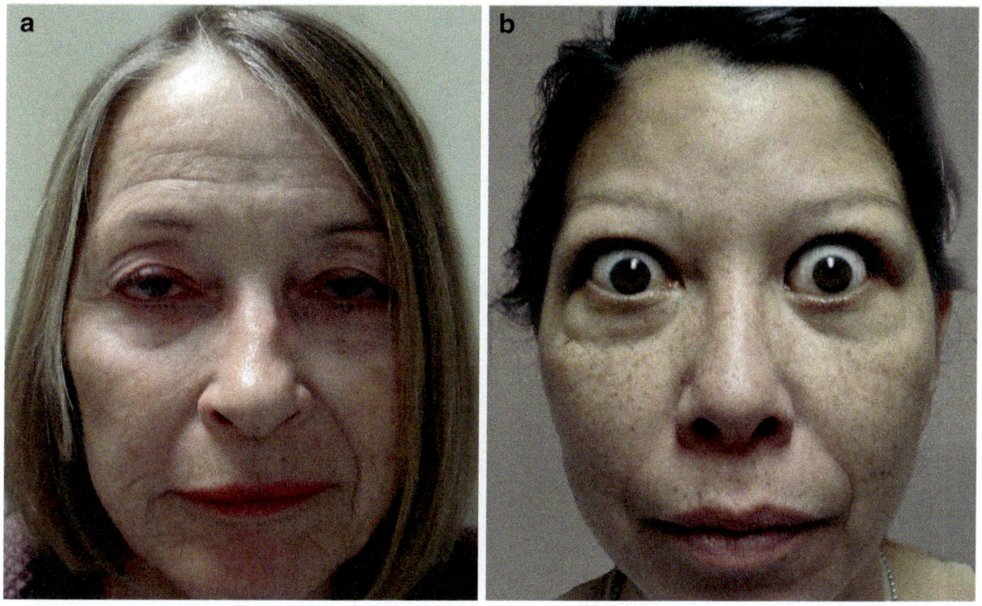

Fig. 4.15 (**a**) Example of a low (0 mm) MRD1 due to levator dehiscence ptosis; (**b**) Example of a high (9 mm) MRD1 due to thyroid related upper eyelid retraction

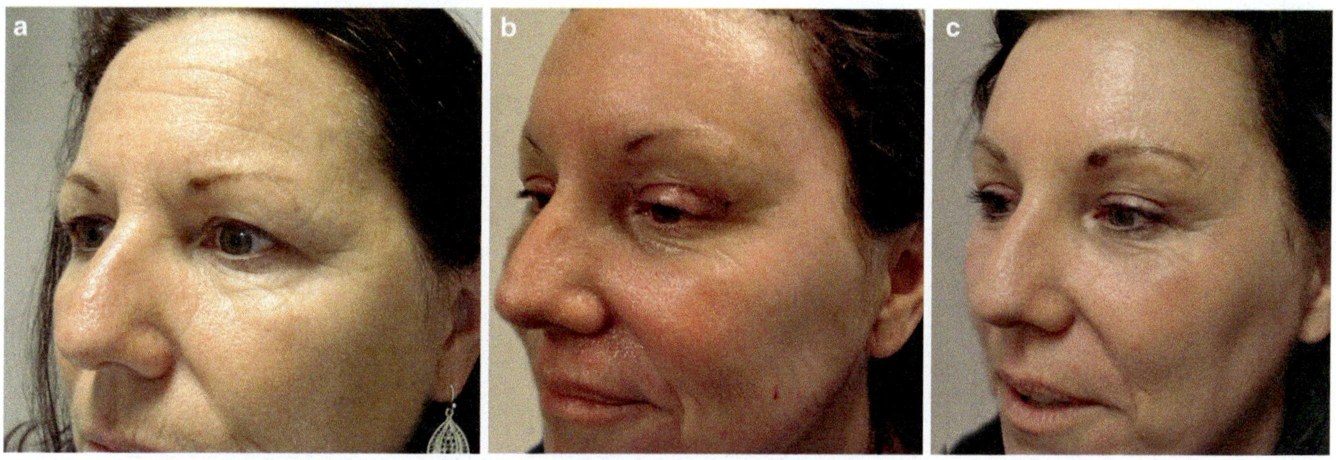

Fig. 4.16 (**a**) Periorbital rhytids with concomitant brow ptosis and dermatochalasis. (**b**) One week following laser skin-resurfacing with brow lift and upper blepharoplasty. (**c**) At 6 weeks after surgery there is excellent improvement of skin quality and rhytids

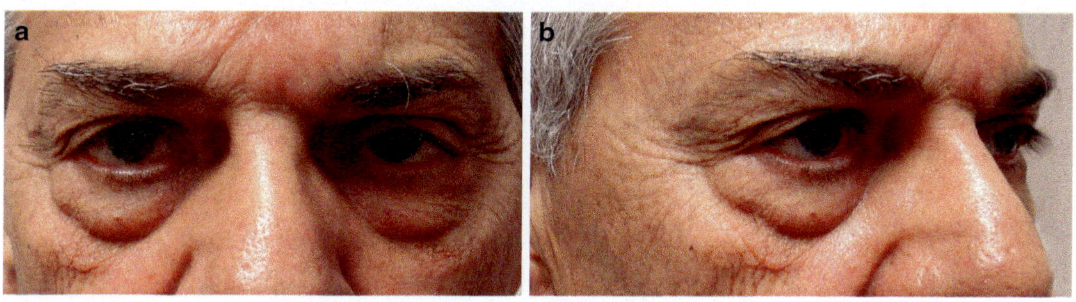

Fig. 4.17 Orbital fat herniation of the lower eyelids. (**a**) Frontal view, (**b**) oblique view

Several relationships and measurements help in the appraisal of the lower eyelid position. The lateral canthus is usually 2–3 mm higher than the medial canthus. The eyelid margin should rest slightly above or at the level of the inferior limbus. Eyes should be assessed for scleral show, which is present when the lid margin rests below the limbus. Scleral show can be present due to lid retraction, exophthalmos, ectropion, or a combination of these. In prominent eyes, scleral show can be a normal variant; however surgical intervention should not increase the amount [20–22].

The space between the lower eyelid margin and pupil light reflex distance is known as margin reflex distance two (MRD_2), which is normally approximately 5 mm. Values higher than 5.5 mm may define lower eyelid retraction. Grave's orbitopathy, surgery, trauma, and senile eyelid flaccidity are common causes of lower eyelid retraction [23].

Lower eyelid palpation may help identify a middle or posterior lamellar cicatrix, especially in patients who have had prior surgery or trauma. A "finger" technique may indicate a need for additional strategies for lower lid support. With index finger repositioning of the lateral canthus and mimicking the effect of canthal anchoring procedures, a persistent low central eyelid position may be suggestive that a spacer graft may be necessary, for example [24]. In addition, manual elevation of the lower lid should be free without restriction. Limitation of this maneuver (a tethering) may indicate a vertical deficiency of eyelid tissue or cicatrix of internal eyelid tissue to the orbital rim. Surgery including scar lysis, midface elevation, eyelid support, and a spacer graft may be needed in this scenario.

Lower eyelid laxity is an important diagnosis. The tarsoligamentous sling, consisting of the tarsal plate and canthal tendons, provides the skeletal support of the lower lids, and descends with age-related losses in elasticity. Floppy eyelid syndrome is a variant that may occur in younger individuals, who are also often overweight, and may have sleep apnea. Floppy eyelids often require horizontal eyelid tightening procedures to avoid or improve eye irritation.

Eyelid laxity can be assessed with the snap-test and distraction tests (Fig. 4.18). Pulling the lower eyelid downward and observing the time it takes to return to a normal position accomplishes the snap-test. A swift return to position without blinking is considered normal. Pinching the lower eyelid and pulling it anteriorly, away from the globe accomplish the lid distraction test. Movement of the lid margin greater than 10 mm is considered abnormal and signifies diminished tone. Significant eyelid laxity may be an indication for canthal anchoring to avoid lower lid malposition, lagophthalmos, and eye fissure shape deformity with periorbital procedures.

The eyelid fissure shape is influenced by canthal laxity. With involutional eyelid laxity there is elongation of the vertical palpebral aperture, rounding of the canthal angle, and increased scleral show. The area of the lateral scleral triangle – the "white" triangle whose confines are the lateral limbus, and the lateral upper and lower eyelid, enlarges as the lateral commissure descends (Fig. 4.19) [25–27].

The lower eyelid and midface continuum is an important concept. In youth, the midface exhibits a single convexity shape on lateral view. With age, a convexity–concavity–convexity develops, as the midface separates from the lower eyelid at the level of the orbital rim. Hence, the single unit is lost in the aging face (Fig. 4.20) [28].

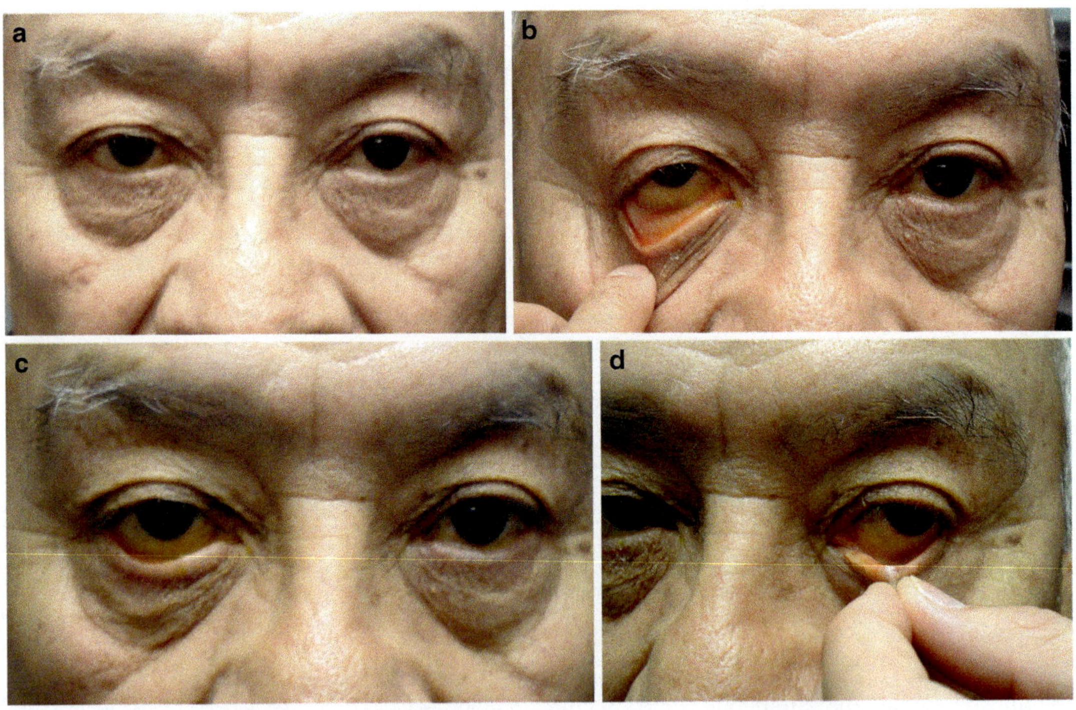

Fig. 4.18 (**a**) Laxity of the lower eyelids and scleral show are risk factors for ocular exposure complications from lower eyelid and midface surgery. (**b**) Snap-test. (**c**) With eyelid laxity, the lid does not promptly return to the normal position against the globe. (**d**) Lid distraction test

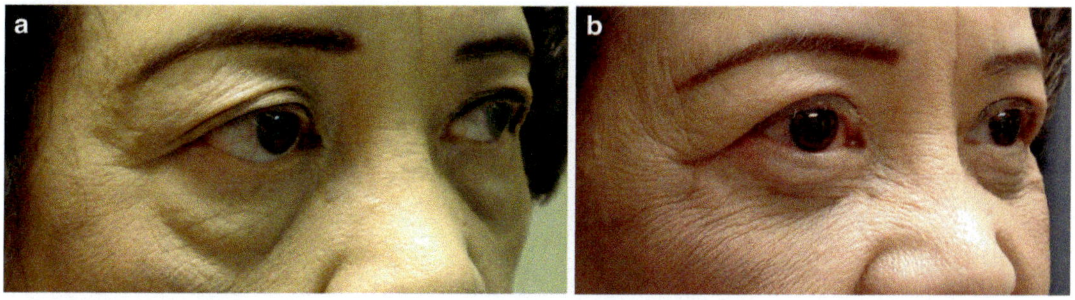

Fig. 4.19 (**a**) Lower eyelid laxity, scleral show, increased lateral scleral triangle, lower eyelid bags, upper dermatochalasis, and ptosis. (**b**) Same patient after undergoing periorbital rejuvenation (upper blepharoplasty, ptosis repair, canthoplasty and midface lift)

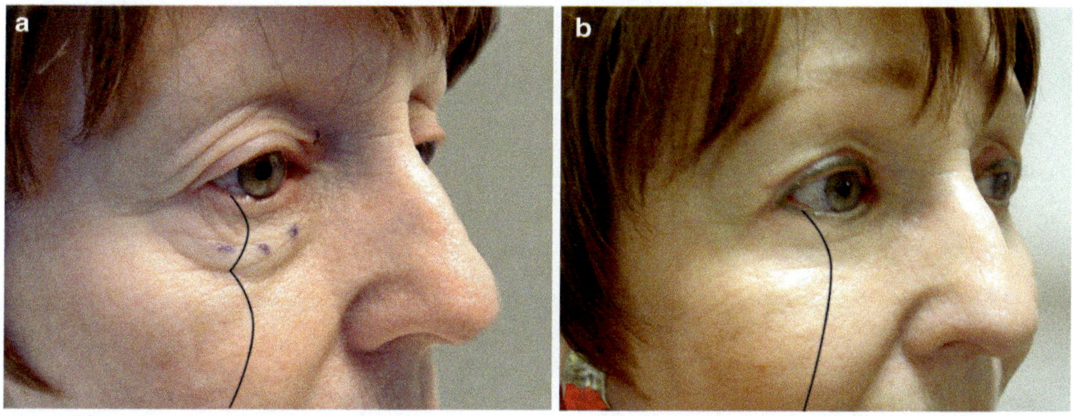

Fig. 4.20 (**a**) The convexity–concavity–convexity in lateral view as a result of lid-cheek segment aging. (**b**) After periorbital rejuvenation, the single unit appearance of the lid-cheek zone is restored

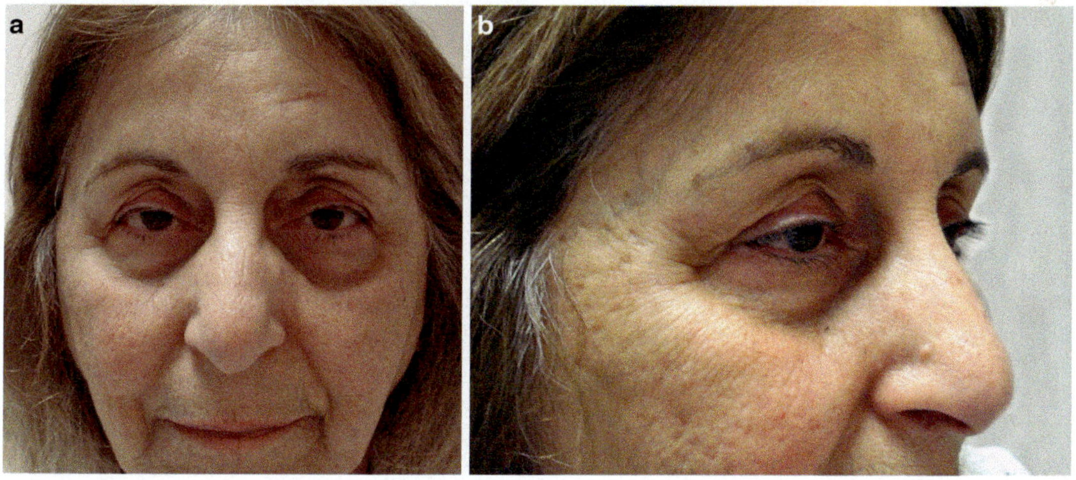

Fig. 4.21 Skeletonization of inferior orbital rim and depletion of orbital volume as part of the aging process. (**a**) Frontal and (**b**) oblique view

Volume depletion and weakened midfacial soft tissue support cause the lower eyelid-cheek junction to descend below the orbital rim (Fig. 4.21). The orbicularis oculi muscle, an integral segment of the superficial musculoaponeurotic system (SMAS), descends and loses tone. Inferiorly displaced midface tissue, in combination with orbital fat prolapse, result in lid-cheek junction contour irregularities: the nasojugal groove medially and the palpebro-malar groove

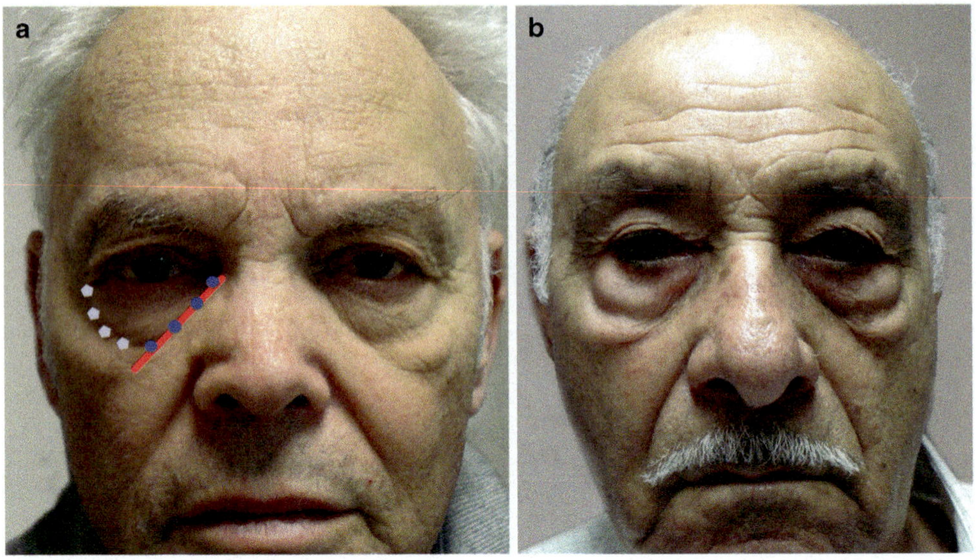

Fig. 4.22 (**a**) Malar mounds. White pentagons demarcate the palpebro-malar groove, red line the nasojugal groove, and blue dots the tear trough deformity. (**b**) Festoons

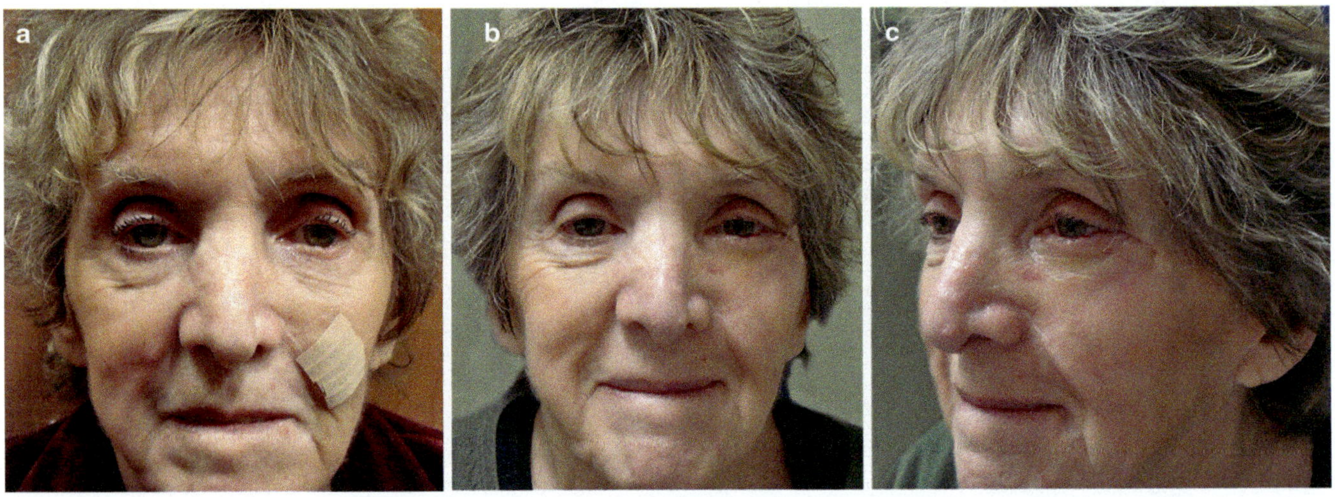

Fig. 4.23 (**a**) Patient with signs of aging process in the lower eyelids. Examination reveals notching and a suspicious pearly lesion affecting left lower eyelid margin. (**b**, **c**) After left lower eyelid basal cell carcinoma excision (with frozen section control) and reconstruction (tarso-conjunctival posterior lamella flap with skin and orbicularis cheek advancement flap). This unilateral reconstructive case demonstrates effect of midface lifting procedures in restoring the single unit appearance of the eyelid and cheek

inferolaterally. The medial half of the nasojugal fold is also referred to as a tear trough deformity. The presence of soft tissue folds (malar mounds) and skin folds (festoons) may be found in the triangular zone formed at the junction of the lateral inferior orbital rim and cheek (Figs. 4.22 and 4.23) [29, 30]. Midface descent also contributes to deepening of the perioral "laugh lines," also known as "marionette lines," which may be corrected with cheek lifting or facial filling strategies.

4.5 Conclusion

The critical aesthetic assessment of the periorbital face includes knowledge of periocular and ophthalmic anatomy, as well as an understanding of morphologic changes that occur with age and variations among sex and race. Consideration of the orbitoskeleton and globe, the forehead and upper eyelid complex, and the lower eyelid and midface complex may assist in delivering aesthetically pleasing and functionally sound interventions. Importantly, the assessment of these units is not limited to inspection but may include palpation and digital manipulation. Additionally, dialogue and patient involvement is essential. With a structured assessment, optimal results can be achieved.

References

1. McCurdy Jr JA. Beautiful eyes: characteristics and application to aesthetic surgery. Facial Plast Surg. 2006;22(3):204–14.
2. Springer IN, Wannicke B, Warnke PH, Zernial O, Wiltfang J, Russo PA, et al. Facial attractiveness: visual impact of symmetry increases significantly towards the midline. Ann Plast Surg. 2007;59(2): 156–62.
3. Rhodes G, Proffitt F, Grady JM, Sumich A. Facial symmetry and the perception of beauty. Psychon Bull Ver. 1998;5(4):659–69.
4. Ho T, Brissett AE. Preoperative assessment of the aging patient. Facial Plast Surg. 2006;22(2):85–90.
5. McCord CD, Codner MA. Aging changes in the eyelid and periorbital area. In: Eyelid and periorbital surgery. St. Louis, MO: Quality Medical; 2008. p. 133–50.
6. Hester Jr TR, Douglas T, Szczerba S. Decreasing complications in lower lid and midface rejuvenation: the importance of orbital morphology, horizontal lower lid laxity, history of previous surgery, and minimizing trauma to the orbital septum: a critical review of 269 consecutive cases. Plast Reconstr Surg. 2009;123(3):1037–49.
7. Hirmand H, Codner MA, McCord CD, Hester Jr TR, Nahai F. Prominent eye: operative management in lower lid and midfacial rejuvenation and the morphologic classification system. Plast Reconstr Surg. 2002;110(2):620–8.
8. Ahmadi H, Shams PN, Davies NP, Joshi N, Kelly MH. Age-related changes in the normal sagittal relationship between globe and orbit. J Plast Reconstr Aesthet Surg. 2007;60(3):246–50.
9. Gunter JP, Antrobus SD. Aesthetic analysis of the eyebrows. Plast Reconstr Surg. 1997;99(7):1808–16.
10. Alex JC. Aesthetic considerations in the elevation of the eyebrow. Facial Plast Surg. 2004;20(3):193–8.
11. McCord CD, Doxanas MT. Browplasty and browpexy: an adjunct to blepharoplasty. Plast Reconstr Surg. 1990;86(2):248–54.
12. Pitanguy I, Radwanski HN. Rejuvenation of the brow. Dermatol Clin. 1997;15(4):623–34.
13. Morton AD. Assessment and management of the eyebrow. In: Albert DM, Jakobiec FA, editors. Principles and practice of ophthalmology. Basic sciences. Philadelphia: Elsevier; 2008. p. 3529–42.
14. Starck WJ, Griffin Jr JE, Epker BN. Objective evaluation of the eyelids and eyebrows after blepharoplasty. J Oral Maxillofac Surg. 1996;54(3):297–302.
15. Ross AT, Neal JG. Rejuvenation of the aging eyelid. Facial Plast Surg. 2006;22(2):97–104.
16. Goldstein SA, Goldstein SM. Anatomic and aesthetic considerations in midfacial rejuvenation. Facial Plast Surg. 2006;22(2):105–11.
17. Perkins SW, Batniji RK. Rejuvenation of the lower eyelid complex. Facial Plast Surg. 2005;21(4):279–85.
18. Logau RG. Systematic evaluation of the aging face. In: Bolognia JL, Jorizzo JL, Rapini RP, editors. Dermatology. 2nd ed. Philadelphia: Elsevier; 2008. p. 2295–9.
19. Goldberg RA, McCann JD, Fiaschetti D, Ben Simon GJ. What causes eyelid bags? Analysis of 114 consecutive patients. Plast Reconstr Surg. 2005;115(5):1395–402.
20. Byrd HS, Burt JD. Achieving aesthetic balance in the brow, eyelids, and midface. Plast Reconstr Surg. 2002;110(3):926–33.
21. Hester Jr TR, Codner MA, McCord CD, Nahai F, Giannopoulos A. Evolution of technique of the direct transblepharoplasty approach for the correction of lower lid and midfacial aging: maximizing results and minimizing complications in a 5-year experience. Plast Reconstr Surg. 2000;105(1):393–406.
22. Goldberg RA. The three periorbital hollows: a paradigm for periorbital rejuvenation. Plast Reconstr Surg. 2005;116(6):1796–804.
23. Holck DEE, Foster JA, Kalwerisky K. Lower eyelid blepharoplasty and midface elevation surgery. In: Albert DM, Jakobiec FA, editors. Principles and practice of ophthalmology. Basic sciences. Philadelphia: Elsevier; 2008. p. 3471–82.
24. Patipa M. Combined hard palate spacer graft, midface suspension, and lateral canthoplasty for lower eyelid retraction: a tripartite approach. Plast Reconstr Surg. 2005;115(7):2115–7.
25. Hamra ST. The role of the septal reset in creating a youthful eyelid-cheek complex in facial rejuvenation. Plast Reconstr Surg. 2004; 113(7):2124–41.
26. Muzaffar AR, Mendelson BC, Adams Jr WP. Surgical anatomy of the ligamentous attachments of the lower lid and lateral canthus. Plast Reconstr Surg. 2002;110(3):873–84.
27. Kikkawa DO, Bradley NL, Dortzback K. Relations of the superficial musculoaponeurotic system to the orbit and characterization of the orbitomalar ligament. Ophthal Plast Reconstr Surg. 1996;12(2):77–88.
28. Atiyeh BS, Hayek SN. Combined arcus marginalis release, preseptal orbicularis muscle sling, and SOOF plication for midfacial rejuvenation. Aesthet Plast Surg. 2004;28(4):197–202.
29. De Cordier BC, de la Torre JI, Al-Hakeem MS, Rosenberg LZ, Costa-Ferreira A, Gardner PM, et al. Rejuvenation of the midface by elevating the malar fat pad: review of technique, cases, and complications. Plast Reconstr Surg. 2002;110(6):1526–36.
30. Kawamoto HK, Bradley JP. The tear "TROUF" procedure: transconjunctival repositioning of orbital unipedicled fat. Plast Reconstr Surg. 2003;112(7):1903–7; discussion 1908–9.

Oculofacial Anesthesia

5

Julie A. Woodward, Usha P. Reddy, Nicholas A. Ramey,
Daniel J. Woodward, and Guy G. Massry

Key Points

- Anesthetic agents utilized in periorbital surgery include topical ophthalmic drops and skin creams, oral and injectable agents, intravenous medications, inhaled anesthetics, and regional nerve blocks. All modalities have risks that the surgeon should be familiar with.
- Modern anesthesia techniques provide surgeons the ability to perform more procedures on conscious patients, avoiding the risks of deeper sedation.
- Management of preoperative anxiety with oral medications is an important element of care. Familiarization with these medications is critical before they are administered.
- Local injectable anesthetics have the potential for significant toxic side effects.
- Local injectable anesthetics can be used effectively alone, or in conjunction with intravenous medications or deeper sedation to provide effective analgesia.
- Conscious sedation must be performed with adequate monitoring in a credentialed setting.
- Postoperative pain management, which is an important part of care, can be accomplished with a variety of oral, injectable, and intravenous medications.
- Intravenous monitored anesthesia care (MAC) or general anesthesia is safe and effective when administered by a trained anesthesia specialist.
- Regional motor and sensory blocks can aid greatly in facilitating surgery and potentially avoiding the need for riskier forms of anesthesia.
- The physician administering any form of anesthesia should be prepared to address all possible complications related to treatment.

J.A. Woodward (✉)
Associate Professor, Chief Division of Oculofacial Surgery,
Department of Ophthalmology, Duke University,
Durham, NC, USA
e-mail: juliewoodward1@mac.com

5.1 Introduction

Aesthetic eyelid and periorbital procedures require particular attention to the appropriate anesthetic choice. The procedures may be performed at the physician's office, a minor procedure room, or an operating room. As such, it is important to evaluate the procedure and patient selection criteria for procedure location and anesthesia type. Options for anesthesia include topical medications (drops, skin creams), local injectable agents, tumescent infiltration, oral medications, intravenous sedation, and general anesthesia. Factors in determining the appropriate type of anesthesia include procedure length, invasiveness, patient comorbidities, age, anxiety level, prior history of similar procedures, and pain tolerance. Selection should reflect a team approach involving the patient, family, and care providers.

5.2 Topical Anesthesia

5.2.1 Eye Drops

Topical ophthalmic drops can be used to anesthetize the ocular surface, place protective shields in the eye for surgery, remove small conjunctival lesions, and epilate lashes. They are also useful when examining patients who are intolerant of light or instruments approaching the eye. In addition, they prevent eye burning from surgical preparation solutions, such as betadine, that may contact the eye. The surgeon should be aware that topical anesthetics break down the hemidesmosomes that attach the corneal epithelium to Bowman's layer of the cornea which predisposes to corneal abrasion [1]. These drops delay corneal wound healing and should be used for procedural and diagnostic purposes only. Anesthetic drops should not be given to patients to take home for pain control, as corneal decomposition, nonhealing abrasions, or ulcers may develop [2].

Proparacaine hydrochloride 0.5% ophthalmic solution is the most commonly used topical medication for surface

G.G. Massry et al. (eds.), *Master Techniques in Blepharoplasty and Periorbital Rejuvenation*,
DOI 10.1007/978-1-4614-0067-7_5, © Springer Science+Business Media, LLC 2011

Table 5.1 Topically applied ophthalmic drops

Type	Available concentrations	Duration of action	Onset	Maximum dosage
Proparacaine hydrochloride	0.5% Solution	15 min	Fast	
Tetracaine hydrochloride	0.5–1% Solution	10–20 min	Fast	
Lidocaine hydrochloride	2% Gel, 1–4% solution	1.5–2 h	Fast	5 mg/kg up to 300 mg

anesthesia. Its high lipid content allows for rapid absorption through the corneal epithelium resulting in fast peak onset. However, the duration of anesthesia is limited to just 15–20 min, making it appropriate for examination techniques or short procedures only [3].

Tetracaine hydrochloride 0.5–1% ophthalmic solution or 0.5% ophthalmic ointment has similar onset and duration of action as proparacaine, but confers more corneal epithelial toxicity. Overuse may cause ocular irritation and pain. The duration of effect for proparacaine and tetracaine may be prolonged by repeat instillation [3].

Lidocaine hydrochloride 1–4% solution or 2% gel may also be applied topically to the ocular surface. It has rapid onset like proparacaine and tetracaine, with a significantly longer duration of action. Lidocaine without preservatives is used routinely inside the anterior chamber (intracamerally) of the eye during cataract surgery. In addition, injectable lidocaine can be dropped on the cornea prior to its local injection for blepharoplasty to minimize the sting of prep agents that may contact the eye (Author's (J.A.W) anecdotal experience).

Table 5.1 reviews and compares these topically applied ophthalmic drops.

5.2.2 Topical Skin Creams

Topical skin creams are used for laser skin resurfacing, laser hair removal, superficial skin surgery, placement of intravenous catheters, suture removal, and neurotoxin and fillers injections. They provide a degree of surface anesthesia for these procedures, and when necessary can be augmented with regional sensory nerve blocks or diffuse local infiltration. These preparations have allowed the performance of appropriate procedures in a less invasive manner (no injections) which has led to higher patient acceptance.

The maximum dose for topical lidocaine is 4.5 mg/kg up to 300 mg [4]. There is a case report of a woman who died from administration of anesthetic cream over one third of her body's surface area for a prolonged period of time [5]. Consequently, many hospitals will not formulate high concentrations of lidocaine creams. They will however allow preformulated preparations such as eutectic mixture of local anesthetics (EMLA™) and LMX™.

EMLA™ consists of lidocaine 2.5% and prilocaine 2.5% in eutectic mixture (5% oil in water). It is applied under an occlusive dressing for 60 min to achieve maximum effect (onset/duration). It is packaged in 5 and 30 g tubes. It also comes in a patch form. LMX™ is a lidocaine cream available in both 4 and 5% that is also applied for 60 min under occlusive dressing.

A compounding pharmacy can be used to manufacture higher concentration creams of local anesthetics (up to 30% lidocaine). These are not recommended for use on areas greater than 5 cm^2, as significant lidocaine toxicity (seizure) can result from larger surface area applications.

5.3 Local Injectable Anesthesia

Local injectable anesthetic agents act internally on neuronal axon sodium channels to prevent conduction of nerve impulses. Smaller and nonmyelinated nerve fibers are affected more quickly than larger or myelinated fibers. The effects are reversible as the local anesthetic diffuses away from the site of injection with no permanent effects on nerve function. Lidocaine, bupivacaine, mepivacaine, and prilocaine are the most commonly used medications. Structurally, these are amides, which are metabolized in the liver, and carry only rare risk of allergic reactions. Esters such as tetracaine and cocaine, which require plasma pseudocholinesterase for breakdown, carry a higher risk of allergy and are less commonly used for infiltration. Locally injected anesthetic agents have potential systemic toxicity directly related to the total dose and the site of administration. This usually manifests with central nervous system signs (drowsiness, paresthesias, and seizures) or cardiovascular issues (dysrhythmias and cardiac arrest). These agents have p*K*a's of approximately 8, but are prepared as ionized hydrochloride salts in a weak acid solution with a pH of 4.5–6 to increase their shelf life and water solubility. This acidic environment leads to variable degrees of pain with injection. The advantage of using local anesthetics is that they can mitigate the need for intraoperative monitoring, significantly lowering patient costs.

Local anesthetics are administered via local infiltration into subcutaneous tissues and also as nerve blocks. Lidocaine hydrochloride 1–2% solution confers the least pain on injection. The maximum dose is 5 mg/kg, but if combined with epinephrine 1:200,000, the maximum dose raises to 7 mg/kg. It confers a rapid onset of action with an effect lasting up to 1–2 h. Bupivacaine hydrochloride 0.5–0.75% solution has a

Table 5.2 Local injectable anesthetics

Type	Available concentrations (%)	Duration of action	Onset	Maximum dosage
Lidocaine hydrochloride	0.5–2	60–120 min	Fast	5 mg/kg (7 mg/kg with 2.5–5 μg/mL Epi)
Bupivacaine hydrochloride	0.25–0.75	4–12 h	Slow	150 mg (2.5 mg/kg with Epi)
Mepivacaine hydrochloride	1.5–2	2–3 h	Fast	500 mg (600 mg with Epi)

slower onset with a longer duration (4–12 h) when compared to lidocaine. Its maximum safe dose is 2.5 mg/kg with epinephrine, and it carries the risk of significant cardiac toxicity with overdose. Mepivacaine 1–3% has a rapid onset of action and intermediate duration of 2–3 h with a maximum safe dose of 7 mg/kg. Lidocaine and bupivacaine are often mixed prior to administration in order to maximize speed of onset and duration of action. In order to decrease the pain on injection, sodium bicarbonate 8.4% (9:1 mixture) is often added. This has the added benefit of deprotonating the local anesthetics, making them able to cross into neurons freely and work more rapidly. Further pain upon injection can be reduced by slow injection and use of small-bore needles.

Table 5.2 reviews and compares the local anesthetics described above.

The addition of epinephrine to these anesthetics decreases the rate of systemic absorption through vasoconstriction, resulting in diminished diffusion of anesthetic away from the injection site. This effect allows greater maximal dosing and potentially extended duration of effect. These anesthetics may be formulated with 1:100,000, 1:200,000, or 1:400,000 epinephrine.

The addition of hyaluronidase (0.5 cc hyaluronidase to 9.5 cc lidocaine) helps improve the spread of the anesthetic and speed of onset. The improved spread allows for fewer needle sticks as gentle massage disperses the solution well. Hyaluronidase acts by depolymerizing hyaluronic acid and facilitating diffusion of local anesthetic agents. However it may reduce duration of anesthesia as the anesthetic diffuses away from the surgical site. Epinephrine should be used with hyaluronidase in the solution mixture to improve its duration. The combination may also help maintain surgical planes [6, 7].

5.4 Tumescent Anesthesia

Significant regional anesthesia of skin and subcutaneous tissue can be accomplished with subcutaneous infiltration of large amounts of dilute lidocaine and epinephrine solution (mixed in saline) until the skin feels hardened (tumesced). The technique is typically used for liposuction, but can also be given for rhytidectomy, laser resurfacing, scalp surgery, and other soft tissue procedures. Prior to the development of this technique, the maximum established safe dose of injectable lidocaine was 5 mg/kg, and 7 mg/kg when mixed with epinephrine. With the tumescent technique, developed by dermatologist Klein [4], the maximum safe dose for lidocaine is 50 mg/kg. This is related to the action of epinephrine and to the mechanical effect of the high volume of dilute solution injected. Both act as a vascular tourniquet preventing spread of lidocaine systemically where it can become toxic. The technique provides excellent hemostasis, pain control, and possibly a decreased rate of infection due to the acidity of the lidocaine [4].

5.5 Oral Sedation

Anxiety can play an important role in anesthetic choices and surgical decision-making. Even minor procedures can be extremely stressful for patients, regardless of adequate pain control. Systemic anxiolytics are useful in these situations, particularly when a healthy patient undergoes a simple procedure that does not require systemic monitoring.

Benzodiazepines such as oral diazepam (Valium) and lorazepam (Ativan) are useful adjuncts to help relax patients. Both bind to the GABA receptor, facilitating influx of chloride, producing membrane hyperpolarization, and decreasing neuronal activity. Care should be taken with benzodiazepines and other drugs such as barbiturates, opioids, and antidepressants, as their effects are often synergistic [8].

Zolpidem tartrate (Ambien®) is a short-acting nonbenzodiazepine that potentiates GABA receptors similarly to benzodiazepines. This medication has benefits over benzodiazepines, including a low risk of habit-formation and an improved safety profile in elderly patients [9].

Table 5.3 reviews the properties of the oral sedatives described earlier. For certain painful procedures, these medications can be given with oxycodone/acetaminophen (Percocet 5/325) or meperidine (Demerol) PO prior to the procedure, for combined pain control and sedation.

5.6 Monitored Anesthesia Care

Monitored anesthesia (conscious sedation) care (MAC) refers to monitored intravenous sedation and analgesia without endotracheal intubation. It can be administered by the surgeon or anesthesia specialist. Certification is required for

Table 5.3 Oral sedatives

Type	Available dosages (mg)	Metabolic half-life	Onset	Maximum dosage
Diazepam	2, 5, 10	20–100 h	1–2 h	20 mg
Lorazepam	0.5, 1, 2	10–20 h	2–4 h	10 mg/day
Zolpidem tartrate	5, 10	2–3 h	15 min	10 mg/day

surgeons to administer this form of sedation. Most surgeons prefer a certified registered nurse anesthetist (CRNA) or anesthesiologist to provide IV sedation so that they can concentrate on the procedure itself. This also minimizes the surgeon's liability. In determining if MAC will suffice or whether deeper sedation with endotracheal intubation is warranted, the surgeon and anesthesia practitioner should work together. This would include a full physical examination and review of the patient's health condition to assess anesthesia risk.

Benzodiazepines are commonly used in MAC. They produce sedation, retrograde amnesia, anxiolysis, and muscle relaxation. Risks include hypotension and respiratory depression. Use benzodiazepines with caution in patients with liver disease as they can be hepatotoxic. They also increase the seizure threshold for lidocaine allowing for safer injection.

Useful IV benzodiazepines include midazolam, diazepam, and lorazepam. Midazolam is a potent amnestic and has short redistribution and elimination half-lives, making it useful during injection of local anesthetics. It has all, but replaced diazepam and lorazepam for outpatient procedures. Diazepam is longer acting but often causes irritation at the injection site and localized thrombophlebitis. Lorazepam is potent but has a delayed onset which makes it less useful in ambulatory surgical cases. Overdose or toxicity from benzodiazepines can be reversed with flumazenil, a benzodiazepine antagonist, which reversibly competes with benzodiazepines at GABA receptor binding sites.

Opioids are useful IV anesthetic agent utilized to provide analgesia. Unfortunately, they carry a long list of side effects including drowsiness, respiratory depression, pruritis, miosis, bradycardia, nausea, and vomiting. Fentanyl (Sublimaze®) is commonly used for the initial phase of sedation to facilitate a short period of deep anesthesia. Morphine or other long-acting opioids can be utilized when postoperative pain is expected. Overdose (sedation and respiratory depression) from opioid use can be reversed with Naloxone (Narcan®), a competitive antagonist which reversibly binds to opioid receptors. It should however be used judiciously since it effectively unmasks the pain for which the opioids were initially administered. Acute pain can significantly increase patient's stress which can result in poor outcome (hypertension, tachycardia, etc.), particularly if they have comorbid cardiovascular disease. To help combat nausea and vomiting associated with opioids, antiemetics such as decadron or ondansetron (Zofran®) can be administered intra- or postoperatively [8, 10].

Propofol (Diprivan®) is a widely used short-acting sedative-hypnotic useful for induction of anesthesia. It has all but replaced barbiturate use in the surgical arena. It is formulated in a 1% egg lecithin and soy lipid emulsion and has rapid onset and recovery. It is not an analgesic and often causes a burning pain upon injection, so it is often preceded by or mixed with IV lidocaine. Opioids such as fentanyl are often administered immediately prior to propofol as well. Propofol is generally well tolerated by healthy patients, but carries side effects including hypotension from vasodilation, or cardiac depression and transient apnea [8].

Dexmedetomidine hydrochloride (Precedex®) is a relatively new centrally acting alpha-2 agonist that controls stress, anxiety, and pain while keeping patients cooperative. It is also desirable because it is not a respiratory or cardiac depressant. This drug has had increasing popularity in recent years [11].

5.7 General Anesthesia

General anesthesia aims to induce reversible amnesia, analgesia, loss of responsiveness, and muscle relaxation. These attributes may be achieved through a careful balance of the above-described anesthetic agents. To be sure, trained anesthetists should be consulted to administer and to manage general anesthesia. These professionals are responsible for patient preoperative evaluations, intraoperative anesthetic management, and postoperative anesthetic recovery. General anesthesia can be useful in a variety of situations. Medically frail, severely anxious, disinhibited, developmentally delayed, and infants or children should be considered for this type of anesthesia. Procedural constraints are also important to consider, as prolonged surgeries or those with the potential for significant blood loss may warrant general anesthesia for strict control of fluids and patient comfort.

Preoperatively, systemic conditions must be evaluated. A history of cardiovascular disease, including myocardial infarction, angina, valvular disorders, and hypertension increases the risk of intra- or postoperative myocardial ischemia. Respiratory disorders such as chronic obstructive pulmonary disease and obstructive sleep apnea are associated with chronic hypoxemia, which could influence anesthetic decision-making. Undertreated asthma can be particularly problematic perioperatively as well. Both cardiovascular and pulmonary disease can present practical problems pre- and postoperatively, as these patients often have difficulty lying flat for surgery and may require supplemental oxygen.

Finally, some agents administered in general anesthesia have particular ophthalmic or systemic side effects that need to be kept in mind. The potent inhaled anesthetics and propofol lower intraocular pressure, while ketamine increases it. Isoflurane and the modern, less soluble agents – sevoflurane and desflurane are the potent inhaled anesthetics utilized in the United States today. They are rapidly exhaled, allowing tight titration of wake-up timing. Nitrous oxide, a nonpotent inhaled anesthetic, is a useful adjunct to the other agents for lowering overall anesthetic concentration demands. It has low blood solubility and is as rapidly exhaled as desflurane [8].

5.8 Issues for Consideration

Anesthesia medications are associated with side effects from minor to life-threatening. Allergic (type 1 hypersensitivity) reactions require previous sensitization to a drug and may range from minor (pruritis, urticaria, and angioedema) at the injection site to severe anaphylaxis (wheezing, hypotension, and cardiovascular collapse). Anaphylactoid reactions are toxic nonimmune mediated reactions to a medication. Treatment for minor reactions includes immediate discontinuation of suspected triggering medications and the prompt administration of antihistamines such as diphenhydramine and glucocorticoids such as dexamethasone. Severe anaphylaxis requires prompt administration of epinephrine and generous IV fluids.

Malignant hyperthermia (MH) is a rare, life-threatening reaction seen only in genetically susceptible patients who have been exposed to either potent inhaled anesthetics or succinylcholine. MH is a medial emergency. Early signs are tachycardia, clenching of jaw muscles, and systemic muscular rigidity. Increased metabolic demand by the musculature causes acidosis, hyperthermia, and free release of myoglobin into the bloodstream. Initial treatments include discontinuation of all volatile anesthetics, conversion to an IV anesthetic, administration of 100% oxygen, and active cooling. It is important to treat any electrolyte imbalances, particularly hyperkalemia, and maintain urine output. Intravenous dantrolene, a muscle relaxant, should be given immediately to depress skeletal muscle excitation. Mortality from episodes of MH has decreased from 90% to less than 10% since the introduction of dantrolene [3, 8].

5.9 Postoperative Care

Anesthesia and pain management does not end with the surgical procedure. Patient perception of pain during and after a procedure varies widely. A basic postoperative method of attaining patient comfort is the use of ice packs for reduction of pain and swelling. Also, keeping the patient's head elevated helps to avoid dependent edema around the face.

Postoperative pain control can be initiated at the conclusion of the case. Local anesthetic injection of long-acting amides, such as bupivacaine, can diminish postoperative pain and is a useful tool to decrease the need for narcotics. Intravenously or intramuscularly administered narcotics, such as fentanyl, morphine, and hydromorphone also bridge patients through the immediate postoperative period. Oral narcotic agents including codeine with or without acetaminophen, oxycodone with or without acetylsalicylic acid, or acetaminophen may provide longer-duration effects, and are excellent agents for responsible outpatient controlled analgesia. Notably, these agents may be associated with frustrating or dangerous side effects, including habit-formation, nausea and vomiting, respiratory depression, and/or orthostatic hypotension. Finally, nonsteroidal anti-inflammatory (NSAID) agents, such as ibuprofen, naproxen, and ketorolac (Toradol®), which inhibit prostaglandin synthesis, are generally well-tolerated and may be useful to avoid narcotic side effects. If all else fails, pain consultation should be considered for refractory patients.

5.10 Regional Nerve Blocks

Regional nerve blocks in the periorbital region are a very useful adjunct to surgery and can be divided into motor or sensory type. The term regional refers to the area supplied by the nerve. A motor block causes akinesia, while a sensory block leads to loss of sensation.

The motor nerve of the face is the facial nerve (seventh cranial nerve). It exits the facial skeleton at the stylomastoid foramen. Its main trunk separates into five component branches within the parotid gland: temporal (frontal), zygomatic, buccal, mandibular, and cervical. The temporal, zygomatic, and buccal branches travel superomedially to innervate the frontalis, orbicularis oculi, corregator supraciliaris, and procerus muscles [11]. The temporal branch innervates the brow and upper lids. The zygomatic and buccal branches contribute to the movement of the lower lids (Fig. 5.1). There are significant anastomoses between these branches [12].

In ophthalmology, regional motor blocks are used to prevent forceful eyelid closure during intraocular surgery [13]. On occasion, these blocks may be useful during eyelid surgery. An example would be an awake patient who is squeezing the lids making surgery more difficult and less precise. This can be encountered with canthal suspension. In this setting, lid squeezing can significantly reduce the surgical field

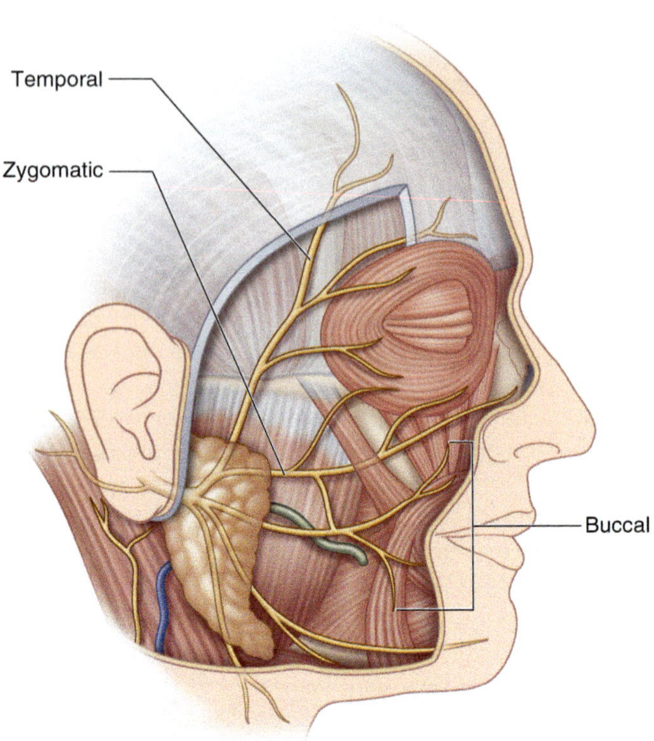

Fig. 5.1 Branching pattern of the facial nerve and innervation of the brow and eyelids. Note that the temporal (frontal) branch innervates the brow and upper lid, while the zygomatic and buccal branches innervate the lower lid

and exposure. These blocks would also be useful when surgery is performed under local anesthesia or MAC in patients with facial dystonia (blepharospasm, hemifacial spasm, or synkinesis).

The most useful regional motor nerve block for eyelid surgery is the Van Lint block [12, 14, 15]. The needle is inserted at the point where a parallel line along the lateral and inferior orbital rims would meet. Approximately 2 cc of local anesthetic is injected along the superotemporal orbital rim. This blocks the temporal branches which supply the upper lids. Another 2 cc is injected along the temporal aspect of the inferior orbital rim. This blocks the zygomatic branches which innervate the lower lid. There may be buccal branches which innervate the medial lower lid which are missed with this block. The Van Lint block is easy to perform, selectively blocks branches of the facial nerve, and has a low risk of iatrogenic nerve damage (as bigger trunks of the nerve are avoided).

The Atkinson block is a more proximal block than the Van Lint, and is less predictable in producing eyelid akinesia, as there are numerous anastomoses between the branches of the facial nerve. The needle is inserted at the inferior edge of the zygomatic arch with 2.5 cc injected superolaterally towards the top of the ear and also in the opposite direction in a linear tract over the zygomatic arch [12, 15].

The O'Brien block is the most proximal of the three blocks. Five cubic centimeter of local anesthetic is injected in front of the tragus of the ear to the condyloid process of the mandible [12, 15, 16].

Figure 5.2 depicts the injection patterns of all three regional motor nerve blocks.

5.11 Sensory Blocks

Sensory blocks are the more useful regional blocks in eyelid and facial surgery. They do not provide the hemostasis (epinephrine effect) from diffuse local injections. These injections are helpful when tissue distortion from diffuse injection is not desired, as in Muellerectomy (posterior approach) ptosis surgery and periorbital laser skin resurfacing.

Sensory innervation of the eyelids and periorbital area is supplied by the ophthalmic (V1) and maxillary (V2) divisions of the trigeminal nerve [11]. The ophthalmic division enters the orbit through the superior orbital fissure and has three branches: lacrimal, frontal, and nasociliary. The maxillary division enters the orbit through the inferior orbital fissure and has two branches: infraorbital and zygomatic nerves. The lacrimal and frontal branches travel outside the muscle cone in the superior orbit, with the frontal branch further dividing into the supraorbital and supratrochlear nerves. The frontal nerve and its branches supply cutaneous innervation to the forehead, scalp medial upper eyelids, and side of the nose. The lacrimal branch innervates the skin overlying the lacrimal gland and temporal eyelid. The nasociliary nerve travels within the muscle cone and contributes sensation to the tip of the nose. The infraorbital branch of V2 travels in the inferior orbit in the infraorbital canal and exits the facial skeleton beneath the inferior orbital rim at the infraorbital foramen. It supplies the skin of the lower lid, cheek, upper lip, and side of the nose. The zygomatic nerve divides into a zygomaticotemporal and zygomaticofacial branch which supply innervation to the cheek and temple. Figure 5.3 demonstrates the sensory nerve branches of the eyelids and periorbital area.

There are various useful regional sensory blocks in the periorbital region. They are as follows:

- Frontal nerve block: The frontal nerve can be blocked by injecting 2 cc of local anesthetic at the level of the

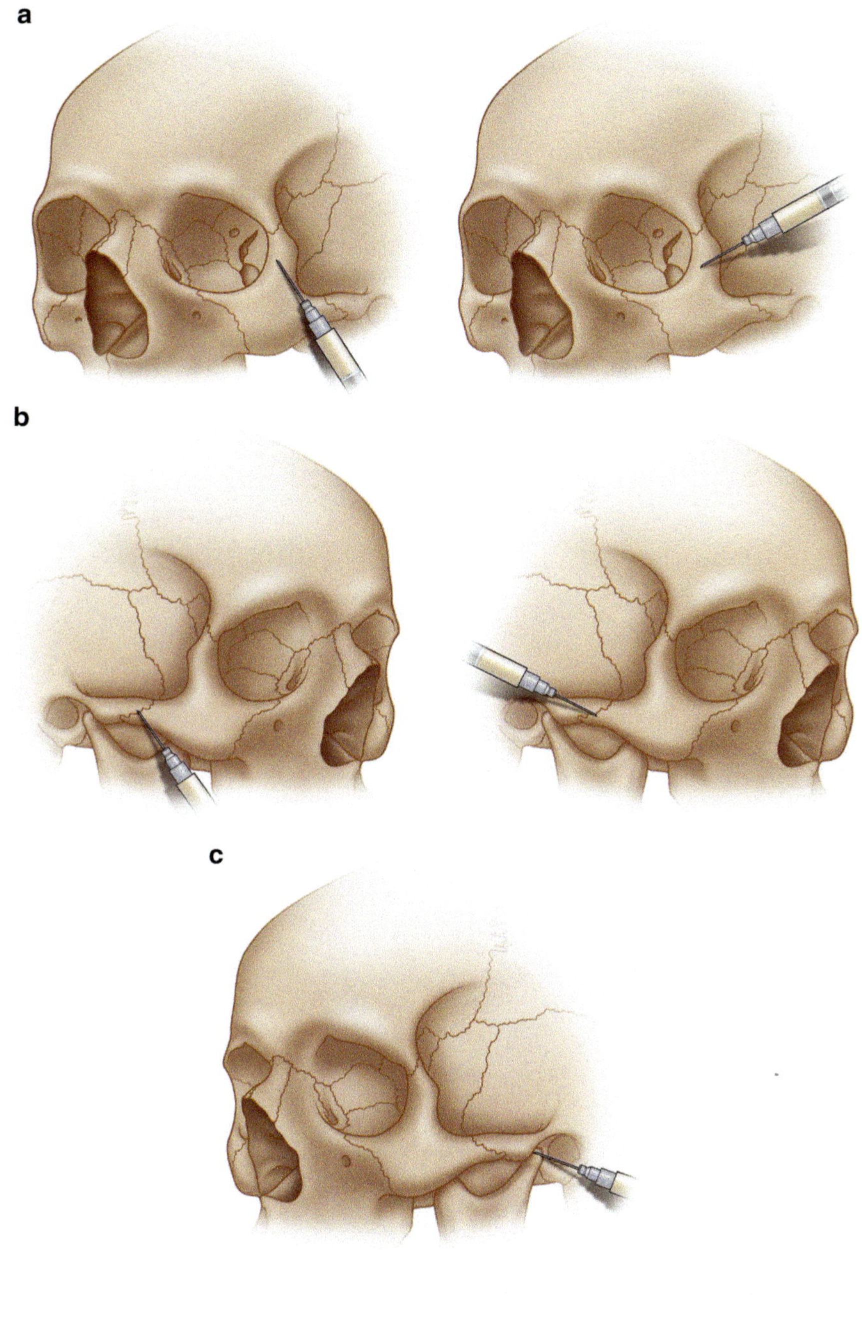

Fig. 5.2 The three regional facial nerve blocks of the eyelids are demonstrated by injection over the facial skeleton: (**a**) Van Lint; (**b**) Atkinson; and (**c**) O'Brien

supraorbital notch 2 cm into the superior orbit, hugging the orbital roof. A safer alternative is to inject the same anesthetic to the superior orbital rim at the level of the supraorbital notch (supraorbital nerve block) and advancing the needle nasally with a second injection to block the supratrochlear nerve.

- Infraorbital nerve block: The nerve is blocked by injecting 1–2 cc of local anesthetic 1.0 cm below the inferior orbital rim in line with the supraorbital notch (junction of medial one third and lateral two third of orbital rim). Alternatively, the nerve can be blocked via an intraoral (gingivobuccal) approach.
- Zygomaticofacial nerve block: This nerve exits a foramen by the same name located in the inferolateral orbital rim just below the canthus. The nerve is blocked by a 1–2 cc direct injection of local anesthesia.
- Zygomaticotemporal nerve block: The nerve exits a foramen near the level of the lateral canthus behind the

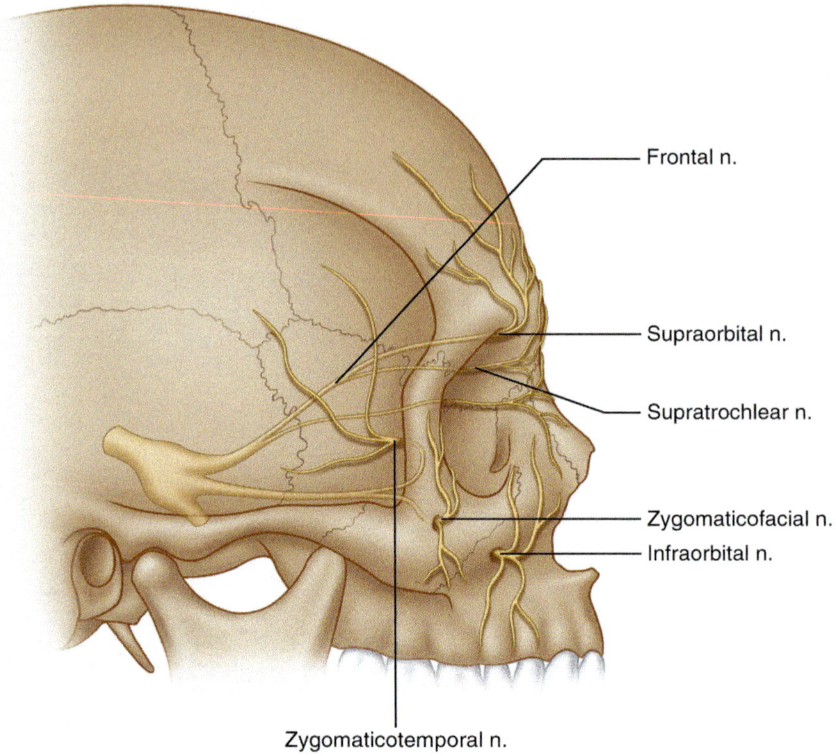

Fig. 5.3 Note the peripheral nerve branches of the ophthalmic (supraorbital, supratrochlear) and maxillary (infraorbital, zygamaticotemproal, zygamaticofacial) divisions of the trigeminal nerve which supply sensation to the eyelids and periorbital region

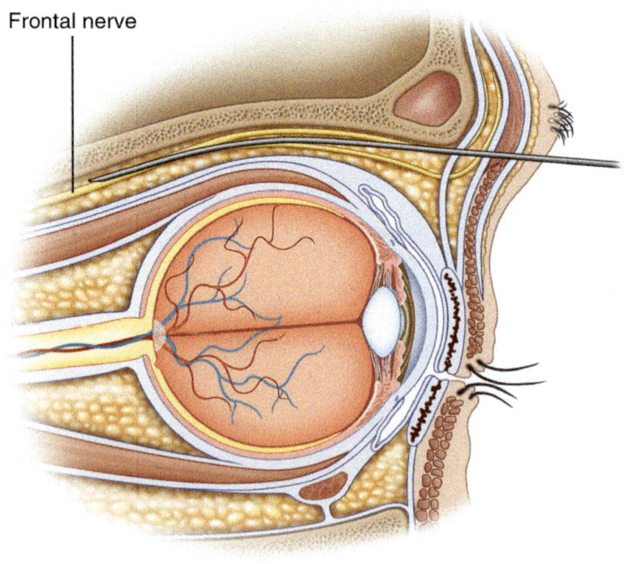

Fig. 5.4 Frontal nerve block: a sagittal view of the orbit detailing the path of the needle along the roof of the orbit

orbital rim. A 1–2 cc injection of local anesthetic is given behind the lateral orbital rim. The injection must follow the posterior rim.

Figures 5.4 and 5.5 demonstrate the injection location for each regional sensory nerve block.

5.12 Conclusion

Aesthetic surgery of the eyelids is both delicate and precise. It is obvious that a detailed knowledge of relevant anatomy, superior surgical skills, and experience are essential in order to attain appropriate surgical results. Often times, as surgeons are focused more on the technical aspects of the procedures, they have given less time and attention to the anesthesia-related issues. When a basic understanding of topical, regional, oral, intravenous, and general anesthesia is attained, the surgery becomes easier and patient safety is significantly increased.

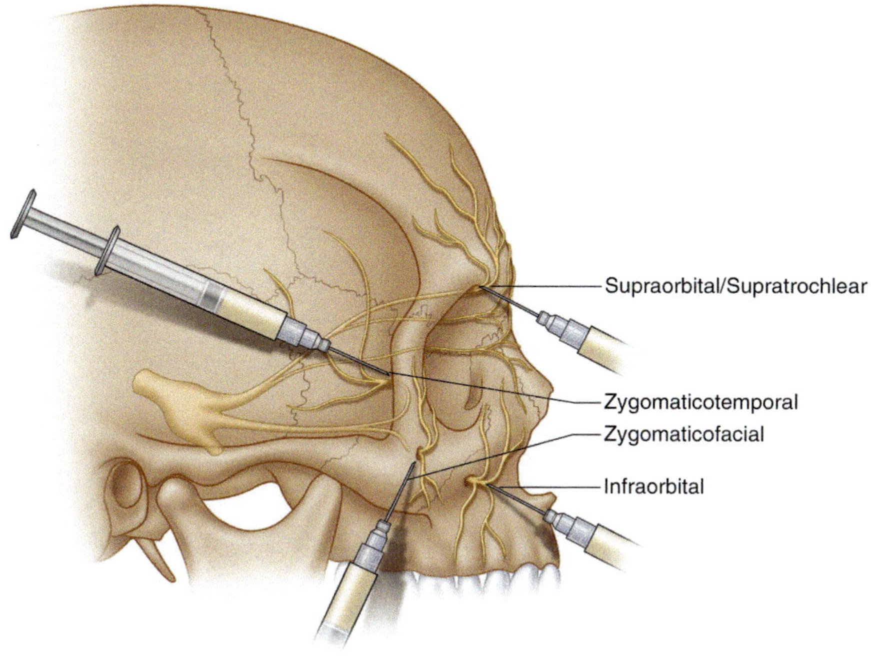

Fig. 5.5 The injection patterns for the remaining important regional sensory nerve blocks of the periorbital area are depicted

References

1. Bruce RA. Local anesthetics. In: Bruce RA, McGoldrick KE, Oppenheimer P, editors. Anesthesia for ophthalmology. Birmingham, AL: Aesculapius; 1982. p. 27–33.
2. Bisla K, Ranelian DL. Concentration-dependent effects of lidocaine on corneal epithelial wound healing. Invest Ophthalmol Vis Sci. 1992;33(1):3029–33.
3. Stewart WB. Surgery of the eyelid, orbit, and lacrimal system, vol. 1. San Francisco: American Academy of Ophthalmology; 1993.
4. Klein JA. The tumescent technique for liposuction surgery. J Am Acad Cosmetic Surg. 1987;4:263–7.
5. U.S. Food and Drug Administration. Topical anesthetics. http://www.fda.gov/Drugs/DrugSafety/DrugSafetyPodcasts/ucm079047.htm. Accessed 23 January 2011.
6. Moody BR, Holds JB. Anesthesia for office-based oculoplastic surgery. Dermatol Surg. 2005;31:766–9.
7. Berde CB, Strichartz GR. Local anesthetics. In: Miller R, editor. Anesthesia. 5th ed. New York: Churchill Livingstone; 2000. p. 491–522.
8. Hemmings HC, Hopkins PM. Foundations of anesthesia: basic sciences for clinical practice. Philadelphia: Mosby Elsevier; 2006. p. 373–403.
9. Reves JG, Glass PSA, Lubarsky DA. Non-barbiturate intravenous anesthetics. In: Miller R, editor. Anesthesia. 5th ed. New York: Churchill Livingstone; 2000. p. 228–72.
10. Bailey PL, Egan TD, Stanley TH. Intravenous opioid anesthetics. In: Miller R, editor. Anesthesia. 5th ed. New York: Churchill Livingstone; 2000. p. 273–376.
11. Shovlin JP, Lemke B. Clinical eyelid anatomy. In: Bosniak S, editor. Principals and practice of ophthalmic plastic and reconstructive surgery. Philadelphia, PA: WB Saunders; 1996. p. 261–80.
12. Schiedler V, Sires B. Motor nerve blocks in oculofacial surgery. In: Hartstein M, Holds JB, Massry GG, editors. Pearls and pitfalls in cosmetic oculoplastic surgery. New York, NY: Springer; 2008. p. 18–21.
13. Greenbaum S. Anesthesia for eye surgery, Chap. 1. In: Tasman W, Jaegar EA, editors. Duane's clinical ophthalmology on CD-ROM, vol. 6. Philadelphia: Lippincott Williams and Wilkins; 2005.
14. Van Lint A. Paralysie palpebrae temporaire par l'operation de la cataracte. Ann Ocul. 1914;151:420.
15. Schimek F, Fahle M. Techniques of facial nerve block. Br J Ophthalmol. 1995;79:166–73.
16. O'Brien CS. Local anesthesia in ophthalmic surgery. JAMA. 1928;90:8.

Part II

Forehead and Eyebrow Rejuvenation

The Open Approach to Forehead Lifting

6

Mark R. Murphy

Key Points

- Open brow lifts have a long history of successful brow rejuvenation.
- There are two open approaches: trichophytic and coronal. The procedure selection depends on the patient's preoperative assessment.
- The open approach allows the best exposure to all key anatomic structures.
- Morbidity associated with this procedure is greatly minimized with proper technique.
- Appropriate beveling of the incision and meticulous closure are vital to the success of the operation.
- The excision of skin, not tissue repositioning, secures an excellent long-term result.
- There is little to no concern of the surgical outcome fading with time.

6.1 Introduction

Surgical forehead rejuvenation began at the turn of the twentieth century [1]. Passot is recognized as an early pioneer in the field [2]. Several other surgeons described their work over the subsequent years [3–6]. The popularity of these operations faded as morbidity was found to outweigh the benefit gained from surgery. However, as with most plastic surgical procedures, interest was renewed in the latter half of the twentieth century, when new techniques evolved and results improved [7–9].

There is an ongoing controversy as to the "correct" technique to rejuvenate the brow, i.e., an open vs. an endoscopic approach. This controversy is now spilling over to rhytidectomy as well. The contention that one operation is superior to the other has left many surgeons unsure of the appropriate approach to employ.

Historically all brow rejuvenation procedures were initially performed via an open approach. And while the open coronal/trichophytic procedures demonstrated excellent long-term results, patients and surgeons were often hesitant to undergo such an involved procedure with extensive incisions and recovery time. With the advent of the endoscopic techniques in the early 1990, surgical rejuvenation of the upper third of the face became increasingly more acceptable to patients [10–14]. This trend, paired with the advent of noninvasive neuroparalytic agents and volume replenishment, has brought brow lifting to the forefront of facial rejuvenation.

6.2 Background

The upper third is perhaps the most important region of the face. This is the focal region of the face during communication with others. Patients are less aware of this region when compared to the neck and jowl as the brow can be elevated by the patient, thus "pseudo-rejuvenating" the area, whereas the corresponding areas on the lower third cannot. Consequently, the patient generally focuses more on the latter regions than the upper third. The patient must be educated on this salient point.

If middle and lower-facial rejuvenation is performed without the addressing the brow, the patient may be left with an overall disharmonious appearance [15]. This is a common omission because these regions, the jowl and neck, can be addressed with the same procedure, the rhytidectomy, whereas the brow lift requires a separate procedure.

The primary reason for brow rejuvenation is the patient's feeling, or being told, that they look tired or angry, especially in the glabellar area. The goals of any brow lifting procedure are to eradicate the depressing effect of the musculature of the glabellar region and to raise the lateral aspects of the brow. A key benefit of the open approach is the excellent

M.R. Murphy (✉)
Director, Palm Beach Facial Plastic Surgery,
Palm Beach Gardens, FL, USA
e-mail: mrm9002@gmail.com

G.G. Massry et al. (eds.), *Master Techniques in Blepharoplasty and Periorbital Rejuvenation*,
DOI 10.1007/978-1-4614-0067-7_6, © Springer Science+Business Media, LLC 2011

exposure which allows for precise handling of these problems. There is no need for overcorrection with the open approach because results remain, as ptotic tissue is excised, not suspended. In addition, the coronal and trichophytic approaches allow for more control of the brow contour by way their differential scalp incision [16].

Though the emphasis in the last decade has been on endoscopic and less invasive nonsurgical brow lifting methods, such as Botox®, the author has found that the open brow lift provides excellent and lasting results with minimal side effects. The open forehead lift allows optimal removal of the corrugator muscles and direct excision of skin, which promotes stability to the surgical outcome [17]. The open brow lift is an excellent operation in patients with severe ptosis of the brows, deep glabellar or mid-forehead wrinkles, or in the patient with a preexisting high forehead when a trichophytic lift is selected. The results achieved with this forehead lift are predictable, natural appearing, long lasting, and aesthetically pleasing with minimal morbidity.

I feel the side effects of the open brow lift techniques have been unduly negative. In a recent, unpublished report on the significance of the side effects of the open brow techniques, the authors found an overwhelming percentage of patients recommend the procedure to a friend or relative (Murphy MR and Johnson CM; unpublished data). Recent reports have also shown that the difference in the rate of alopecia between the open and endoscopic techniques is small, that sensory loss is higher with the endoscopic procedure, and that patient satisfaction is higher with the open technique [18, 19].

The other issue of concern when discussing the open approach to forehead rejuvenation is the extent of the incision. This is predominantly a matter of proper patient education. When comparing the length of the open incision vs. the combined length of the endoscopic incisions, the difference is negligible, and the patient can be comfortably reassured. Certainly, if the patient feels they are going to be "scalped" they will not consent to the procedure [20].

The coronal incision can be completely camouflaged with the patient's hair. In the case of the trichophytic incision, only the anterior aspect of the incision is exposed. Additionally, this segment of the incision can also be masked with hair when the patient wears their bangs forward. In both instances, the incision generally heals imperceptibly when proper beveling and meticulous technique are employed during incision and closure. The patient must be counseled as to the amount of time it requires for the wound to heal completely. If the patient does not wish to have an open procedure because of the incision, the endoscopic approach should be explored.

The open technique via the pretricheal route enables the surgeon to manipulate certain aesthetic variables in unique ways. For example, the trichophytic lift allows for shortening of an elongated forehead. A long forehead disrupts the harmony of the face and adds to the perception of the patient's age [21]. The forehead shortening capabilities of the trichophytic brow lift cannot be obtained with the endoscopic technique [22, 23]. Detractors argue that the incision in this location is prohibitive. However, with proper planning and execution this approach yields an excellent aesthetic result [22]. This is not to say that this procedure is appropriate in all patients with an elongated forehead. If the patient is overly conscious of any scar, or whose hairstyle requires the hair being placed posteriorly, the surgeon should avoid this approach. The decision as to which open incision to use (coronal vs. trichophytic) has been discussed extensively in the literature and will be further elaborated in this chapter [24].

The purpose of this chapter is not to argue over the superior brow lifting technique. That is an individual decision for the patient and surgeon. The open brow lift and endoscopic procedures should be familiar to all aesthetic surgeons who rejuvenate the upper third of the face, and should be discussed with all patients. What will be presented is a detailed review of the open brow lift procedure and its inherent risks and benefits.

6.3 Anatomy

To appropriately rejuvenate the brow, the surgeon must be cognizant of its anatomy (see Chap. 2). The position and movement of the brow is determined by several factors. First among these are the paired frontalis muscles. The frontalis is the sole elevator of the brow. These paired muscles have a definitive midline separation [25]. Each of these muscles originates from the galea aponeurotica. The muscles are encased by fascia, and insert onto the orbicularis oculi muscles, which in turn insert to the dermis of the eyebrow. Only the lower 20% of the frontalis muscle is mobile [26].

The brow has four depressor muscles: the procerus, corrugator supercilli, depressor supercilli, and the orbital portion of the orbicularis oculi. The depressor supercilli is located on the medial arc of the orbicularis and is considered by some to be part of the orbicularis [27]. This muscle aids the corrugator in depressing the medial head of the brow. The corrugator muscles originate from the frontal bone near the superior-medial orbital rim, and insert into the dermis of the forehead skin behind and immediately superior to the middle third of the brow [25]. Contraction of the corrugator complex results in depression of the medial brow and the formation of deep vertical glabellar rhytids. The procerus originates from the nasal bone and inserts into the lower medial skin of the forehead. Its contraction leads to the most inferior horizontal rhytid over the radix of the nose [27]. The orbital fibers of the orbicularis oculi muscle arise from the medial canthal tendon, arch along the orbital rim, and meet laterally at the zygoma. The superior division of the muscle acts as an accessory brow depressor. The galea is contiguous with the superficial temporalis fascia laterally. The periosteum of the frontal bone is contiguous with the deep temporalis fascia. These respective fascial layers converge just medial to the temporal fusion line of the skull.

The sensory innervation to the forehead and scalp is derived from two nerves, the supraorbital and supratrochlear, with the supraorbital nerve being the main contributor. The supraorbital nerve has two divisions, superficial (medial) and deep (lateral) [28]. The deep division courses in the subgaleal plane, over the periosteum towards the superior temporal line before turning superficially through the galea, on its way to the skin of the frontoparietal scalp. The superficial division courses from the orbital rim, through and over the frontalis muscle, and terminates on the anterior scalp [26], supplying this area and the forehead skin. The supratrochlear nerve accompanies the superficial branch of the supraorbital nerve over the surface of the frontalis muscle. Motor innervation of the forehead/eyebrow muscles is supplied by the frontal branch of the facial nerve. It runs within the superficial temporalis fascia on its way to innervate the frontalis, currugator, and the orbicularis muscle.

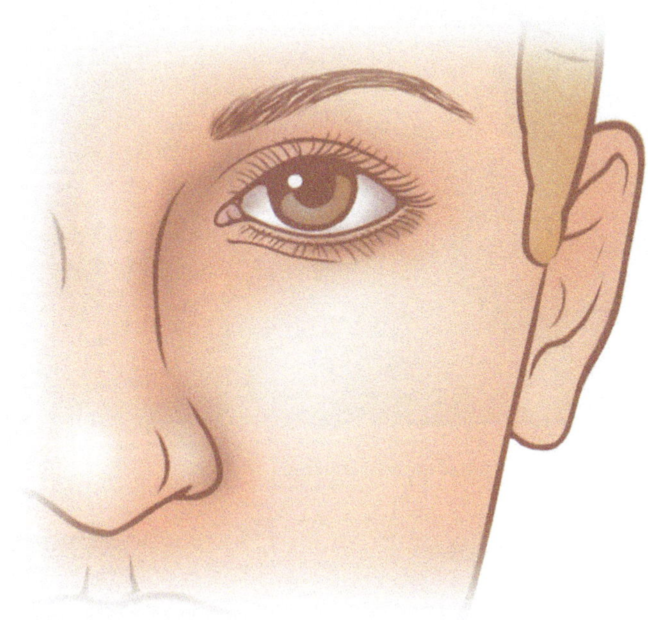

Fig. 6.1 The continuous line from the brow to the dorsal line of the nose is a key anatomic feature

6.4 Preoperative Assessment

There have been numerous studies on the ideal aesthetic of the female eyebrow [24, 29–34]. An individual's ethnicity, age, sex, culture, and adjacent structures all influence the perceived beauty of the brow. Though opinions vary, there are certain characteristics that commonly recur: (1) the medial brow should lie at, or below, the level of the supraorbital rim, (2) the brow should have an apex lateral slant, (3) the medial brow should begin in the vertical plane of the medial canthus and lateral extent of the ala, (4) the brow ends laterally in line with a tangent drawn from the lateral ala through the lateral canthus, (5) the apex of the brow should lie above either the lateral limbus or lateral canthus [24, 29–32, 35]. An additional feature of facial beauty is the relationship of the medial brow to the dorsal aesthetic lines of the nose (Fig. 6.1). The soft and uninterrupted shadow effect, as the medial brow transitions to the dorsal nasal aesthetic line, can add inherent attractiveness to the face [7, 29].

The decision of utilizing a trichophytic vs. coronal incision is discussed with the patient before surgery. This judgment is based on the position of the hairline (low vs. high) and the manner in which the patient wears his or her hair [36]. Of course, the personal preferences of the patient must also be taken into account.

The key to an accurate preoperative assessment is the relaxation, manual if necessary, of the brow. It is in repose that the patient must objectively view the resting position of the brow. The patient reflexively raises his or her brow when placed in front of a mirror or when a photo is taken. The surgeon can manually position the brow as it appears at rest with the patient's eyes closed and then instruct them to open their eyes slowly.

6.5 Technique

The sequence of procedures for facial rejuvenation usually begins with the forehead lift. Rarely is the brow lift the sole procedure performed. In the author's practice, it is most often combined with an upper and lower lid blepharoplasty and deep plane facelift. The brow lift is performed first because it allows for a more conservative, and accurate, upper lid blepharoplasty. In selected cases, such as those with deep-set eyes, previous blepharoplasty or those with minimal excess upper lid skin, the brow lift is all that is needed for rejuvenation of the upper third of the face.

Marking and shaving of the hair can be performed prior to or after the administration of the anesthesia method of choice. The patient is often very anxious during this time and the marking and shaving of hair can magnify these feelings. When performed under anesthesia, anxiety is reduced. However, in an arena where cost management is a priority, this can be done prior to the anesthetic.

For a coronal approach, a fusiform segment of tissue is shaved and marked for excision (Fig. 6.2). The markings for the tissue excision should lay 5–6 cm posterior to the anterior hairline. The lateral extent of the incision should terminate

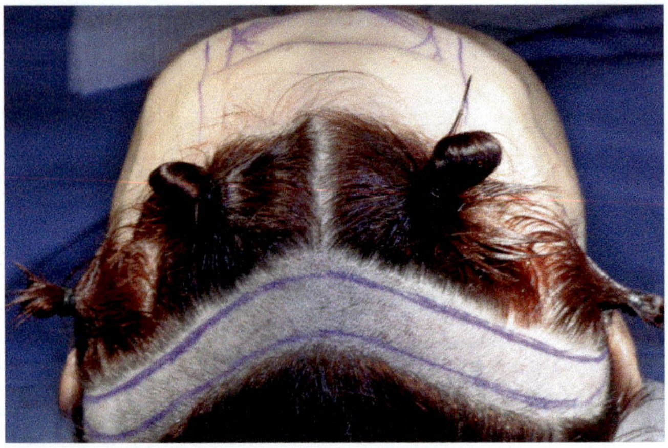

Fig. 6.2 The standard coronal markings

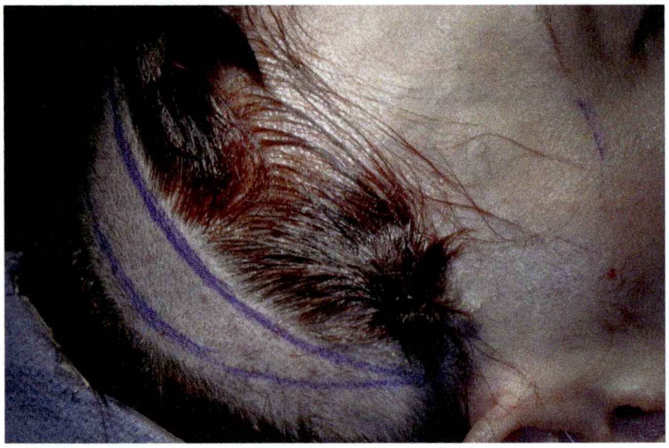

Fig. 6.3 The coronal markings mimic the anterior hairline and taper laterally

approximately 1–2 cm above the superior insertion of the auricle to the skull, in an attempt to incorporate the superficial temporal vessels within the flap. It is preferable to preserve this vasculature. However, if it is compromised, the blood supply to the flap is relatively robust. The surgeon should insure that an adequate amount of temporal hair is left behind, especially if this procedure is being performed in conjunction with a facelift where a portion of the sideburn is shaved as well (Fig. 6.3). The incision should parallel the anterior hairline tapering at the lateral aspects to a point. The surgeon can reliably gauge the amount of tissue to resect by assessing the mobility of the scalp and its associated effect on brow position prior to incision. One can also decide on the exact amount of skin to be excised after raising the flap. However, precise incising of the tissue, as is desired when trying to preserve as many hair follicles as possible, is very challenging when incising this thick tissue after it has been mobilized. With adequate experience, the surgeon will be proficient in anticipating the total skin excision prior to the initial incision. Generally speaking, the amount of skin lies

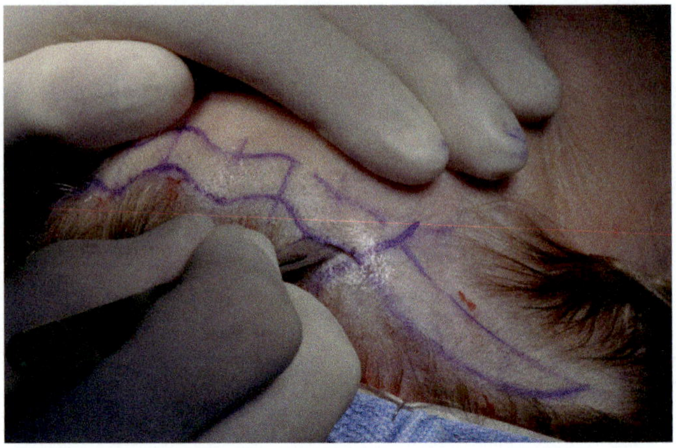

Fig. 6.4 The markings for the trichophytic lift are similar to that of the coronal but have undulations in the center and the angles are slightly different

between 1 and 2 cm. If the surgeon discovers that he or she has miscalculated and resected too much tissue, a posterior scalp elevation can be performed to reduce tension and aid in the closure. Obviously, it is better to err on the side of caution and remove less skin if the surgeon is uncertain as to the exact amount to be removed.

The trichophytic incision is more difficult to plan and perform; however, this approach yields excellent results when the procedure is executed in a meticulous manner. The marking begins with scissor trimming of the first two to three rows of hair in the anterior aspect of the hairline. Laterally the hair is shaved as an elongated, curved triangle with its apex above the superior insertion of the auricle to the scalp (Fig. 6.4). This area is generally 4–5 cm in length and should not be placed too inferior so as to encroach on the temporal hairline. This termination point varies from patient to patient depending on the position of the hairline and the contour of the patient's skull. Once the incision is created a flap must be mobilized to allow access to the glabellar musculature. This often requires folding the flap upon itself so an adequate rotation point must be chosen laterally. In the midline, the incision has gentle undulations closely following the hairline. This undulation allows for improved camouflage of the incision over a simple straight-cut. This posterior aspect of the incision should be placed in the transition zone between the thick posterior hair of the scalp and the fine hairs that constitute the anterior hairline (Fig. 6.4).

The hair is secured with rubber bands anteriorly and with a circumferential band of tape posteriorly. In the trichophytic incision the only hair that is secured with rubber bands is the lateral temporal hair. The hair is shaved. The surgeon should be mindful not to place the posterior tape too tightly around the circumference of the head as to create a "false" lift leading to an under-correction at the conclusion of the case.

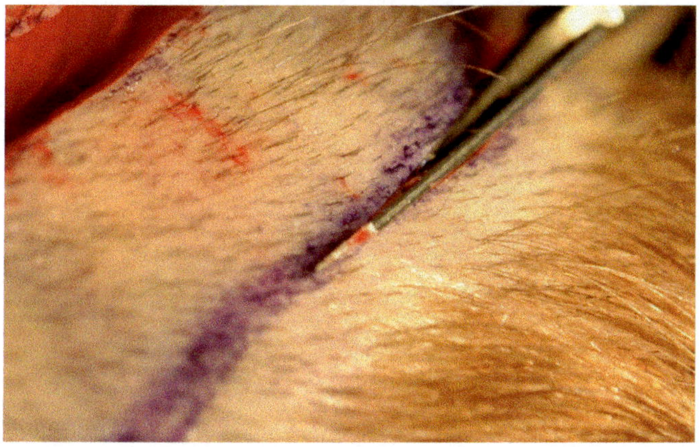

Fig. 6.5 The incision is beveled with the hair follicles in the coronal approach

The incisions are remarked and injected with local anesthetic. I prefer a mixture of equal parts of 0.5% lidocaine with 1:100,000 epinephrine with 0.5% bupivacaine with 1:200,000 epinephrine. The injection should be in the galeal, where most of the vessels run their course, and the subgaleal planes. Bilateral supraorbital and supratrochlear nerve blocks are administered. Lastly, the corrugator and procerus muscles are directly injected to aid in pain management as well as hemostasis. The patient is then prepped and draped in the standard fashion. A sterile towel is gently stapled around the head in a parallel course to the previous hair taping, being mindful not to place the towel too tightly.

The incisions are performed with a ten blade. This blade is preferred for its increased surface area, which allows for less blunting (and changing) of blades. The forehead skin is thick and will quickly dull smaller blades, requiring numerous replacements, increased cost, and operating time. Proper beveling of both the pretricheal and coronal incisions is vital to attaining maximal hair regrowth and scar camouflage. In the coronal incision the bevel parallels the follicles throughout the length of the incision (Fig. 6.5). The entire amount of shaved hair is removed leaving a hair-to-hair closure and preventing a noticeable region of alopecia postoperatively. The incision traces further laterally than the pretricheal incision and the orientation of hair at the end point of the incision is almost perpendicular to the skin; the blade must mimic this orientation.

The pretricheal incision requires alternating beveling techniques, and the surgeon must be cognizant of three separate incision areas (Fig. 6.6). The first is the anterior, visible hairline (Fig. 6.7). In this area the beveling transects the follicles to allow them to grow through the incision as it heals over time. This hair generally grows anteriorly and the incision is almost perpendicular to the follicles. When the surgeon chooses this approach, he or she should assess the growth pattern of these vital hairs preoperatively. If they grow posteriorly, masking of the incision by wearing the

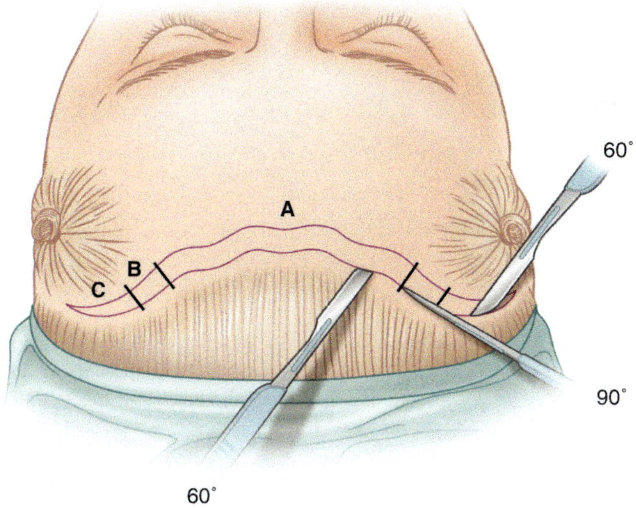

Fig. 6.6 This graphic depicts the varying angles of the blade during the trichophytic incision

bangs forward may not be possible. This should be discussed with the patient.

The second aspect of the incision is the interface of the anterior region of the incision with the hair bearing areas laterally (Fig. 6.8). At this juncture the beveling must be altered from one transecting the follicles to one running almost parallel to them. This is a brief transition and should quickly evolve into the standard follicle sparing angle seen with the coronal lift (Fig. 6.9). It should be noted that the surgeon must utilize the same angle of incision for both the posterior and anterior portions of the incision to ensure the best possible closure. The importance of proper beveling technique cannot be overemphasized. When done improperly, alopecia and noticeable, unattractive scars result. Lack of attention to detail in this step of the surgery, with resultant loss of hair and scars, are what have substantiated the criticisms of these techniques.

For the entire coronal incision and the lateral aspects of the pretricheal incision, the blade is advanced with a pushing motion, instead of the classical method of pulling the knife towards oneself. This technique allows for better control of the knife through the thick skin of the forehead. It also enhances the surgeon's ability to follow the hair follicles correctly as one can see where the knife is directed instead of being masked by the hand. This is vital when one considers the exacting manner in which the knife must be beveled for these procedures. The incision is carried down to the level of the subgaleal plane of dissection. After the incisions have been created, the excess skin is removed. This is done one side at a time, so that blood loss is kept to a minimum. As all surgeons who operate in this area know, the blood supply to the scalp is robust. By removing half of the excess skin and obtaining hemostasis, complications can be avoided and

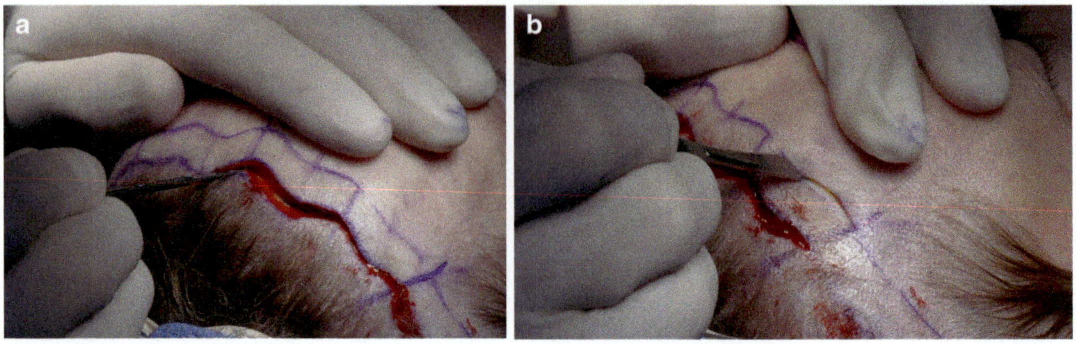

Fig. 6.7 (**a**) The posterior aspect of the trichophytic incision is made through the first few anterior hairs. This incision transects the follicles so that they grow through, and thus mask the healing wound. (**b**) The trichophytic incision is completed. Please note the angle of the bevel must be identical to that of the posterior portion of the incision to optimize wound healing

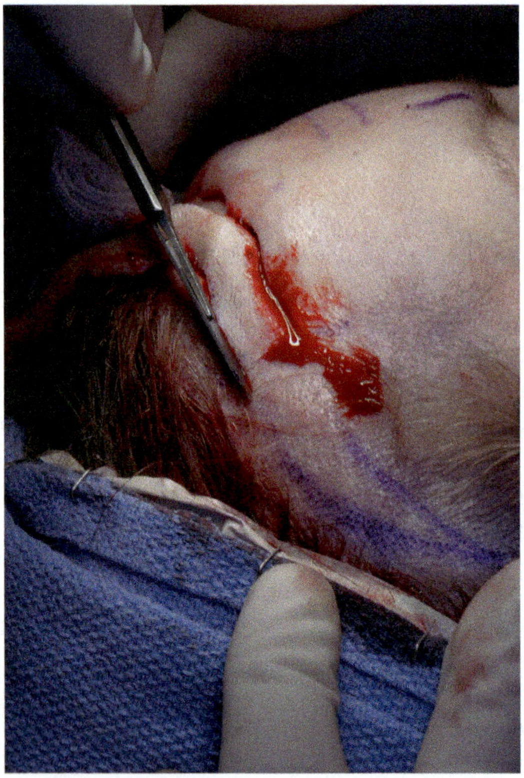

Fig. 6.8 The angle of the blade transitions as the incision moves laterally

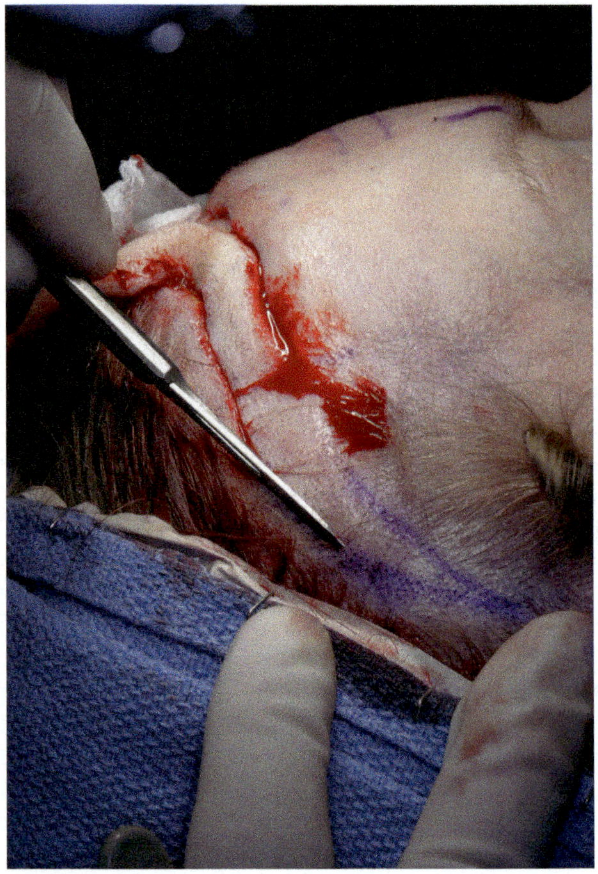

Fig. 6.9 The lateral aspect of the trichophytic incision parallels the coronal incision

surgery is better controlled. Frequently, the superficial temporal vessels are transected laterally and bleeding should be immediately controlled. Bipolar cautery should be used to reduce thermal damage to adjacent hair follicles. To further prevent hair loss, the surgeon should control bleeding superficial to the galea with cold compresses rather than electrocautery, as the region lacks any major blood vessels. A complete examination of the incision should be performed prior to placing a cool, moist compress on the posterior portion of the incision. Bleeding can persist in the lateral aspects of the incisions and go unnoticed by the surgeon for extended periods of time as he or she is focused elsewhere. The surgeon must check both lateral aspects of the incision periodically throughout the case to insure adequate hemostasis. The contralateral skin is removed, hemostasis is obtained, and the anterior flap is then elevated.

A subgaleal dissection is performed using a ten blade and Anderson bear claw retractor. The dissection is carried down to the superior aspect of the orbital rim (Fig. 6.10).

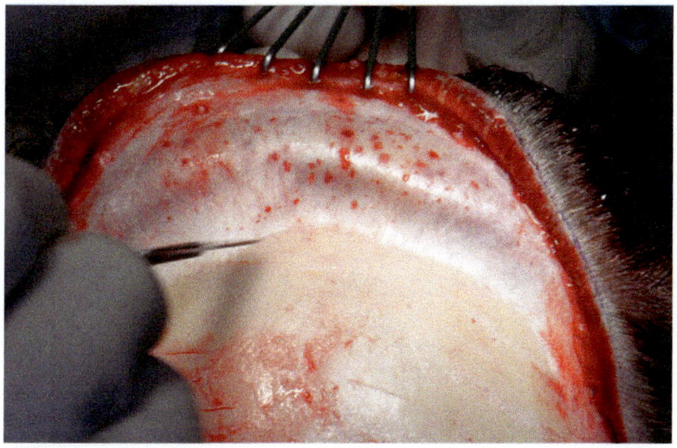

Fig. 6.10 The subgaleal dissection is performed with the ten blade

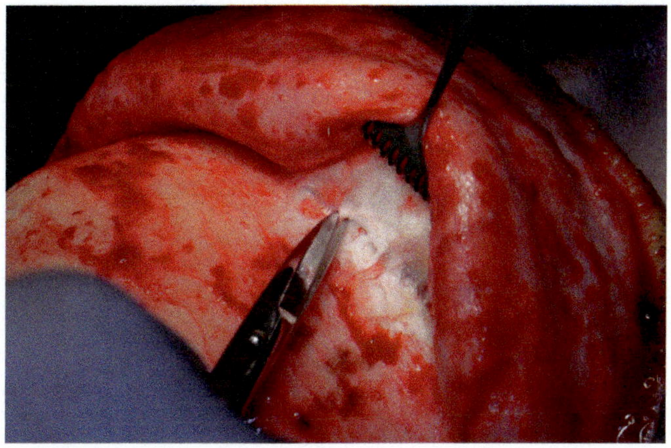

Fig. 6.12 A sharp scissor and non-penetrating retractor is used in the lateral component of the dissection

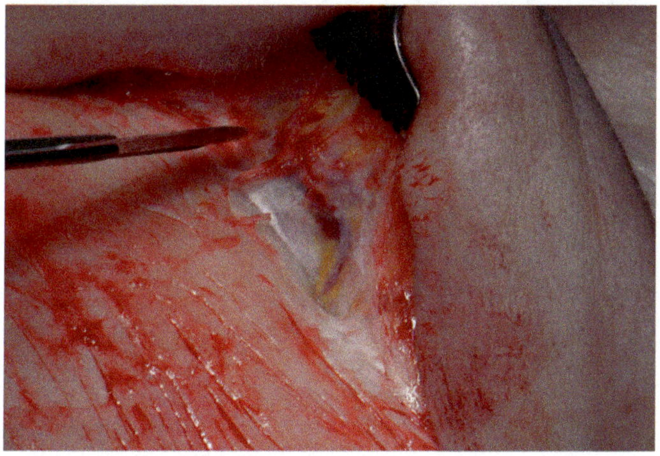

Fig. 6.11 A non-penetrating retractor is employed when approaching neurovascular structures

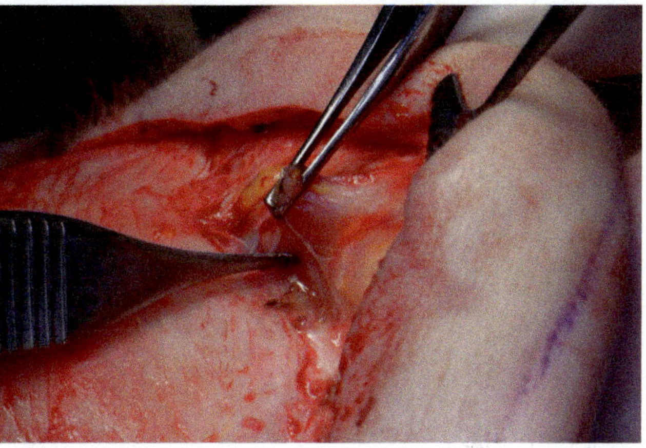

Fig. 6.13 The corrugator excision is performed with the bipolar after transecting the muscle. This maneuver is aided by retraction in the vector of the muscle

This "sliding plane" is preferable compared to the subperiosteal plane due to the ease of dissection [18]. With the excision of tissue in the open technique, we do not need to relay upon the periosteum adhering to the cranium to ensure longevity. A non-penetrating retractor is used when approaching the supraorbital and supratrochlear nerves medially, and the frontal branch of facial nerve laterally (Fig. 6.11). The supraorbital and supratrochlear bundles are preserved at the orbital rim, or notch, depending on the patient's anatomy. The frontal branch is preserved by dissecting directly on the superficial aspect of the deep temporalis fascia.

When approaching the zygomatic arch, I change dissecting instruments from a ten blade to fine sharp scissors and cotton tip applicator for blunt dissection (Fig. 6.12). The dissection is carried down to the zygomatic arches bilaterally. Monopolar cauterization is avoided in this area to prevent potential thermal injury to the facial nerve. Judicious bipolar cautery is advised if necessary.

With the flap completely mobilized, attention is directed to the glabellar musculature. The flap is raised to the radix. Using an Adsen forceps and sharp, fine dissecting scissors, the corrugator muscles are mobilized. This dissection is greatly aided by the assistant using a non-penetrating retractor in the natural vector of the corrugator to help expose the muscle (Fig. 6.13). Care must be taken to avoid inadvertent trauma to the supratrochlear neurovascular bundle during this phase of the operation. There is often a large vein encountered in the region. The medial 2–3 cm of the muscle is dissected free from the galea and it is transected and cauterized at its medial attachment to the bone.

The excision of the corrugator muscles leads to a long-term benefit unattainable with other methods of muscle weakening such as Botox. The concern over muscle resection leading to a deficit of expression is exceedingly rare. Even with aggressive muscle resection the patient usually has adequate expression postoperatively.

With the flap elevated the procerus is scored horizontally with a monopolar cautery (Fig. 6.14). This is performed gently

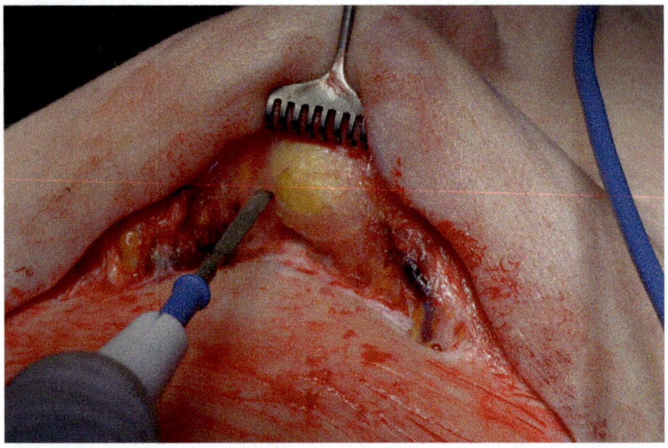

Fig. 6.14 The procerus is scored horizontally with monopolar cautery

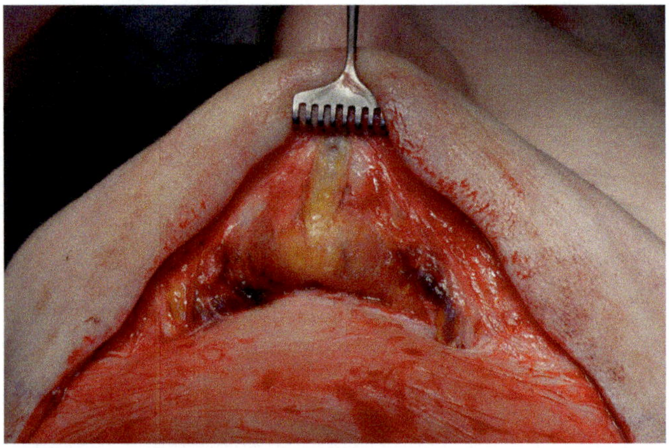

Fig. 6.15 In selected cases, the glabellar region is scored vertically to alleviate excessively heavy brows

through muscle only. If done too aggressively, the patient will be left with a soft tissue depression in the glabellar region. The scoring should center on the medial aspect of the muscle to insure the supratrochlear neurovascular bundles are left undisturbed. Occasionally, in the heavy brow, I will perform a vertical myotomy to allow for lateral spread of the glabella (Fig. 6.15).

In most cases, a galeotomy and midline myotomy of the frontalis at the level of the most prominent mid-forehead rhytid is performed with monopolar cautery (Fig. 6.16). By performing this maneuver in the midline only (up to the medial aspects of the orbital rims), the surgeon allows the patient to retain muscle function laterally with lateral brow elevation. This technique however, should be used judiciously to avoid creating a "surprised" appearance.

A suction drain is then placed above the superior orbital rims and the field is copiously irrigated with antibiotic solution. The drain is brought out through a puncture in the posterior, non-elevated flap. Care should be exercised not to traumatize the temporal vessels during placement of the drain. Both open techniques are closed in a two-layer fashion.

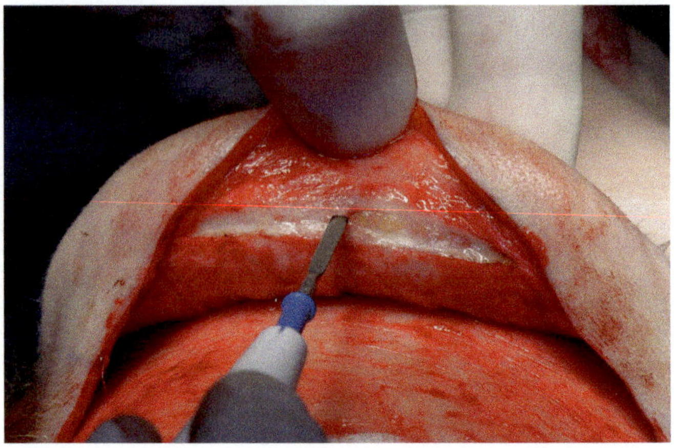

Fig. 6.16 The frontalis is scored horizontally at the foremost forehead rhytid in most cases

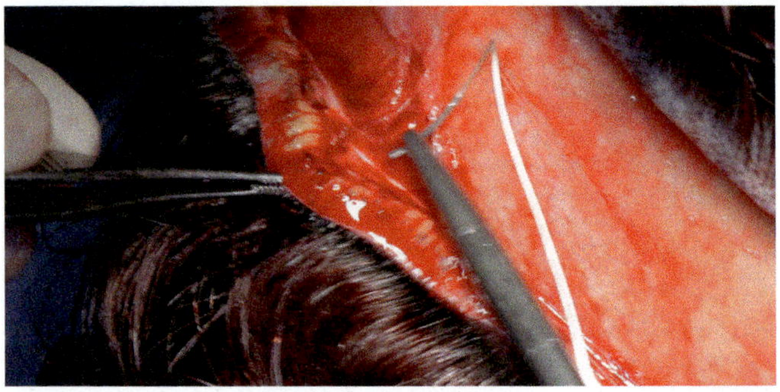

Fig. 6.17 The galeal closure is performed with buried, absorbable suture with the coronal technique

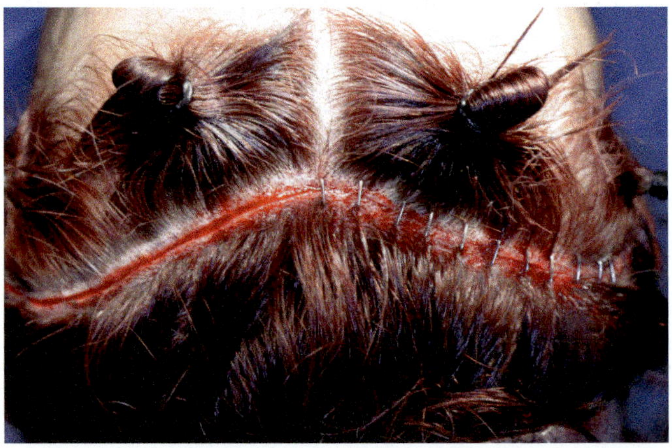

Fig. 6.18 The coronal closure is complete with staples at the skin level. Please note the hair-to-hair apposition, a frequently misunderstood concept with this technique

For the coronal incision, a galeal closure is performed with interrupted 2–0 Dexon suture (Fig. 6.17). This is followed by skin closure with wide staples (Fig. 6.18). The pretricheal lift closure is more detailed. The deep layer closure is with 4–0 Maxon suture (Fig. 6.19). These deep sutures

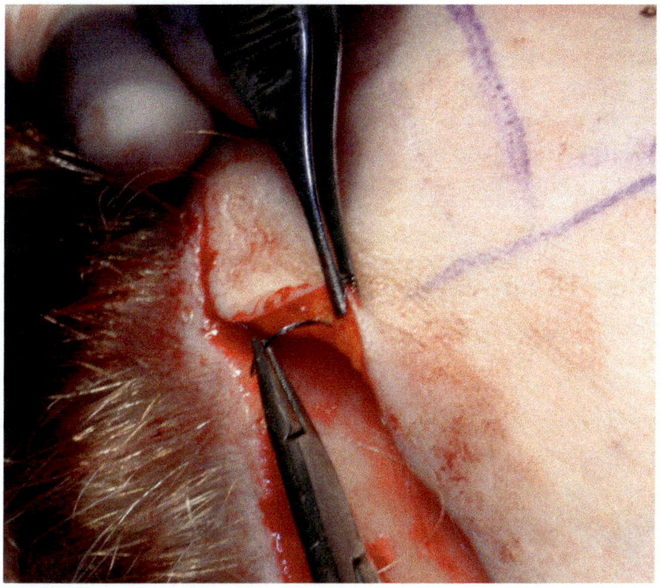

Fig. 6.19 The trichophytic closure is begun with buried, absorbable sutures at the galeal level

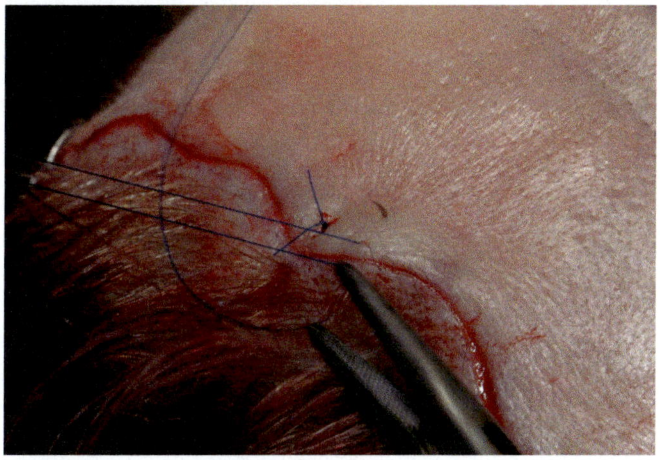

Fig. 6.20 The skin closure is accomplished with vertical mattress sutures. We prefer nonabsorbable suture at the skin level to minimize the inflammatory response

will cause a dimpling of the tissue immediately inferior to the incision in the midline. The patient should be informed preoperatively that this will resolve when the sutures dissolve. The skin in the visible region of the incision is then closed with interrupted 5–0 Prolene suture in a vertical mattress fashion (Fig. 6.20). Skin eversion is vital and must be attained with these sutures. The vertical mattress suture line is further enhanced with the use of a running, locking 6–0 Nylon to maximize the wound approximation (Fig. 6.21). The hair bearing areas are closed with larger staples on the lateral components and smaller staples in the medial aspect of the incision (Fig. 6.22). Though time consuming, this elaborate closure greatly enhances the patient's wound

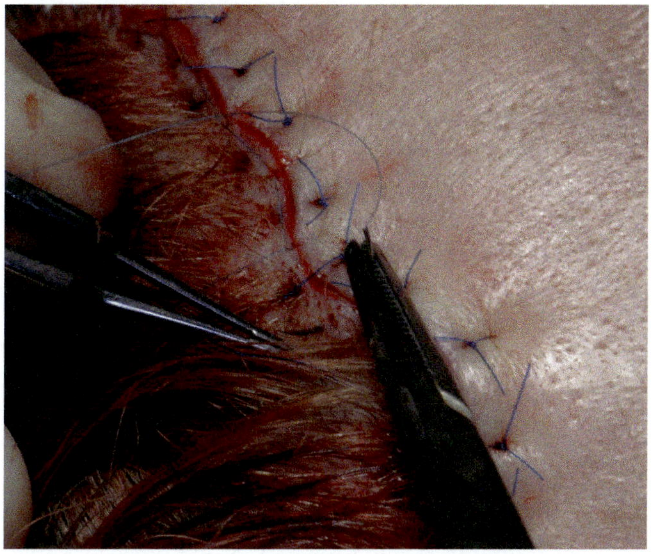

Fig. 6.21 A running, locking 6–0 nonabsorbable suture is used to maximize wound closure and thus, the postoperative result

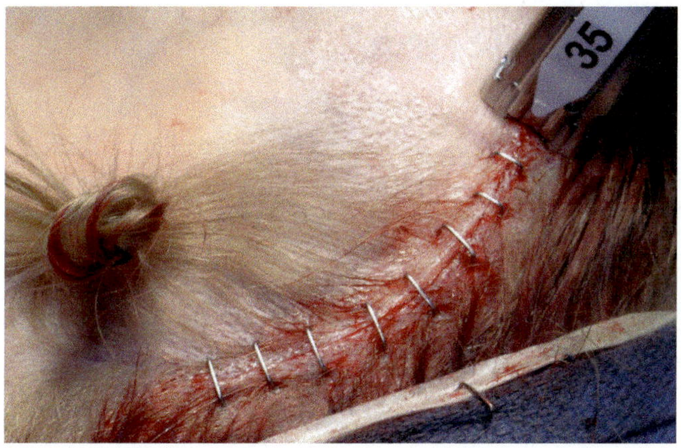

Fig. 6.22 The lateral portions of the trichophytic incision are closed with large staples laterally and smaller ones medially

healing. The wound is then coated with antibiotic ointment and a nonadhesive telfa is placed over the incision. A light compressive dressing is then applied.

6.6 Postoperative Care

The drain is often removed in the recovery room on the evening of the procedure to decrease the headache and nausea that often accompanies drains in this area.

The dressing is removed on postoperative day 1 and no further dressing is necessary. The patient may immediately begin using hydrogen peroxide to keep the incision free of crusts. Showering with baby shampoo is allowed 48 h after the procedure. The sutures for the pretricheal lift are removed on postoperative day 3–5 depending on the nature of the healing and logistics of removing sutures from other surgical procedures that may have been performed. The staples are removed at 1 week postoperatively. The pretricheal incision is immediately taped in the non-hair bearing area after application of adhesive. The tape is worn continuously for 1 week after the removal of the sutures. After this point, the tape is kept every night for approximately 1 month. The tape minimizes tension on the skin encouraging excellent camouflage of the wound. In the coronal approach, all staples are removed 1 week postoperatively.

The patient is advised that the edema in the forehead will be most significant 2–3 days after the procedure. This edema can be quite uncomfortable for the patient. The patients are advised that this will gradually resolve and they may commence strenuous activity 3–4 weeks after the procedure. They are also advised to avoid using a curling iron or a blow-dryer on a hot setting in the first 6 weeks of the procedure since they may have poor sensory perception during this period. This paresthesia is rarely an issue in the author's practice.

6.7 Complications

Despite the recent advances of endoscopic techniques, the open brow lifting method remains an excellent option for brow rejuvenation as it leads to excellent surgical outcomes and high patient acceptance. The complication profile for the open brow lift is excellent with a 0.4% incidence of hematoma formation, permanent alopecia, and "nerve damage" [37]. Others have found similar complication rates.

I have rarely encountered hematomas after surgery. They are treated as with hematomas elsewhere on the face with drainage, or rarely reexploration. The most common and troubling complication I see after open brow lifting is paresthesia. The patient must be aware, preoperatively, that the forehead and scalp will be numb for several months, and possibly permanently. When discussed extensively in the preoperative phase this issue is managed adequately and usually resolves in the appropriate time period. Scarring can occur after surgery but its incidence is greatly reduced with appropriate surgical technique. When it does occur it can be managed with steroid injections. Alopecia is directly related to incision technique, tension on wound closure, tissue trauma, and overzealous use of cautery. Its occurrence cannot be eliminated, but certainly reduced, with adhering to sound surgical principals. In my practice, as well as those of other highly experienced surgeons, alopecia, numbness, and scarring have been of limited impact [36, 38, 39].

A very troublesome complication from surgery is the creation of a "surprised look," evidenced by a widened, elevated medial brow complex [1]. This is minimized by judicious removal of tissue and an appropriate resection of the glabellar musculature.

An occasional issue that arises postoperatively is pruritus along the incision line. If the patient aggressively scratches and rubs this area, focal alopecia may develop. This can be avoided with patient education. If the alopecia has already occurred, the patient is advised not to disturb the area further and the hair often returns.

6.8 Conclusion

The open brow lift remains as the standard by which brow rejuvenation techniques are measured. All surgeons should be familiar with, and competent in utilizing these procedures as they may be the only option for certain patients. With adequate experience, the open brow lift approach can be performed with limited morbidity and high patient satisfaction.

References

1. Lexer E. Zur Geischsplastik. Arch Klin Chur. 1910;92:749.
2. Passot R. La Churugie Esthetique des Rides du Visage. Presse Méd. 1919;27:258.
3. Hunt HL. Plastic surgery of the head, face and neck. Philadelphia: Lea & Febiger; 1926.
4. Noel A. La Chirurgie Esthetique et son Role Socia. Paris: Masson; 1926.
5. Joseph J. Nasenplastik und Sonstige Gesichtplastik Nebst Einen Anhang Uber Mammaplastik. Leipzig: Kabitzch; 1931.
6. Paul M. The evolution of the brow lifting. Aesthetic plastic surgery. Plast Reconstr Surg. 2001;108:1409.
7. Brennan GH. The forehead lift. Otolaryngol Clin North Am. 1980;13:209.
8. Connell BF. Eyebrow, face and necklifts for males. Clin Plast Surg. 1978;5:15.
9. Kaye BL. The forehead lift: a useful adjunct to facelift and blepharoplasty. Plast Reconstr Surg. 1977;60:161.
10. Core GB, Vasconez LO, Askren C, et al. Coronal facelift with endoscopic techniques. Plast Surg Forum. 1992;15:227.
11. Liang M, Narayanan K. Endoscopic ablation of the frontalis and corrugator muscles: a clinical study. Plast Surg Forum. 1992;15:58.
12. Vasconez LO, Gore GB, Gamboa-Bodadilla M, et al. Endoscopic techniques in coronal brow lifting. Plast Reconstr Surg. 1994; 94:788.
13. Isse NG. Endoscopic facial rejuvenation. Endoforehead, the functional lift: case reports. Aesthet Plast Surg. 1994;18:21.
14. Ramirez OM. Endoscopic techniques in facial rejuvenation. An overview: part I. Aesthet Plast Surg. 1994;18:141.
15. Wojtanowski MH. Bicoronal forehead lift. Aesthet Plast Surg. 1994;18:33.
16. Yarenchuk MJ. Subperiosteal and full-thickness skin rhytidectomy. Plast Reconstr Surg. 2001;107:1045.
17. Hamra ST. A study of the long-term effect of malar fat repositioning in face lift surgery: short term success but long-term failure. Plast Reconstr Surg. 2002;110:940.
18. Elkwood A, Matarasso A, Rankin M, et al. National plastic surgery survey: brow lifting techniques and complications. Plast Reconstr Surg. 2001;108:2143.
19. Godek CP, Buckey LP, Whitaker LA. Endoscopic versus open coronal forehead surgery: surgeon preference and patient satisfaction. Plast Surg Forum. 1999;22:182.

20. Koch RJ. Endoscopic browlift is the preferred approach for rejuvenation of the upper third of the face. Arch Otolaryngol Head Neck Surg. 2001;127:87.
21. Guyuron B, Behmand RA, Green R. Shortening of the long forehead. Plast Reconstr Surg. 1999;103:218.
22. Marten TJ. Hairline lowering during foreheadplasty. Plast Reconstr Surg. 1999;103:224.
23. Michelow BJ, Guyuron B. Rejuvenation of the upper face: a logical gamut of surgical options. Clin Plast Surg. 1997;24:199.
24. McKinney P, Mossie RD, Zukowski ML. Criteria for the forehead lift. Aesthet Plast Surg. 1991;15:141.
25. Knize D. An anatomically based study of the mechanism of eyebrow ptosis. Plast Reconstr Surg. 1996;97:1321.
26. Knize D. Limited-incision forehead lift for eyebrow elevation to enhance upper blepharoplasty. Plast Reconstr Surg. 1996; 97:1334.
27. Romo III T, Jacono AA, Sclafani AP. Endoscopic forehead lifting and contouring. Facial Plast Surg. 2001;17:4.
28. Knize DM. A study of the supraorbital nerve. Plast Reconstr Surg. 1995;96:564.
29. Gunter J, Antrobus SD. Aesthetic analysis of the eyebrows. Plast Reconstr Surg. 1997;99:1808.
30. Whitaker LA, Morales Jr L, Farkas LG. Aesthetic surgery of the supraorbital ridge and forehead structure. Plast Reconstr Surg. 1986;78:23.
31. Cook TA, Brownrigg AJ, Wang TD, et al. The versatile midforehead browlift. Arch Otolaryngol Head Neck Surg. 1989;115:163.
32. Matarasso A, Terino EO. Forehead-brow rhytidoplasty: reassessing the goals. Plast Reconstr Surg. 1994;93:1378.
33. Freund RM, Nolan III B. Correlation between brow lift outcomes and aesthetic ideals for eyebrow height and shape in females. Plast Reconstr Surg. 1996;97:1343.
34. Ellenbogen R. Transcoronal eyebrow lift with concomitant upper blepharoplasty. Plast Reconstr Surg. 1983;71:490.
35. Roth JM, Metzinger SE. Quantifying the arch position of the female eyebrow. Arch Facial Plast Surg. 2003;5:235.
36. Adamson PA, Johnson CM, Anderson JR, Dupin CL. The forehead lift: a review. Arch Otolaryngol Head Neck Surg. 1985;111:325.
37. Vinas JC, Caviglia C, Cortinas JL. Forehead rhytidoplasty and brow lifting. Plast Reconstr Surg. 1976;57:445.
38. Adamson PA, Cormier R, McGraw BL. The coronal forehead lift: modifications and results. J Otolaryngol. 1992;21:1.
39. Kerth JD, Torimui DM. Management of the aging forehead. Arch Otolaryngol Head Neck Surg. 1990;116:1137.

7 Endoscopic Brow and Forehead Rejuvenation

Christian L. Stallworth and Tom D. Wang

Key Points

- The forehead and brows are an integral part of aesthetic rejuvenation of the upper face.
- Traditional brow lifting procedures involve large dissections, predispose to sensory deficits, and can lead to visible scars.
- The endoscopic brow lift offers a less invasive alternative to open brow lifting procedures.
- With appropriate training and experience, the procedure results in reliable and reproducible surgical outcomes.
- A detailed knowledge of relevant anatomy, especially the temporal dissection, is critical to avoiding complications.
- Surgical success is dependent on appropriate patient selection, familiarity with endoscopic equipment and techniques, and an understanding of forehead/brow aesthetics.
- The main variable in surgery is the method of brow fixation to the calvarium. The authors prefer the bone bridge technique.
- The endoscopic approach to brow lifting reduces the likelihood of complications when compared to open approaches.
- Complications such as hematoma formation, alopecia, and sensory or motor nerve deficit can be avoided with strict maintenance of hemostasis and meticulous surgical dissection.

7.1 Introduction

The gamut of human emotions, whether joy, surprise, anger, or grief, is written in our eyes. With age, that expression may be misconstrued. The aged brow, with its prominent rhytids, lateral hooding, and lid redundancy, tends to convey fatigue, anger, suspicion, or disinterest – all despite the fact that the person may not truly harbor any of these sentiments. In this way, our expression is no longer a reflection of our true emotion. The result is an adverse effect on communications, personal interactions, and self-image.

The weight of these factors was the impetus for development of brow rejuvenation techniques over the last century [1]. Starting with direct and mid-forehead techniques in the early 1900, forehead and brow rejuvenation evolved to include the traditional coronal approach. The latter is still viewed by some to be the gold standard [2, 3]. For many surgeons and their patients however, the disadvantages outweigh the potential gains from all three. The mid-forehead and direct brow approaches invariably result in visible, and sometimes detracting, scarring. The coronal lift requires greater dissection, has an increased risk of hematoma formation, and may cause alopecia or elevate the hairline. The trichial and pretrichial modifications of the coronal approach have been used as alternatives, but still carry many of the same potential risks. And this says nothing of the fact that all three carry varied risks of interrupted forehead or scalp sensation.

These are but a few of the reasons many surgeons worked to incorporate endoscopic techniques into their armamentarium once technology, cost, and their skill set permitted. First reported by Isse in 1992, the endoscopic brow lift has since gained wide acceptance, having proven to provide lasting cosmetic results [4]. Now, the greatest variability among surgeons appears to lie with the method used for brow fixation. Here, we present our technique for endoscopic brow rejuvenation with emphasis placed on salient points that have helped the senior author's (TDW) results reproducibly stand the test of time.

7.2 Forehead and Temporal Anatomy

The goals of endoscopic lifting are to provide reproducible and lasting restoration of the brow but to do so while concealing scars, preserving forehead and scalp sensation,

T.D. Wang (✉)
Professor and Chief, Division of Facial Plastic and Reconstructive Surgery, Department of Otolaryngology – Head and Neck Surgery, Oregon Health and Science University, Portland, OR, USA
e-mail: wangt@ohsu.edu

G.G. Massry et al. (eds.), *Master Techniques in Blepharoplasty and Periorbital Rejuvenation*, DOI 10.1007/978-1-4614-0067-7_7, © Springer Science+Business Media, LLC 2011

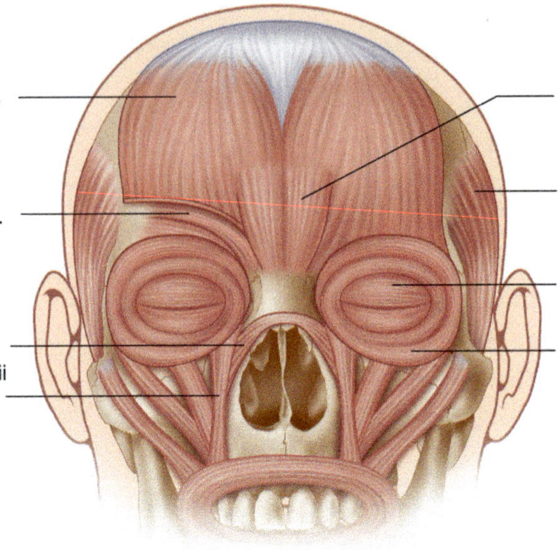

Fig. 7.1 Brow musculature. Contraction of the primary brow elevator, the frontalis muscle, causes formation of prominent horizontal rhytids. The depressors include the procerus muscle, the corrugator supercilii muscle, and the orbicularis oculi muscle. The procerus' action results in horizontal glabellar rhytids, and the corrugator in vertical medial brow rhytids

maintaining facial nerve function, and minimizing the potential complications found in each of the other operations. Meeting these objectives helps to set this technique apart from the other approaches. A detailed understanding of the associated anatomy is necessary to achieve these goals [5].

The brow and forehead fall within the superior horizontal third of the face and are delineated by the area lying between the trichion and the supraorbital rim. The organization of skin and soft tissue here is identical to that found in the scalp. The superficial skin overlies an underlying layer of subcutaneous tissue, which then rests upon the galea aponeurotica. The galea is a broad tendinous sheet that spans the scalp and connects the frontalis with the occipitalis posteriorly. Loose areolar connective tissue separates the galea from the deepest layer, the pericranium, which then densely adheres to the skull.

The brow musculature can be divided into those that elevate and those that depress the brow (Fig. 7.1). Each independently contributes to the formation of rhytids perpendicular to their respective vector of contraction. The frontalis muscle is the primary brow elevator and is responsible for deep, prominent horizontal rhytids. Originating from the galea, it descents the forehead with insertions into the dermis. Brow depressors include the procerus muscle, the corrugator supercilii muscle, and the orbicularis oculi muscle. The procerus originates from the nasal bones and cephalic margin of the upper lateral cartilages. It ascends the nasal dorsum spanning across the radix to insert into the caudal frontalis muscle from below. The procerus' contraction depresses the glabella, yielding finer horizontal rhytids in this area. The corrugators are responsible for drawing the brow medially and inferiorly. They originate from the nasal process of the frontal bone and extend obliquely over the supraorbital rim where they interdigitate with fibers from the frontalis and orbicularis. When contracted, they cause vertical, paraglabellar furrows. Finally, the orbicularis oculi serves as the palpebral sphincter, and with contraction, will depress the brow along with closure of the upper lid. This is a minor depressor mechanism, but cannot be forgotten [5–7].

The temporal branch of the facial nerve provides voluntary and involuntary motor innervation to the brow musculature and the superior divisions of the orbicularis oculi muscle. Upon leaving the substance of the parotid gland, the nerve passes deep to the superficial aponeurotic muscular system (SMAS) and then passes over the middle third of the zygomatic arch in a plane between the SMAS and the zygomatic periosteum. Above the arch, the nerve continues its course within the substance of the temporoparietal fascia (TPF) before entering its respective musculature on the deep undersurface. The nerve enters the undersurface into the frontalis approximately 1 cm above the supraorbital rim [8]. A line drawn between a point 0.5 cm anterior to the tragus and a point 1.5 cm lateral to the taper of the lateral brow approximates the course of the nerve. This line typically crosses the middle third of the zygomatic arch, or "danger zone" for the nerve [5]. Here, the nerve is confined within tightly adherent tissue planes that are relatively immobile leaving the nerve prone to injury.

Sensation of the forehead, brow, and upper lids is conveyed via afferent branches of the ophthalmic division of the trigeminal nerve. The lacrimal nerve innervates the lateral upper lid and brow. The supraorbital and supratrochlear nerves both branch from the frontal nerve to provide afferent innervation to the remaining upper lid, forehead, and scalp. These nerves leave their respective supraorbital notches and pass through the periosteum where they then course in a supramuscular plane along the superficial surface of the frontalis muscle. Knowledge of this plane is critical to the understanding of postoperative brow, forehead, and scalp sensation following any of the brow rejuvenating techniques.

The forehead and brow tissues receive their blood supply from both the external and internal carotid systems. The external carotid artery terminally branches into the superficial temporal artery, and its arborization supplies the temple and lateral forehead. A primary branch responsible for the lateral brow is the zygomaticotemporal artery. The internal carotid artery terminally branches into the ophthalmic artery. Its distal branches, the supraorbital and supratrochlear arteries, supply the medial and central forehead and anterior scalp. Cadaveric studies have found the supraorbital and supratrochlear arteries reliably located approximately 2.5 and 1.8 cm, respectively, lateral to the midline [9].

Venous drainage mirrors the arterial supply. One specific vessel, the zygomaticotemporal vein receives branches that span the potential space between the superficial temporoparietal fascia (STPF) and the deep temporal fascia (DTF). A prominent branch encountered during the endoscopic approach is commonly referred to as the *sentinel vein* because of its apparent proximity to the temporal branch of the facial nerve. Identified within temporal fat at the approximate level of the frontozygomatic suture, Quatela and colleagues found this vessel to consistently lie within 2 mm of the temporal branch of the facial nerve. In addition, they demonstrated that when *multiple* temporal vessels are seen endoscopically, *each* is associated with one of several temporal motor branches that appear to traverse the superficial fascia immediately above the vein [10]. Thus, cautery and manipulation of these vessels should be done along the dissection floor, directly on top of the DTF to prevent nerve injury.

Lastly, but arguably most important is an understanding of the fascial planes and compartments in the forehead, brow, and temple (Fig. 7.2). The superficial musculoaponeurotic system (SMAS) that envelops the musculature of the lower and middle thirds of the face extends above the zygomatic arch as the superficial TPF. The TPF then merges with the galeal layer in the brow and scalp. Below the TPF lies the DTF. Superficial and deep layers of the DTF envelop the temporalis muscle, and an intermediate layer helps to partition the temporal fat pad above the zygomatic arch. Superiorly, the deep and superficial layers of the DTF fuse with the frontoparietal periosteum at the origin of the temporalis muscle. This delineates the temporal line. Anterior, the DTF becomes densely adherent to the frontal and zygomatic periosteum at the lateral orbital rim and along the medial zygomatic arch. The lateral margin of the galea joins here as well, forming the conjoined tendon. Along the supraorbital rim, the fusion of the galea and frontal periosteum creates the arcus marginalis, an anchor for the brow that impedes brow elevation [8, 11]. As we shall discuss, an understanding of these layers is key to operative success and safety.

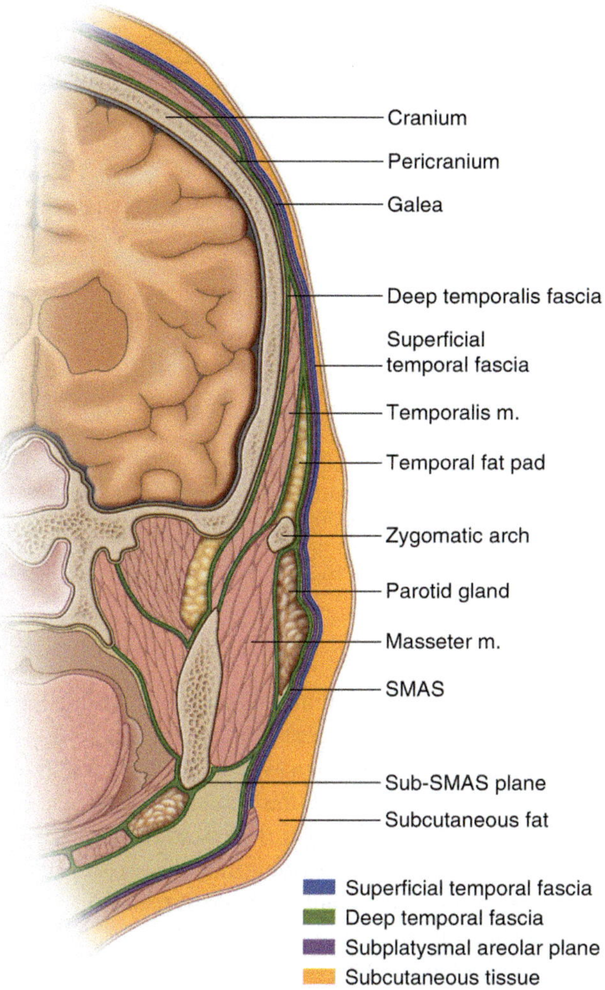

Fig. 7.2 Fascial planes. The superficial musculoaponeurotic system (SMAS) of the lower and mid-face is contiguous with the superficial TPF above the zygomatic arch. The temporal branch of the facial nerve runs within the substance of the TPF. The TPF merges with the galeal layer in the brow and scalp. The deep temporal fascia (DTF) lies below the TPF. Superficial and deep layers of the DTF envelop the temporalis muscle, and an intermediate layer helps to partition the temporal fat pad above the zygomatic arch. The temporal line represents the fusion of the deep and superficial layers of the DTF with the frontoparietal periosteum at the origin of the temporalis muscle

7.3 Aesthetics and Aging

The shape and position of the eyebrow itself is key for brow aesthetics. Medially, the brow should be clubbed and rounded, and approximate a line drawn vertically tangent to the nasal ala. The brow should then arch superolaterally with its apex at the level of, or just lateral to, the lateral limbus. The brow should taper and end at an oblique line drawn from the nasal ala through the lateral canthus. In general, the youthful brow is positioned higher over a well-demarcated supraorbital rim. The supratarsal crease should also be visible. In the female patient, the brow should be arched and

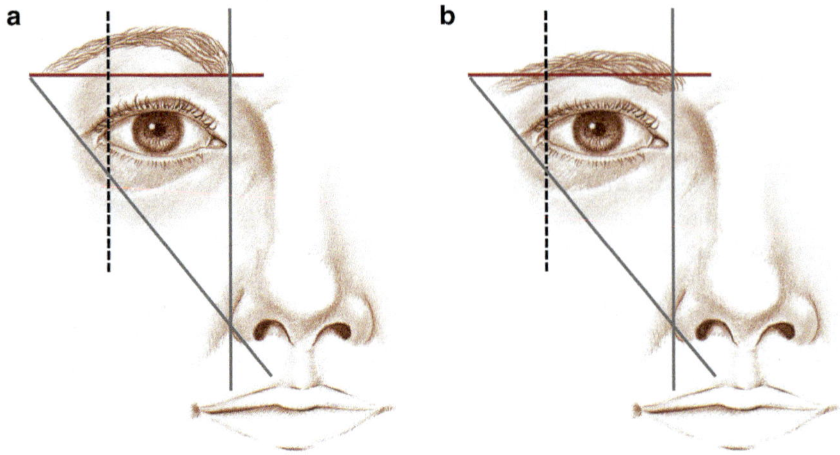

Fig. 7.3 Ideal brow position. (**a**) In the female patient, the brow should reside above the supraorbital rim and arch between the lateral limbus and lateral canthus. (**b**) The male brow should be less arched and lie at the level of the supraorbital rim. Medially, both brows should be clubbed and rounded, and in an approximate line drawn vertically tangent to the nasal ala. The brow should then arch superolaterally with its apex at the level of, or just lateral to, the lateral limbus. The brow should taper and end at an oblique line drawn from the nasal ala through the lateral canthus

reside above the supraorbital rim. Male patients, on the other hand, have more prominent frontal bossing. Their brow shape should be less arched and lie at the level of the supraorbital rim (Fig. 7.3). At rest, the youthful forehead is smooth without horizontal or vertical rhytids, and has a gentle convexity [5, 12, 13]. Aging is a multifactorial process that leads to deterioration of the youthful brow over time.

Aging results from the cumulative effects of both internal and external factors. Our skin inherently loses elasticity and there is regression of buoyant subcutaneous tissue as we grow older. Bone remodeling results in contour changes and an overall increase in bone resorption. Together, these processes contribute to tissue deflation and laxity. Other internal influences include genetics, gender, and skin type. External factors including gravity, ultraviolet light exposure, diet, sleep habits, unique personal facial expression, and smoking further compound these factors [13].

Brow aging typically progresses from lateral to medial, starting first in the lateral third of the brow. Ptosis initially manifests as lateral brow hooding, but as aging migrates medially, the brow, glabella, and forehead fall victim to deteriorating aesthetics as well. Early on, evolving tissue ptosis is countered by compensatory muscular contraction of the brow elevators. However, with subcutaneous tissue loss and progressive elastosis, pleating of the underlying muscles and fascia leads to wrinkle formation. The aged brow, with its prominent rhytids, lateral hooding, and lid redundancy, then conveys fatigue, anger, suspicion, or disinterest. In addition, the combination of brow ptosis in conjunction with frontal and temporal hairline recession leads to an increase of the vertical height of the upper facial third. This also detracts from overall facial harmony.

7.4 Patient Selection

As with any cosmetic procedure, patient selection and identification of the appropriate indications for a given technique are keys to surgical success and patient satisfaction. Endoscopic lifting of the brow is no different.

The preoperative assessment begins with an understanding of a patient's concerns, preferences, and expectations. It should also include an extensive critical facial analysis and exam [8, 11]. Skin type and evidence of photo aging are documented using the Fitzpatrick and Glogau classifications, respectively. This should include not only the extent but also the orientation of rhytids present. Attention is paid to evaluation of brow ptosis, differentiating between true brow ptosis and hooding that results from upper lid skin redundancy. Dynamic and static asymmetries should be noted in order to avoid the alteration of dynamic asymmetries that come from an individual's unique facial expressions. The position and shape of the hairline must be documented, along with a history and exam for the presence of balding. And bony contours are assessed, noting any prominent frontal bossing or convexity that may impede visualization and dissection through the endoscopic approach. Additionally, a thorough past medical and family history is taken, specifically looking for a history of dry eyes, previous blepharoplasty, androgenic hair loss, and alopecia [6]. Finally, preoperative photographs are taken. This assessment is crucial because it will influence the ultimate surgical approach and help predict surgical outcome and overall patient satisfaction.

In general, patients with brow ptosis, lateral brow and eyelid hooding, forehead or glabellar rhytids, and/or visual field deficits that result from these meet criteria for brow and/or periocular rejuvenation. The "ideal" patient for the application of the endoscopic technique is a Caucasian patient with medium to thin skin thickness, glabellar rhytids, minimal brow ptosis, and minimal skin redundancy. At the same time, relative contraindications exist for women with high hairlines and men with male pattern baldness, patients with thick, densely adherent skin, and patients with extensive bone attachments and protuberances [6, 8, 11]. Blepharoplasty is not a topic addressed in this discussion, but it should be noted that determination of the need for concomitant eyelid or ptosis surgery is necessary prior to brow rejuvenation. If needed, lid skin excision should follow after elevation and fixation of the brow to avoid untoward postoperative lagophthalmos.

The prospective benefits of the endoscopic technique include the use of smaller incisions with subsequently less scarring, decreased risk of sensory neuropathy, decreased risk of alopecia, less bleeding, and reportedly decreased recuperative time. On the other hand, the use of this approach requires more specialized training, a steeper learning curve, and costly operative equipment. It also does not permit the excision of brow or scalp skin redundancy, and may be limited by any of the less than ideal patient characteristics previously mentioned.

7.5 Instrumentation

The senior author prefers endoscopic browlift instruments by Snowden Pencer® (Table 7.1) and:

- Endoscopy tower with telescopic input and video display
- Storz Hopkins® II 30° Telescope, 7228 BA (Karl Storz Endoscopy-America, Inc., El Segundo, CA, USA)
- Synthes drill bit 1.5×4 mm with stop (Synthes, Inc., West Chester, PA, USA; http://us.synthes.com)
- Stryker TPS (Total Performance System) Drill (Stryker Craniomaxillofacial, Portage, MI, USA)

Table 7.1 Endoscopic browlift instruments by Snowden Pencer®

Catalog No.	Manufacturer	Manufacturer's description
88–5086	Snowden-Pencer®	Ramirez EndoForehead Curved Dissector
88–5080	Snowden-Pencer®	Ramirez EndoForehead Spreader
88–5084	Snowden-Pencer®	Ramirez EndoForehead Parietal Elevator
88–5076	Snowden-Pencer®	Midface Fascia Dissector
88–5077	Snowden-Pencer®	Ramirez EndoForehead T Dissector
88–5075	Snowden-Pencer®	Ramirez EndoForehead Dissector
88–5081	Snowden-Pencer®	Ramirez EndoForehead A/M Dissector
88–5052	Snowden-Pencer®	Daniel EndoForehead Nerve Dissector

Distributed by CareFusion (San Diego, CA, USA and http://www.cardinal.com/legacy/vmueller/vmcatalog/vmueller.html)

7.5.1 Technique

Once the patient is secure in the operating room with the desired level of anesthesia induced, the head of the bed is turned away from anesthesia. This permits positioning of the endoscopic tower at the foot of the table where it lies in direct line of sight to the operating surgeon at the head of the bed. The plane of the bed is then placed in 5–10° of reverse Trendelenburg or a beach chair configuration to maintain slight elevation of the head.

First, a topographical line predicting the course of the facial nerve is drawn as a point of reference. Then, five access incisions, none greater than 2 cm in length, are marked for creation of the optical pockets. The midline incision is drawn approximately 1.5 cm posterior to the hairline and oriented in the coronal plane, paralleling the anterior hairline. Two lateral incisions are placed just medial to the temporal line approximating both the position of anticipated greatest brow height and the vector of brow suspension. These lay equidistance from the hairline, but are drawn in a sagittal plane. Finally, right and left temporal access incisions are drawn in the temporal hair tuft. These are drawn in the coronal plane and approximate the vertical level of the lateral canthus. These typically are 2–3 cm behind the anterior hairline and should be well behind the previously drawn anticipated course of the facial nerve. Hair is then parted at each of the planned incisions and secured in small, twisted tufts using dental elastic rubber bands (Fig. 7.4).

Next, each incision and the brow is injected with the authors' preferred local anesthetic mixture consisting of a 50:50 blend of 1% lidocaine, 0.5% bupivacaine, and epinephrine in a 1:100,000 concentration. Care is taken to inject precisely within the anticipated plane of dissection. Each access point is injected in the subcutaneous plane with approximately 0.5 cc of local anesthetic. The forehead is then injected in a ring-block fashion in the subgaleal or subperiosteal plane, injecting the inferior margins of dissection across the supraorbital rim, medially over the glabella, the lateral orbital rim at the conjoined tendon, laterally along each temporal line, and superiorly along the hairline. The patient is then prepped and draped in the standard sterile fashion.

At the start of the case, the forehead and brow are first examined and manipulated. An attempt is made to manually elevate the brow to demonstrate its ideal position and arching shape. In doing so, it is easy to appreciate the anatomic

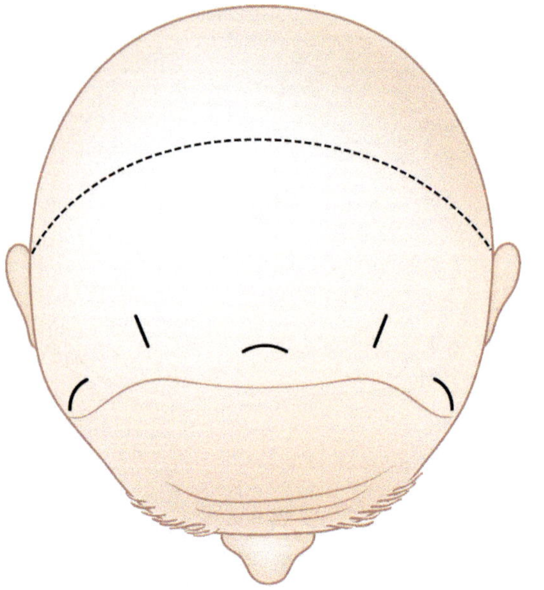

Fig. 7.4 Endoscopic access incisions. Five access incisions, none greater than 2 cm in length, are used to create optical pockets needed for elevation and suspension. These include a midline incision approximately 1.5 cm posterior to the hairline and oriented in the coronal plane, two lateral incisions in a sagittal plane medial to the temporal line approximating the desired position of greatest brow height and the vector of brow suspension, and bilateral temporal incisions in the temporal hair tufts. The latter are drawn in the coronal plane and approximate the vertical level of the lateral canthus

separation between the brow and upper lids due to fixation of the arcus marginalis. With elevation of the brow, the lids will remain in repose. This provides a reference point for adequate arcus release later in the case.

Starting with the left temporal access point and continuing to the right, all five points are incised using a No. 15 blade. Each incision is superficial and deep enough to only break through the dermis. Then, with the aid of an assistant, narrow, double skin hooks are used to retract the incision margins to reveal the underlying subcutaneous tissue and hair follicles. Blunt scissors are then spread perpendicular to the long axis of the wound to gently separate the underlying fascial attachments. To avoid injury to adjacent hair follicles, distinct bleeding vessels are judiciously cauterized only when necessary. Similarly, dissection within the temporal tuft proceeds cautiously to avoid injury to the superficial temporal vessels. Dissection in the three central access points is carried down to the pericranium, which is then incised with electrocautery. Dissection in the lateral temporal incisions is taken to the level of the superficial layer of the DTF.

Elevation of the optical pockets begins first at the midline incision and progresses from territory known to unknown. Using the nondominant hand to stabilize the head at nasal root, a curved periosteal elevator is used to elevate the midline and superior forehead pericranium. This subperiosteal pocket is extended laterally to, but not through, the temporal line using the temporoparietal access points. If the temporal line were violated from the medial pocket, the dissection plane would become uncertain. Initially, the caudal extent of the dissection is limited due to the curvature of the skull. This can be overcome using instruments with progressively greater angulation. However, the surgeon will find that the farther posterior the incisions are placed, the greater the restriction in caudal dissection. Direct visualization is not used at this point. Rather, the surgeon relies on tactile and auditory feedback to ensure dissection immediately on top of bone. The inferior extent of the dissection ceases once elevation progress to the arcus marginalis and the conjoined tendon. In addition, palpating the supraorbital notch provides the mind's eye with the anticipated location of the sensory nerves. Dissection within a 1 cm radius about this point is avoided as well.

Next, the temporal optical pockets are generated using the temporal tuft incisions, starting again on the left side of the patient. Using the spatula-shaped "T-Dissector," the STPF is swept from the underlying DTF. This delineates the floor of the pocket. The elevator is used as a fulcrum to *lift* the STPF from the underlying DTF and then slowly advanced in a path aiming for the ipsilateral temporoparietal incision. The elevator is never blindly advanced, ensuring that it never violate an adjacent and inappropriate fascial plane. Once the pocket becomes constrained at the temporal line, the elevator is advanced through the temporal line, into the subperiosteal pocket, and visualized through the temporoparietal incision. The elevator is then withdrawn and replaced, again ensuring dissection directly on the floor of the pocket. Dissection then progresses along a new radius slightly inferior to the previous plane, the temporal line is again encountered, and the elevator advances through the line into the subperiosteal pocket. This method is continued until the entire pocket is open from an inferior margin that approximates the lateral canthal height, and medial to the zygomaticofrontal buttress and the conjoined tendon. The temporal line now contains postage stamp breaks that can now be connected by sweeping the elevator superiorly and inferiorly. In this way, both optical pockets are connected, while at the same time preserving the temporal branch of the facial nerve within the fascia superficial to the pocket. An identical method is used then to open the temporal pocket on the right.

Once each temporal compartment is connected to the central subperiosteal dissection, release of the arcus and conjoined tendon may commence. First, the lateral brow is palpated with the nondominant hand and an elevator is used to free the arcus and conjoined tendon from the superior outer orbital rim. The surgeon realizes the appropriate plane when

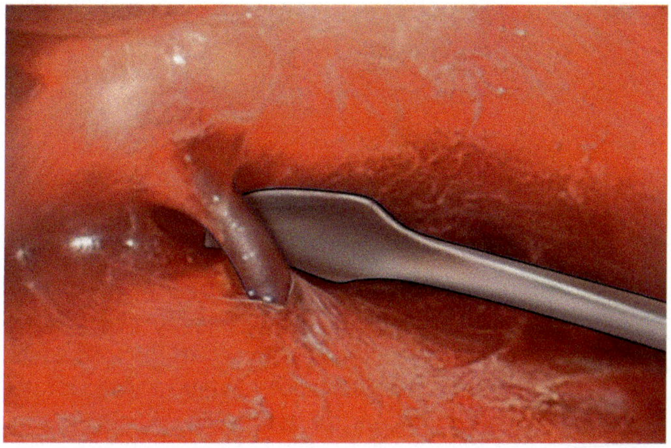

Fig. 7.5 Identification of the sentinel vein. Following release of the arcus and conjoined tendon, the sheathed 30° endoscope and dissector are inserted via adjacent temporal and temporoparietal incisions, respectively. Remaining attachments are visualized and released, elevating the TPF laterally to identify the sentinel vein. Here, the dissector is shown carefully freeing associated fascial bands without injury to the vein itself

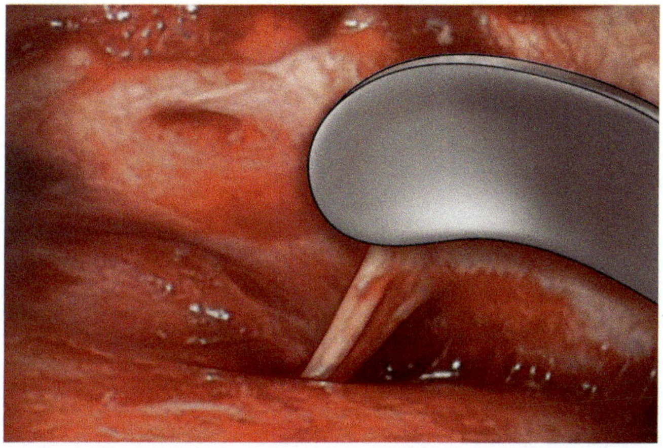

Fig. 7.6 Arcus marginalis release. Here, the arcus marginalis is shown elevated above the supraorbital rim as a back elevator demonstrates the more medial supraorbital neurovascular bundle. Retroorbicularis oculi fat (ROOF) is seen inferior to the arcus line, denoting adequate elevation is complete

the elevator leaves the thicker, denser brow tissue and is appreciated beneath the thinner soft tissue of the upper lid. Next, the sheathed 30° endoscope is inserted into the left temporal optical pocket and a dissector introduced via the adjacent temporoparietal incision. Under direct visualization, the remnants of the broken temporal line and conjoined tendon are examined. Remaining attachments are freed, sweeping and elevating the overlying scalp from superior to inferior. As this tissue is elevated laterally, the surgeon should work to identify the sentinel vein. Care is taken to preserve this vessel in order to prevent surrounding postoperative venous engorgement that may lead to visible temporal varicosities. However, an attempt is also made to free any associated dense fascial bands that may hinder adequate release and elevation. Once the level of the lateral canthus is reached, within approximately one fingerbreadth of the zygomatic arch, the dissection is complete (Fig. 7.5).

The arcus marginalis is viewed as a condensed fascial line that parallels the orbital bony contour. With elevation, underlying retroorbicularis oculi fat (ROOF) is seen inferior to this well-demarcated line. More aggressive release is required at this point to ensure significant brow elevation. A back-elevator is useful here to draw the arcus up and onto the supraorbital rim. Continuing with the dissection from lateral to medial, the arcus is released completely from the lateral two-thirds of the orbital margin. Approaching the midline, the supraorbital and then supratrochlear neurovascular bundles are encountered. The periosteum is freed about these as well (Fig. 7.6). Arcus elevation does not continue medial to the bundles in order to prevent excessive medial brow elevation that leads to a "disappointed" appearance.

Once bilateral arcus marginalis release is complete, corrugator and procerus muscle fibers are identified over the glabella. The muscle fibers are typically sectioned and teased apart with an elevator. However, the fibers are occasionally more robust, particularly in male patients. They may also bleed. In either case, sectioning and hemostasis can be achieved using endoscopic electrocautery forceps.

At this point, the entire forehead and brow should be free and mobile as a single unit. This can be tested with reexamination of the brow itself. Manual elevation of the forehead should now draw the brow with it, and in turn, secondarily elevate the upper lids. This is evident by either the reduction of upper lid skin redundancy or lagophthalmos and resulting upper lid lash eversion. It is for this reason that blepharoplasty should follow rather than precede brow elevation and fixation.

Our preferred method of brow fixation involves anchoring the scalp with 2–0 resorbable suture to the outer table of the calvarium using a bone bridge located beneath the superior-most margin of the right and left temporoparietal access incisions. First, the right incision is splayed apart using two wide, double pronged skin hooks. An assistant then not only holds the incision open but also pulls the brow superior, posterior, and approximately 10° lateral. This mimics the vector of suspension force and provides not only brow elevation but also a brow arch as well. Next, the underlying periosteum is incised with electrocautery and the bony cortex is exposed. A Stryker TPS Drill creates the actual tunnel using a 1.5 × 4 mm bit with a stop. The bit must engage the bone in a line nearly tangent to the surface, drilling first the superior and then the inferior limb of the tunnel. These must communicate beneath an intervening bridge of bone that is

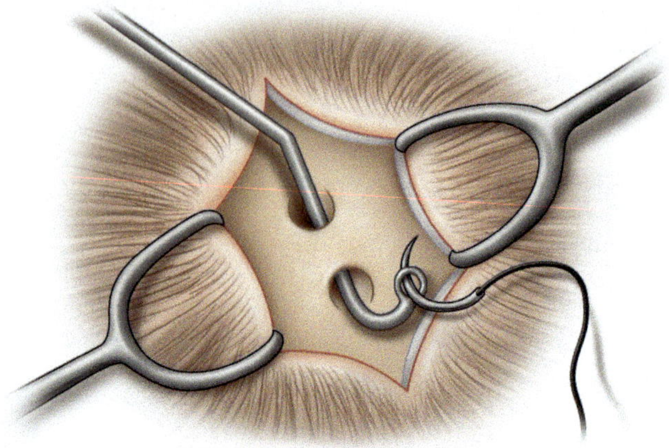

Fig. 7.7 Brow fixation using bone bridges. Wide-double skin hooks retract a temporal incision and simultaneously elevate the brow. The completed bone bridge is shown while 2–0 Vicryl suture is threaded through the tunnel using wire

2–3 mm wide by 2 mm deep. If the bit enters the cortex at a more acute angle or the entry points are too distant from one another, the limbs will not communicate. And if the entry points are too close, the bridge will be thin and fracture during the suspension. A 26-guage wire is then folded on itself and fashioned into the letter "J," passing the curled end through the tunnel. A 2–0 Vicryl suture is threaded through the wire and the wire is withdrawn, pulling the suture beneath the bone bridge (Fig. 7.7). With the hooks released, the suture is placed in a buried fashion into the dermis, galea, and periosteum approximately 2–3 cm *inferior* to the inferior apex of the incision. Retraction on the suture should dimple the overlying dermis. The right and left suspension sutures are tied simultaneously while an assistant manually elevates the brow and reduces the tension on the flap. A smooth Webster needle driver may be used, if needed, to clasp the suture's first throw so that it is less apt to recoil under tension before the knot is locked. Ideally, 1–2 mm of lagophthalmos will be present once the fixation is complete.

Lastly, the temporal suspension is performed, again using an inverted, buried 2–0 Vicryl suture. Grasping the same layers of the scalp anterior to the temporal access incisions, the right and left temporal flaps are anchored back to the DTF. When placing this suture, the surgeon must remain mindful of the facial nerve course and the underlying superficial temporal vessels. Once both sides are complete, all incisions are closed with 5–0 Vicryl Rapide suture in run-lock fashion. If blepharoplasty is planned, it is done at this time. At the completion of the case, the elastics bands are removed from the hair, antibiotic ointment applied to the incisions, and a Kerlix™ gauze head wrap applied to help eliminate optical pocket dead space. Drains are not used.

7.5.2 Complications

There are number of potential complications inherent to brow lifting. For the most part, the endoscopic approach reduces the likelihood of them all. The risk is never completely eliminated, though. In general, bleeding and resultant hematoma formation is possible with any of the techniques. The greater the dissection, elevation, and dead space created below the flaps, the greater the risk [5–7]. When bleeding does occur, the superficial temporal or zygomaticotemporal vessels are the typical culprits. Endoscopic lifting carries these same potential risks, only eliminating the risk of scalp bleeding associated with coronal lifting. Preoperative injection and meticulous dissection help avert this risk in our procedure. In addition, the postoperative head dressing helps to compress the dead space and reduce the possibility of hematoma formation.

Lagophthalmos is also a potential risk that may follow brow elevation. Particularly, susceptible patients are those who have previously undergone blepharoplasty. The probability also rises when blepharoplasty is done prior to brow elevation and suspension. As previously discussed, we have minimized this risk by adhering to conservative lid skin resection *following* all brow procedures [7, 8, 11].

Alopecia is also worth mentioning. This, too, is more often experienced in larger dissections, particularly the coronal approach. Even so, local follicle loss can occur at each of the incision sites. The key to prevention in this case is limited use of electrocautery. Again, local injection with epinephrine and precise dissection help to reduce the chances of hair loss.

Most feared of all is the risk of nerve injury. Temporary or permanent hypesthesia or anesthesia typically results from severing sensory nerve rootlets. Although temporary loss of sensation may occur with the endoscopic approach, this appears to result from traction neuropraxia, and in the senior author's experience, has never resulted in permanent loss of sensation. Making the patient aware of this potential transient loss during the preoperative discussion will help to allay their concerns. Temporal nerve damage, on the other hand, is not expected. Risk to this nerve can be avoided with comprehensive knowledge of the facial nerve's path and the associated fascial compartments. Together with the operative technique submitted above, the surgeon may then circumvent permanent injury to this nerve and its branches. If dissection is meticulous and weakness is recognized immediately following surgery, the weakness is more commonly the result of residual local anesthetic effects.

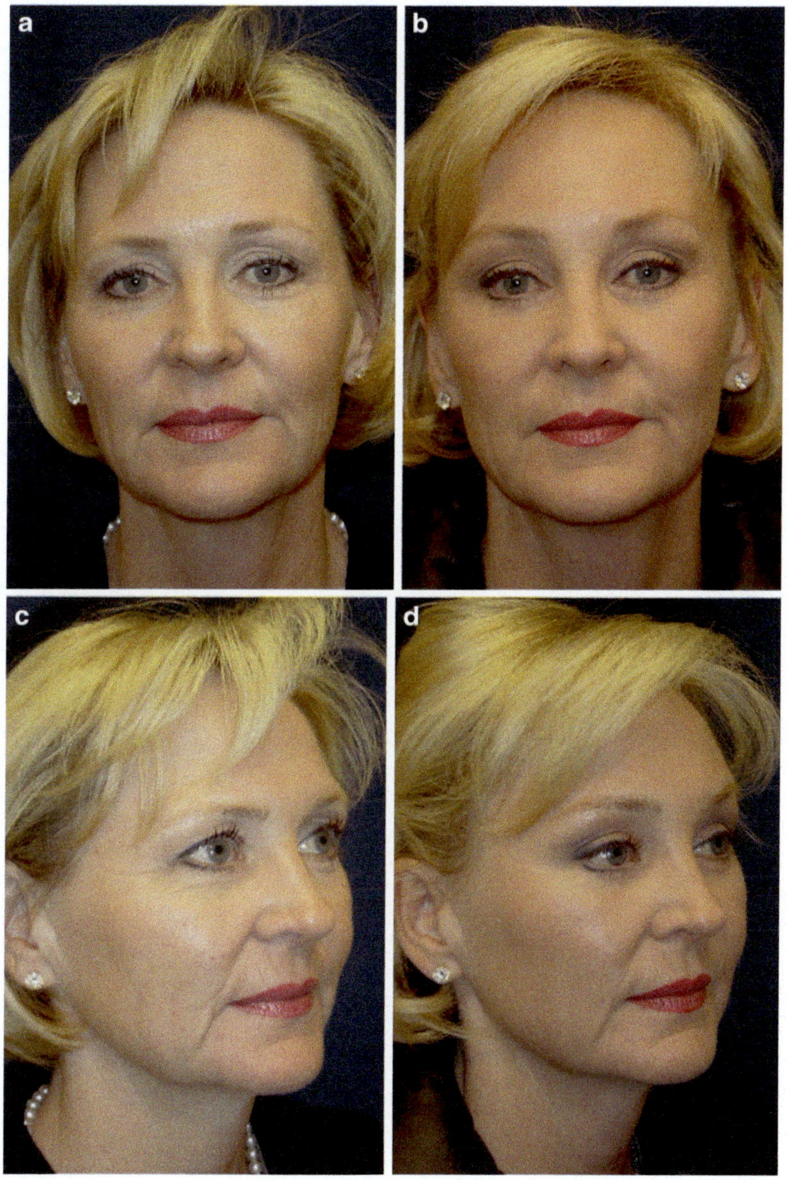

Fig. 7.8 Frontal and oblique pre- and postoperative views of two patients who underwent endoscopic brow lift and conservative upper blepharoplasty

7.6 Conclusion

The human experience is garnered and conveyed through the window of the eyes.

With the wear of age though, this window becomes erroneously reflective rather than transparent. Rejuvenation of the periorbita then not only restores cosmesis and self-image but also facilitates improved personal interactions and ensures the communication of one's true emotions to others. While many techniques exist to aid in this, the restorative process, none is as comprehensive and relatively free of morbidity as the endoscopic brow lift. It remains our operation of choice to return aesthetics to this area of the aging face (Fig. 7.8).

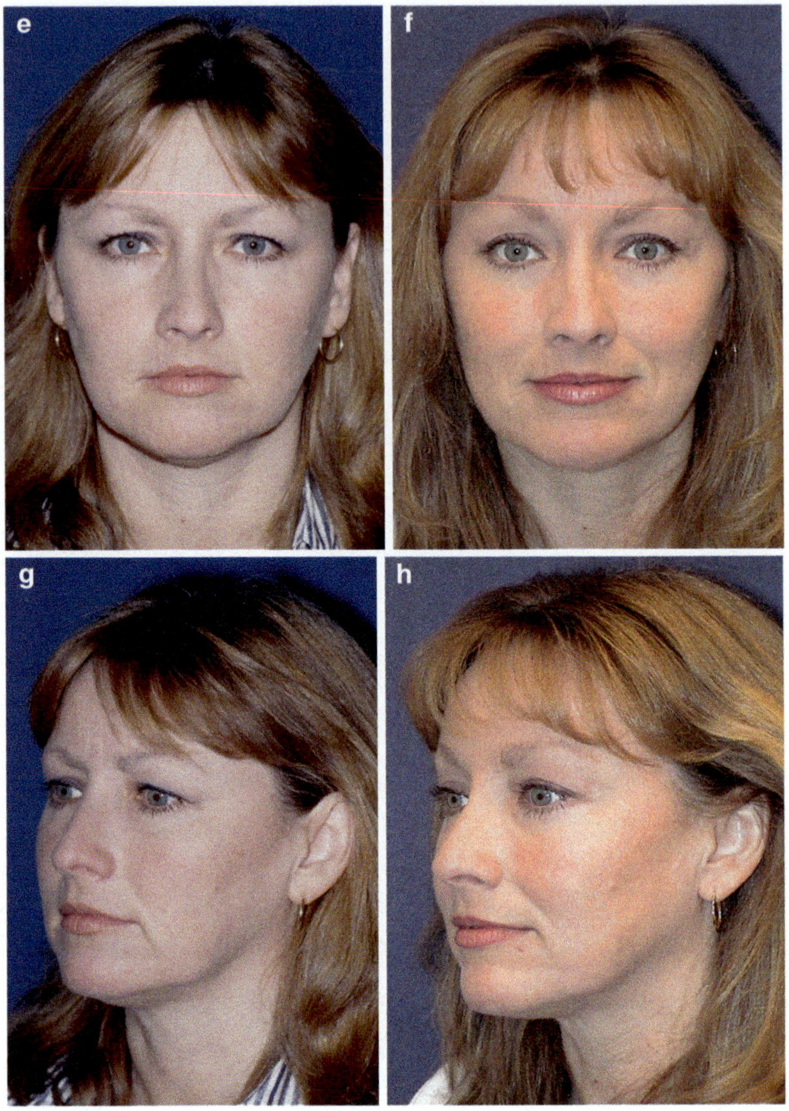

Fig. 7.8 (continued)

References

1. Brennan HG. The forehead lift. Otolaryngol Clin North Am. 1980;13(2):209–23.
2. Paul MD. The evolution of the brow lift in aesthetic plastic surgery. Plast Reconstr Surg. 2001;108(5):1409–24.
3. Cilento BJ, Johnson CJ. The case for open forehead rejuvenation. Arch Facial Plast Surg. 2009;11(1):13–7.
4. Isse NG. Endoscopic forehead lift. In: Presented at the Annual meeting of the Los Angeles County Society of Plastic Surgeons, Los Angeles, CA, 12 September 1992.
5. Friedman O, Wang TD, Cook TA. Management of the aging periorbital area, Chap. 32. In: Cummings otolaryngology – head and neck surgery. Philadelphia: Mosby; 2005. p. 764–89.
6. Larrabee WF. Brow lifts: coronal, tricophytic, pretrichial. In: Atlas of head and neck surgery – otolaryngology. Philadelphia: Lippincott Williams & Wilkins; 2001. p. 520–3.
7. Quatela VC, Graham HD, Sabini P. Rejuvenation of the brow and midface, Chap. 16. In: Facial plastic and reconstructive surgery. 2nd ed. New York: Thieme; 2002. p. 171–84.
8. Keller GS, Hutcherson RW. Browlift: a facial plastic surgeon's perspective, Chap. 14. In: Aesthetic facial plastic surgery – a multidisciplinary approach. New York: Thieme; 2000. p. 226–35.
9. Shumrick KA, Smith TL. The anatomic basis for the design of forehead flaps in nasal reconstruction. Arch Otolaryngol Head Neck Surg. 1992;118:373.
10. Sabini P, Wayne I, Quatela VC. Anatomical guides to precisely localize the frontal branch of the facial nerve. Arch Facial Plast Surg. 2003;5:150–2.
11. Goldberg RA. Browlift: an oculoplastic surgeon's perspective, Chap. 13. In: Aesthetic facial plastic surgery – a multidisciplinary approach. New York: Thieme; 2000. p. 211–23.
12. Zimbler MS, Jongwook H. Aesthetic facial analysis, Chap. 21. In: Cummings otolaryngology head and neck surgery. 4th ed. Philadelphia: Elsevier Mosby; 2005. p. 513–28.
13. Adamson PA, Brunner E, Pearson DC. The aging forehead, Chap. 182. In: Bailey's head and neck surgery – otolaryngology. 3rd ed. Philadelphia: Lippincot Williams & Wilkins; 2001. p. 2355–71.

8 Direct Brow Lift: An Aesthetic Approach

Gregory J. Griepentrog and Mark J. Lucarelli

Key Points

- With aging, the lateral brow descends more than the medial brow.
- A direct eyebrow lift provides significant lift per millimeter of excised tissue.
- The limited lateral supraciliary eyebrow lift provides excellent functional improvement and a reasonable aesthetic outcome.
- In mid-forehead lifting, dividing the incision between rhytids of differing vertical levels on each side of the hemiface avoids a longer, less natural, more visible scar that traverses the width of the forehead.
- Visible scarring is the most significant drawback of both direct eyebrow and mid-forehead lifting.
- Silicone sheeting and intralesional corticosteroid injections are excellent treatment options available to manage early surgical scarring.

8.1 Introduction

Eyebrow position intimately influences eyelid position and architecture. In particular, eyebrow position may affect the height of the upper eyelid. For example, some cases of apparent upper eyelid ptosis and dermatochalasis result from eyebrow ptosis. The eyebrows are also important to facial expression. Complex changes of expression are possible due to a superficial eyebrow musculo-cutaneous plane that slides over bone and rigidly anchored periosteum.

The ideal aesthetic contour of the eyebrow has been debated and refined during the past 4 decades. In 1974, Westmore described the ideal eyebrow as having an arch where the brow apex rests above the lateral limbus, with the medial and lateral ends of the brow at the same horizontal level [1]. In general, the youthful eyebrow complex has easily appreciated three-dimensional fullness. Gender differences play an important role in our perception of ideal eyebrow position. For example, the male eyebrow tends to ride lower and flatter than the female brow. For either a man or woman, an eyebrow that has dropped partially or wholly below the supraorbital rim may be classified as ptotic.

Aging changes of the eyebrow region result from descent and deflation. Solar damage to this region is often less pronounced than in the remainder of the periorbita due to the relative thickness of the eyebrow skin and camouflaging effects of the eyebrow hairs. The supraorbital rim tends to become more prominent with aging due to a loss of eyebrow fullness [2]. Deflation of the eyebrow complex is likely due to fat atrophy [2]. Descent of facial tissues due to gravitational forces plays another important role in the aging brow. With aging, the lateral brow descends more than the medial brow owing to a number of anatomic factors. Lateral to the temporal fusion line, beyond the action of the frontalis muscle, there is no upward vector to counteract the gravitational forces on the temporal brow or the depressor action of the lateral orbicularis oculi muscle [3]. Also, dense fibrous attachments anchor the eyebrow to the supraorbital ridge on the medial one-third to one-half of the eyebrow. Finally, the lateral brow fat pad's lack of this same degree of underlying support may facilitate its descent relative to the medial brow [4].

M.J. Lucarelli (✉)
Professor, Director, Oculofacial and Orbital Surgery, Department of Ophthalmology and Visual Sciences, University of Wisconsin-Madison, Madison, WI, USA
e-mail: mlucarel@wisc.edu

G.G. Massry et al. (eds.), *Master Techniques in Blepharoplasty and Periorbital Rejuvenation*, DOI 10.1007/978-1-4614-0067-7_8, © Springer Science+Business Media, LLC 2011

Several nonsurgical and surgical options are available to correct eyebrow ptosis. Selective chemical denervation of the eyebrow depressors with botulinum toxin may allow unopposed action of the frontalis muscle to lift the eyebrow position [5]. Volume augmentation of the brow with facial fillers or autologous fat has been advocated to address brow deflation [6, 7]. For many patients, surgical eyebrow lifting procedures remain the treatment of choice. Options include coronal or pretrichial brow lift, mid-forehead lift, temporal lift, endoscopic brow lift, trans-blepharoplasty browpexy, and direct supraciliary brow lift. In this chapter, we describe an aesthetic surgical approach to direct eyebrow and mid-forehead lifting.

8.2 Direct Eyebrow Lift

A direct eyebrow lift provides significant lift per millimeter of excised tissue. Due to the proximity of the incision to the eyebrow, it also provides ability to control brow contour. Direct eyebrow lifting has traditionally been used in older men with heavy brows as an alternative to coronal or temporal eyebrow-lifting procedures. Direct brow lifting is especially considered in patients with a receding hairline where scars from other techniques may be more visibly noticeable. Other advantages include a brief operating time, technical ease, and a favorable complication profile along with reasonable long-term results.

The greatest drawback of direct brow lifting is visible scarring. Although meticulous wound closure technique may minimize scarring, patients must be willing to accept visible scarring as a potential outcome. Scarring is often most visible in the medial extent of the incision, while the lateral incision is more easily camouflaged into the eyebrow hairs and thinner brow skin. Our surgical technique has evolved to limit substantially the medial extent of our incision. For most patients with predominantly lateral eyebrow ptosis, this limited lateral supraciliary eyebrow lift usually provides excellent functional improvement and a reasonably aesthetic outcome. Also, this refined technique has allowed us to expand the pool of appropriate surgical candidates.

Other potential risks to direct eyebrow lifting include damage to the hairs of the upper eyebrow as well as the supraorbital nerve. Facial nerve injury to the temporal (frontal) branch during direct eyebrow-lifting is extremely rare. Injury is avoided by keeping the depth of the lateral portion of the incision relatively superficial [8].

In the properly selected and counseled patient, acceptance of direct eyebrow lifting is excellent. A recent retrospective review of patients undergoing direct brow lift for involutional brow ptosis or facial nerve palsy revealed excellent efficacy and patient satisfaction [9]. Fifty-four direct eyebrow lift procedures were performed on 36 patients (M:F 17:19). With a mean follow-up period of 11 months (3–44), the most common documented complications were temporary paresthesias and numbness in 22 cases. Four patients were unhappy with their final scar appearance. In this study, the authors used a traditional direct eyebrow technique that included an incision that extended across the full width of the eyebrow.

8.3 The Limited Lateral Supraciliary Eyebrow Lift Procedure

Preoperative markings are performed with the patient in an upright position. With the frontalis muscle fully relaxed, the eyebrow is manually elevated to the desired level while a marking pen is held over the skin at the superior edge of the eyebrow. Once the eyebrow is released and allowed to fall to its native position, a mark is made on the skin above the brow (Fig. 8.1). This mark on the skin will serve as a guide for the superior incision line. This is repeated in the lateral, central, and medial portions of the desired incision site. Natural rhytids should be used when possible. The keys to achieving aesthetically pleasing results with this operation are selecting patients with predominantly lateral brow ptosis and limiting the medial extent of the incision. The inferior portion of the incision marking may include a few eyebrow hairs, thus helping to conceal the postoperative scar (Fig. 8.2). Local infiltrative anesthesia is achieved with 2% lidocaine with 1:100,000 units epinephrine (American Regent, Inc.) mixed in equal parts of 0.5% bupivacaine (APP Pharmaceuticals, LLC).

Incision along the previously placed markings is performed with a No. 15 Bard-Parker blade. The incision adjacent to the brow should be beveled parallel to the direction of the eyebrow cilia in order to avoid hair follicle damage (Fig. 8.3). A similarly beveled incision should be made on the superior incision line to provide normal wound apposition during closure. A microdissection needle (Megadyne) on a monopolar unit (ConMed Corporation) may be used to remove the skin/brow fat flap. The frontalis muscle is left undisturbed (Fig. 8.4).

The wound is closed with deep, buried sutures of either 4–0 chromic or 4–0 polyglactin. At the medial aspect of the crescent, a few interrupted, vertical mattress sutures of 4–0 nylon or polypropylene are used to reapproximate the wound edges and provide excellent wound eversion. The lateral aspect of the wound may be closed with running 5–0 or 6–0 nylon or polypropylene (Fig. 8.5). Antibiotic ointment is placed at the end of the procedure and no dressings are necessary. The sutures should be removed at the first postoperative visit 5–7 days later (Fig. 8.6).

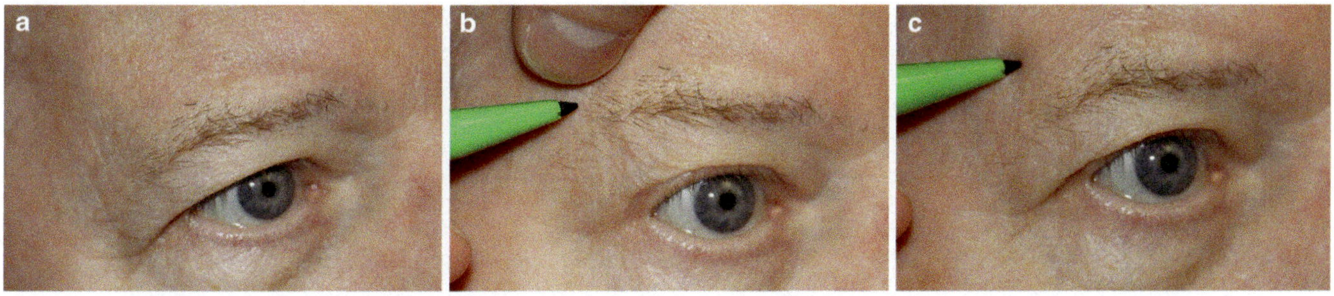

Fig. 8.1 (**a**) Preoperative eyebrow ptosis. (**b**) The eyebrow is elevated to the desired level while a marking pen is held over the skin at the superior edge of the eyebrow. (**c**) The eyebrow is released and allowed to fall to its native position, and a mark is made on the skin above the brow

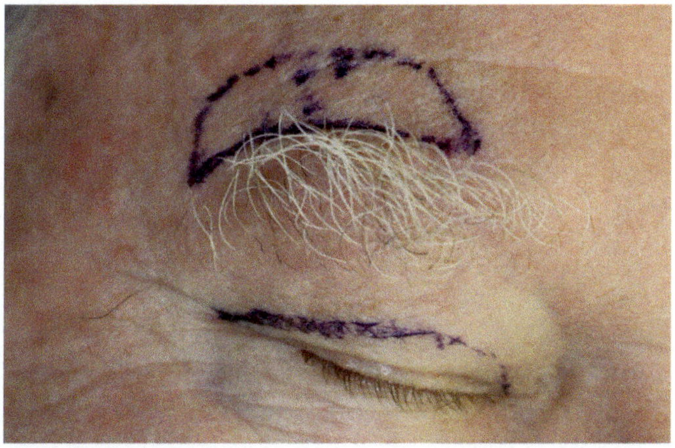

Fig. 8.2 Completed limited lateral supraciliary eyebrow lift and blepharoplasty markings, right eye

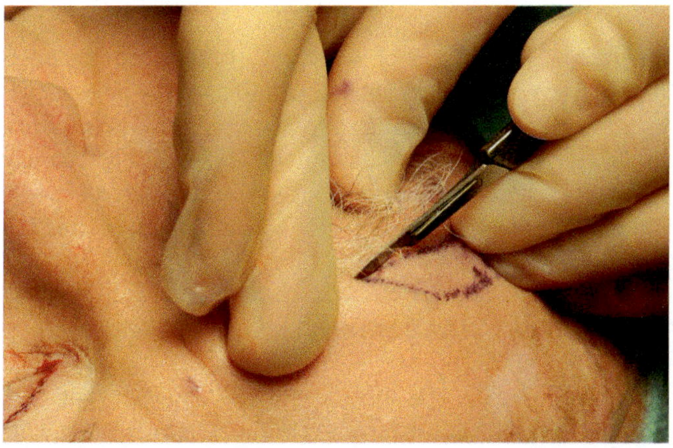

Fig. 8.3 The eyebrow incision is beveled in the direction of the upper brow hairs to minimize damage to the follicles

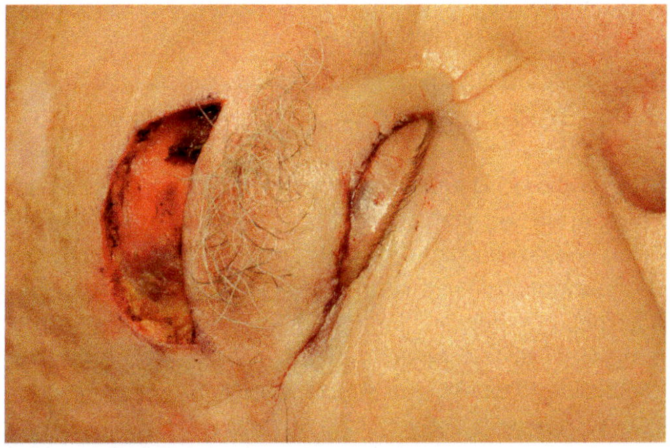

Fig. 8.4 The frontalis muscle is left undisturbed

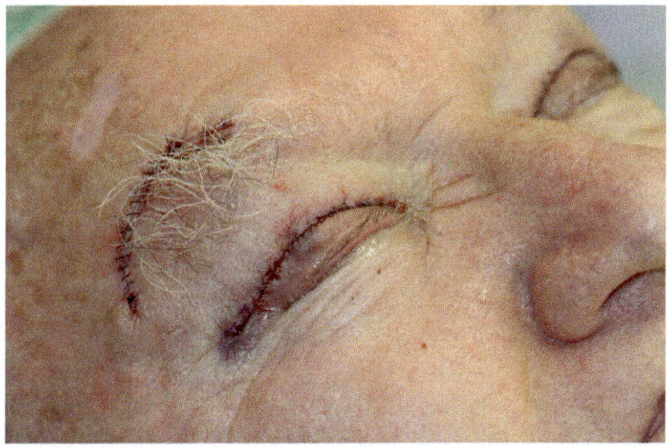

Fig. 8.5 Proper suturing technique is used to create wound eversion. In this example, a few vertical mattress sutures of 5–0 Nylon are placed medially and continued laterally in a running fashion

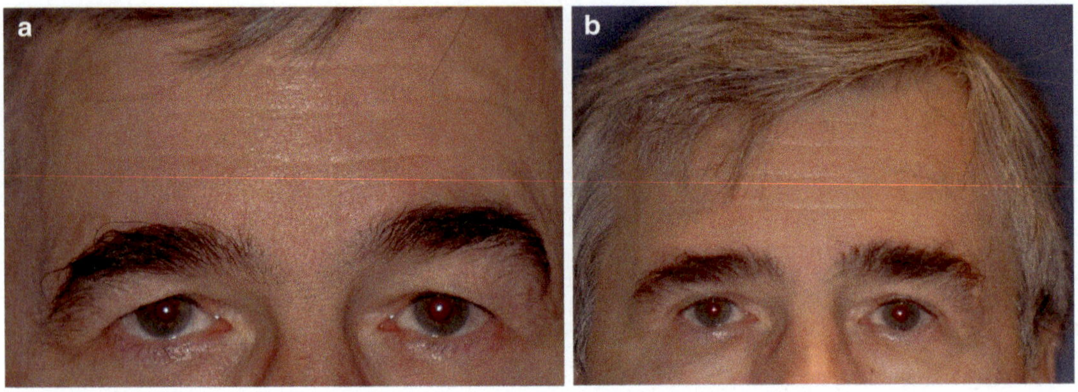

Fig. 8.6 (**a**) Preoperative photo of a patient undergoing limited lateral supraciliary eyebrow lift combined with a blepharoplasty. (**b**) Postoperative photo 12 weeks after surgery. The incisions have healed well and are concealed by the patient's eyebrows

8.4 Mid-forehead Lift

Mid-forehead lifting is most effective for patients with combined brow and glabellar ptosis with sufficiently tall foreheads and prominent horizontal brow rhytids. This technique has traditionally been used in men with heavy brows, deep horizontal rhytids, and high frontal hairlines. It may also be considered in select elderly female patients with prominent forehead rhytids. As with direct eyebrow lifting, visible scarring is a significant potential drawback. Although some authors have described the incision as traversing the entire width of the forehead, we routinely divide the incision between rhytids of differing vertical levels on each side of the hemiface, respecting the midline (Fig. 8.7) [8, 10]. This avoids a longer, less natural, more visible scar that traverses the width of the forehead (Figs. 8.8 and 8.9). Careful wound eversion techniques should again be employed to help minimize visible scarring.

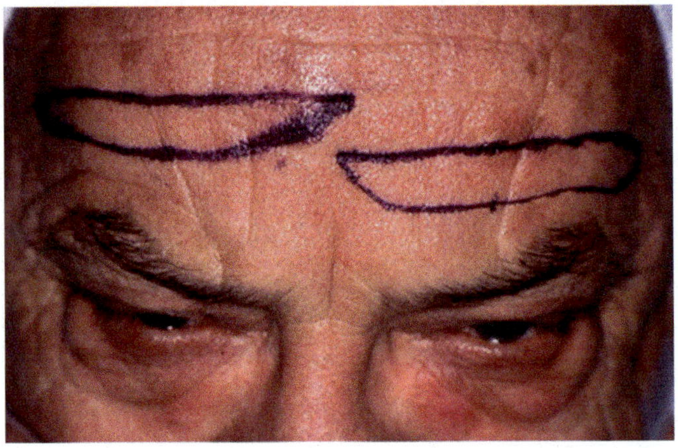

Fig. 8.7 Mid-forehead lift markings divide the incision between differing rhytids on each side of the hemiface, respecting the midline

8.4.1 The Mid-forehead Lift Procedure

Preoperative marking are made bilaterally with the use of natural forehead rhytids. The bilateral markings do not cross the midline or do so with minimal overlap. Local infiltrative anesthesia is achieved with 2% lidocaine with 1:100,000 units epinephrine (American Regent, Inc.) mixed in equal parts of 0.5% bupivacaine (APP Pharmaceuticals, LLC).

Incision along the previously placed markings is performed with a No. 15 Bard-Parker blade. A microdissection needle (Megadyne) on a monopolar unit (ConMed Corporation) may be used to remove the skin/brow fat flap. The frontalis muscle is left undisturbed. Laterally, the dissection may be taken down to just above the superficial temporalis fascia. Meticulous hemostasis is achieved with monopolor cautery and when necessary, gelatin foam soaked in thrombin. The wound is closed with deep, buried sutures of either 4–0 chromic or 4–0 polyglycan. Multiple interrupted, vertical mattress sutures of 4–0 nylon or polypropylene are used to reapproximate the wound edges. Alternatively, the lateral aspect of the wound may be closed with running 5–0 or 6–0 nylon or polypropylene suture. The sutures should be removed at the first postoperative visit 5–7 days later.

8.5 Scar Management

Visible scarring is the most significant drawback of both direct eyebrow and mid-forehead lifting. Even normal mature scars which are flat and not hyperpigmented may be noticeable. More concerning, though, are erythematous, hyperpigmented or hypertrophic scars. In our experience, hypertrophic scarring with these procedures has been exceedingly rare. These scars result from excessive wound tension, infection, or delays in healing.

Both surgical and nonsurgical treatments are available to manage surgical scarring. A wide range of nonsurgical treatments has been evaluated. These are summarized in

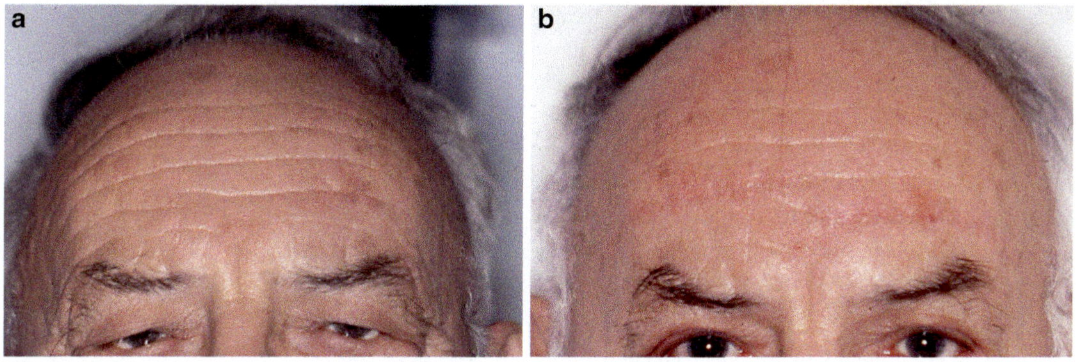

Fig. 8.8 (**a**) Preoperative photo of an excellent candidate for mid-forehead lift and upper eyelid blepharoplasty. Note the severe brow and glabellar ptosis, deep horizontal rhytids, and tall forehead. (**b**) Erythema still present in the wounds 12 weeks after mid-forehead lift. Note that the incisions are staggered at different vertical levels. The brow ptosis and the horizontal rhytids are markedly improved. The overall shape and contour of the eyebrow remain similar to the preoperative state

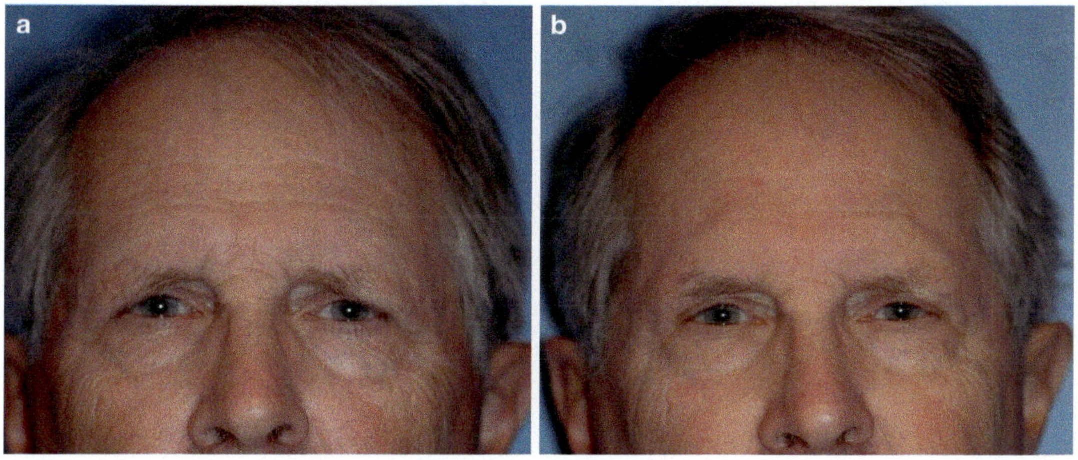

Fig. 8.9 (**a**) Preoperative photo of a patient undergoing a lateral mid-forehead lift and upper eyelid blepharoplasty. Note the severity of the lateral brow ptosis. (**b**) Postoperative photo 6 months after surgery. Some medial and central brow ptosis remains as expected, but the severe lateral ptosis has been substantially improved

Table 8.1 Summary of nonsurgical therapies currently used for the management of scarring

Therapy	Modality
Massage starting 3–4 weeks postoperatively	Mechanical
Vitamin E	Topical preparation
Onion extract (Mederma)	Topical preparation
Topical or intralesional corticosteroids	Pharmaceutical
Compression garments	Wound dressing
Adhesive microporous paper tape	Wound dressing
Hydrogel sheeting	Wound dressing
Silicone sheeting	Wound dressing
Nonablative lasers	Laser
Ablative lasers	Laser (removes scar surface or whole scar)
Chemical peel	Chemical (removes scar surface)

Partially adapted from Occelston et al. [11]

Table 8.1 [11]. We often manage eyebrow or forehead wounds beginning at 3 weeks postoperatively with commercially available silicone sheeting, which has been demonstrated to be safe and effective [12, 13]. Intralesional corticosteroid injections (triamcinolone 10 mg/mL; Bristol-Squibb Company) are employed at approximately 6 weeks postoperatively when needed, although they do carry a small risk of skin atrophy, depigmentation, and telangiectasia [14]. Finally, scar revision techniques such as dermabrasion, excision, or laser may be necessary subsequently in rare cases.

8.6 Conclusion

In conclusion, direct eyebrow and mid-forehead lifting are effective long-lasting management options in the treatment of brow ptosis of carefully selected and well-counseled patients.

Modifications in technique, such as the limited lateral supraciliary eyebrow lift as well as a staggered approach to the placement of mid-forehead lift incisions, allow for both satisfactory aesthetic and functional outcomes.

References

1. Westmore MG. Facial cosmetics in conjunction with surgery. In: Presented at the Aesthetic plastic surgical society meeting, Vancouver, BC, Canada, May 1974.
2. Cuici PM, Obagi S. Rejuvenation of the periorbital complex with autologous fat transfer: current therapy. J Oral Maxillofac Surg. 2008;66(8):1686–93.
3. Knize DM. An anatomically based study of the mechanism of eyebrow ptosis. Plast Reconstr Surg. 1996;97(7):1321–33.
4. Lemke BN, Stasior OG. The anatomy of eyebrow ptosis. Arch Ophthalmol. 1982;100:981–6.
5. Foster JA, Proffer PL, Proffer LH, et al. Modifying brow position with botulinum toxin. Int Ophthalmol Clin. 2005;45:123–31.
6. Carruthers JD, Carruthers A. Facial sculpting and tissue augmentation. Dermatol Surg. 2005;31:1604–12.
7. Berman M. Rejuvenation of the upper eyelid complex with autologous fat transplantation. Dermatol Surg. 2000;26(12):1113–6.
8. Green JP, Goldberg RA, Shorr N. Eyebrow ptosis. Int Ophthalmol Clin. 1997;37:97–122.
9. Booth AJ, Murray A, Tyers AG. The direct brow lift: efficacy, complications, and patient satisfaction. Br J Ophthalmol. 2004;88:688–91.
10. Johnson CM, Waldman SR. Midforehead lift. Arch Otolaryngol. 1983;109:155–9.
11. Occelston NL, O'Kan S, Goldspink N, et al. New therapeutics for the prevention and reduction of scarring. Drug Discov Today. 2008;13:973–81.
12. Mustoe TA, Cooter RD, Gold MH, et al. International clinical recommendations on scar management. Plast Reconstr Surg. 2002;110:560–71.
13. Poston J. The use of silicone gel sheeting in the management of hypertrophic and keloid scars. J Wound Care. 2000;9:10–6.
14. Sproat JE, Dalcin A, Weitauer N, et al. Hypertrophic sternal scars: silicone gel sheeting versus kenalog injection treatment. Plast Reconstr Surg. 1992;90:988–92.

Part III

Upper Eyelid Rejuvenation

9 Upper Eyelid Blepharoplasty

Asa D. Morton

Key Points

- Upper blepharoplasty is one of the oldest described treatments of the aging face.
- Surgery is commonly performed to improve both appearance and field of vision.
- A detailed knowledge of eyelid function and anatomy is critical to achieving appropriate surgical outcomes.
- The preoperative evaluation should focus on identifying patients not suitable for surgery as a result of ocular pathology (dry eye, etc.) or unrealistic expectations.
- Preoperative brow ptosis and true eyelid ptosis must be pointed out to the patient.
- To achieve the best surgical results a brow lift and ptosis repair are added when necessary.
- While surgery is generally straightforward, complications can be severe and lead to significant discomfort and visual compromise.
- Complications are avoided with appropriate patient selection and surgical technique.
- In experienced hands, upper blepharoplasty surgery is a very rewarding procedure.

9.1 Introduction

Initial historical reference to upper eyelid blepharoplasty dates back to the tenth and eleventh centuries [1], when the functional impairment of eyelid skin relative to vision was recognized. The first cosmetic references to the procedures were described in the early part of the twentieth century [2, 3]. It was not until the 1950s that the traditional techniques of upper lid blepharoplasty that are still used today were described in detail [4]. In contemporary times, upper lid blepharoplasty has become an accepted and common cosmetic procedure. The procedure is relatively straightforward and safe, is performed by physicians in many specialties, and yields high patient satisfaction. However, when performed improperly and poor outcome is attained, more than appearance can be affected. Patients may experience significant discomfort, visual difficulty, and dissatisfaction. When this occurs in functional surgery, it may be tolerated until resolution is achieved. Conversely, when surgery is cosmetic in nature, the postoperative expectation is high and the patient less forgiving. As most aesthetic facial surgeons consider this a "bread and butter" procedure, and because it is so commonly performed, mastering the technique is essential. In addition, there are a host of reasons for which patients pursue blepharoplasty and it is incumbent upon the surgeon to identify patient expectations and determine if they can be met.

In this chapter I will review the essential components of the preoperative evaluation of the blepharoplasty patient. In addition the surgical technique will be reviewed in detail. Finally, the postoperative care for patients undergoing the operation and the common complications encountered will be described.

A.D. Morton (✉)
Director of Oculoplastic and Facial Reconstruction,
Eye Care of San Diego, San Diego, CA, USA
e-mail: admorton@aol.com

9.2 Anatomic Eyelid and Periorbital Considerations

The anatomy of the eyelids and periorbital structures is discussed in Chap. 2. The eyelid surgeon is well advised to review normal anatomy prior to performing eyelid surgery. In brief, the upper eyelid is composed of skin and orbicularis muscle, the orbital septum, two fat compartments, the levator muscle and aponeurosis, Mueller's muscle, tarsus, and conjunctiva (Fig. 9.1). The skin overlying the septum is loosely attached to underlying tissue, is generally above the eyelid crease, and is the skin which becomes redundant with age and is excised in surgery. The pretarsal skin is firmly attached to underlying tissue, is below the crease, is not excised during surgery, and forms the pretarsal lid platform of the eyelid.

G.G. Massry et al. (eds.), *Master Techniques in Blepharoplasty and Periorbital Rejuvenation*,
DOI 10.1007/978-1-4614-0067-7_9, © Springer Science+Business Media, LLC 2011

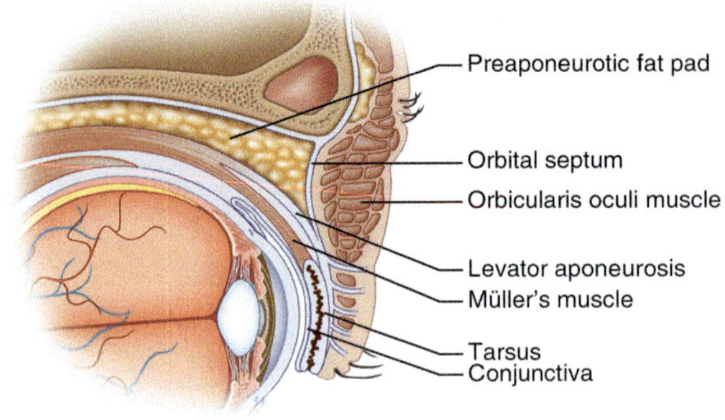

Fig. 9.1 Key anatomic components of the upper lid

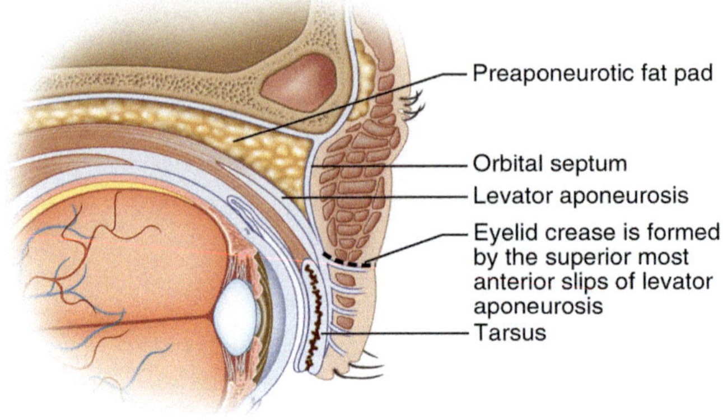

Fig. 9.2 The levator aponeurosis attaches to the anterior surface of the tarsus and sends slips of tissue forward through the orbicularis muscle to the pretarsal skin (*dotted black line*). This creates a pull on the eyelid skin and the formation of the crease

Just posterior to the orbital septum are the nasal and central (preaponeurotic) fat pads of the upper lid. These fat pads differ in color and constitution (see Chap. 2) [5–7] which may give rise to the typical involutional changes seen in the eyelids. The preaponeurotic fat is a critical landmark in surgery. The fat pad may be debulked as needed, and it directly overlies the levator aponeurosis (the main eyelid elevator), a structure which must be preserved in surgery. Posterior to the levator muscle and intimately associated with it is Mueller's muscle, the accessory (and sympathetically driven) eyelid elevator. Unlike the lower eyelid, the upper lid does not have a third (temporal) fat pad. If fullness is present in this area, consideration should be given to an anteriorly displaced or translocated lacrimal gland [8, 9]. This should be addressed by repositioning the gland into its associated fossa, not excision, as to avoid potentially significant postoperative dry eye complications. The tarsus is the cartilaginous skeleton of the upper lid and provides it with rigid support. Its superior edge is the general location of the eyelid crease, and it acts as the anchor point for the levator aponeurosis.

The eyelid crease is an anatomic structure essential to blepharoplasty surgery. The creases of the two lids should be symmetric. In occidental eyes, the lid crease generally forms between 8 and 12 mm above the lash margin. This varies and is a function of where the levator aponeurosis and orbital septum fuse, and at what level the distal levator fibers adhere to the skin. The levator aponeurosis attaches to the anterior surface of the tarsus and sends slips of tissue forward through the orbicularis muscle to the pretarsal skin. This creates a pull on the eyelid skin and the formation of the crease (Fig. 9.2). The level at which the orbital septum fuses with the levator aponeurosis limits descent of preseptal fat into the eyelid and defines the eyelid crease. In the Asian eyelid, the septum fuses much lower on the levator allowing descent of the eyelid fat. This blunts the anterior fibers of the levator aponeurosis from which adhering to the skin, and creates a low or nonexistent lid crease (Fig. 9.3).

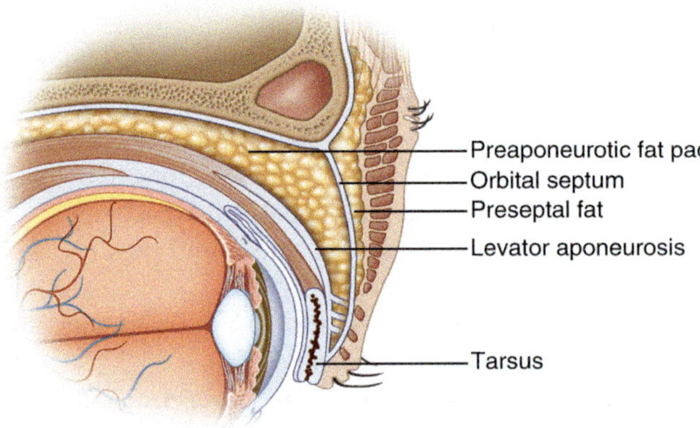

Fig. 9.3 In the Asian eyelid, the septum fuses much lower on the levator allowing descent of the eyelid fat. This blunts the anterior fibers of the levator aponeurosis from adhering to the skin and creates a low or nonexistent lid crease. Also note that the Asian eyelid has a preseptal fat pad, normally absent from the Caucasian eyelid, which also (in addition to lower riding postseptal fat) adds fullness to the lid

Normally, the eyelashes are directed anteriorly so as not to obstruct the visual axis. With advancing age, the crease elevates, reducing its support of lash position (the attachments of the levator to the skin/orbicularis), and advancing dermatochalasis mechanically rides on the lashes. These events may redirect the lashes into the visual axis adversely effecting vision and appearance. In addition, the overhanging lid fold can trap bacteria and skin debris, inducing blepharitis. These issues can be addressed surgically with tissue debulking and crease reformation when necessary.

The position of the brow is important in performing appropriate upper lid blepharoplasty. In general, the male brow is flat and sits just at, or slightly above, the orbital rim. The female brow is arched above the orbital rim and slopes inferio-laterally out over the lateral canthus (Fig. 9.4). Significant horizontal rhytids of the forehead suggest

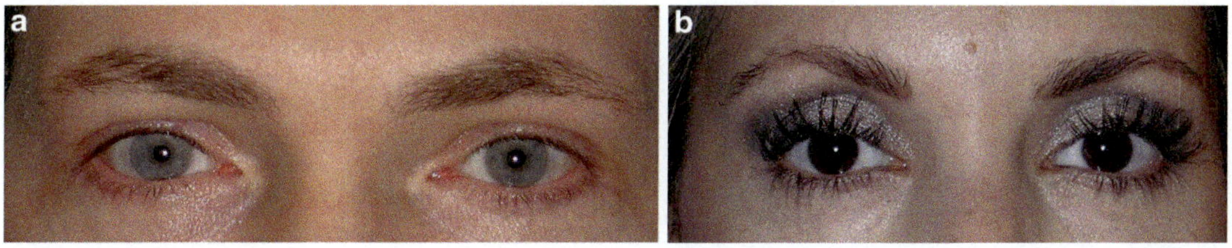

Fig. 9.4 The male brow follows the orbital rim and is relatively flat. The female brow arches over the lateral limbus of the eye and then descends slightly into the temporal region

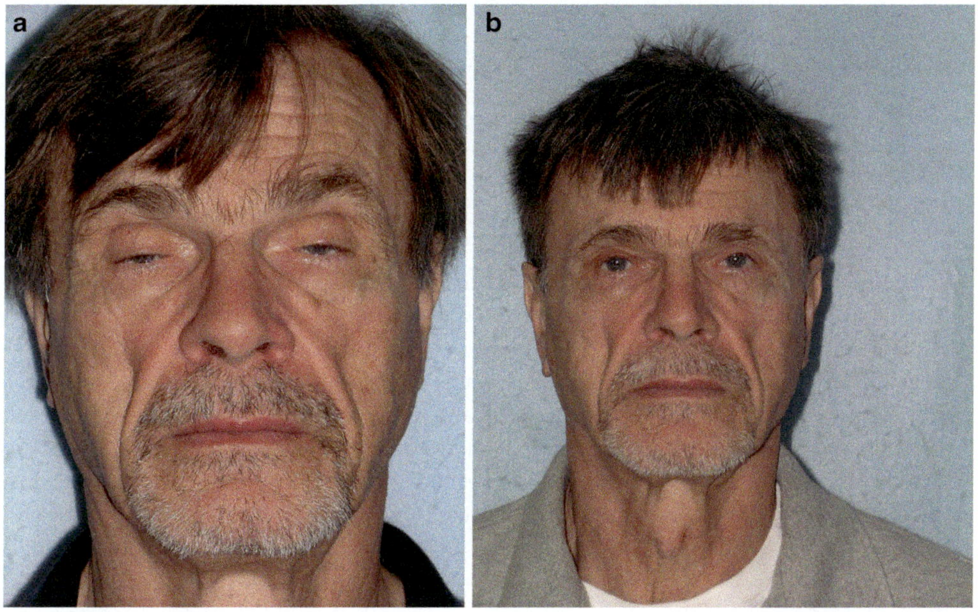

Fig. 9.5 (**a**) Patient with significant blepharoptosis and dermatochalasia. Deep forehead rhytids indicate prominent frontalis contraction to elevate heavy brows off of ptotic lids. This contraction is subconscious and represented the patients' normal preoperative facies. (**b**) Patient declined a brow lifting procedure and underwent blepharoplasty and ptosis repair. The postoperative photo demonstrates dramatic change in brow position. Due to appropriate preoperative counseling, the patient accepts this change

compensation for brow ptosis. Patients subconsciously will elevate their brows to reduce the weight on the eyelids and improve super temporal visual fields. This compensation can be negated by eyelid surgery resulting in postoperative brow ptosis (Fig. 9.5).

9.3 Assessing Patients' Concerns

The initial consultation may be the most important part of the surgical relationship. It is incumbent upon the surgeon to understand the concerns and goals of the patient. The following questions will help to reveal the patient's intentions and assess how reasonable their goals are:

- How is it that I can best help you?
- What is it that you would like to change?
- How do you feel your eyelids affect your appearance or vision?
- Are there any life circumstances that effect your decision to proceed with surgery now?

A mirror held by the patient will encourage them to accurately demonstrate areas of concern. Patients are encouraged to describe what they wish to change and not comment on the surgical procedure they feel is needed. Prospective patients often arrive with preconceived notions on how their aesthetic goals will be realized and these should be carefully reviewed and corrected if necessary.

It is difficult with instruments or fingers to demonstrate expected outcomes. A Q-tip or bent paperclip can be utilized to indent the lid crease and elevate redundant skin to simulate the intended result. Patients should be cautioned as to the accuracy of these techniques. Ideally, the patient is photographed directly before the consultation so that a series of standard photographs are available for reference. A moderately sized flat screen monitor positioned for shared viewing is ideal (Fig. 9.6). Areas of concern can be enlarged for greater clarification during the discussion. Digital morphing programs are available to simulate postoperative results, but increase the risk for unrealistic patient expectations. A portfolio of pre- and postoperative photos of actual patients demonstrates true results and speaks to the surgical skills of the surgeon.

To ensure an accurate assessment of patient goals, it is useful to conclude with a review statement such as, "I hear

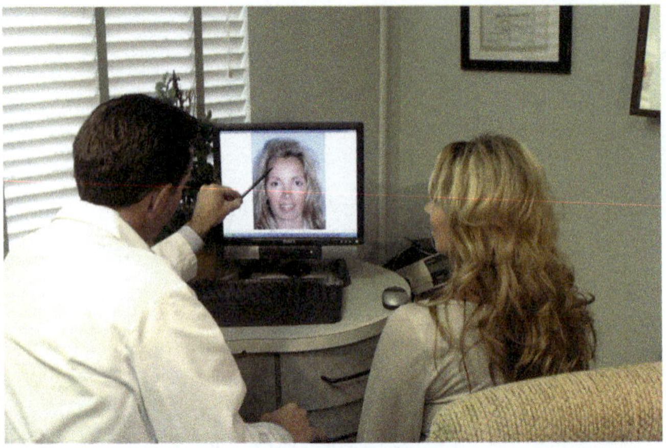

Fig. 9.6 A flat screen computer monitor is used to project the patients photos. Areas of concern can be visualized from full face, oblique, and side view images. Representative pre- and postoperative images from consenting patients can be shared

you saying that you would like to accomplish the following." The patient confirms understanding and the accuracy of communication is verified. It cannot be overemphasized that time spent carefully listening and explaining the course of events, recovery phase, and risks of surgery, is crucial and should never be rushed. Not every patient is a candidate for surgery. This is the time to identify mismatches in expectations and reality and politely decline to participate if necessary.

9.4 Patient History

Prior to consultation the patient completes the history form. This is an opportunity to discover and assess key relevant medical information before surgery. The information is reviewed with the patient during the interview. A thorough discussion of medications, especially those that increase intraoperative bleeding time, should be obtained. Anticoagulation for various maladies is becoming more and more common as the patient population lives longer. The risk of stopping these agents versus the risk of intraoperative bleeding with their continued use must be carefully assessed and reviewed with their primary physician. This is an elective surgery which should not create undo risk to the patient.

The patient is questioned about chronic systemic diseases and autoimmune processes. Patients with increased periorbital edema and prominent eyes or swelling should be evaluated for thyroid-related orbitopathy. A history of dry eye or frequent artificial tear use should be solicited.

A careful record of drug allergies and medication sensitivities should be obtained. Anesthesia complications during prior surgeries should be noted. In all but the healthiest of patients, it is advisable to request a medical clearance from the patient's primary physician.

9.5 Patient Examination

A careful and thorough preoperative examination is essential to attaining a good surgical result and a vital reference should postoperative problems develop. The surgeon must be careful to ensure that preexisting problems are documented and not credited postoperatively to the surgical procedure they perform.

With all eyelid surgery, the patient's best-corrected visual acuity should be recorded. The presence of an afferent pupillary defect, ocular misalignment, or limitations in ocular motility is noted. Standardized eyelid measurements are very useful and necessary to document pre- and postoperative findings. These should include the vertical palpebral fissure measurement from upper lid margin to lower lid margin (typically 10 mm). Levator excursion is measured by immobilizing the brow with the thumb and measuring the excursion from full down-gaze to full up-gaze. Normal levator function is 15 mm of excursion. This is an especially important measurement in the presence of true eyelid ptosis. The lid crease height is measured by having the patient look down and measuring from the lid margin to the lid crease. A normal Caucasian crease is approximately 10 mm, and significantly lower in Asians. Pretarsal show is measured in primary gaze from the inferior aspect of the lid fold to the lid margin. This is an important measurement in blepharoplasty surgery as it defines the visible lid platform after surgery. Negative numbers can be used to represent a lid fold that hangs below the lid margin. The margin reflex distance (MRD) is measured as the distance from mid-pupil to the lid margin with the patient fixating in primary gaze. This can be measured for both the upper (MRD1 - an assessment of ptosis) and lower eyelid (MRD2 – assessment of lid retraction or sclera show). If ptosis is noted, neurological disease must be ruled out (Myasthenia Gravis, Horner's syndrome, etc.) before proceeding (see Chap. 12). The term "pseudo MRD" can be used to measure the distance from the hanging lid fold to mid-pupil in cases where the fold drops below the lid margin. These "pseudo" measurements can also be applied to the vertical palpebral fissure. Also important is an assessment of orbicularis oculi strength. The patient is asked to close the eyes with force. The examiner then attempts to open the eyes. This should be difficult when lid strength is normal. The strength is measured from 1 to 4, with 4 being normal and decreasing numbers gradations of weakness. Even with conservative skin excision, patients may develop reduced lid closure after surgery. This can be related to preexisting muscle weakness which can be exacerbated by the trauma of surgery. Finally, the Bells' phenomenon can be assessed. This is globe supraduction (elevation) that occurs with lid closure. It is a normal protective mechanism of the cornea. If this is deficient, patients are at greater risk of postoperative exposure or dry eye symptoms. Any other significant findings, such as the presence of an epicanthal fold, scar form previous surgery or trauma, lid lesion, or other irregularities, should be noted.

One of the more common risks of upper lid blepharoplasty is dry eye and this can be exacerbated by lower lid function. Lower lid tone, lid margin disease, lagophthalmos, and punctal position should all be recorded. Lax lower eyelids with an ineffective blink can place the patient at increased risk for dry eye postoperatively. A basic tear secretion test can be performed using Schirmer's strips. These tests can be affected by environmental conditions in the exam room and other extraneous factors, making their results somewhat unpredictable. While they may be useful, a thorough clinical exam is essential. A slit lamp examination with the use of fluorescein drops and cobalt blue illumination is a valuable tool in determining the presence of punctate epithelial staining. Any preexisting corneal scarring should be noted. In patients with preexisting signs of dry eye and lower lid laxity, consideration for coincident lower lid tightening may be prudent to provide the patient with appropriate postoperative corneal protection.

When examining the upper eyelid, the presence of a lateral lid mass may represent lacrimal gland ptosis and could require repair during surgery. The examiner should note the brow position relative to the superior orbital rim and assess the potential for new or worsening postoperative brow ptosis. Aggressive blepharoplasty in a patient with preexisting brow ptosis, and significant compensatory forehead rhytids, is a recipe for dissatisfaction. These patients should be encouraged to have appropriate brow surgery in conjunction with upper lid blepharoplasty. If the patient declines brow surgery, a conservative blepharoplasty should be performed. The goal is to maintain the patient's subconscious drive for frontalis contraction, minimizing the risk of postoperative brow descent. The patient must understand that this approach will not remove all of the redundant skin from their lids but is necessary to keep the brow from drooping and creating an unnatural appearance. Normal aging brow descent creates greater temporal upper lid fullness than that seen more medially. Patients with significant temporal hooding should be advised that blepharoplasty alone has limited ability to correct this condition.

Visual field testing may be necessary if the surgical procedure is to be considered a medically necessary one. Improvements in superior visual field testing between untaped and taped eyelids are a standard for this approval process. Photographs are generally taken prior to the consultation to be utilized during the patient interview. These photographs generally involve a full face, bilateral 45 and 90° profiles. Carefully taken standardized photographs are essential to the entire process. They are utilized preoperatively for discussion, at surgery as a reference, and postoperatively to demonstrate change. As the surgeon frequently deals with postoperative concerns associated with cosmetic patients, there is no more useful tool than a good preoperative photograph.

9.6 Preparation for Surgery

Appropriately marking the patient may be one of the most significant preparatory steps for a successful outcome. Many authors recommend marking the patient in a sitting position. My preference is to have the patient supine, with the surgeon sitting at the head of the bed. This allows for more accurate placement of intended surgical incisions.

Several patient instructions and techniques will help to increase the accuracy and sustainability of your marks. Prior to marking, a drop of topical anesthetic is placed into each eye. The eyelids are then cleaned with alcohol wipes (Fig. 9.7). This cleansing removes skin oils and eyelid debris, which may cause marking lines to spread. Prior to marking, the patient is instructed to gently close their eyes and to maintain closure, even if asked a question.

If existing eyelid creases are symmetric, and at the desired height, they are marked as the base of the proposed surgical excision. Frequently asymmetry in lid creases exists. A compass caliper can be very useful to create symmetric marks. The position of the surgical incision, which will create the postoperative lid crease, should be determined based upon ethnicity and patient desires, but there are some standard precepts. Using the calipers four reference points are placed to define the lower incision. Medially, a small dot is

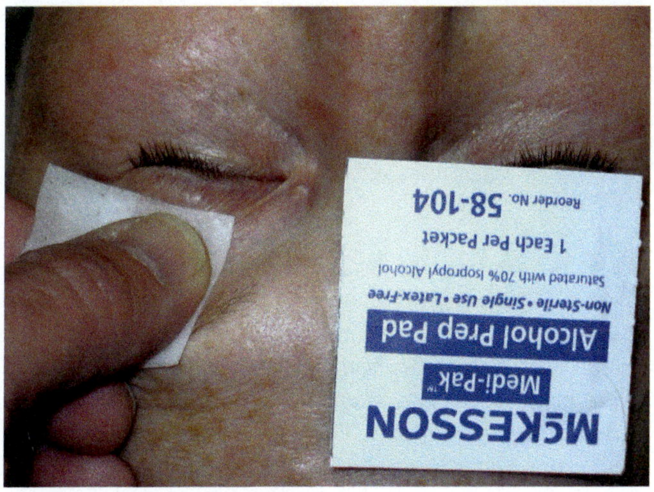

Fig. 9.7 Alcohol wipes are used to clean skin oils in preparation for eyelid marking. This improves the accuracy of the markings and reduces surgical marker ink "bleed" along natural skin lines. Alcohol vapor may be irritating to the eye so a drop of topical ophthalmic anesthetic is first applied to the eye

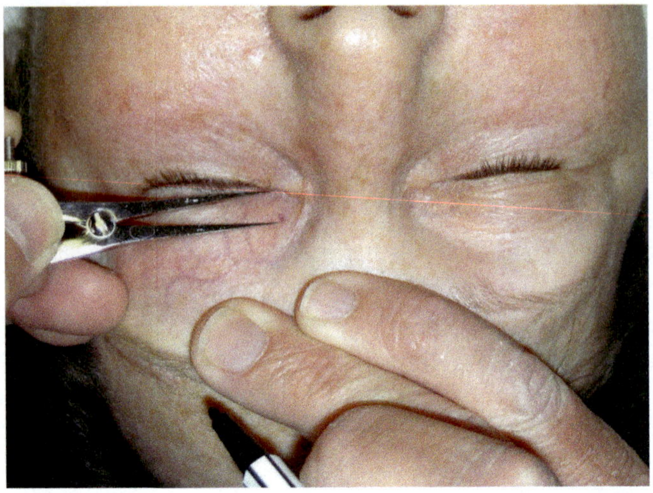

Fig. 9.8 Compass calipers are useful to create symmetric cardinal points between the eyelids. This is not necessary in patients with well-defined and symmetric lid creases that are positioned at the desired height

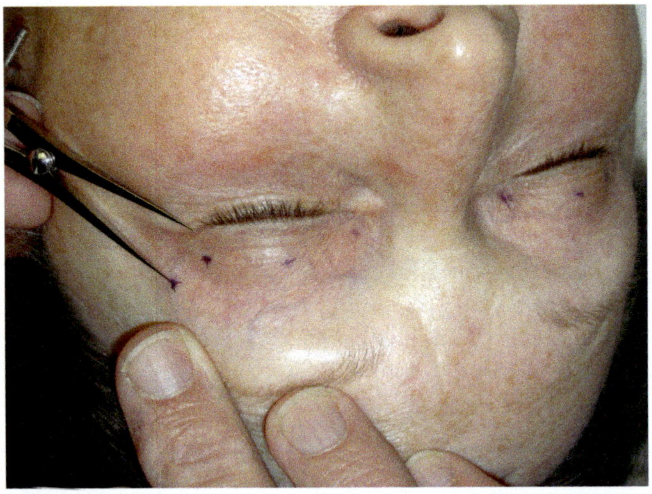

Fig. 9.9 To ensure symmetry of the lateral extent of the lid crease incision, the calipers are used. The calipers are set between 12 and 15 mm, with one tip placed at the lateral commissure and the other directed superolateral. The calipers can be rotated based on the lateral flare desired. This technique helps to create incisions that are symmetric

made 5–7 mm above the medial commissure (Fig. 9.8). Centrally, a small dot is made 9–11 mm above the lid margin at mid-pupil. Laterally, a mark is made 8–10 mm above the lateral canthal angle. To ensure symmetry of the lateral extent of the incision, the calipers can also be used to measure the terminus of this marking. The calipers are set between 12 and 15 mm, with one tip placed at the lateral commissure and the other end directed superolateral. The calipers can be rotated up or down based on the lateral flare desired. This technique helps to create incisions that are bilaterally symmetric (Fig. 9.9). The markings are then drawn through each of these four reference points. To increase the accuracy of the

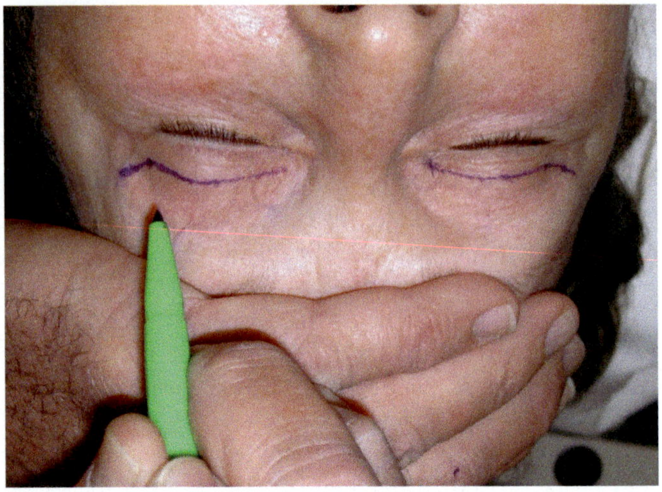

Fig. 9.10 The nondominant hand is placed on the brow, elevating the brow and stretching the eyelid skin against gentle closure by the patient. The drawing hand is placed on top of the nondominant hand which provides an excellent point of stabilization, improving incision accuracy

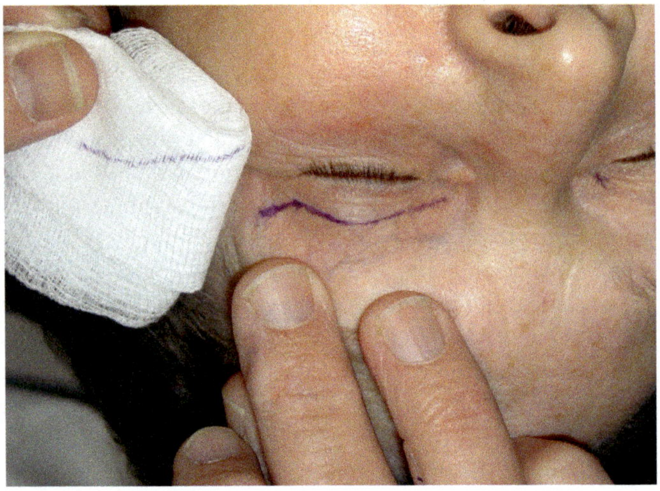

Fig. 9.11 Each line is dried three times. Most surgical markers leave excess ink and tend to dry slowly. This creates widening and rubber-stamping of the marks

surgical marks, the surgeon sits above the patient's head. The nondominant hand is placed on the brow and serves to elevate the brow and stretch the eyelid skin against gentle closure by the patient. The drawing hand is placed on top of the nondominant hand which provides an excellent point of stabilization (Fig. 9.10). Finally, after each line is drawn, it is dried three times. Most surgical markers leave excess ink and tend to dry slowly. This leads to widening and rubber-stamping of the marks. As each line is drawn, the assistant is instructed to dry by dabbing three times with gauze (Fig. 9.11). This technique establishes the placement of the inferior incision and will ultimately decide the postoperative lid crease position and symmetry (Fig. 9.12).

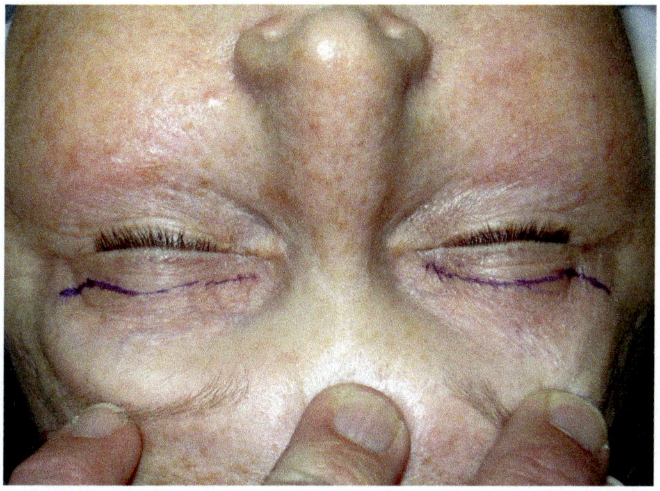

Fig. 9.12 Eyelid creases are compared for symmetry

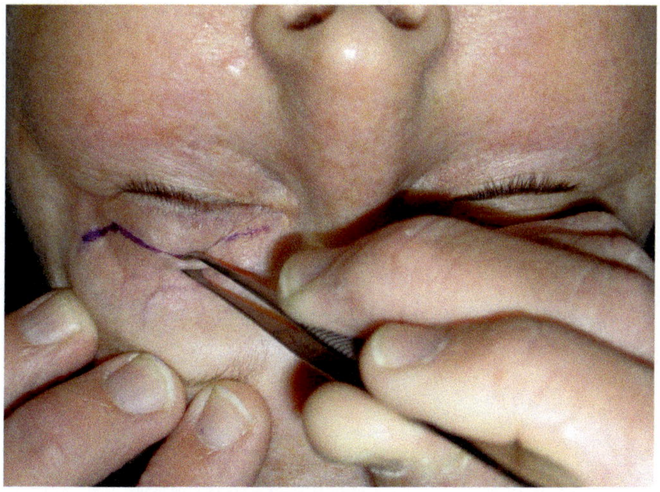

Fig. 9.13 A Graffe fixation forceps is used to determine the amount of excess skin above the lid crease. Several measurements are made across the eyelid to insure adequate skin is left for eyelid closure. A conservative excision is favored

The forceps pinch technique is utilized at three or four locations across the upper eyelid to determine the amount of skin to be excised, and to define the position of the superior incision. This maneuver confirms an appropriate amount of skin excision without undue risk of lagophthalmos (Fig. 9.13). Preoperative photos, taken in an upright position, are used during the drawing process to help refine the markings. Excess medial skin can be addressed with a wider angle where the superior incision meets the inferior lid crease incision. Conversely, patients with less dermatochalasis medially would benefit from a narrower angle (Fig. 9.14). Although temporal hooding is best corrected with brow elevation, it may be partially remediated by a more aggressive lateral superior marking before descending to meet the inferior marking. A minimum of 1 cm of lid skin must be preserved between the inferior most brow cilia and the superior aspect of the incision.

Patients with significant brow ptosis who decline correction should have conservative upper lid blepharoplasty. While the patient is supine, the brow rests higher than when they are sitting upright. As such, the markings should be more conservative in the supine position.

Finally, the patient is placed in a sitting position and symmetry is assessed with eyes open and closed (Fig. 9.15). Forceps are used to reconfirm that the proposed skin excision is appropriate.

9.7 Anesthesia

The choice of anesthesia is driven by patient preference, patient health, financial concerns, and other simultaneous procedures performed. Local injection is always utilized for comfort (even under general anesthesia) and the hemostatic effect of the added Epinephrine. Systemic anesthesia may vary from mild to deep sedation requiring airway control with laryngeal masked airway or endotracheal intubation. For office-based blepharoplasty, oral sedation will reduce anxiety and improve comfort during the injection of local anesthetic. Monitored intravenous sedation anesthesia is best performed by appropriately trained personnel, allowing the surgeon to concentrate on the procedure. While general anesthesia is rarely necessary for an isolated blepharoplasty, it may be useful when other, more invasive procedures are also being performed.

For local anesthesia, Lidocaine (Xylocaine hydrochloride 1%) with epinephrine 1:100,000 is mixed in a 1:1 ratio with bupivacaine (Marcaine 0.5%) without epinephrine. This combination provides prolonged anesthesia with an epinephrine dilution of 1:200,000. The Lidocaine allows for a quick onset of anesthesia while the epinephrine and Marcaine help to prolong its effect.

The technique used to inject the local anesthetic is crucial to patient-comfort. This can easily be done without sedation or oral agents in appropriately chosen patients. If inappropriately performed, the patient will remember this portion of the procedure above others. Despite an excellent result, it may affect their referral of other patients. The use of 1 cc syringes with 30-gauge needles allows for a very slow infusion and accurate placement of the local anesthetic. By verbally preparing the patient for a brief sting, followed by spreading numbness, they will be more tolerant of the experience. With this technique it is not necessary to use bicarbonate with the local anesthetic. A useful technique in patients who are anxious or sensitive is to dilute 1 cc of the local anesthetic mixture noted above with 9 cc of normal saline. This one-tenth dilution is then placed into 1 cc syringes and utilized as the initial block to the eyelid. The normal saline dilution

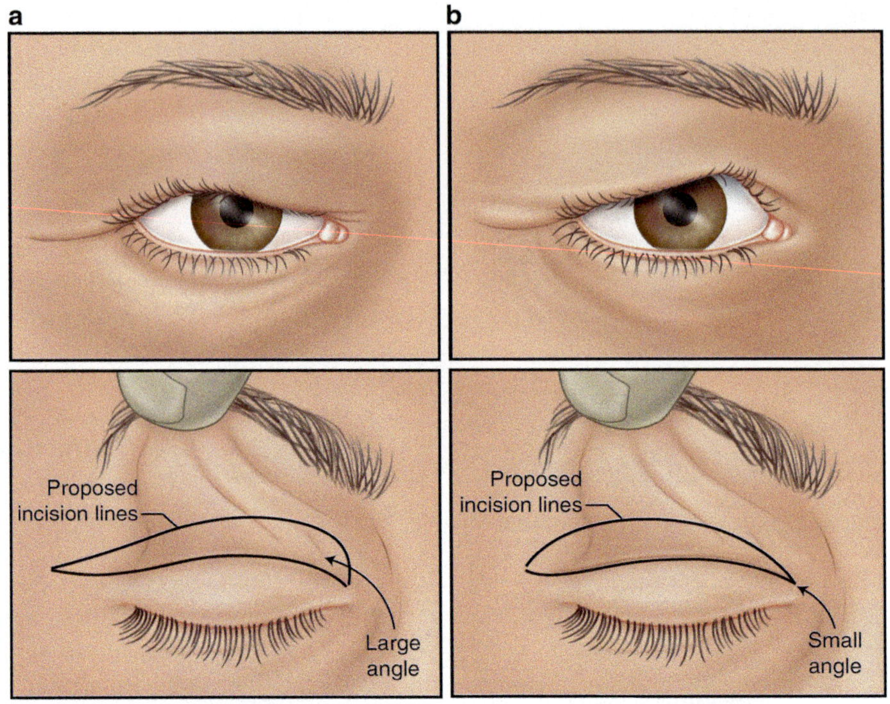

Fig. 9.14 (**a**) Excess medial skin can be addressed with a wider angle where the superior incision meets the inferior lid crease incision (*arrow*). (**b**) Conversely, patients with less dermatochalasis medially would benefit from a narrower angle where the superior incision meets the inferior lid crease incision (*arrow*)

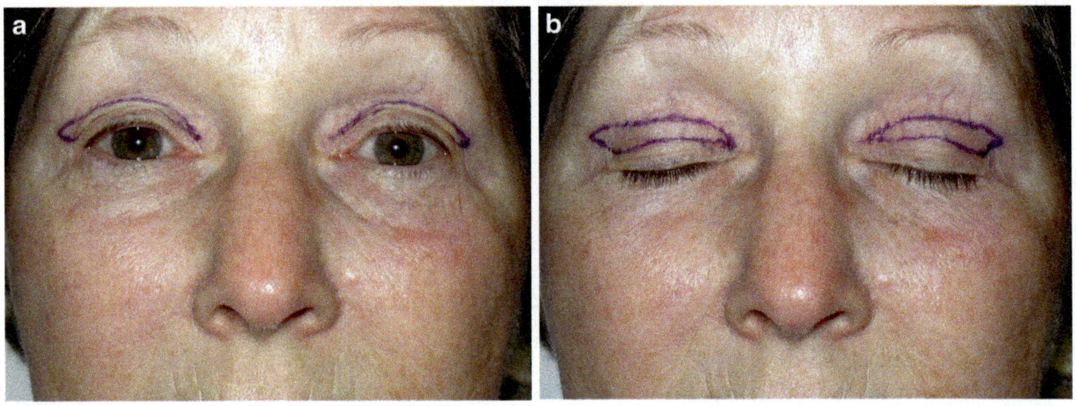

Fig. 9.15 Marking symmetry is assessed with the patient sitting upright. Comparisons are made with eyes (**a**) open and (**b**) closed

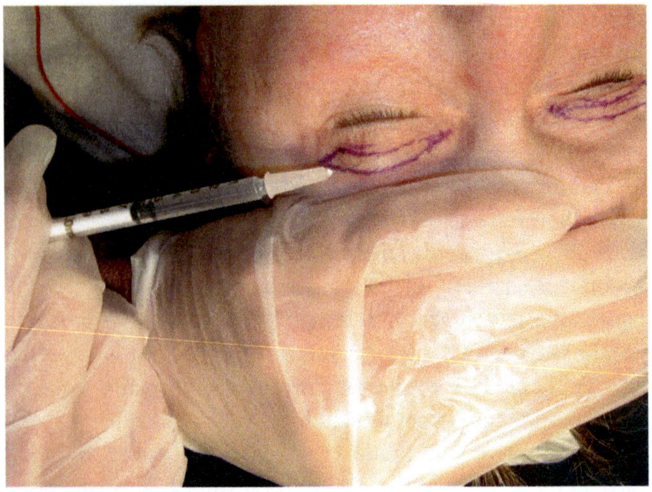

Fig. 9.16 A superficial injection into eyelid skin will ease dissection and encourage vasoconstriction

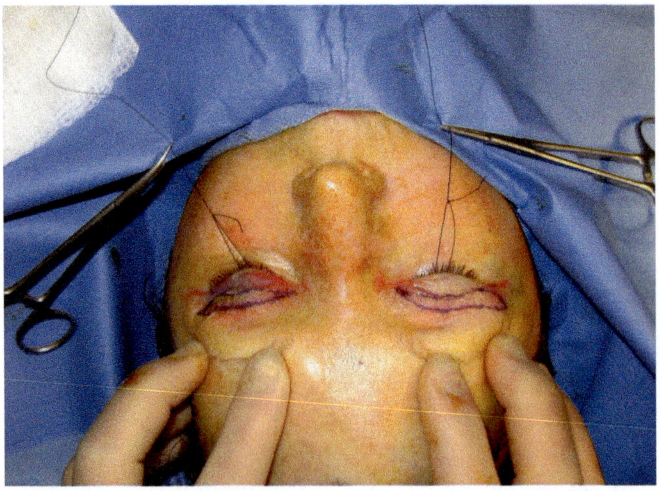

Fig. 9.17 A 4–0 silk traction suture helps to position the eyelid for surgical incisions

decreases the acidity and minimizes discomfort. This is done before the surgical prep and additional full-strength local anesthetic anesthetic is added, without discomfort, prior to the surgical incision. Generally, 1–3 cc of local anesthetic per eyelid is adequate. The initial injection is placed superficially into the eyelid skin to ease dissection and to encourage vasoconstriction (Fig. 9.16). Additional local anesthetic is injected into the medial fat pad with care taken to direct the needle away from the eye. Blocks to the supratrochlear and supraorbital nerves are an option, but rarely necessary.

9.8 The Surgical Prep

A full-face prep from below the jaw line up to the hairline is performed using Betadine solution (paint). Betadine scrub (soap) is toxic to the cornea and is never used for the face. A cotton tipped applicator dipped in Betadine is used to prep the lash line. The prep is always preceded by a topical anesthetic drop to block ocular irritation. Prep sponges are used in a dabbing fashion over the eyelids so as not to erase the carefully crafted surgical markings. The remainder of the face is painted with the Betadine solution and blotted dry. The patient is draped with the mouth and nose left open in the surgical field. Full face exposure decreases the risk of oxygen tenting, which can result in a fire hazard, and is less claustrophobic.

9.9 The Surgery

Incisional options include a #15 scalpel blade, electrosurgical radio frequency or monopolar cutting devices ,or laser. While any of these options allow for an accurate incision, it is the author's preference to use radio frequency or monopolar instrumentation. Prior to incision a 4–0 silk suture is placed through the lid margin and placed on traction (Fig. 9.17). The lower lid crease incision is performed first. The hands are positioned as described for drawing of the surgical markings. Using the nondominant hand to elevate the brow, and as a rest for the operating hand, improves control. A right-handed surgeon has more control when sweeping the cutting instrument backhand from left to right. The surgeon's hand applies gentle counter traction against the lid margin suture and minimal cutting energy is necessary to observe wound separation (Fig. 9.18). This minimizes the risk of incising beyond the very thin eyelid skin and injuring other lid structures or the cornea. It is prudent to use a corneal protector.

After the lid crease incision is completed, the superior incision is opened in a similar fashion. Using cautery a skin flap is then dissected from the orbicularis (Fig. 9.19). Several bleeding vessels will be encountered and should be cauterized.

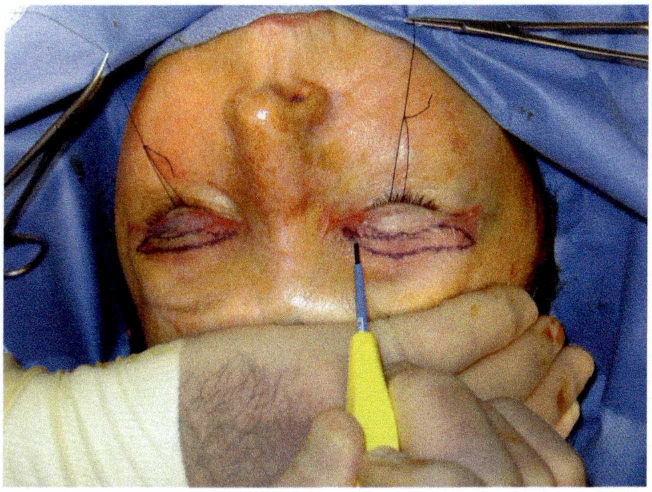

Fig. 9.18 The surgeon's nondominant hand applies gentle counter traction against the lid margin suture. Minimal cutting energy is necessary to observe wound separation. This keeps incision depth to a minimum, protecting deeper structures

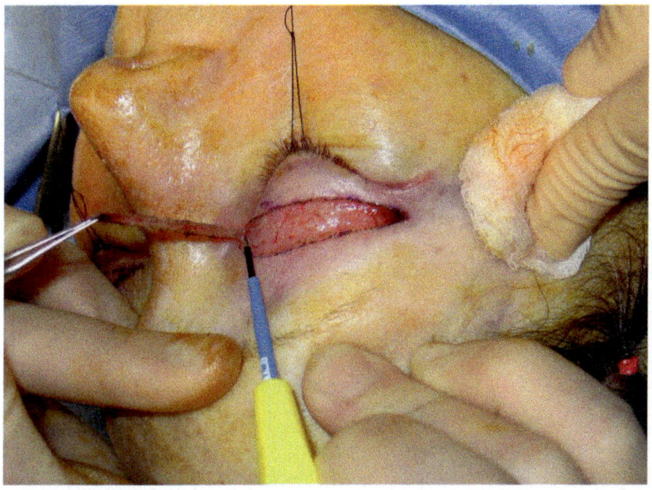

Fig. 9.19 Gentle cautery is used to separate the thin eyelid skin from the underlying orbicularis oculi muscle

The surgeon now has a view of the orbicularis oculi muscle across the wound bed. Preservation of all or some of the orbicularis muscle will decrease the potential for lagophthalmos and dry eye [10]. In patients with full lids, partial debulking of the orbicularis may be necessary to create a more aesthetic result. If no lid crease fixation is to be performed, then a higher opening in the orbicularis medially and centrally will allow access to the fat pockets while preserving orbicularis oculi muscle. If lid crease fixation to the levator aponeurosis is anticipated, the opening should occur lower in the wound bed with excision of a small band of orbicularis.

The orbicularis muscle is opened at its most medial extent with the incision extended to approximately mid-pupil. This should allow adequate access to the nasal (medial) and

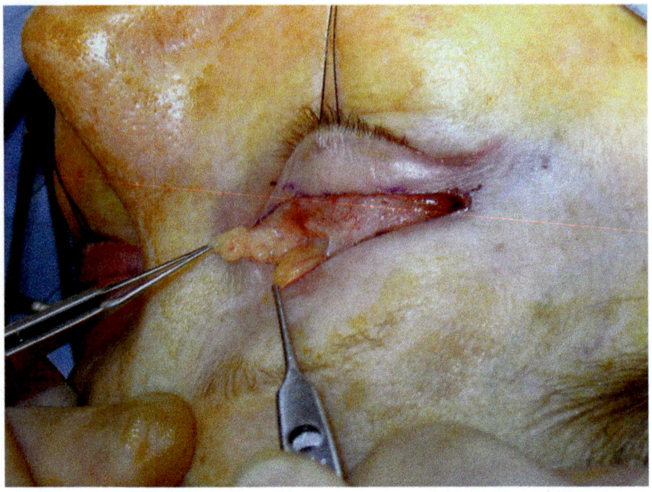

Fig. 9.20 A horizontal incision is made through the orbicularis oculi muscle and orbital septum exposing the nasal and central fat pads. A conservative excision of fat is performed based upon the amount of fat present and the degree of lid sculpting desired

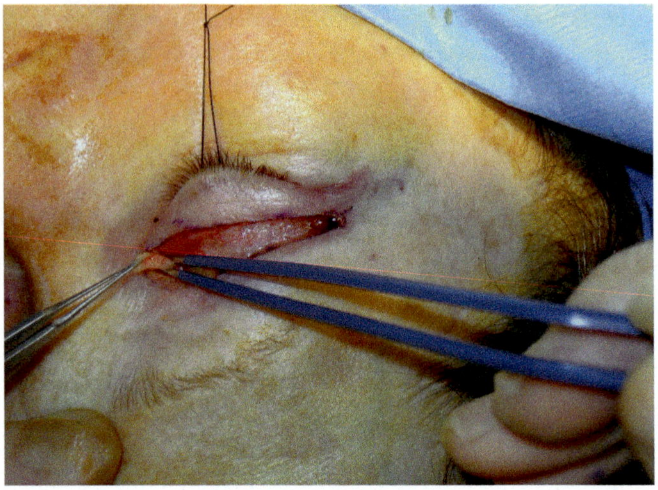

Fig. 9.21 Bipolar cautery is applied to the more vascular nasal fat pad prior to excision. Bleeding vessels in the area can be more difficult to identify when the fat pad retracts into the orbit

central (preaponeurotic) fat pads (Fig. 9.20). The nasal fat is often paler than the preaponeurotic fat, which is more yellow in color. The preaponeurotic fat is relatively avascular and minimal cautery is necessary during excision. The nasal fat pad is more vascular and it is prudent to apply bipolar cautery to its base prior to excising the exposed fat (Fig. 9.21). Gentle spreading in the medial pocket with tenotomy scissors may help to better expose the more fibrotic fat in this area. It is common for the minimally sedated patient to experience greater discomfort in this area and require injection of additional local anesthesia. Gentle globe pressure may also help to identify the fat pockets for excision. Care should be taken not to overexcise fat and create a hollow, gaunt appearing upper eyelid. It is important to remember that generally patients lose fat in the periorbital area with age and overexcision will result in even greater hollowing of the eyes later in life.

Care must be taken when exposing the anterior surface of the levator aponeurosis to avoid disinsertion from the tarsal plate with resultant blepharoptosis. The levator aponeurosis will be identified just posterior to the preaponeurotic fat. If the orbital septum is opened more superiorly, the potential for injury to the levator aponeurosis is minimized. This will also provide excellent access to the nasal and central fat pads, which can be excised in accordance with the preoperative plan and the amount of visible fat prolapsed.

Lid crease fixation is not performed in every patient. It may be indicated when the surgeon is attempting to balance preexisting lid crease asymmetry or to create a more defined pretarsal area beneath the lid fold. When utilized, it is performed as the last step prior to wound closure. Small bites of aponeurosis, positioned at the desired lid crease position, can be incorporated into the running skin closure. Greater accuracy may be achieved with the use of separate interrupted fixation sutures. A 7–0 Vicryl (polyglactin) works well for this purpose. Three to five interrupted sutures are spread across the wound opening where it spans the aponeurosis. The knot is buried by first placing the suture, in a forehand fashion, through the levator aponeurosis at the appropriate height for the lid crease. This is determined by using forceps to elevate the inferior lip of the incision to the desired height. The suture is then placed through the orbicularis muscle, just deep to the skin, at the inferior wound margin. When securing the suture, it is tightened slowly to the point that the pretarsal skin is elevated to an appropriate height. Overtightening should be avoided, as this may create an overly deep lid crease. Identical sutures are placed across the eyelid as necessary (Fig. 9.22). Having the patient look up will allow the surgeon to assess the lid crease position as the levator elevates the wound margin.

Final wound closure is performed with a running 6–0 Prolene suture. The suture is placed through skin approximately 10 mm medial to the incision. It exits from the skin on the superior aspect of the wound where it begins medially. It is then run in a continuous fashion across the wound. The last bite enters the skin adjacent to the lateral most aspect of the wound, and the needle is directed 1 cm lateral to the wound where it exits the skin. This continuous suture is not tied at its medial or lateral extent (Fig. 9.23). Three small Steri-Strips, over Mastisol, are used at each end to fold the suture over in a fashion that will keep it from slipping (Fig. 9.24). This technique allows for some tissue expansion during healing which helps to improve the final appearance of the wound. The technique also facilitates suture removal as it can be snipped centrally with the medial and lateral halves each removed in one gentle pull. At the conclusion of

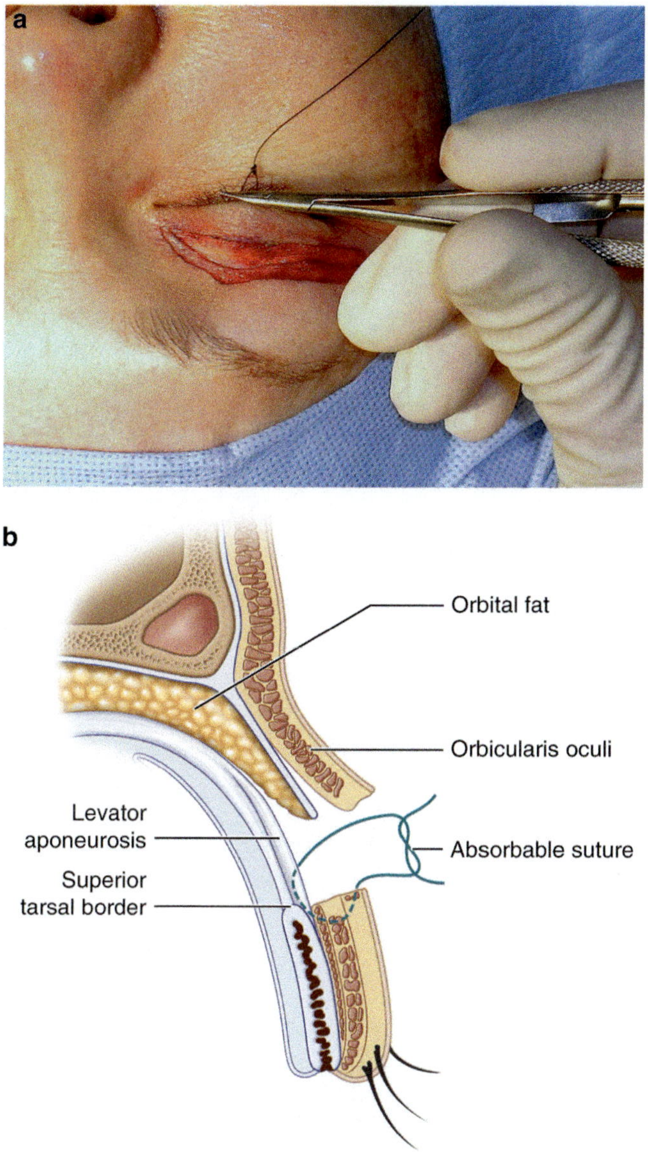

Fig. 9.22 (**a**) Lid crease fixation is defined with 7–0 Vicryl suture. The knot is buried by first placing the suture, in a forehand fashion, through the levator aponeurosis at the appropriate height for the lid crease. The suture is then placed through the orbicularis muscle, just deep to the skin, at the inferior wound margin. When securing the suture, it is tightened slowly to the point that the pretarsal skin is elevated to an appropriate height. Identical sutures are placed across the eyelid as necessary. (**b**) Artists drawing of lid crease fixation suture

the case, antibiotic ophthalmic ointment is applied to the wound.

9.10 Postoperative Management

Patients are instructed in routine postoperative care. Cold compresses are applied to the eyes as tolerated for the first two to three postoperative days. Commercial gel masks are available and easy to use. Alternatively, small zip lock bags

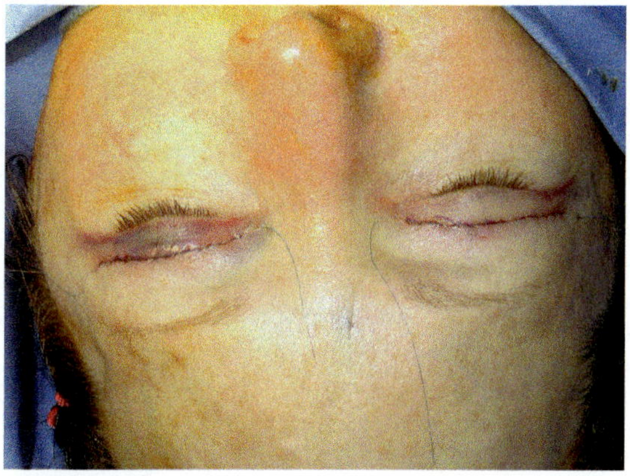

Fig. 9.23 (Photo and illustration) The suture is placed through skin approximately 10 mm medial to the incision. It exits from the skin on the superior aspect of the wound where it begins medially. It then runs in a continuous fashion across the wound. The last bite enters the skin adjacent to the lateral most aspect of the wound, and the needle is directed 1 cm lateral to the wound where it exits the skin

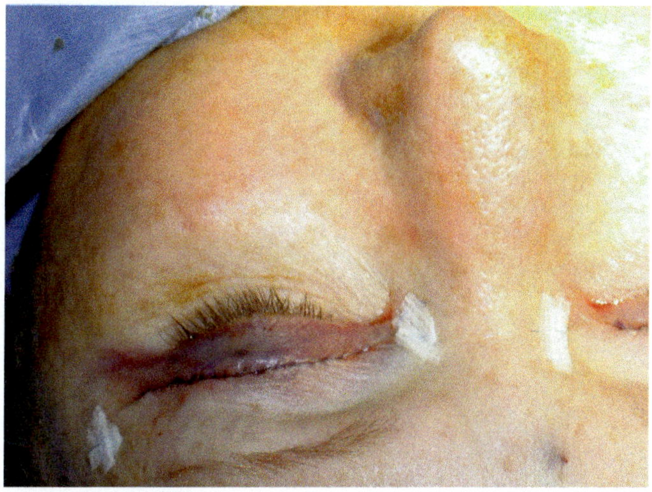

Fig. 9.24 Three small Steri-Strips, over Mastisol, are used at each end of the wound. The free suture ends are folded and locked over small segments of Steri-Strips. This technique allows for tissue edema during healing and helps to minimize scarring

of frozen peas work nicely and can be rotated through the freezer for reuse. Patients are instructed to keep their head elevated using pillows, or a recliner chair, for the first 3 days postoperatively. Patients are advised to not bend at the waist or lift anything over five pounds. Antibiotic ophthalmic ointment is applied to the wounds twice a day. During the first few days the eyelids may not close completely, and it may be necessary to place antibiotic ointment in the eye as well. Patients should be advised that the ointment will blur their vision.

After 3 days, patients are instructed to use warm compresses. This will soften dried blood at the wound and allow for gentle cleaning of the area. On postoperative day 7, the wound will be cleaner, allowing for easier suture removal.

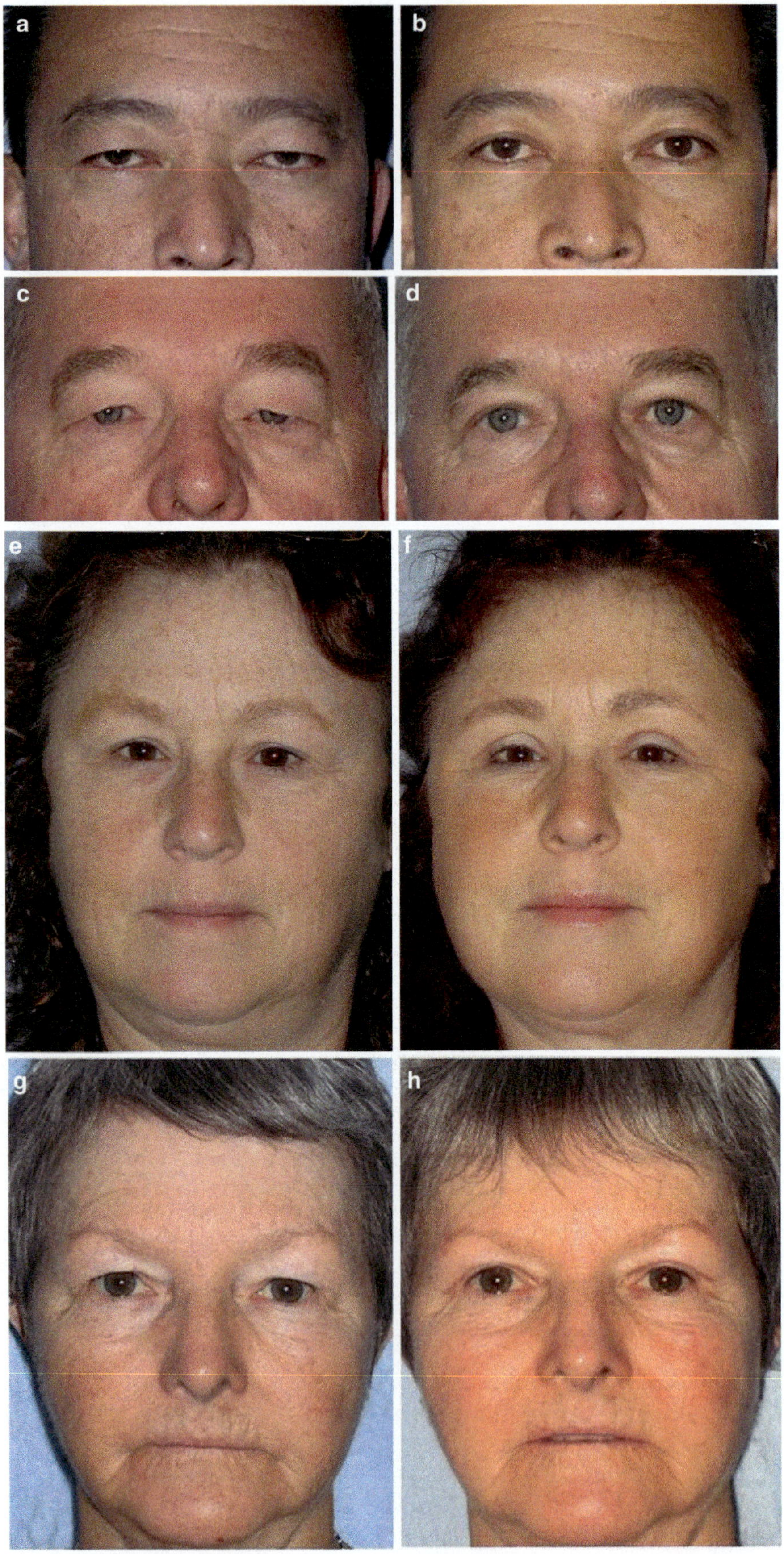

Fig. 9.25 (**a**) Forty-five-year-old male with dermatochalasia causing pseudoptosis. (**b**) Postoperative photo shows symmetric pretarsal show and lid creases. Notice that the patient is still exerting brow elevation (creases) to maintain brow in acceptable position. (**c**) Sixty-seven-year-old male also with significant pseudoptosis. Hanging skin fold causes lash ptosis and blepharitis. (**d**) Postoperatively, this conservative result shows the lid margin and improved function and appearance. A small drop in brow position is evident but the patient was prepared for this during preoperative counseling. (**e**) Forty-two-year-old lady with familial history of heavy lid skin. (**f**) Postoperatively, she is pleased to be able to wear eyeliner and shadow. (**g**) Sixty-five-year-old lady with pseudoptosis and significant temporal hooding. (**h**) Reasonable resolution is achieved postoperatively although greater improvement with a brow lifting procedure would have been possible

Following suture removal, patients are instructed to avoid rubbing the eyelids as this may result in wound dehiscence. Patients should also be cautioned of hypesthesia below the incision line. As recovery progresses and patients return to the use of eyeliner, they may abruptly discover the hypesthetic lid margin, prompting an urgent call to the surgeon. The patient's cornea is assessed and the presence of lagophthalmos or punctuate corneal staining should encourage the aggressive use of artificial tears and ointment until such time that it resolves. If the patient is doing well at the 1 week postoperative check, they are instructed to return for a final examination 6–8 weeks following surgery. Pre- and postoperative photographs are compared for every case and help the surgeon to refine their technique (Fig. 9.25).

9.11 Complications

As mentioned previously, stand alone upper eyelid blepharoplasty in the hands of an experienced eyelid surgeon is a generally straightforward procedure. As such, most complications are not severe, respond to conservative care such as eyelid lubricants and reassurance, and are mostly self-limiting. These complications include prolonged bruising and swelling, mild lagophthalmos, exposure keratitis with dry eye symptoms, and lid tightness. Oral steroid can be used if swelling persists, and typically allow quick resolution. On rare occasion, vision threatening complications can develop, such as intraoperative or postoperative hemorrhage. Please refer to Chap. 11 for a detailed discussion of these issues.

Other, nonvision threatening, but more significant complications [11] include postoperative ptosis, wound issues, eyelid crease asymmetry, over or undercorrections, and allergic reactions to medications. Most cases of postoperative ptosis are related to edema and resolve over the first few weeks after surgery, with or without oral steroids. When ptosis persists, or is associated with reduced levator function, levator injury should be suspected. In these cases, the wound may require exploration to address muscular or aponeurotic lacerations. Wound infection, dehiscence, and epithelial suture cysts can occur. These are managed with antibiotics, resuturing, and cyst removal as needed. Eyelid crease asymmetry should be followed for 6 months, and only revised should it be an issue to the patient. Patients typically are more concerned with the symmetry of the pretarsal lid show (lid fold to lid margin distance) than with the height of the crease. In either instance, skin re-excision or formal crease formation may be necessary. Undercorrection of skin removal requires re-excision, while overcorrection may require excision on the opposite side if excess skin exists. Finally, allergic skin and conjunctival reactions to topical medications can be very bothersome to patients. Treatment involves removing the offending medication and adding topical anti-inflammatory agents as needed.

9.12 Conclusion

Upper lid blepharoplasty can be a very satisfying surgical procedure for both surgeon and patient. With appropriate counseling, planning, and surgical technique, a very predictable result can be achieved. Recognizing that the eyelids are affected by other facial structures, and being sensitive to the effects of brow position, lid margin position, dry eyes, and lower lid laxity will help the surgeon to achieve the best results possible.

References

1. Dupuis C, Rees TD. Historical notes on blepharoplasty. Plast Reconstr Surg. 1971;47:246–51.
2. Miller CC. Cosmetic surgery: the correction of featural imperfections. 2nd ed. Chicago: Oak; 1908. p. 40–2.
3. Miller CC. Cosmetic surgery: the correction of featural imperfections. Philadelphia: FA Davis; 1924. p. 30–2.
4. Costaneras S. Blepharoplasty for herniated intraorbital fat: anatomic basis for a new approach. Plast Reconstr Surg. 1951;8(1):46–58.
5. Korn BS, Kikkawa DO, Hicok KC. Identification and characterization of adult stem cells from human orbital adipose tissue. Ophthal Plast Reconstr Surg. 2009;25:27–32.
6. Sang-Rog Oh, Weerawan C, et al. Analysis of upper eyelid fat pad changes with aging. San Francisco: ASOPRS; 2009.
7. Sires BS, Saari JC, Garwin GG, et al. The color difference in orbital fat. Arch Ophthalmol. 2001;119:868–71.
8. Morley AM, Malhotra R. Subconjunctival prolapse of the palpebral lobe of the lacrimal gland occurring in association with occult orbital fat herniation. Orbit. 2009;28(6):430–2.
9. Beer GM, Kompatscher P. A new technique for the treatment of lacrimal gland prolapse in blepharoplasty. Aesthet Plast Surg. 1994 Winter;18(1):65–9.
10. Saadat D, Dresner SC. Safety of blepharoplasty in patients with preoperative dry eyes. Arch Facial Plast Surg. 2004;6(2): 101–4.
11. Schiller JD, Bosniak S. Blepahroplasty: conventional and incisional laser techniques. In: Mauriello JA, editor. Unfavorable results of eyelid and lacrimal surgery: prevention and management. Boston: Butterwoth-Heinemann; 2000. p. 3–26.

Adjunctive Procedures in Upper Eyelid Blepharoplasty: Internal Brow Fat Sculpting and Elevation, Glabellar Myectomy, and Lacrimal Gland Repositioning

10

Dan Georgescu, Geeta Belsare, John D. McCann, and Richard L. Anderson

Key Points

- The upper eyelid blepharoplasty incision provides direct access to those brow, glabellar, and orbital structures that may contribute to brow ptosis and upper eyelid crowding and fullness.
- Adjunctive procedures that can be performed via the upper eyelid blepharoplasty incision at the same setting as blepharoplasty include internal brow fat sculpting and elevation, glabellar myectomy, and lacrimal gland repositioning.
- Internal brow elevation can be achieved by releasing the brow retaining ligaments (orbital ligament and the anterior leaf of the deep galea) that tether the brow to the lateral orbital rim. This allows the lateral and central brow to slide upward under the action of frontalis muscle. Internal brow fat pad sculpting lightens the brow tissues, further improving the position of the brow over the supero-lateral orbital rim.
- Although not as effective as those procedures that lift the brows from above, internal brow elevation and brow fat pad sculpting can be excellent options for those patients concerned with postoperative morbidity, operative time, and surgery costs. In addition, these procedures offer the advantage of ease of access as they are performed through the same blepharoplasty incision.
- Internal browpexy is performed by securing the brow to the periosteum above the orbital rim. This procedure is best used in patients with involutional brow ptosis, brow asymmetry, or even facial paralysis, who are concerned with the cosmetic result. Care must be taken to prevent skin dimpling and irregularities in brow contour with this technique.
- To permanently improve the glabellar furrows and to elevate the medial brow, a glabellar myectomy can be performed by excising the corrugator and the depressor supercilii muscles via the upper eyelid blepharoplasty incision. The procerus muscle is undermined and stretched but not excised.
- We have found the trans-eyelid glabellar myectomy to be the most effective procedure for elevating the medial brow.
- The main complication of corrugator muscle removal is temporary damage to the supratrochlear nerves and the superficial branches of the supraorbital nerve. This results in transient anesthesia to the central forehead that usually resolves over a period of several months and should be discussed with the patients preoperatively.
- Corrugator and depressor supercilii muscle extirpation may be the best treatment for migraine and tension-type headaches originating in the glabellar region that are refractory to other treatment modalities.
- There are two surgical techniques utilized to correct lacrimal gland prolapsed at the time of blepharoplasty surgery: resection of the prolapsed gland and repositioning/resecuring the gland to the lacrimal fossa. Repositioning/resecuring of the gland is our favored technique, as it does not damage the gland parenchyma or the excretory ducts, which can result in dry eyes postoperatively.

10.1 Introduction

Upper blepharoplasty is the most common eyelid surgery performed today. When a patient presents with excess tissue and heaviness in the upper eyelids, it is imperative that the surgical procedure chosen takes into consideration all factors that may contribute to the fullness of the upper lids. Factors which may aggravate upper eyelid appearance and heaviness include brow ptosis, glabellar muscle activity with secondary medial brow depression and rhytid formation, and lacrimal gland dislocation with associated temporal lid fullness.

D. Georgescu (✉)
Clinical Assistant Professor, Wilmer Eye Institute, Johns Hopkins Medical Center, Baltimore, MD, USA
e-mail: dan.oculoplastics@gmail.com

G.G. Massry et al. (eds.), *Master Techniques in Blepharoplasty and Periorbital Rejuvenation*,
DOI 10.1007/978-1-4614-0067-7_10, © Springer Science+Business Media, LLC 2011

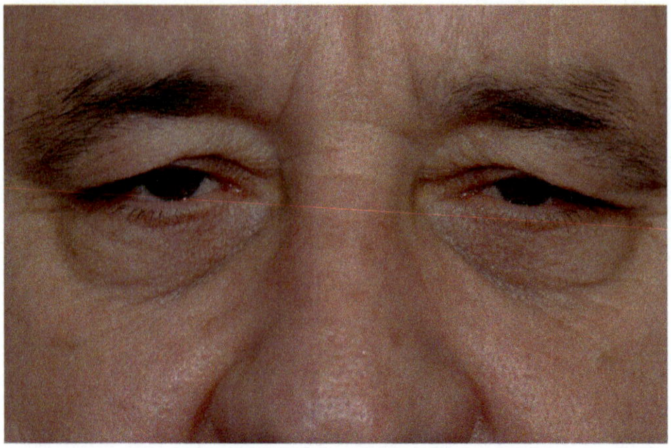

Fig. 10.1 Preoperative clinical photograph of a 55-year-old man with brow ptosis and dermatochalasis, resulting in a tired facial appearance

When one, or all, of these deficits is present in association with dermatochalasis of the upper lids, they can be addressed simultaneously at the time of the upper blepharoplasty. Three adjunctive procedures: brow sculpting and elevation, glabellar muscle extirpation, and lacrimal gland repositioning can be performed through the same incision to improve upper eyelid cosmesis and function.

The effects of gravity and aging work at least as much on the brows and the forehead as they do on the eyelids. It is common for patients to have brow ptosis, dermatochalasis, and eyelid ptosis simultaneously (Fig. 10.1). A typical, yet preventable error of aesthetic eyelid surgeons is failing to recognize the brow ptosis component when evaluating patients with upper eyelid dermatochalasis, herniated fat, and eyelid ptosis [1–6].

In the presence of significant brow ptosis, upper eyelid blepharoplasty performed alone can result in further lowering of brow position and worsening of brow ptosis. This occurs as the distance between the two structures is narrowed, and because the action of the frontalis muscle, the main elevator of the brow, is reduced as the forehead no longer has the stimulus to raise the brows in order to clear the superior field of vision [2, 7–9]. In addition, blepharoplasty, performed alone in the setting of brow ptosis, may lead to excessive skin excision. This can drag the thick skin of the brow into the upper eyelid, impairing lid dynamics and narrowing the space between the eyelashes and the brow hairs. This can worsen the appearance and make future brow lifting difficult [3, 10].

Understanding the pathophysiological mechanisms associated with brow ptosis is critical in determining the best surgical correction [7–9, 11–16]. This provides the framework for attaining the best cosmetic and functional results. Age-related brow ptosis does not occur in isolation. It is part of the general aging process of the upper face. The soft tissues of the forehead, skin, frontalis muscle, galea, and fat, slide downwards with time, as they lack deep attachments to the underlying periosteum. This causes the brows to fall, a process further influenced by an imbalance between the depressor and the elevator muscles of the brow.

Internal brow sculpting and elevation is not as effective as the direct, open coronal or endoscopic brow lift. However, with appropriate patient selection, good brow elevation can be achieved, which makes it a useful adjunctive procedure to blepharoplasty [11–17].

Often times, brow ptosis may have a significant medial component associated with heavy glabellar rhytids. When necessary, weakening the glabellar musculature may benefit the final outcome. The medial brow is depressed by the corrugator, procerus and depressor supercilii muscles, and to some degree by the medial segment or the orbicularis oculi muscle [2, 11–13]. Medial brow depression is seen clinically as frowning. People who frown frequently develop hypertrophy and hypertonicity of these depressor muscles with resultant downward slanting of the medial brow. This is seen in both men and women, although more commonly in men, and in those who spend considerable time outdoors and use the brows to protect their eyes from the sun. Corrugator muscle contraction produces vertical furrow lines in the glabellar region while procerus muscle contraction is responsible for the horizontal glabellar lines. Depressor supercilii muscle contraction adds inferior displacement of the medial brow. For those patients concerned with vertical furrowing and medial brow ptosis, glabellar myectomy can be performed at the time of upper eyelid blepharoplasty to enhance cosmetic results. This consists of extirpating the corrugator and depressor supercilii muscles and elevating the procerus muscle from its deep ligamentous attachments in the glabellar area. This procedure can be performed best via the upper eyelid blepharoplasty incision due to excellent access and visualization of these muscles.

Finally, in patients presenting with temporal upper eyelid fullness, a prolapsed lacrimal gland can sometimes be found at the time of blepharoplasty. This finding is typically involutional in nature and is seen in approximately 10% of patients at the time of surgery [18–20]. Less frequently, a prolapsed lacrimal gland can be seen in congenital ptosis, thyroid eye disease, lacrimal gland tumors, lacrimal gland inflammation, trauma, and infection. A prolapsed lacrimal gland can be resuspended to the periosteum inside the superolateral orbital rim via the blepharoplasty incision, to decrease the temporal fullness and enhance the cosmetic result.

In this chapter, we will elaborate on these three surgical procedures: internal brow fat sculpting and elevation, glabellar myectomy, and lacrimal gland repositioning, which can be performed at the time of blepharoplasty to improve the outcome of eyelid surgery. All three procedures have the advantage of being performed via the blepharoplasty incision. This not only cuts down on costs and operative time but also increases patient acceptance and cosmetic results.

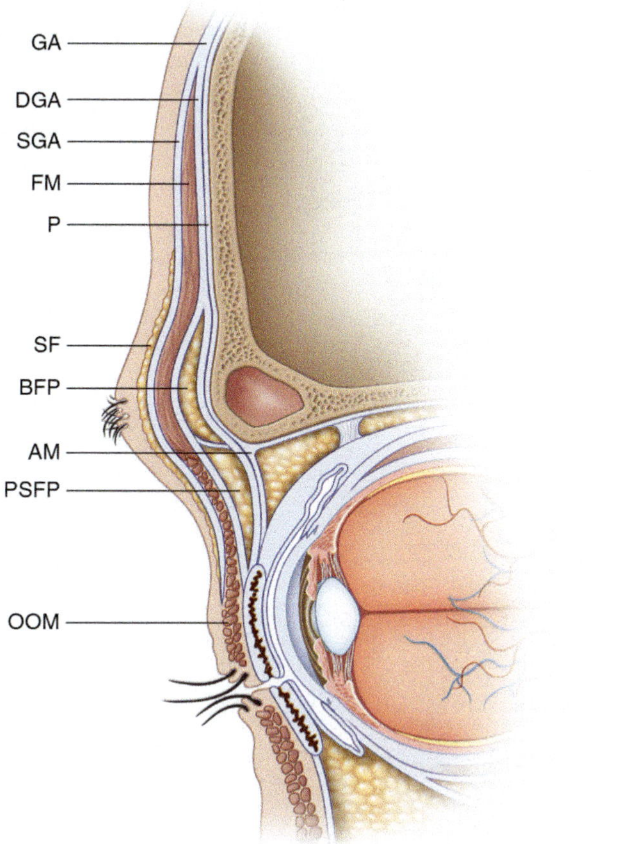

Fig. 10.2 Superior orbital rim anatomy (artist's rendition of a sagittal section at the level of the pupil). *GA* galea aponeurotica; *DGA* deep galea aponeurotica; *SGA* superficial galea aponeurotica; *FM* frontalis muscle; *P* periosteum; *SF* subcutaneous fat; *BFP* brow fat pad; *AM* arcus marginalis; *PSFP* preseptal fat pad; *OOM* orbicularis oculi muscle

10.2 Anatomical Considerations and Preoperative Evaluation

The brow is a complex structure composed of a muscular layer sandwiched between two layers of fat [2, 7–9]. Most superficially, under the thick forehead skin, the subcutaneous fat lies on top of an interdigitation of the frontalis and the orbicularis oculi muscles. The muscle layer is covered anteriorly by the superficial galea and posteriorly by the anterior leaf of the deep galea (Fig. 10.2). Laterally, beneath the muscular layer, above the orbital rim, and between the leafs of the deep galea sits the brow fat pad which continues inferiorly, below the rim, as the retro-orbicularis oculi fat (ROOF) [2, 7–9]. The ROOF is situated above and anterior to the orbital septum and should not be confused with the preaponeurotic fat pad of the eyelid which is situated behind the orbital septum. Medially, the anterior leaf of the deep galea gives rise to the fascia that covers the corrugator muscle.

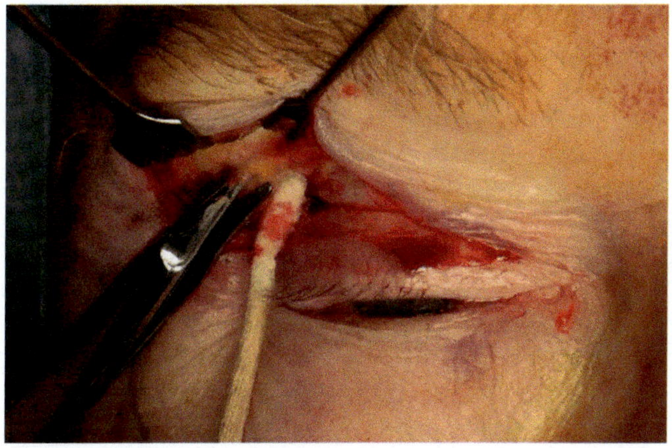

Fig. 10.3 Intraoperative photograph showing the release of the orbital ligament at the supero-lateral orbital rim with Stevens scissors to enter the plane between the posterior leaf of the deep galea and periosteum. Release of the orbital ligament allows the brow to elevate under the action of the frontalis muscle

Laterally, the anterior leaf of the deep galea has a dense attachment to the orbital ligament, which is fused to the lateral orbital rim periosteum and the lateral canthal tendon. It is the orbital ligament and the anterior leaf of the deep galea that must be released to allow the brow to move upward under the action of the frontalis muscle (Fig. 10.3).

In addition to brow height, two other issues need to be addressed in the preoperative evaluation of the patient with brow ptosis: brow symmetry and brow contour. The brow height is apparent to the patient and addressed with the elevation inherent to surgery. However, many patients with asymmetrical brows may not be aware of it. It is important to point out brow and facial asymmetry and give patients reasonable expectations of what improvements can be made. In general, eyebrow and forehead surgery can be expected to reduce but not completely correct asymmetry. Brow contour, on the other hand, is not something patients usually complain of, as opposed to height or symmetry. However, the contour is an important variable of brow aesthetics. Most women prefer a higher lateral than medial brow position. This is particularly important in patients who have downward slanting brows preoperatively. Once the patient's expectations have been determined, a treatment plan can be carefully formulated and presented.

10.3 Internal Brow Fat Sculpting and Elevation

This procedure was initially described by McCord et al. who recommended internal brow sculpting followed by reattachment of the brow to a higher position [6]. Attaching the brow to the periosteum above the orbital rim is now commonly performed by many surgeons [3, 4, 6, 14]. This can be very useful in the treatment of involutional brow ptosis, brow asymmetry, and even facial palsy, when there is significant concern with postoperative scarring. However, for patients with an intact facial nerve it can actually prevent the action of the frontalis muscle and limit the natural elevation and animation of the brow. In addition, it can result in skin dimpling and an irregular brow contour, if sutures are placed too superficially. These problems usually resolve when the anchoring sutures dissolve. However, if nonresorbable sutures are used, these complications can be longer lasting and unsightly.

Our group has reported on 15 years of experience of a modified internal brow elevation technique that achieves excellent results with minimal side effects and no restriction in voluntary brow elevation [3, 10]. Our standard technique avoids fixating the frontalis muscle to periosteum and instead releases the brow retaining ligaments, the anterior leaf of the deep galea, and the orbital ligament that tether the brow down laterally. If the brow has an excessive fat pad, some of the fat is sculpted to decrease brow heaviness [17]. However, care is taken to leave enough fat over the lateral orbital rim to prevent the skin from adhering to the bone. Also it is the brow fat pad, and not the frontalis muscle, which is secured to periosteum in order to avoid the complications mentioned above.

In our technique, the orbicularis oculi muscle is removed together with the skin at the time of blepharoplasty. Excision of the lateral orbicularis oculi muscle helps raise the temporal brow, much like the effect obtained with neurotoxin injection into this site. This not only weakens this brow depressor but also thins and lightens the eyelid tissue. Interestingly, we have found that, in moderate brow ptosis with good frontalis muscle function, the lateral brow is equally elevated after internal brow sculpting regardless of whether suture fixation is performed or not [10]. However, in patients with severe brow ptosis, marked brow asymmetry, or facial palsy, fixation sutures are essential to outcome. In patients in whom the brow fat pad is not in excess, it is not sculpted, but only resuspended superiorly with sutures.

In selected cases, a lateral canthal resuspension and a midface elevation can also be performed via the same upper blepharoplasty incision to further reduce inferior traction on the brow and aid in elevation. The brow, the lateral canthus, and the midface should be regarded as one functional and aesthetic unit, and should be treated at the same setting.

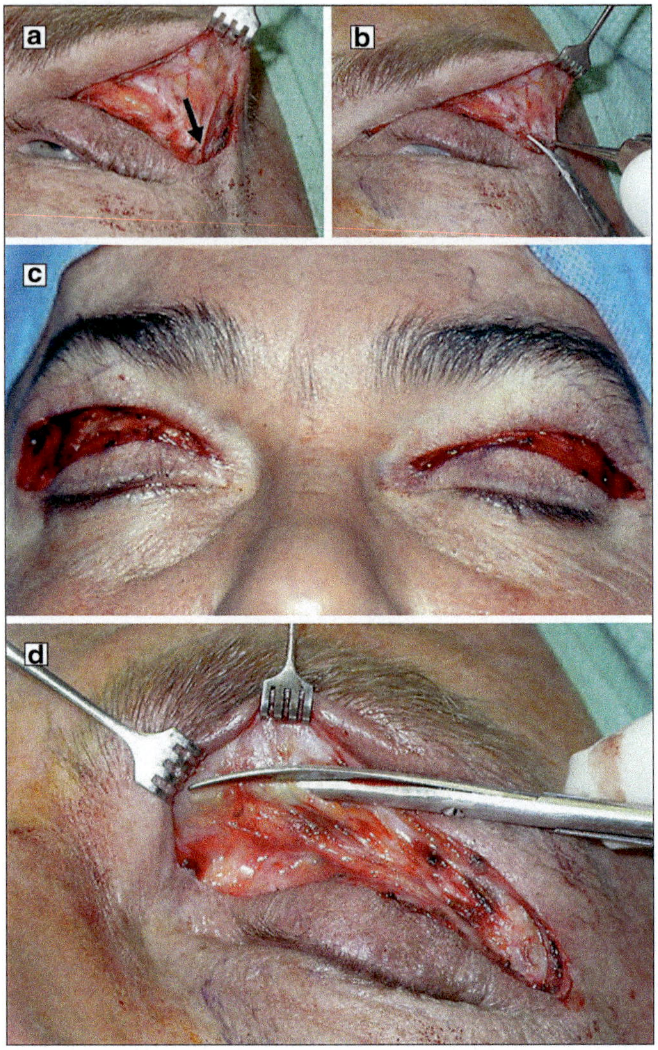

Fig. 10.4 Intraoperative photographs showing the internal brow fat sculpting and release procedure. (**a**) Upward traction with a lacrimal rake shows the anterior leaf of the deep galea (*arrow-tight band*) and the orbital ligament tethering the brow down to the lateral orbital rim. (**b**) The brow retaining ligaments are sharply incised with Stevens scissors, starting laterally. (**c**) The lateral and central part of the right brow move to a higher position immediately after the brow retaining ligaments are released on the *right side*. (**d**) The anterior leaf of the deep galea is sharply incised with Stevens scissors to expose the brow fat pad laterally and the depressors medially

10.3.1 Surgical Technique

This procedure is performed following an upper skin-muscle blepharoplasty. After the orbicularis oculi muscle is retracted superiorly, Stevens scissors are used to incise the brow retaining ligaments (Fig. 10.4a, b). This results in immediate release of the lateral and central brow (Fig. 10.4c). The anterior leaf of the deep galea and the orbital ligament are grasped with toothed forceps at the lateral orbital rim and incised across the superior orbital rim to expose the brow fat pad laterally and the depressor muscles medially (Fig. 10.4d). To further mobilize the brow, dissection is continued for 2 cm above the superior orbital rim, between the posterior leaf of the deep galea and the periosteum, using a vertical spreading technique. The excess brow fat pad is sculpted and cauterized conservatively to avoid hollowing, as brow fullness is a sign of youthfulness. In cases where midface suspension is added, dissection proceeds inferiorly at the lateral canthus, undermining the orbicularis oculi muscle in the preperiosteal plane. The orbicularis

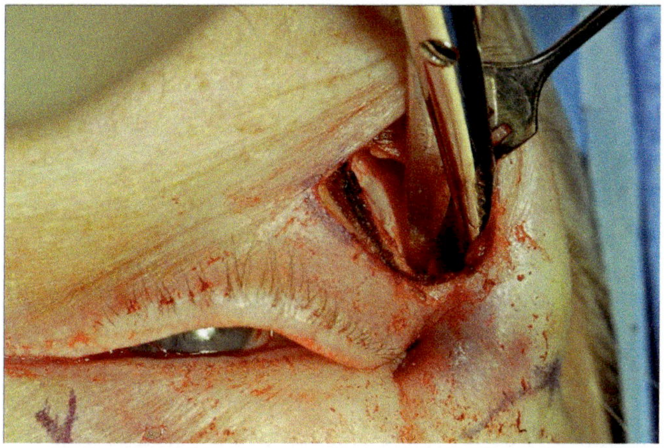

Fig. 10.5 Intraoperative photograph showing the elevation of the orbicularis oculi muscle from its deep ligamentous attachments at the lateral orbital rim using a vertical spreading technique with Stevens scissors. The orbitomalar and zygomaticomalar ligaments are released, creating a large myocutaneous flap all the way from the brow to the cheek

oculi muscle is elevated from its deep ligamentous attachments using a vertical spreading technique with Stevens scissors (Fig. 10.5). Dissection proceeds downward below the suborbicularis oculi fat (SOOF), releasing the orbitomalar and the zygomaticomalar ligaments. The lateral canthal tendon is not detached from Whitnall's tubercle. The brow fat pad is then suspended to the periosteum 1–2 cm above the lateral orbital rim with one or two interrupted 4.0 PDS or 4–0 polyglactin sutures. Care must be taken to avoid dimpling the skin. A canthopexy and a midface lift can be performed at the same setting via the upper eyelid incision using the same suture type as for the browpexy.

10.4 Glabellar Myectomy

Based on the anatomy of brow elevation, the current belief is that procedures that elevate the brow from below, through a blepharoplasty incision, are not as effective as those that elevate the brow from above [3–6]. While overlooked by many surgeons, the depressor supercilii muscle is the strongest depressor of the medial brow [21]. In our experience the medial brow is maximally and most permanently elevated by removal of the brow depressor muscles, which can be effectively performed via a blepharoplasty incision [3, 10]. Elevating the brow from above without releasing the depressor muscles will not achieve the same result on the medial aspect of the brow. We have also found that corrugator and depressor supercilii muscle extirpation is an excellent treatment for migraine and tension-type headaches originating in the glabellar region [22]. This surgery has improved more than 90% of headaches refractory to other forms of treatment. Finally, from a cosmetic standpoint, the trans-blepharoplasty glabellar myectomy effaces the vertical furrows between the brows in a reliable and reproducible manner.

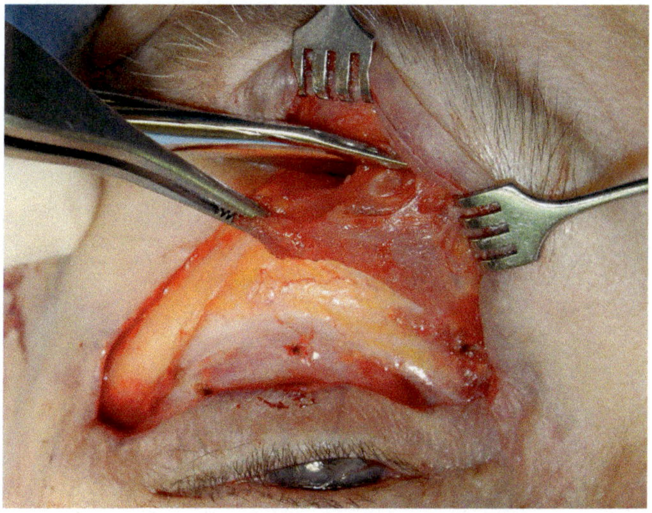

Fig. 10.6 Intraoperative photograph showing the *en block* resection of the corrugators superciliaris muscle with Stevens scissors via an upper eyelid blepharoplasty incision. The orbicularis oculi muscle is retracted superiorly with two lacrimal rakes

The main complication of corrugator muscle removal is damage to the supratrochlear nerves and the superficial branches of the supraorbital nerve, which travel through and above this muscle. This results in transient anesthesia to the central forehead that usually resolves over a period of several months [10]. Patients should be informed of this expected complication in their preoperative evaluation.

10.4.1 Surgical Technique

The corrugator and depressor supercilii muscles are excised while the procerus is undermined and stretched. This procedure can be performed in isolation, or in conjunction with upper lid blepharoplasty, using the same upper eyelid incision. The anterior leaf of the deep galea is released across the superior orbital rim to the medial canthus while the orbicularis oculi muscle is elevated with two lacrimal rakes (Fig. 10.4d). Dissection proceeds superior to the orbital rim and the corrugator muscle fascia is sharply incised with Stevens scissors to expose the muscle belly. A number of sensory nerve branches are usually seen overlying this fascia. The muscle is grasped with a heavy forceps and elevated anteriorly and superiorly over the supraorbital notch, to avoid damage to the supraorbital neurovascular bundle. The corrugator muscle is then excised en bloc to its medial attachments on the frontal bone (Fig. 10.6). The depressor supercilii muscle is then pulled from underneath the orbicularis oculi muscle at the medial canthus and excised sharply with scissors (Fig. 10.7). This results in immediate release and elevation of the medial brow (Fig. 10.8). Scissors dissection is used to further elevate the medial brow by undermining the procerus muscle and releasing its deep attachments to the bone

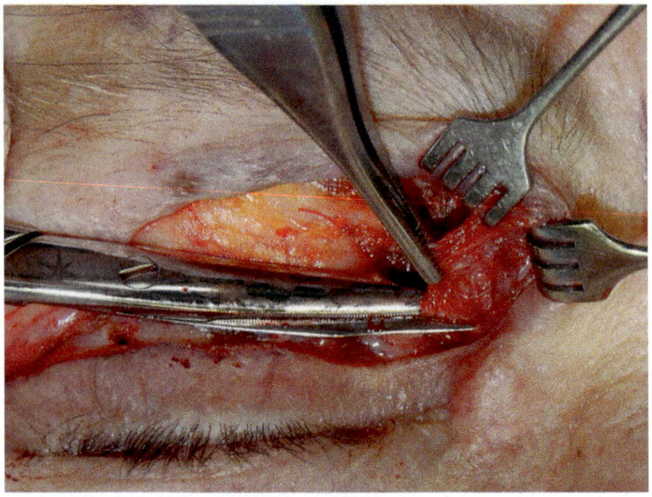

Fig. 10.7 Intraoperative photograph showing the excision of the depressor supercilii muscle with Stevens scissors via the upper eyelid blepharoplasty incision after the corrugator superciliaris muscle has been removed. The orbicularis oculi muscle is retracted medially with two lacrimal rakes. The depressor supercilii muscle is pulled from under the orbicularis oculi muscle with a heavy forceps

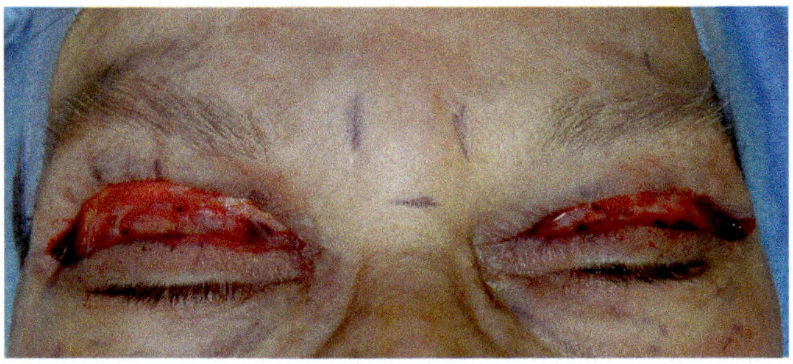

Fig. 10.8 Intraoperative photograph showing the immediate elevation of the medial and central brow on the right side after excision of the medial brow depressors: corrugators and depressor supercilii muscles

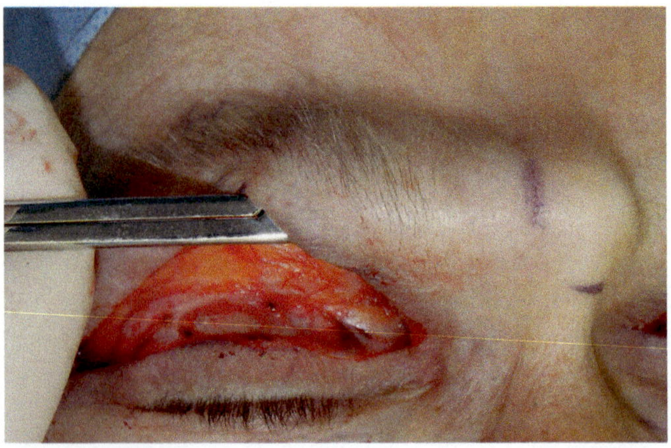

Fig. 10.9 Intraoperative photograph showing the undermining of the procerus muscle. The muscle is elevated from its deep attachments to the glabellar area with Stevens scissors

(Fig. 10.9). A tearing type release is felt at the base of the nose ("the sound of beauty"), and can be heard by both the surgeon and the patient, confirming the full release of the procerus muscle.

10.5 Lacrimal Gland Prolapse

The preoperative examination of the patient with lacrimal gland prolapse shows fullness in the temporal upper lid, which is firmer to palpation than the adjacent fat (Fig. 10.10). The lacrimal gland prolapse can be made more apparent with retropulsion of the globe and can be easily visualized with eversion of the upper eyelid. The lacrimal secretory complex is composed of the main lacrimal gland and the additional accessory glands of Krause and Wolfring [18–20]. The lacrimal gland proper is further composed of the smaller palpebral lobe and the larger orbital lobe, which normally adheres to the lacrimal gland fossa. Four ligaments suspend the gland in the lacrimal fossa. Anteriorly, bands of fascia connect the

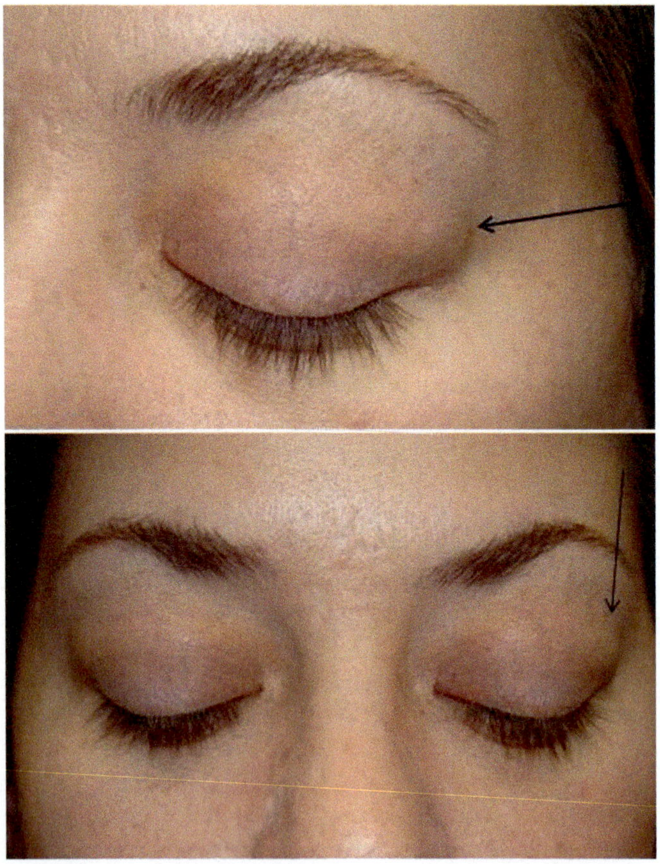

Fig. 10.10 Photograph of patient at oblique angle (*above*) and frontal view (*below*) demonstrating temporal upper lid fullness associated with lacrimal gland prolapse (*arrows*) (Photo courtesy of Guy G. Massry, MD)

lacrimal gland to the lateral margin of the levator aponeurosis. Posteriorly and superiorly, the gland is supported by fascial bands connected to periosteum. Medially, a fascial band connects the gland to Whitnall's ligament [2, 7].

There are two surgical techniques utilized to address lacrimal gland prolapse: the resection technique which removes the prolapsed part of the gland, and the repositioning technique which reinforces the prolapsed part of the gland [18–20]. Resecting the prolapsed part of the lacrimal gland has lost favor due to dry eye consequences. The accessory glands are insufficient for basal tear production. Repositioning and reinforcing the lacrimal gland to the lacrimal fossa is the generally accepted technique employed today. This simple procedure poses minimal risks for decreasing tear production since it does not violate either the lacrimal gland parenchyma or the excretory ducts.

10.5.1 Surgical Technique

As with the aforementioned procedures described in this chapter, repositioning the prolapsed lacrimal gland is performed at the time of standard upper lid blepharoplasty, through an eyelid crease incision. The skin and underlying orbicularis oculi muscle are excised and the septum is opened. The medial and central fat compartments are sculpted. The lacrimal gland is identified by its tan color and firmer consistency than the surrounding orbital fat (Fig. 10.11a). A double-armed 5.0 chromic or 5.0 PDS suture is passed through either the anterior or the inferior part of the lacrimal gland capsule (Fig. 10.11b). The gland is secured to the periosteum inside the lacrimal fossa (Fig. 10.11c). One should avoid passing the sutures through the lacrimal gland parenchyma, as this may cause bleeding and postoperative dacryoadenitis.

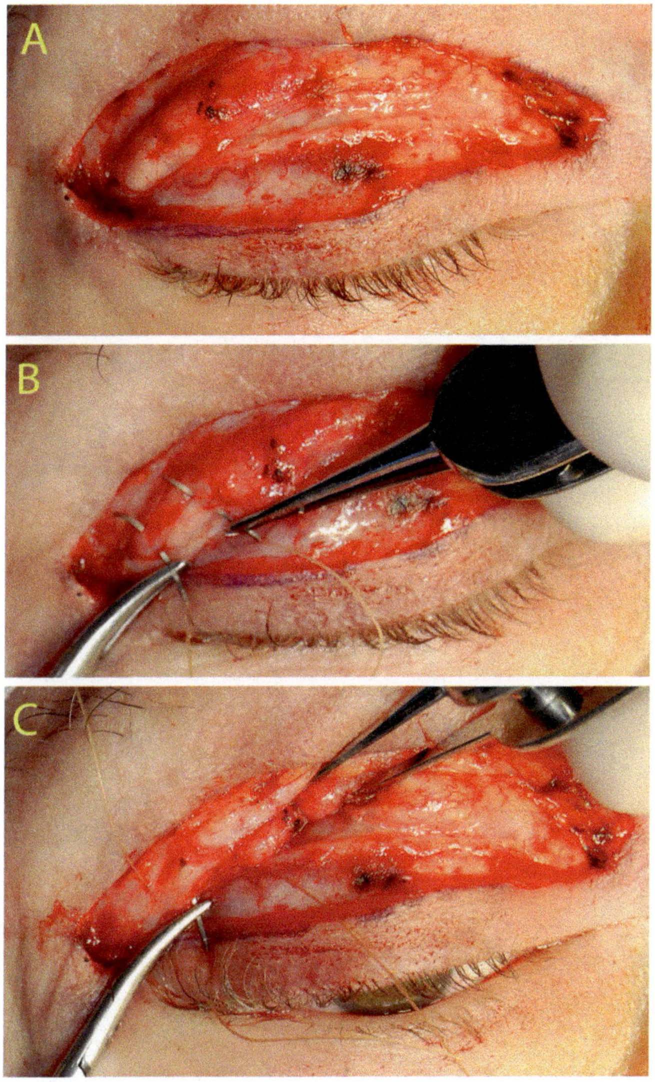

Fig. 10.11 Lacrimal gland resuspension technique. (**a**) Intraoperative photograph showing a prolapsed lacrimal gland after the orbital septum had been opened. (**b**) A double-armed 5.0 chromic gut suture is passed through the inferior aspect of the lacrimal gland capsule. (**c**) The gland is then secured to the periosteum inside the lacrimal fossa

10.6 Conclusion

Understanding the mechanisms responsible for "heavy lids" is critical in choosing the best therapeutic approach for surgical upper lid rejuvenation. It is not uncommon for brow ptosis, dermatochalasis, glabellar furrowing, and lacrimal gland prolapse to simultaneously contribute to the fullness of the upper lids. It is essential to identify all contributing factors and select the surgical plan that best suits the patients' needs. In this chapter we have reviewed how, via an upper blepharoplasty incision, the eyebrow fat can be sculpted, the brow elevated, the glabellar muscles weakened, and the displaced lacrimal gland repositioned. These are useful procedures that provide the surgeon with an effective means of directly addressing all associated deficiencies at the time of blepharoplasty via one incision.

References

1. Rafaty FM, Goode RL, Abramson NR. The brow-lift operation in a man. Arch Otolaryngol. 1978;104(2):69–71.
2. Standring S. Gray's anatomy: the anatomical basis of clinical practice. 39th ed. Philadelphia: Churchill Livingstone; 2004. ISBN ISBN-10: 0443071683.
3. Georgescu D, Anderson RL, McCann JD. Brow ptosis correction: a comparison of five techniques. Facial Plast Surg. 2010;26(3): 186–92.
4. Johnson Jr CM, Anderson JR, Katz RB. The brow-lift 1978. Arch Otolaryngol. 1979;105(3):124–6.
5. Goldstein SM, Katowitz JA. The male eyebrow: a topographic anatomic analysis. Ophthal Plast Reconstr Surg. 2005;21(4):285–91.
6. McCord CD, Doxanas MT. Browplasty and browpexy: an adjunct to blepharoplasty. Plast Reconstr Surg. 1990;86(2):248–54.

7. Lemke BN, Stasior OG. The anatomy of eyebrow ptosis. Arch Ophthalmol. 1982;100(6):981–6.
8. Knize DM. An anatomically based study of the mechanism of eyebrow ptosis. Plast Reconstr Surg. 1996;97(7):1321–33.
9. Presti P, Yalamanchili H, Honrado CP. Rejuvenation of the aging upper third of the face. Facial Plast Surg. 2006;22(2):91–6. Review.
10. Burroughs JR, Bearden WH, Anderson RL, McCann JD. Internal brow elevation at blepharoplasty. Arch Facial Plast Surg. 2006;8(1):36–41.
11. Michelow BJ, Guyuron B. Rejuvenation of the upper face. A logical gamut of surgical options. Clin Plast Surg. 1997;24(2):199–212.
12. Levine MR. Manual of oculoplastic surgery. 3rd ed. Philadelphia: Butterworth Heinemann; 2003.
13. Tyers AG. Brow lift via the direct and trans-blepharoplasty approaches. Orbit. 2006;25(4):261–5. Review.
14. Walden JL, Orseck MJ, Aston SJ. Current methods for brow fixation: are they safe? Aesthet Plast Surg. 2006;30(5):541–8.
15. McKinney P, Mossie RD, Zukowski ML. Criteria for the forehead lift. Aesthet Plast Surg. 1991 Spring;15(2):141–7.
16. Pedroza F, dos Anjos GC, Bedoya M, Rivera M. Update on brow and forehead lifting. Curr Opin Otolaryngol Head Neck Surg. 2006;14(4):283–8. Review.
17. May Jr JW, Fearon J, Zingarelli P. Retro-orbicularis oculus fat (ROOF) resection in aesthetic blepharoplasty: a 6-year study in 63 patients. Plast Reconstr Surg. 1990;86(4):682–9.
18. Morley AM, Malhotra R. Subconjunctival prolapse of the palpebral lobe of the lacrimal gland occurring in association with occult orbital fat herniation. Orbit. 2009;28(6):430–2.
19. Jordan DR, Germer BA, Anderson RL, Morales L. Lacrimal gland prolapse in craniosynostosis syndromes and poor function congenital ptosis. Ophthal Surg. 1990;21:97–101.
20. Beer GM, Kompatscher P. A new technique for the treatment of lacrimal gland prolapse in blepharoplasty. Aesthet Plast Surg. 1994 Winter;18(1):65–9.
21. Cook Jr BE, Lucarelli MJ, Lemke BN. Depressor supercilii muscle: anatomy, histology, and cosmetic implications. Ophthal Plast Reconstr Surg. 2001;17(6):404.
22. Bearden WH, Anderson RL. Corrugator superciliaris muscle excision for tension and migraine headaches. Ophthal Plast Reconstr Surg. 2005;21(6):418–22.

11 Management of Complications of Upper Eyelid Blepharoplasty

Craig N. Czyz, Vincent B. Lam, and Jill A. Foster

Key Points

- An appropriate preoperative assessment and plan minimizes the risk of postoperative complications after blepharoplasty.
- Patient selection is critical to surgical outcome. It is important to avoid surgery on high-risk patients or those with unrealistic expectations.
- Identifying preoperative ocular or systemic conditions that can hinder surgical outcome is necessary to prevent postoperative adverse events.
- It is necessary to review the use of all systemic medications and anticoagulation risks with patients prior to surgery.
- The surgeon should create a plan for the amount of skin/muscle/fat to be excised/preserved prior to proceeding with surgery.
- Detailed intraoperative measurements are important to achieve postoperative symmetry.
- Eyelid symmetry should be evaluated at various points of the procedure.
- Meticulous attention to homeostasis during surgery, and at the conclusion of the case, is essential.
- Wound closure should be performed under minimal tension.
- Be prepared to manage all potential postoperative complications, including those that you cannot prevent.

11.1 Introduction

Blepharoplasty is one of the most common aesthetic cosmetic procedures performed. In 2009, the American Society for Aesthetic Plastic Surgery stated that it was the third most common cosmetic surgical procedure performed after breast augmentation and lipoplasty [1]. As the procedure is so common and performed by many different surgical subspecialties, it is important to recognize the potential complications and appropriate management techniques to effectively reduce the risk of adverse sequelae. There are multiple potential complications that may occur after upper blepharoplasty [2–5], ranging from self-limited annoyances to severe complications resulting in permanent loss of vision.

This chapter will discuss the complications that may occur in association with upper blepharoplasty. The appropriate medical management and surgical interventions will be reviewed for each potential complication.

11.2 Complications

11.2.1 Hemorrhage

11.2.1.1 Eyelid Hematoma

An eyelid hematoma may occur during or after upper blepharoplasty and is commonly associated with anticoagulant therapy (Fig. 11.1), uncontrolled high blood pressure, trauma to the orbicularis muscle during surgery, and/or violation of the arcade vessels or deeper vasculature. Intraoperatively, visualization and cauterization of the tissues is imperative for hemostasis. Bleeding can lead to a collection of blood in tissue, which can be diffusely distributed (interstitial blood), or can manifest as a localized collection, or hematoma. It is important to distinguish between the two entities and treat each appropriately to avoid short- and long-term problems. Long-term side effects of eyelid hematomas can include fibrosis of the eyelid (malposition and/or decreased function) or pigmentary changes to the eyelid skin.

More importantly, if bleeding is extensive or progressive, it is important to assess for the presence of a retrobulbar hemorrhage by checking vision and pupillary reaction, testing retropulsion of the globe, measuring intraocular pressure,

J.A. Foster (✉)
Associate Clinical Professor, Director, Division of Oculofacial Plastic and Reconstructive Surgery, Department of Ophthalmology, Ohio State University, Columbus, OH, USA
e-mail: fosterj@jillfoster.com

G.G. Massry et al. (eds.), *Master Techniques in Blepharoplasty and Periorbital Rejuvenation*,
DOI 10.1007/978-1-4614-0067-7_11, © Springer Science+Business Media, LLC 2011

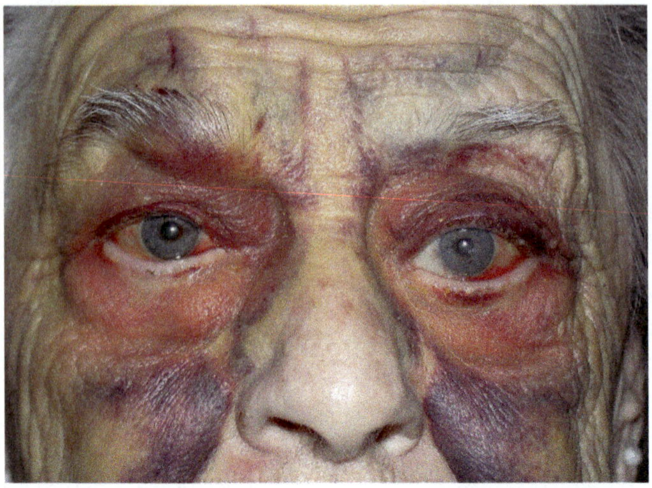

Fig. 11.1 Diffuse superficial hemorrhage following bilateral upper blepharoplasty in a patient who did not discontinue his daily 81 mg aspirin

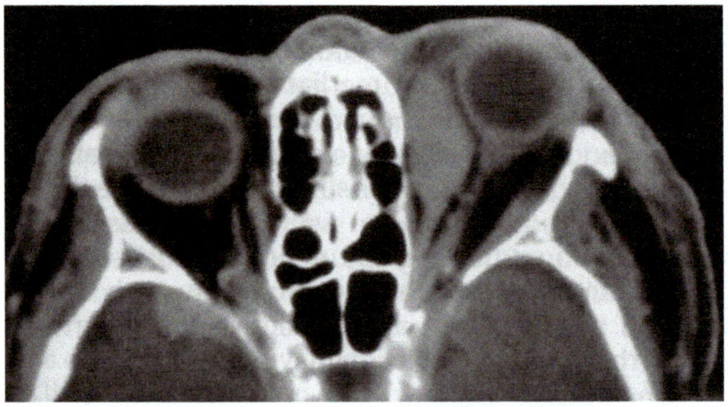

Fig. 11.2 Computed tomography of the orbits (axial) shows proptosis and a compartmentalized intraorbital hemorrhage posteromedial to the left globe

and evaluating for proptosis, as a collection of blood in the orbit is more likely to threaten vision than a similar collection in the eyelid. If there is clinical uncertainty, a computed tomography (CT) scan of the orbits may be performed to confirm or help exclude the diagnosis of orbital hemorrhage (Fig. 11.2). In the absence of a retrobulbar hematoma, treatment should begin with conservative medical management.

Medical Management

The first step in the management of intraoperative hemorrhage is to identify and control any source of active bleeding. Small leaks may be initially controlled with direct pressure held over a period of time. For bleeding at the skin edge, this is sometimes preferable as cautery may cause thermal damage to the epithelium. If the surgical wound is closed and active bleeding is noted, this may necessitate reopening the wound, identifying the source of bleeding, and reapplying cautery. For actively "pumping" arteries, a forceps or hemostat is used to grasp the vessel and stop the flow of blood. Cautery is then applied to the metallic instrument and transmitted to the tissue. In the rare circumstance that cautery is unsuccessful, thrombin, or gelfoam soaked in thrombin may be applied to the area to aid in hemostasis. If bleeding persists the vessel can be ligated with a suture when possible.

When a patient returns for a postoperative visit with an eyelid hematoma, and in the absence of active bleeding, treatment involves cold or warm compresses depending on the timing. For a diffuse (interstitial) collection of blood in the first 24–36 h after surgery, a cold compress will vasoconstrict blood vessels and decrease swelling, bleeding, and bruising. After this time, heat may speed up the breakdown and resorption of the blood. Small sequestered hematomas can be followed clinically (with compresses as above) until liquefaction has occurred. If the hematoma is localized and larger, needle aspiration should proceed. Patients who report bleeding after surgery should suspend anticoagulant therapy if medically possible. There are also many supplements and foods that affect the natural clotting process and should be discontinued until resolution of the hematoma [6] (Table 11.1).

Surgical Management

In severe or refractory cases, surgical exploration is necessary to identify and control the source of bleeding. Hematomas that continue to expand can be worrisome and lead to orbital compartment syndrome with possible permanent loss of vision.

11.2.1.2 Retrobulbar/Intraorbital Hemorrhage

Retrobulbar or intraorbital hemorrhage (Figs. 11.2 and 11.3) is one of the most feared complications of blepharoplasty. Retrobulbar hemorrhage causing orbital compartment syndrome is the most common cause of postoperative permanent vision loss. Presentation is commonly within the first 3 h after surgery, with the risk diminishing substantially after 24 h. Although less likely, hemorrhage can occur on a delayed basis. [7, 8]. In a questionnaire of members of the American Society of Ophthalmic Plastic and Reconstructive Surgery (ASOPRS), Hass et al. noted the incidence of retrobulbar hemorrhage after blepharoplasty to be 0.05% and retrobulbar hemorrhage associated with permanent vision loss 0.0045% [9]. The mechanism of permanent vision loss from retrobulbar hemorrhage is believed to be elevated intraocular and intraorbital pressure caused by the space-occupying hematoma. The rise in pressure can lead to compressive optic neuropathy or vascular ischemia of the optic nerve or retina [10–12].

Risk factors for retrobulbar hemorrhage are: thyroid associated orbitopathy, blood dyscrasias, hypertension, atherosclerosis, vascular disease, and anticoagulation [13]. Careful assessment of the patient's risk factors for hemorrhaging

Table 11.1 Medications and supplements that have effects on the natural clotting process

Advil	Daypro	Lanorinal	Ponstel
Aggrenox	Diflunisal	Lioresal	Relafen
Aleve	Di-gesic	Lodine	Robaxisal
Alka-Seltzer	Dipridacot	Magan	Rufin
Anacin	Dipyridamole	Magsal	Ru-Tess
Anaprox	Disalcid	Marnal	S-A-C
Anadynos	Dolobid	Meclofenamate	Salatin
Ansaid	Dolpm	Meclomen	Saleto
APC	Dong quai root	Mefenamic	Saliflex
Argesic	Dristan	Meloxicam	Salicylamide
Arthropan	Duoprin	Mendomen	Salocol
Arthrotec	Durgesic	Melomen	Salsalate
Arthritis pain formula	Durasal	Methocarbamol with Aspirin	Selenium
ASA	Easprin	Micrainin	Sine-aid
Axriptin	*Echinacea*	Midol	Sine-off sinus
Asocdeen-30	Ecotrin	Mobic	Sinutab
Aspergum	Emagrin	Mobidin	SK-65
Aspirin	Emprazil	Mobigesic	Soma
Atromid	Empirin with codeine	Momentum backache formula	Stanback
Axotal	Encaprin	Monacet with Codeine	Stendin
Azolid	*Ephedra* (ma huang)	Motrin	St. John's Wort
Bayer products	Equagesic	Nabumetone	St. Joseph's products
B.C. tablets/powder	Etodolac	Nalfon	Sulindac
Bextra	Etraqfon	Naprelan	Supac
Bilberry	Excedrin	Naprosyn	Synalgos-DC
Bufferin products	Feldene	Naproxen	Talwin compound
Buffets II	Fenoprofen	Neocylate	Ticlid
Buffinol	Feverfew	Norgesic	Ticlopidine
Buf-tabs	Fiorinal	Novnaproxen	Tolectin
Butalbital	Fish oil	Novodipiradol	Tolmetin
Butazolidin	Flaxseed	Nuprin	Toradol
Cama products	Flurbiprofen	Oraflex	Triaminicin
Carisoprodol	Four way cold tabs	Orudis	Trigesic
Cataflam	Gaysal-S	Oruvail	Trilisate
Chamomile	Garlic	Oxaprozin	Valdecoxib
Cheracol	Gelprin	P-A-C	Valerian
Cilostazol (Pletal)	Gemnisin	Pabalate-SF	Vanquish
Clinoril	Ginger	Pabrin buffered tabs	Vitamin E
Clopidogrel	*Ginkgo biloba*	Pamprin	Vivarin
Congesprin chewable	Ginseng	Panalgesic	Voltaren
Contac	Goody's	Parnate	Warfarin
Cope	IBU	Pepto-BiPercodan	Willow bark
Coricidin	Ibuprofen	Persantine	Yohimbe
Cosprin	Indocin	Persistin	Zactrin
Coumadin	Indomethacin	Phenylbutaxone	Zomac
CP-s	Kava kava	Plavix	Zomax
Damason P	Ketoprofen	Pletal	Zorprin
Darvon	Ketorolac	Piroxicam	

should be performed prior to performing blepharoplasty. Any patient who complains of a constellation of symptoms including pain, asymmetric swelling, proptosis, dimming of vision, or loss of vision following blepharoplasty may have a retrobulbar hemorrhage and must be evaluated and treated promptly. A complete ophthalmic examination, including visual acuity, pupil assessment, intraocular pressure, and dilated fundus examination is performed. However, if the clinical suspicion is high, none of these assessments should delay emergent surgical exploration. Clinical examination is usually sufficient for diagnosis, but as mentioned previously, orbital CT may be a useful adjunct.

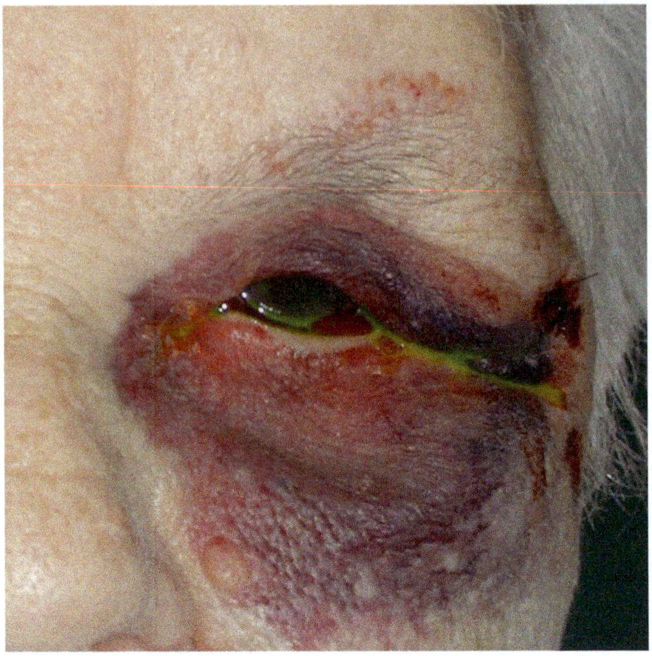

Fig. 11.3 Eyelid, subconjunctival and orbital hemorrhage

Medical Management

Intraoperatively, achievement of hemostasis is crucial in prevention of retrobulbar hemorrhage. In the postoperative period, one may consider the use of antiemetics and antitussives to help prevent Valsalva, a possible trigger for bleeding [9]. Conservative management may include the use of systemic corticosteroids to reduce soft tissue edema. If intraocular pressure is elevated, the use of topical or systemic medications to control intraocular pressure may be used to temporarily protect the optic nerve. However, treatment of elevated intraocular pressure may not be useful as the elevated intraocular pressure is due to transmitted intraorbital pressure from the space-occupying hematoma. Decreasing the intraocular pressure in the face of increased orbital pressure may further diminish intraocular blood flow. In cases where vision is intact and the hematoma is felt to be stable, progression can be followed with monitoring of the pupils, color plates, exophthalmometry, intraocular pressure, and serial Humphrey or Goldmann visual field testing.

Surgical Management

Ultimately, to prevent permanent vision loss from a retrobulbar hematoma with orbital compartment syndrome, urgent surgical intervention is required. The blepharoplasty incision is opened and the tissues are explored, cauterizing or ligating any potential sources of bleeding. Any visualized clots are excised and compartmentalized blood evacuated. If the patient's presenting condition is severe or worsens, then a lateral canthotomy and cantholysis with or without orbital decompression may be performed to decrease intraorbital pressure [14, 15]. Often, the canthotomy and cantholysis are adequate to control the intraorbital pressure and protect vision. If not, decompression of the orbit proceeds with fracture of the orbital floor and rarely the medial wall depending on the amount of volume expansion required for adequate pressure reduction. The canthus can be repaired days later to allow for further drainage if there is concern of additional hemorrhage. Conversely, the canthus may be allowed to heal spontaneously with future revision if necessary.

Following surgical intervention, adequate reduction of intraorbital pressure must be assessed. As discussed in the previous section, the patient is closely followed with monitoring of visual acuity, pupillary reactions, color plates, exophthalmometry, intraocular pressure, and serial Humphrey or Goldmann visual field testing. The obvious goal is restoration of vision and all measured parameters to the preoperative state. The key to success in all cases is the early recognition of the signs and symptoms of retrobulbar hemorrhage and aggressive immediate intervention, which provides the best chance of regaining vision [16].

11.2.2 Vision Loss

11.2.2.1 Orbital Compartment Syndrome

Orbital compartment syndrome describes a condition where there is an increase in intraorbital pressure within the confined orbital volume [17]. When the intraorbital pressure exceeds the arterial pressure, optic nerve or choroidal ischemia may lead to irreversible vision loss. In upper blepharoplasty, orbital compartment syndrome can occur secondary to a space-occupying retrobulbar/intraorbital hemorrhage. Retrobulbar/intraorbital hemorrhage and treatment options are discussed in the previous section.

11.2.2.2 Globe Rupture/Perforation

Globe rupture or perforation can occur during any periocular surgery. When performing upper blepharoplasty, the globe is at risk for perforation during injection of local anesthetics, incision, dissection, and suturing. Globe rupture is an ophthalmic emergency and can lead to permanent vision loss. Perforation risks can be decreased by the use of plastic or metallic corneoscleral protective shields (OculoPlasik, Montreal, Canada), placed prior to surgery. A topical ocular anesthetic, such as tetracaine ophthalmic, should be placed in each eye prior to insertion of the shields. If the case is prolonged, anesthetic should be applied approximately every 45 min or when the patient complains of ocular discomfort. If using laser for incision or dissection, a nonreflective metallic scleral shield is useful for corneal and globe protection.

Medical Management

The placement of a corneoscleral shield at the start of surgery and proper injection and surgical technique can help decrease the chances of globe perforation, but the shield will only protect the area it covers. It is possible for the conjunctiva, sclera, and/or cornea to be lacerated without perforation. Seidel testing can be performed to evaluate for a leak of aqueous or vitreous humor from the wound. Seidel testing involves applying topical flourescein to the cornea and then viewing the cornea with a cobalt blue light. In a positive Seidel test, a "waterfall" within the flourescein is seen emanating from the wound. However, puncture wounds can be self-sealing. Therefore, an ophthalmic evaluation should be performed in the event of any suspected perforation, laceration, or rupture.

Surgical Management

Globe rupture is an ophthalmic emergency; if suspected, any procedure and manipulation of the eye should immediately be stopped. Broad-spectrum antibiotics are given topically and intravenously, and an eye shield placed over the eye. An ophthalmic evaluation must be performed immediately with emergent surgical intervention if indicated.

11.2.2.3 Corneal Abrasion

Corneal abrasions are related to inadvertent damage to the corneal epithelium during surgery from harsh sterilization chemicals, exposure and drying, or mechanical abrasion. In addition, in the absence of direct corneal damage, an abrasion can result from general anesthesia as the cornea is exposed when the patient is insensate and unable to blink. Patients can experience eye pain, discomfort with blinking, foreign body sensation, photophobia, tearing, or decreased vision. The abrasion is diagnosed by symptoms and instillation of topical flourescein to the cornea. The cornea is then evaluated under cobalt blue light. If a corneal abrasion is present, the flourescein will stain the site of injured corneal epithelium [18]. Undiagnosed, or improperly treated, corneal abrasions can progress to corneal ulceration, scarring, or perforation, with associated visual loss.

Medical Management

Corneal abrasions usually heal rapidly, but patients should be medically managed to prevent corneal infection and to control pain and discomfort. Once the diagnosis of corneal abrasion is made, the patient should be seen by an ophthalmologist and treated accordingly with the application of ophthalmic antibiotic ointment or drops, and corneal coverage with a contact lens or patching. The patient is followed daily, and the abrasion typically resolves within 24–48 h depending on its size.

Surgical Management

In the unlikely event that a corneal abrasion results in scarring or opacification, or progresses to an ulcer, the patient should be referred to a corneal specialist for evaluation and treatment. A delay in referral should be avoided as surgical intervention, such as a patch graft or corneal transplant may be required.

11.2.3 Infection

Infection after blepharoplasty is exceptionally rare, occurring at a rate of approximately 0.04% [19]. Periocular infection can be divided into preseptal and orbital cellulitis. Preseptal cellulitis, also known as periorbital cellulitis, is infection that is confined to the eyelid skin and subcutaneous tissues anterior to the orbital septum (Fig. 11.4). On examination the eyelids are warm, edematous, erythematous, and tender to palpation. The extraocular motility is normal, and there is no proptosis. The most common organisms causing preseptal cellulitis are *Streptococcus pyogenes*, *Staphylococcus aureus*, and *Haemophilus influenza* type B [20]. Suture abscess is a mild expression of preseptal cellulitis (Fig. 11.5).

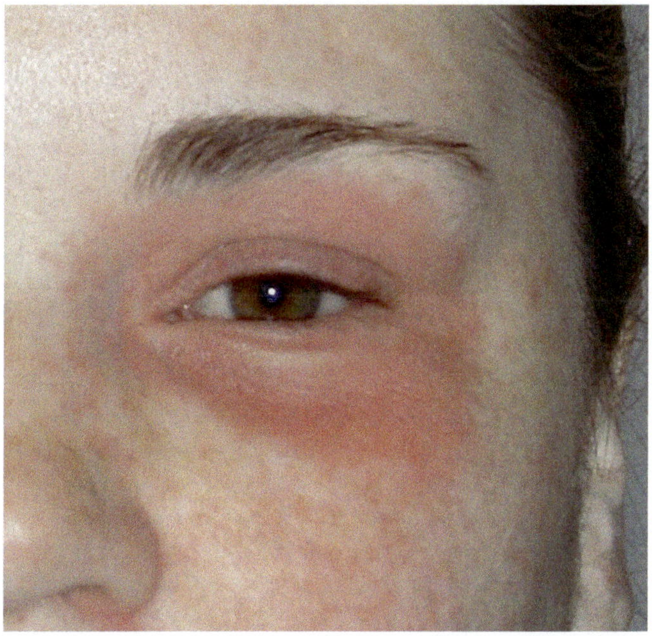

Fig. 11.4 Preseptal cellulitis. Note erythematous eyelid skin. No signs of orbital involvement were noted

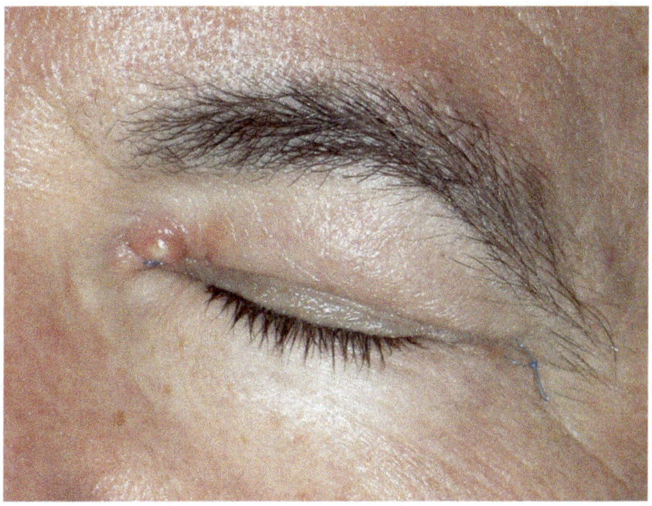

Fig. 11.5 Suture abscess evident to the nasal upper lid

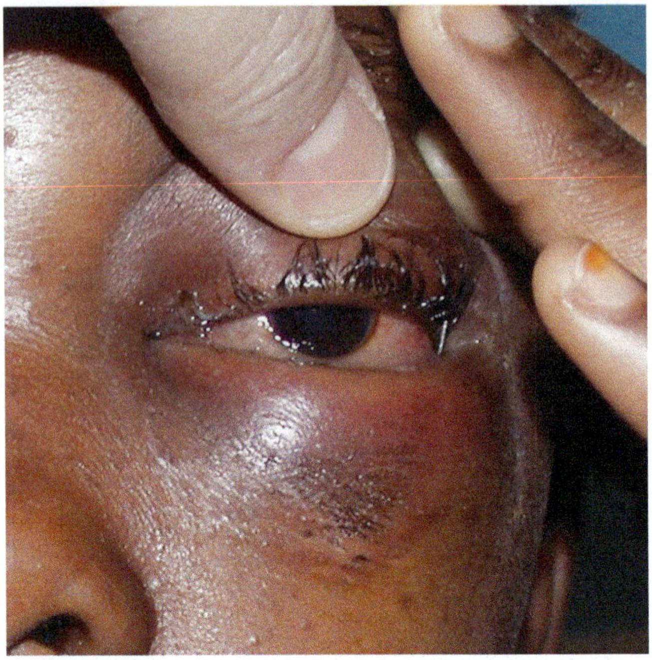

Fig. 11.6 Orbital cellulitis with proptosis and chemosis

Orbital cellulitis occurs when the infectious process involves the tissues posterior to the orbital septum. The clinical presentation differs from preseptal cellulitis by the hallmarks of increased pain, proptosis, restriction of ocular motility, chemosis, pupillary defects, dyschromatopsia, and loss of vision in addition to the findings seen in preseptal cellulitis (Fig. 11.6). The alterations in globe position and pupillary function should not be seen if the process is isolated to the preseptal space. The common organisms involved in orbital cellulitis are the same as those involved in preseptal cellulitis [20].

11.2.3.1 Medical Management

Preseptal cellulitis is initially managed with oral antibiotics and clinical monitoring. The patient typically shows signs of improvement in the first 24–36 h. If patients with preseptal cellulitis do not improve within the expected time frame, or if they progress to orbital involvement, they are managed as a case of orbital cellulitis.

Orbital cellulitis is a more serious infection, and early recognition and treatment is important to prevent further complications, such as subperiosteal abscess, orbital abscess, cavernous sinus thrombosis, optic nerve compression, meningitis, panophthalmitis, brain abscess, or vision loss [21]. In cases of orbital cellulitis, the patient is admitted to the hospital for close observation, CT imaging of orbits and brain, blood cultures, and immediate initiation of intravenous (IV) broad-spectrum antibiotics [13, 20]. It is important that any other aspect of the patient's treatment does not delay the administration of antibiotics. The patient is monitored for clinical improvement with serial measurements of visual acuity, pupillary evaluation, and motility and confrontation (or automated if available) visual field testing. In the absence of noticeable improvement within 24–48 h, CT scanning is repeated and antibiotic modification considered. Radiologic identification of an orbital abscess, particularly in an adult, usually mandates surgical intervention.

11.2.3.2 Surgical Management

Surgical intervention is indicated when there is inadequate improvement with antibiotics and/or evidence of an orbital abscess or progressive visual loss [21]. Surgical approaches for drainage of orbital abscess include opening the upper eyelid blepharoplasty incision, a Kronlein-Burke approach (lateral orbitotomy), an inferior transconjunctival incision, or a transantral (Cladwell Luc) approach [22]. The medial orbit may also be accessed through a transnasal endoscopic approach, but an abscess in this location is more likely to be related to sinus disease than blepharoplasty. In general, orbital abscess after blepharoplasty is very rare [23].

11.3 Surgical Complications

11.3.1 Lagophthalmos

Incomplete closure of the eyelids, lagophthalmos, can be a temporary or permanent sequela of upper blepharoplasty (Fig. 11.7). Transient lagophthalmous is related to postoperative edema and/or a reduction in orbicularis muscle tone secondary to local anesthetic or manipulation. The condition typically resolves spontaneously within the first 1–2 weeks postoperatively. Persistent lagophthalmous can be caused by excessive skin removal, incarceration of the orbital septum into the wound closure with resultant septal adhesions, or trauma to the orbicularis muscle or peripheral seventh cranial nerve. Symptoms of lagophthalmos may include foreign body sensation, blurred vision, burning, tearing, and red eye. The clinical findings can include conjunctival injection, lid edema, corneal staining with fluorescein (superficial punctate keratopathy), or rarely, corneal ulceration. When the eyelids do not close completely, the cornea is partially exposed, and in severe cases, exposure can give rise to corneal ulceration with infection and/or scarring. Prior to performing upper blepharoplasty surgery, patients are assessed for dry eye syndrome, history of previous laser in situ keratomileusis (LASIK), and adequacy of Bell's reflex. Patients with preexisting dry eye syndrome or previous LASIK are at greater risk from the complications of lagophthalmos [24].

11.3.1.1 Medical Management

Initial treatment for lagophthalmos should consist of gentle massage/stretching of the eyelids and aggressive lubrication

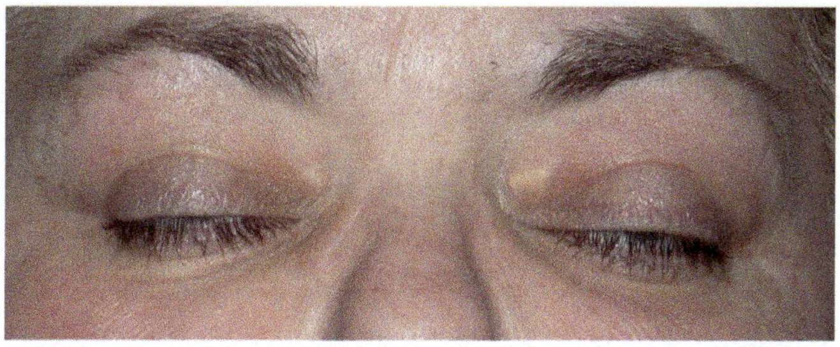

Fig. 11.7 Bilateral lagophthalmos

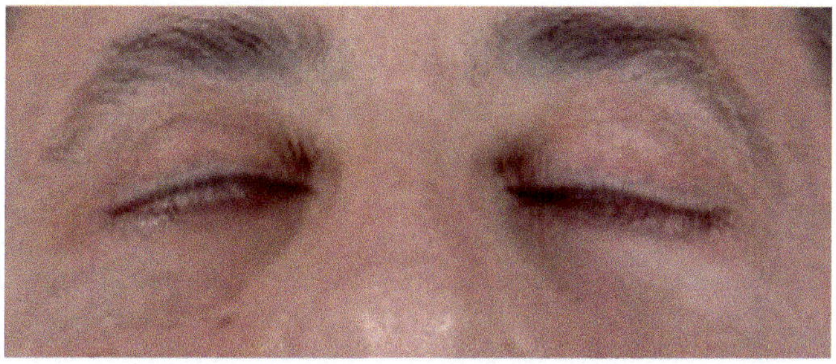

Fig. 11.8 Lagophthalmos on the right resulting from levator incorporation into the wound at time of upper blepharoplasty

of the ocular surface. Ophthalmic ointment or topical artificial tear supplements in drop or gel form can be used protect the cornea. Forced orbicularis closure via taping of the eyelids may reduce mild to moderate postoperative lagophthalmos.

11.3.1.2 Surgical Management

If conservative management fails, then surgery designed to correct the underlying process that created the lagophthalmos is indicated. In instances where the orbital septum is tethered, the operative wound is opened and the orbital septum released. If ptosis repair was performed with the blepharoplasty, or in cases where the levator complex has been inadvertently shortened or incorporated into the wound closure, lagophthalmos may result from the tightening of the levator muscle complex (Fig. 11.8). To improve the lagophthalmos, these attachments are released until full eyelid closure is achieved. Rarely, the good results of surgery are reversed by the secondary release of tissues to protect the patient's cornea and vision, and improve comfort.

Some patients with symptomatic lagophthalmos may have vertical shortening of the eyelid skin (anterior lamellar deficiency) as the primary etiology. In these cases, a full thickness skin graft (FTSG) is the best mechanical way of improving eyelid closure. The skin graft should be harvested from skin that is similar in texture and color. The contralateral upper eyelid skin is the preferred donor site, but preauricular, retroauricular, or supraclavicular skin can also be used. It is important to size the graft with a slight overcorrection in order to account for intraoperative and postoperative contraction [25].

11.3.2 Dry Eye Syndrome

Patients experiencing dry eye syndrome will complain of ocular irritation, foreign body sensation, redness of the conjunctiva, and potentially blurred vision. Individuals with preexisting dry eye syndrome can experience an increase in symptoms following blepharoplasty. Dry eye predominantly results from inadequate tear production, instability of the tear film, or a deficiency in quality of the any tear film component. In postblepharoplasty patients, dryness may be caused or exacerbated by lagophthalmos, alteration of blink, or rarely, lacrimal gland injury. Patients with a history of laser vision correction are at an increased risk of developing dry eye after blepharoplasty, with some authors suggesting that blepharoplasty not be performed for a minimum of 6 months after refractive surgery [26]. Patients in this population should be identified during the preoperative assessment and informed of the potential for increased risk of complications. Also at risk are older patients, related to involutional reduction in tear production, orbicularis weakness, reduced Bell's reflex, eyelid closure, and lower lid deficiencies. These patients require a detailed assessment of the factors which may lead them to symptomatology after surgery.

11.3.2.1 Medical Management

Dry eye syndrome is managed with ocular lubrication such as artificial tears and lubricating ointment. Postoperative dryness may occur even in the absence of lagophthalmos. Patients with preexisting conditions of dry eye syndrome should be lubricated more aggressively in the early postoperative recovery period. In patients who are refractory to simple eye lubrication, punctal occlusion is sometimes beneficial in alleviating symptoms of dryness [27]. Topical cyclosporine (Restasis, Allergan, Inc., Irvine, CA) has been used to increase tear production, but is better suited as a long-term intervention for chronic dry eye syndrome than as an immediate postoperative medication. Symptoms of dryness may abate as the normal speed and frequency of the blink returns when orbicularis function normalizes.

11.3.2.2 Surgical Management

Surgical management of dry eye syndrome is limited to correction of concomitant complications such as lagophthalmos and eyelid retraction. In cases where punctal occlusion is clinically beneficial, permanent surgical punctal occlusion can be performed. However, this should only be performed after evaluation and recommendation by an ophthalmologist.

11.3.3 Lacrimal Gland Injury

Injury to the lacrimal gland can occur during upper blepharoplasty, especially in patients whose lacrimal gland(s) is/are

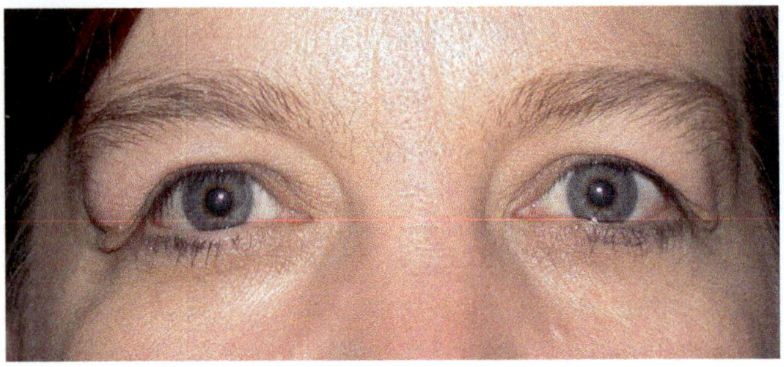

Fig. 11.9 Bilateral prolapsed temporal lacrimal gland. The prolapse is more evident on the right side

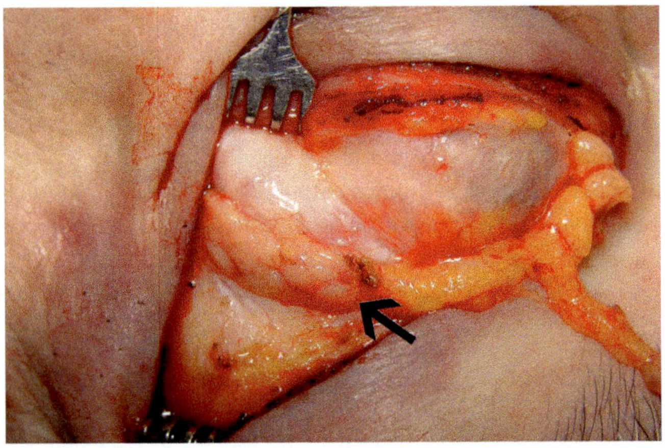

Fig. 11.10 Surgeon's view of a prolapsed lacrimal gland. Black arrow points to lacrimal gland. (Photograph courtesy of Guy Massry, MD)

prolapsed (Fig. 11.9). It is estimated that a minimum of one out of ten patients have unilateral or bilateral prolapsed lacrimal glands [28]. The upper lid has no lateral fat pad, but if a prolapsed lacrimal gland is mistaken for this, it can be inadvertently resected (Fig. 11.10). The lacrimal gland sometimes prolapses posterior to a lateral extension of the preaponeurotic (central) fat pad. This can also lead to mistaken excision or damage if/when the central fat pad is resected. Prior to excision of fat in the temporal lid, it is important to identify if the lacrimal gland is present. This will prevent inadvertent injury to the gland.

11.3.3.1 Medical Management

When lacrimal gland tissue is mistakenly excised there is an increased risk of dry eye syndrome [29]. Medical treatment of resultant dry eyes is discussed within the "dry eye syndrome" section of this chapter (eyelid lubrication with tears, lubricants, punctual occlusion, etc.).

11.3.3.2 Surgical Management

Recognition and protection of the lacrimal gland is crucial in maintaining normal of tear production. When the gland is prolapsed, it is possible to improve the contour of the eyelid

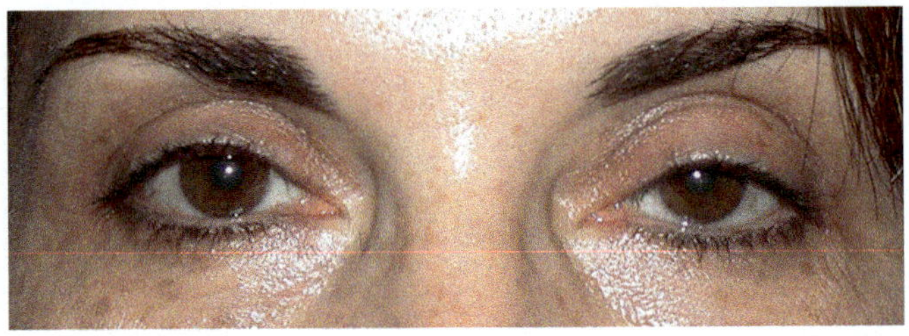

Fig. 11.11 Disruption of the levator aponeurosis during upper blepharoplasty resulting in left upper eyelid ptosis

while still protecting the integrity of the lacrimal gland. Resuspension of a prolapsed lacrimal gland is possible and adds to the cosmetic outcome of upper blepharoplasty. A 4–0, nonabsorbable polypropylene suture (Prolene, Ethicon, Somerville, NJ) can be passed through the capsule surrounding the lacrimal gland. The suture is then passed through the periosteum of the lacrimal gland fossa and secured. Generally, one or two sutures are sufficient for resuspension. Alternatively, there are surgeons who resect portions of the lacrimal gland; however, this greatly increases the risk of dry eye syndrome and should typically be avoided [30].

11.3.4 Ptosis

Ptosis present after blepharoplasty is often due to preexisting ptosis that is "unmasked" after surgery. New onset of ptosis is typically transient in nature and related to postoperative edema weighing the lid down. Ptosis may also occur if the levator aponeurosis sustains injury during blepharoplasty (Fig. 11.11). Anesthetic toxicity to the levator muscle and internal scarring of the surgical site has also been implicated in postoperative ptosis [31].

Postoperative ptosis is closely monitored and measured. As long as there is continued improvement, eyelid repositioning surgery should be deferred. However, if significant ptosis develops immediately after surgery, without significant lid edema, or if there is poor levator excursion, and no improvement of lid position with conservative therapy (see below), an injury to the elevator muscle or aponeurosis is suspected.

11.3.4.1 Medical Management

When ptosis is caused by persistent eyelid edema or presumed to be due to local anesthetic, the patient should be reassured and instructed to continue with the standard postoperative care. If cosmesis is a concern, the edema can be treated with increased ice application, elevation of the head at nighttime, oral diuretics with potassium replacement (Lasix, 40 mg daily), and oral steroids. If there is no improvement of ptosis with resolution of edema, then surgical exploration should be considered.

11.3.4.2 Surgical Management

When the surgeon feels that ptosis seen after blepharoplasty is a preexisting condition that was unmasked by the excision of the redundant skin, then the ptosis may be repaired by conventional methods at a time that is convenient for the patient and the surgeon. It is best to wait for resolution of the edema and inflammation from the blepharoplasty surgery. A retrospective review of the preoperative photos may be helpful in identifying this problem.

When levator injury is suspected or unexpected postoperative ptosis does not improve with conservative management, surgical exploration is warranted. Having the patient conscious during revision, and looking up and down, helps to delineate the levator complex. Violation of the levator aponeurosis is the likely cause of ptosis. The surgical wound is opened, the levator aponeurosis is identified, and its edges and reapproximated with 7–0 Silk or Prolene suture. If the aponeurosis is disinserted from the tarsus, it should be secured to the superior border of the tarsus with the same suture. Ptosis repair is a technically challenging surgery and should be performed by someone with specialized training or experience, especially when transection of the levator muscle is suspected. Early diagnosis is important as these anatomic changes will be easier to correct in the first 2 weeks following surgery before significant wound scarring occurs.

11.3.5 Diplopia

As with ptosis, the presence of diplopia following blepharoplasty can be a transient or persistent complication, usually resulting from interference with extraocular muscle function. Persistent diplopia following blepharoplasty is estimated to occur in 0.003% of cases [32], with a greater incidence in lower than upper blepharoplasty [33]. Transient diplopia may be caused by edema or local anesthetic effects on the extraocular muscles [31]. Persistent diplopia is the result of injury to the extraocular muscles, their tendons, or neurovascular supply.

It is important to clinically differentiate monocular versus binocular diplopia. Monocular diplopia related to blepharoplasty is generally benign and usually caused by corneal tear film abnormality, such as seen in dry eye syndrome. Binocular diplopia is more worrisome warranting detailed assessment of ocular alignment and extraocular muscle function. Syniuta et al. [33] have shown that diplopia after upper blepharoplasty is most commonly associated with dysfunction of the superior oblique complex. The mechanism of superior oblique palsy after upper blepharoplasty is unknown, but it is believed to be related to direct trauma to the superior oblique muscle, formation of a hematoma, or anesthetic toxicity [34]. The superior oblique muscle, trochlea, or tendon can be injured when dissecting or sculpting the nasal fat pad. Therefore, it is important to avoid sharp or blind dissection and/or aggressive cauterization of the nasal fat pad.

11.3.5.1 Medical Management

Initial management of diplopia is conservative. Improvement is often spontaneous and should be monitored by an ophthalmologist or someone versed in the evaluation of strabismus. Diplopia that is monocular, likely caused by tear film inadequacy, should be treated as previously outlined for dry eye syndrome. Persistent monocular diplopia requires evaluation by an ophthalmologist for potential intraocular or corneal pathology. Patients with binocular diplopia should be observed closely for continued improvement. Oftentimes, a trial of oral steroids may hasten recovery. While waiting for resolution, a pair of glasses with built-in or stick-on prisms allow better tolerance of bothersome symptoms.

11.3.5.2 Surgical Management

When binocular diplopia does not improve after a period of observation, then permanent lens prism correction or strabismus surgery is warranted. In all cases of persistent diplopia, consultation with an ophthalmologist specializing in strabismus surgery should be obtained.

11.3.6 Sulcus Deformity

Hollowing or deepening of the superior sulcus may occur from senescent orbital volume changes or iatrogenically as a result of blepharoplasty. Extensive sculpting of the orbital fat in the upper eyelid sulcus may lead to a "skeletonized" or sunken appearance (Fig. 11.12). Similarly, asymmetrical sculpting may produce an irregular contour within and between the sulci. Some patients have a preexisting deep sulcus that appears to be more prominent once eyelid skin and muscle are debulked. In all cases, the cosmetic result is undesirable and particularly so in males as it imparts a more feminine appearance.

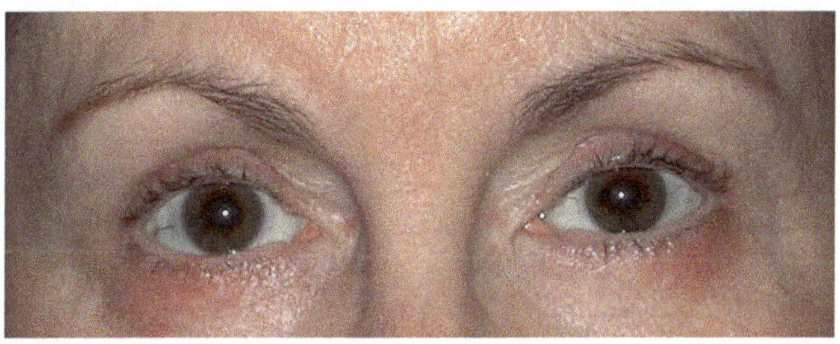

Fig. 11.12 Hollow bilateral superior sulci after upper blepharoplasty

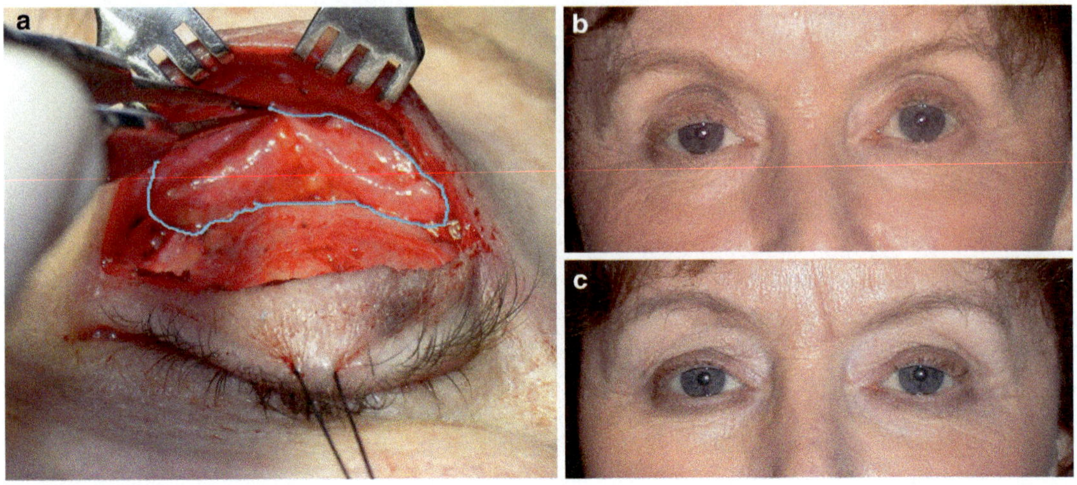

Fig. 11.13 Dermis fat grafting to the superior sulcus. (**a**) The dermis fat graft is outlined in blue. The forceps are shown grasping the dermis side with the underlying fat in the sulcus. (**b**) Preoperative. (**c**) Postoperative

11.3.6.1 Medical Management

The management options for correction of superior sulcus deformities are all procedural in nature. The least invasive option is the use of hyaluronic acid (HA) soft tissue fillers. Volume augmentation with HA fillers can be used as a primary or secondary method of volume correction [35]. A lower viscosity HA, such as Restylane™ (Medicis, Scottsdale, AZ) should be used as "thicker" fillers may interfere with eyelid function. Serial depot injections are placed posterior to the orbicularis and anterior to the orbital fat, below the orbital rim. A volume of 0.2–0.5 cc is usually sufficient for initial correction. Due to the highly vascular nature of this region, intravascular injection is a concern especially in the nasal eyelid region. While minimally invasive with predictable results, HA filler treatment is transient and must be repeated to maintain appropriate volume.

11.3.6.2 Surgical Management

Correction of a sulcus deformity can be achieved by replacing the lost volume with alloplastic implants, autologous free fat grafts, or dermis fat grafts. Alloplastic implants convey the best longevity, outcome, and volume control, but require the most invasive surgical approach. Also, these implants provide minimal tissue integration and do not adapt to the continued processes of facial aging. Free fat grafts provide increased biocompatibility; however, longevity and control of contour can be issues. Dermis fat grafting has long been used for orbital volume correction, and recent variations in technique have been reported for correction of cosmetic sulcus deformities [36–38]. Dermis fat grafts offer less variability in fat absorption and increased control over final volume when compared to free fat grafts [38]. Results to fat grafting vary greatly amongst different surgeons. As such, any method of fat grafting should be undertaken with care and by a surgeon familiar with the techniques.

In brief, the dermis fat graft is implanted in the sulcus via a standard blepharoplasty incision. The anterior surface of the preaponeurotic and nasal fat pads are identified with their capsules intact. The length and width of the required graft is measured and harvested from the donor site. After preparation of the graft, it is placed in the sulcus with the dermis facing anteriorly and the fat in apposition to the exposed eyelid fat pads (Fig. 11.13a). A 6–0 polygalactin suture on a P-1 needle is used to anchor the superior 180° of the dermis border to the superior edge of the fat capsule. The inferior 180° of the dermis fat graft is not sutured. The graft is further trimmed and adjusted to fit the available space as needed. The upper lid skin and orbicularis are draped over the dermis fat graft to assess volume. Initial overcorrection of the superior sulcus defect by 20–30% is the goal at the time of surgery [38]. Figure 11.13b,c illustrates a typical sulci deformity patient preoperatively and postoperatively.

11.4 Incision Irregularities

11.4.1 Canthal Webbing

Webbing after upper blepharoplasty may appear in the medial canthus and/or lateral canthus. Medial canthal webbing is caused by excessive excision of nasal skin, from placing the incision too far medially or too close to the lid margin

(Fig. 11.14). Lateral canthal webbing is the result of poor separation of upper and lower blepharoplasty incisions, poor incision design, or improper closure of a canthoplasty incision (Fig. 11.15a). Webbing results primarily with cosmetic concerns, but may, in unusual cases, cause lagophthalmos and functional problems.

11.4.1.1 Medical Management

In addition to the normal postoperative protocol, the patient is instructed to massage the area of webbing gently. Frequency and duration should be set to the maximal tolerance of the patient. Injection of steroids into area may be of value if the mechanism is cicatricial in nature, rather than lack of skin surface area. Triamcinolone acetonide injectable suspension (Kenalog®, Bristol-Myers Squibb, New York, NY), 10 mg per milliliter, is injected directly into the area of webbing. Care should be taken to avoid intravascular injection as rarely, this can precipitate visual loss. The patient continues massage of the area as tolerated. If the webbing does not resolve to functional and cosmetic standards, then surgical intervention is required.

11.4.1.2 Surgical Management

To correct medial canthal webbing, a V–Y plasty, M plasty, or Z plasty can be performed. In cases with significant traction and skin deficiency, an FTSG may be incorporated into the repair. The correction of lateral canthal webbing (Fig. 11.15b) is approached in a similar manner.

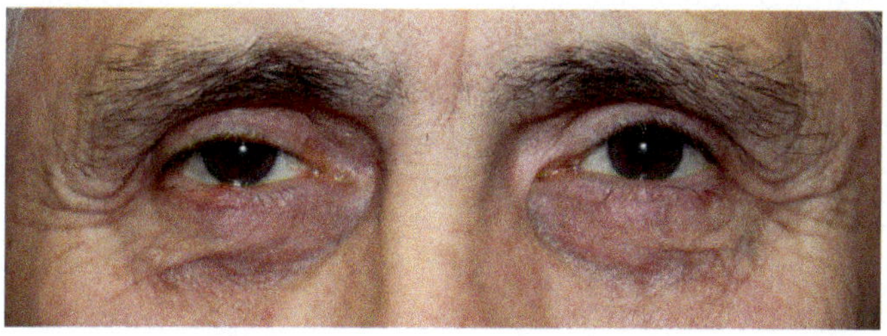

Fig. 11.14 Medial canthal webbing of the left upper eyelid. (Photograph courtesy of Kevin Michels, MD)

11.4.2 Scarring

Hypertrophic scarring or suture "tracts" of the incision line can occur after blepharoplasty from inadequate wound closure or reaction to the suture material. Failure to remove suture material within the proper time frame can also promote incision irregularities. Using fast-absorbing gut or Prolene sutures has been shown to decrease the incidence of scar formation [39]. In African-American and Hispanic patients, keloid formation is possible, but very unusual in the eyelids [40]. Keloid formation can often be diminished by reducing skin tension through taping, corticosteroid injections, or immediate placement of silicone elastomer sheeting [41].

11.4.2.1 Medical Management

There are numerous treatment options for scarring and keloid formation; however, no single therapeutic modality has been determined experimentally to be most effective. Treatments include pressure dressing, corticosteroid injections, silicone sheeting, cryotherapy, and laser. Topical vitamin E and zinc oxide may also be of benefit [42].

11.4.2.2 Surgical Management

Surgical management consists of scar excision with appropriate wound reconstruction. If conservative resection of eyelid skin was performed initially, direct scar excision with meticulous closure using a monofilament suture may be attempted. Subcuticular placement of the sutures will help reduce suture tract formation by diminishing the number of puncture sites along the wound edges. Sutures should be removed 5–7 days after placement. Alternatively,

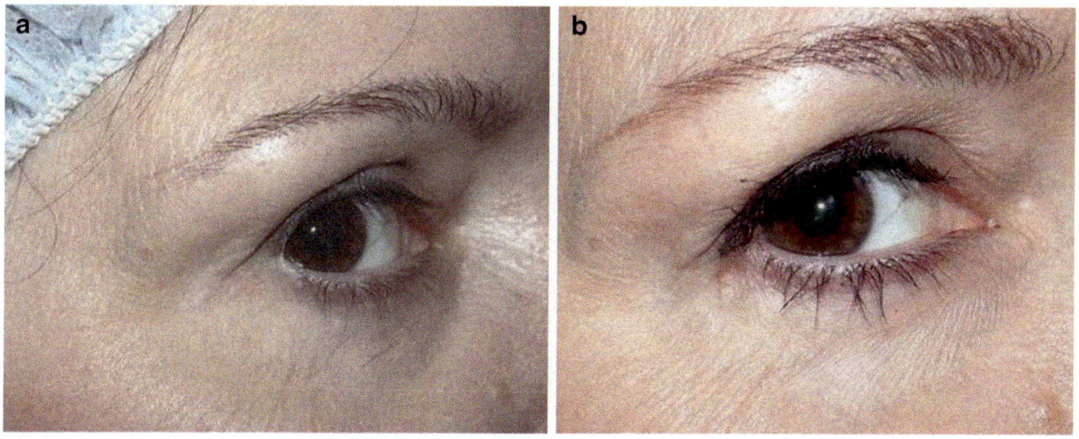

Fig. 11.15 Lateral canthal webbing. (**a**) Prominent lateral canthal web. (**b**) Following repair of the lateral canthal web with a combination of Y-V and Z-plasty (Photograph courtesy of Guy Massry, MD)

tissue adhesives, such as autologous fibrin glue or *N*-butyl-2-cyanoacrylate, can be used for wound closure, in place of, or to reduce the amount of, sutures required. This option may not be applicable for cosmetic blepharoplasty due to poor eversion of wound edges and higher rates of wound dehiscence [39].

11.4.3 Suture Milia

Suture milia are cystic elevations that appear approximately 7 days postoperatively at the sites of suture skin penetration (Fig. 11.16). Milia occur with most suture material, including silk, mild chromic gut, and polypropylene. Joshi et al. [39] have demonstrated that a running/locking Prolene suture had the highest percentage of milia formation, followed by running plain gut, subcuticular Prolene, running fast-absorbing gut, and interrupted Prolene.

11.4.3.1 Medical Management

Suture milia may spontaneously resolve over a period of weeks to months [43]. Subcuticular closure and/or early suture removal may reduce the occurrence of milia.

11.4.3.2 Surgical Management

In the rare instance when milia persist, they can be treated surgically similar to other types of irregular scarring. Typically one waits 4–6 months after the primary surgery before intervening. Individual milia may be removed in the office with minimal local anesthesia. Wescott scissors are used to make "snip" excisions of the milia, which are allowed to heal by granulation.

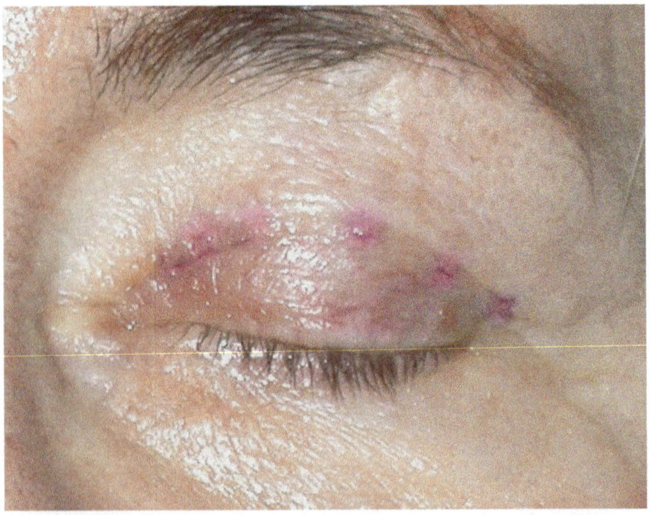

Fig. 11.16 Suture milia of the left upper eyelid marked with purple surgical marker

11.5 Asymmetry

11.5.1 Lid Crease and Fold

A symmetrical and correctly positioned lid crease is crucial for the successful outcome of cosmetic upper blepharoplasty. The surgeon must have an understanding of the correct position of a natural eyelid crease in men and women, and be aware of racial variations in crease height. Men have a low and less distinct lid crease, while women have a high and more definitive lid crease. Poorly positioned and asymmetrical lid creases or folds can result from poorly positioned lid crease markings, preexisting asymmetry, asymmetric lid tissue debulking, improper incision placement, or dissimilar wound healing on the two sides (Fig. 11.17). Brow asymmetry is often a factor in lid fold asymmetry and should be recognized during the surgical planning stage.

11.5.1.1 Medical Management

When lid crease or fold asymmetry occurs, a period of at least 6 months should pass before revision, especially if surgery involved formal crease formation or was on Asian patients. Postoperative swelling and inflammation can be prolonged and persistent in these instances, and any intervention can only occur when stability has been reached. A trial of oral or injectable steroids may be of benefit in these cases.

11.5.1.2 Surgical Management

Surgical correction can include a combination of skin excision, fat excision or grafting, and crease formation depending on the findings (crease asymmetry, fold asymmetry, or both). A lid crease can be formed by incorporation of the levator aponeurosis into the eyelid incision closure (supratarsal fixation – see Chap. 9). When closing the skin incision, the needle pass should engage the levator aponeurosis at the desired location of crease placement before exiting the skin. Alternatively, buried suture can secure the orbicularis muscle

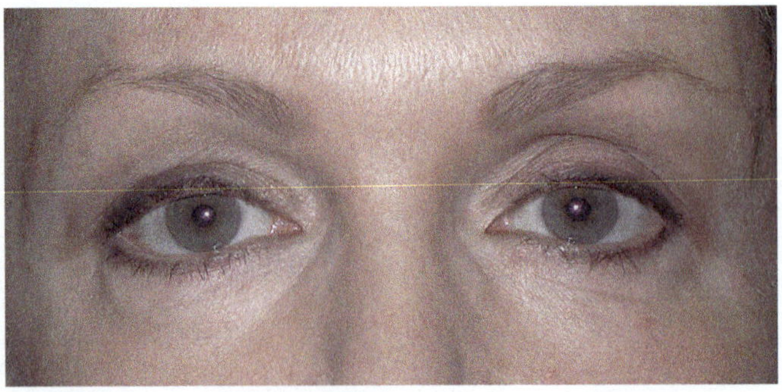

Fig. 11.17 This patient has asymmetric lid creases and also asymmetric lid folds following upper blepharoplasty

to the levator aponeurosis at the desired crease height. Ideally a crease suture is placed nasally, centrally, and temporally. The aponeurosis can also be engaged at these points in a running skin closure.

11.5.2 Skin

Asymmetry in the amount of eyelid skin after surgery results from preexisting asymmetries and/or disproportionate skin excision during surgery. This can be avoided with attention to preoperative differences between the two sides, and careful eyelid markings. If asymmetry of the amount of skin between the eyelids is significant or leads to an unacceptable cosmetic result, revision is appropriate.

11.5.2.1 Medical Management

Prior to performing any additional procedures, the surgeon should observe the patient and allow postoperative edema to resolve. Complete resolution of postoperative edema may take up to a full year depending on the invasiveness of the procedure(s) [44]. Aggressive postoperative icing and oral corticosteroids may hasten the resolution of edema. On rare occasion, an overresection of skin can lead to asymmetry and poor corneal coverage. In these instances, more immediate surgical intervention may be required to protect the cornea (see Sect. 11.5.5).

11.5.2.2 Surgical Correction

Surgical correction of asymmetry usually involves a quick "touch-up" skin excision from one eyelid. These are typically performed in the office under local anesthesia.

11.5.3 Fat

Asymmetric sculpting or excision of the upper eyelid fat pads can lead to an asymmetric cosmetic result between the eyes. As discussed previously, excessive removal of fat can result in deep superior sulci and an undesirable appearance. Overresection of the central fat pad often yields an abnormal configuration of the upper eyelid fold (A-frame deformity). When removing fat in upper eyelids, only the amount that protrudes anterior to the supraorbital rim when gentle pressure is applied to the orbit should be removed. Also, the amount of fat removed from each side should be monitored to ensure that symmetric amounts are being removed, or in the case of preoperative asymmetry, the desired amount of excision is accomplished.

11.5.3.1 Medical Management

As with postoperative skin asymmetry, patience is critical before a revision is planned. At least 6 months should pass before another surgery is performed.

11.5.3.2 Surgical Management

Additional fat excision is performed as with standard blepharoplasty. When there is a hollow sulcus from fat overresection, correction involves volume augmentation (as discussed previously) with filler or autologous or alloplastic material.

11.5.4 Brow Position

Brow ptosis or deflation can give the appearance of a blepharoplasty undercorrection, particularly in the temporal region (Fig. 11.18). A thorough preoperative evaluation should include noting brow position and counseling the patient on the limitations of stand-alone upper blepharoplasty if there is preexisting brow ptosis (which could become worse after surgery) and brow position is not to be concurrently addressed at the time of surgery.

11.5.4.1 Medical Management

If surgery has created new or worsening brow ptosis which is bothersome to the patient, surgical options should be discussed.

11.5.4.2 Surgical Treatment

The addition of a formal browlift (endoscopic, direct, etc.) or brow stabilization (browpexy through the blepharoplasty incision) can be added to any planned eyelid revision. If no further lid surgery is to be considered, an isolated brow lift can be suggested.

11.5.5 Undercorrection/Overcorrection

While not a "true" complication of upper blepharoplasty, surgical undercorrection can be an issue to the cosmetic patient. When referenced to blepharoplasty, the term undercorrection refers to inadequate skin, muscle, or fat removal. Undercorrection should not be confused with asymmetry

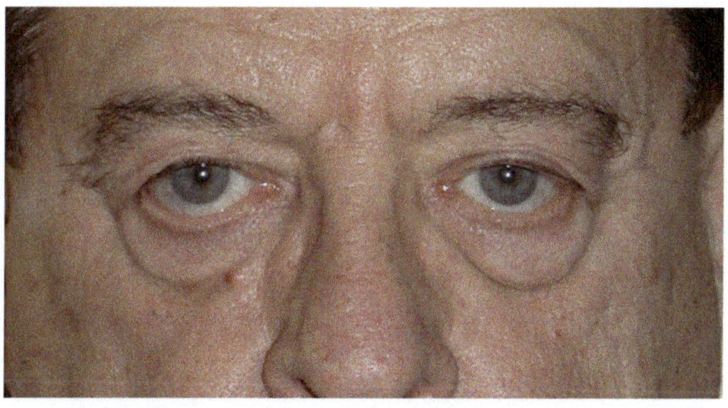

Fig. 11.18 Bilateral involutional brow ptosis. Pre-existing brow ptosis will limit the improvement seen with upper blepharoplasty if the brow position is not addressed concurrently

(see above) as there can be symmetric undercorrection. However, undercorrection can cause asymmetry.

Overcorrection (too much tissue excised) can lead to significant problems (see lagophthalmos). It can be common for the novice blepharoplasty surgeon to underresect skin as the complications associated with overresection are far more significant.

11.5.5.1 Medical Management

If undercorrection is the problem, the patient is treated as previously described for postoperative asymmetry. If an overcorrection occurs with corneal exposure, aggressive ocular lubrication with drops and ointment, eyelid massage, and possibly punctal occlusion are initiated.

11.5.5.2 Surgical Management

Once swelling has resolved and eyelid stability has been reached, surgical revision can be planned. In undercorrections, it is important to assess if there is sufficient anterior lamella to be excised so as not to cause lagophthalmos or brow ptosis. In cases of overcorrection, an FTSG is the only option to improve both function and cosmesis. This is discussed in the previous section on lagophthalmos.

11.6 Unrealized Patient Expectations

Unrealized patient expectations can lead to significant patient dissatisfaction after surgery, and may be the most difficult problem to resolve. A good result to surgery is when the patient is happy. As such, prevention is the best solution. It is critical that the surgeon understands the underlying motivations for which the patient is seeking surgery, and that those expectations can be met. For example, a patient who wants redundant eyelid skin removed and less protrusion of the eyelid fold can benefit from upper eyelid blepharoplasty. However, periorbital dynamic wrinkles, true lid ptosis, brow ptosis, and a deep sulcus will not be addressed with only upper blepharoplasty. It is incumbent upon the surgeon to identify any unrealistic expectations prior to performing surgery. If the patient is unwilling to modify his or her expectations, surgery should not be performed.

11.7 Conclusion

Upper eyelid blepharoplasty is a commonly performed surgery for both aesthetic and functional reasons. It is a generally safe and reliable procedure with high patient satisfaction. However, like all surgery, there are a myriad of potential postoperative complications. Most of these complications can be avoided with proper patient evaluation and counseling, preoperative planning, and sound intraoperative technique. On occasion, adverse events occur in the best of hands under normal circumstances. The surgeon must be prepared to manage such events to prevent potential permanent loss of vision (i.e., orbital compartment syndrome), and deal with less severe but still stressful issues (dry eye, lagophthalmos, asymmetry, etc.). The preoperative assessment is crucial to exclude unrealistic patients, and those whose risks prevent proceeding with surgery.

References

1. American Society for Aesthetic Plastic Surgery. [Online] 2009. http://www.surgery.org/media/statistics. Accessed 7 May 2010.
2. Lelli GJ, Lisman RD. Blepharoplasty complications. Plast Reconstr Surg. 2010;125(3):1007–17.
3. Morax S, Touitou V. Complications of blepharoplasty. Orbit. 2006;25(4):303–18.
4. Lowry JC, Bartley GB. Complications of blepharoplasty. Surv Ophthalmol. 1994;38(4):327–50.
5. Pacella SJ, Codner MA. Minor complications after blepharoplasty: dry eyes, chemosis, granulomas, ptosis, and scleral show. Plast Reconstr Surg. 2010;125(2):709–18.
6. Violi F, Pignatelli P, Basili S. Nutrition, supplements, and vitamins in platelet function and bleeding. Circulation. 2010;121(8):1033–44.
7. Teng CC, Reddy S, Wong JJ, Lisman RD. Retrobulbar hemorrhage nine days after cosmetic blepharoplasty resulting in permanent visual loss. Ophthal Plast Reconstr Surg. 2006;22(5):388–9.
8. Cruz AA, Ando A, Monteiro CA, Elias Jr J. Delayed retrobulbar hematoma after blepharoplasty. Ophthal Plast Reconstr Surg. 2001;17(2):126–30.
9. Hass AN, Penne RB, Stefanyszyn MA, Flanagan JC. Incidence of postblepharoplasty orbital hemorrhage and associated visual loss. Ophthal Plast Reconstr Surg. 2004;20(6):426–32.
10. Wolfort FG, Vaughan TE, Wolfort SF, Nevarre DR. Retrobulbar hematoma and blepharoplasty. Plast Reconstr Surg. 1999;104(7):2154–62.
11. Dolman PJ, Glazer LC, Harris GJ, et al. Mechanisms of visual loss in severe proptosis. Ophthal Plast Reconstr Surg. 1991;7(4):256–60.
12. Anderson RL, Edwards JJ. Bilateral visual loss after blepharoplasty. Ann Plast Surg. 1980;5(4):288–92.
13. Holds JB. Orbit, eyelids, and lacrimal system. San Francisco: Lifelong Education for the Ophthalmologist; 2007.
14. Yung CW, Moorthy RS, Lindley D, et al. Efficacy of lateral canthotomy and cantholysis in orbital hemorrhage. Ophthal Plast Reconstr Surg. 1994;10(2):137–41.
15. Zoumalan CI, Bullock JD, Warwar RE, et al. Evaluation of intraocular and orbital pressure in the management of orbital hemorrhage: an experimental model. Arch Ophthalmol. 2008;126(9):1257–60.
16. Lee KY, Tow S, Fong KS. Visual recovery following emergent orbital decompression in traumatic retrobulbar haemorrhage. Ann Acad Med Singapore. 2006;35(11):831–2.
17. Lima V, Burt B, Leibovitch I, Prabhakaran V, Goldberg RA, Selva D. Orbital compartment syndrome: the ophthalmic surgical emergency. Surv Ophthalmol. 2009;54(4):441–9.
18. Sutphin Jr JE. Toxic and traumatic injuries of the anterior segment. In: Basic and clinical science course, external disease and cornea. San Francisco: Lifelong Education for the Ophthalmologist; 2007. p. 406–7.
19. Lee EW, Holtebeck AC, Harrison AR. Infection rates in outpatient eyelid surgery. Ophthal Plast Reconstr Surg. 2009;25(2):109–10.

20. Tovilla-Canales JL, Nava A, Tovilla Y, Pomar JL. Orbital and periorbital infections. Curr Opin Ophthalmol. 2001;12(5):335–41.
21. Chiu ES, Capell BC, Press R, Aston SJ, Jelks EB, Jelks GW. Successful management of orbital cellulitis and temporary visual loss after blepharoplasty. Plast Reconstr Surg. 2006;118(3):67e–72.
22. Risk SS, Papageorge A, Liberatore L, et al. Bilateral simultaneous orbital decompression for Graves' orbitopathy with combined endoscopic and Caldwell-Luc approach. Otolaryngol Head Neck Surg. 2000;122(2):216–21.
23. Siracuse-Lee DE, Kazim M. Orbital decompression: current concepts. Curr Opin Ophthalmol. 2002;13(5):310–6.
24. Korn BS, Kikkawa DO, Schanzlin DJ. Blepharoplasty in the post-laser in situ keratomileusis patient: preoperative considerations to avoid dry eye syndrome. Plast Reconstr Surg. 2007;119(7):2232–9.
25. Moses JL, Tanenbaum M. Blepharoplasty: cosmetic and functional. In: Tanenbaum M, Nunery WR, McCord CD, editors. Oculoplastic surgery. New York: Raven; 1995. p. 313–4.
26. Lee WB, McCord CD, Somia N, Hirmand H. Optimizing blepharoplasty outcomes in patients with previous laser vision correction. Plast Reconstr Surg. 2008;122(2):587–94.
27. Stevenson D, Tauber J, Reis BL. Efficacy and safety of cyclosporin A ophthalmic emulsion in the treatment of moderate to severe dry eye disease: a dose-ranging randomized trial. Ophthalmology. 2000;107(5):967–74.
28. Smith B, Lisman RD. Dacryoadenopexy as recognized factor in upper lid blepharoplasty. Plast Reconstr Surg. 1983;71(5):629–32.
29. Horton CE, Carraway JH, Potenza AD. Treatment of lacrimal bulge in blepharoplasty by repositioning the gland. Plast Reconstr Surg. 1978;61(5):701–2.
30. Lemke BN, Lucarelli MJ. Anatomy of the ocular adnexa, orbit, and related facial structures. In: Lisman RD, Levine MR, Nesi FA, editors. Smith's ophthalmic plastic and reconstructive surgery. St. Louis: Mosby; 1997. p. 1–75.
31. Rainin EA, Carlson BM. Postoperative diplopia and ptosis: a clinical hypothesis base on the myotoxicity of local anesthetics. Arch Ophthalmol. 1985;103(9):1337–9.
32. Hayworth RS, Lisman RD, Muchnick RS, Smith B. Diplopia following blepharoplasty. Ann Ophthalmol. 1984;16(5):448–51.
33. Syniuta LA, Goldberg RA, Thacker NM, Rosenbaum AL. Acquired strabismus following cosmetic blepharoplasty. Plast Reconstr Surg. 2003;111(6):2053–9.
34. Sachs ME, Bosniak SL. Nonsurgical fat removal in cosmetic blepharoplasty: a new technique. Ann Plast Surg. 1986;16(6):516–20.
35. Czyz CN, Foster JA. Neurotoxins and soft tissue fillers. In: Albert DM, Lucarelli MJ, editors. Clinical atlas of procedures in ophthalmic surgery. 2nd ed. London: Oxford University Press; 2011.
36. Maniglia JJ, Maniglia RF, Jorge Dos Santos MC, Robert F, Magniglia FF, Magniglia SF. Surgical treatment of the sunken upper eyelid. Arch Facial Plast Surg. 2006;8(4):269–72.
37. Proffer PL, Czyz CN, Cahill KV, Kavanagh MC, Everman KR, Burns JA, et al. Addition of dermis-fat graft to diminish cable visibility in frontalis suspension for patients with pre-existing deep superior sulci. Ophthal Plast Reconstr Surg. 2009;25(2):94–8.
38. Phoenix AZ, Czyz CN, Foster JA, Cahill KV, Kavanagh MC, Everman KR. Orbital superior sulcus volumetric rejuvenation utilizing dermis fat graft. In: AACS: 25th Anniversary scientific meeting, American Academy of Cosmetic Surgery, Phoenix, AZ, 18 January 2009.
39. Joshi AS, Janjanin S, Tanna N, Geist C, Lindsey C. Does suture material and technique really matter? Lessons learned from 800 consecutive blepharoplasties. Laryngoscope. 2007;117(6):981–4.
40. Alhady SM, Sivanantharajah K. Keloids in various races. A review of 175 cases. Plast Reconstr Surg. 1969;44(6):564–6.
41. Jucket G, Hartman-Adams H. Management of keloids and hypertrophic scars. Am Fam Physician. 2009;80(3):253–60.
42. Wilhelmi BJ. Wound healing, widened and hypertrophic scars. Emedicine. [Online]. http://emedicine.medscape.com/article/1298541-treatment. Accessed 17 December 2008.
43. Baylis HI, Goldberg RA, Wilson MC. Complications of upper blepharoplasty. In: Warren LA, Putterman AM, editors. Cosmetic oculoplastic surgery. Philadelphia: WB Saunders; 1999. p. 411–28.
44. Czyz CN, Beisman BS, Foster JA. Periorbital rejuvenation utilizing blepharoplasty and adjunctive surgical techniques. In: Lupo M, Narukar V, Beer K, editors. Cosmetic Bootcamp Primer: comprehensive aesthetic management. London: Informa Healthcare; 2011.

12 Levator Ptosis Repair in the Aesthetic Patient With and Without Blepharoplasty

Morris E. Hartstein

Key Points

- Patients presenting for blepharoplasty may have concurrent true eyelid ptosis.
- If present, ptosis should be evaluated and pointed out to each patient, and its repair discussed.
- Aponeurotic/involutional ptosis is the most common etiology encountered.
- The surgeon should be aware of the medical conditions which cause ptosis (myasthenia gravis, Horner syndrome, etc.) which require further workup before proceeding with surgery.
- Dry eye status and corneal protective mechanisms must be evaluated before surgery to prevent potentially significant postoperative complications.
- A thorough knowledge of eyelid anatomy and significant experience with eyelid surgery are prerequisites for successful surgery.
- Levator ptosis repair is performed with blepharoplasty through the same eyelid incision.
- The preaponeurotic fat is a useful surgical landmark as it lies behind the orbital septum and anterior to the levator aponeurosis – the critical anatomic structure identified in surgery.
- The surgical outcome is maximized when patients are awake.
- Intraoperative adjustments in eyelid height and contour are a normal part of surgery.
- Patients should be counseled preoperatively about the potential for postoperative revision of under/overcorrections.

M.E. Hartstein (✉)
Clinical Associate Professor, Department of Ophthalmology and Division of Plastic Surgery, St. Louis University School of Medicine, St. Louis, MO, USA

Director, Oculoplastic Surgery, Department of Ophthalmology, Assaf Harofeh Medical Center, Beer Yaacov, Israel
e-mail: mhartstein@earthlink.net

12.1 Introduction

When evaluating the potential upper eyelid blepharoplasty patient, it is important to determine whether a component of true eyelid ptosis is present, and whether or not it should be addressed [1]. For example, if a patient has mild ptosis, but is primarily bothered by upper eyelid fullness (excess skin/muscle and fat), he/she may only chose to undergo blepharoplasty. Alternatively, marked dermatochalasis may mask significant ptosis, which can become more apparent postoperatively if not corrected. In this instance, ptosis correction may be desired. Even if ptosis is not to be addressed surgically, its presence should be pointed out to the patient before surgery with a mirror or photos, so that there are no surprises after surgery.

There are varied etiologies of ptosis [2–4], and their discussion is beyond the scope of this chapter. The most common form of ptosis is involutional, or aponeurotic in nature [2, 3]. If an etiology other than typical involutional ptosis is suspected, further workup by a specialist (oculoplastic surgeon, neuro-ophthalmologist) is recommended before proceeding with surgery. Also, there are two basic approaches to ptosis repair: an anterior (transcutaneous) approach with levator aponeurotic advancement (with or without resection) [5], or a posterior approach [6], which is discussed in detail in Chap. 13. For the purpose of this chapter, I will focus on involutional ptosis and levator aponeurotic ptosis repair only.

12.2 Ptosis Repair: Which Approach?

When ptosis is identified, and correction is planned, a decision on which surgical procedure to perform is important. As stated above, there are two standard ways to address upper eyelid ptosis: an anterior transcutaneous approach involving levator advancement and reattachment, or a variety of posterior eyelid approaches. Posterior ptosis surgery can be accomplished by a graded resection of Muller's muscle/conjunctiva,

G.G. Massry et al. (eds.), *Master Techniques in Blepharoplasty and Periorbital Rejuvenation*,
DOI 10.1007/978-1-4614-0067-7_12, © Springer Science+Business Media, LLC 2011

tarsus, or a combination of the two. A positive response (eyelid elevation) to the administration of preoperative phenylephrine drops is needed before performing a Muller's muscle/conjunctival repair [6]. This approach is quick, easier than levator surgery, requires no skin incision, yields generally reproducible results, and requires no patient cooperation. This has made posterior approach ptosis repair popular amongst eyelid surgeons. Its main drawbacks are that it is nonanatomic, carries a risk of corneal abrasion, and does not allow intraoperative adjustment of lid height.

Anterior, or levator, ptosis surgery is a more complex procedure which requires a detailed knowledge of eyelid anatomy. In addition, the surgery involves an intricate dissection of the various layers of the eyelid, is time intensive, requires patient participation, is best performed with the patient awake, and carries a higher incidence of postoperative adjustment than its posterior counterpart [7]. It is advantageous in that it is powerful, anatomic, can be employed when posterior surgery is not indicated (poor response to phenylephrine drop testing), and can be titrated during surgery.

Which procedure is better is up for debate and the preference of the ptosis surgeon. As posterior ptosis repair is quick, simpler, and useful in most mild/moderate ptosis patients; the novice ptosis surgeon should be comfortable with the surgery. In this chapter I will review levator ptosis repair. Familiarization with this procedure is essential to the ptosis surgeon. However, this can be a difficult procedure to perform and attain acceptable outcomes, and has a steep learning curve. The noneyelid specialist should pursue appropriate training before undertaking this form of surgery.

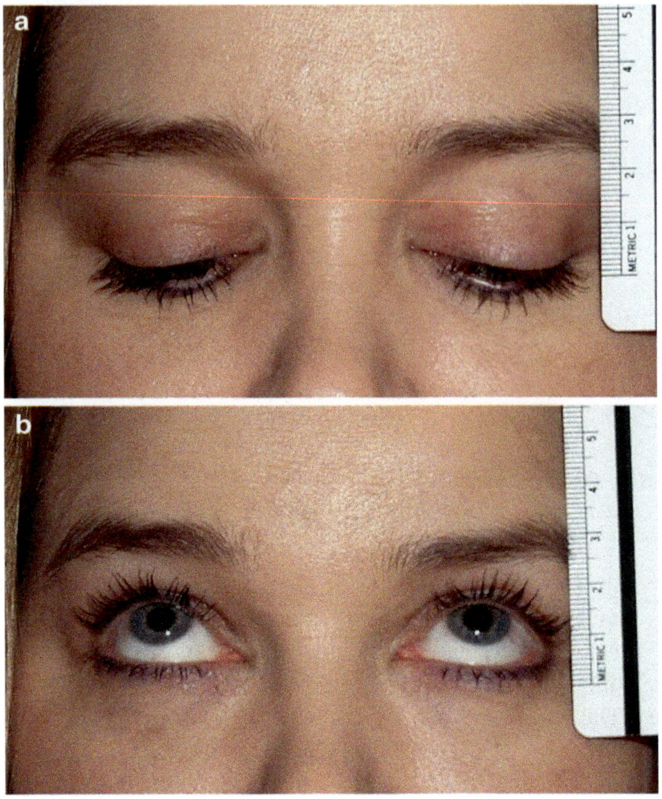

Fig. 12.1 Levator excursion is measured by having the patient look down (**a**) and up (**b**) and measuring the excursion of the upper lid in millimeters

12.3 Patient Evaluation

Patients with ptosis may have a tired look, complain of reduced field of vision, and have headaches from chronic brow elevation. These symptoms can also be present with dermatochalasis, with or without ptosis. As stated previously, noting what lid pathology is present (ptosis, excess lid skin, fat) and to what degree it affects field of vision and appearance will help the surgeon and patient determine what procedures are necessary to attain the desire outcome.

Upper lid ptosis can be an early finding of a potentially serious neurological problem such as myasthenia gravis, third nerve pathology, or Horner syndrome [2–4]. These disorders must be ruled out prior to proceeding with any form of surgery. All patients should be questioned as to the duration and onset of the problem. In general, long-standing ptosis is more likely to have a benign etiology. On the other hand, a sudden onset of ptosis may be an early indicator of a more serious problem. Diplopia is a concern with the ptosis patient. It can be seen in myasthenia gravis and third nerve paresis. Patients with myasthenia gravis may also manifest variability of their ptosis. An enlarged (dilated) pupil can be present in third nerve paresis and a miotic (constricted) pupil in Horner syndrome. A severe headache and decreased facial sweating are a few of a variety of symptoms which may manifest in Horner syndrome. If any of these findings/complaints are identified on the history or examination, a prompt referral to a specialist is warranted. Once serious ptosis pathology has been ruled out, surgery can be considered.

In general, patients with involutional ptosis have a high lid crease and normal levator function [2, 4]. A normal lid crease is at approximately 10 mm above the lid margin. As the levator aponeurosis is attenuated/disinserted in involutional ptosis, the aponeurosis retracts and the crease elevates. However, while the aponeurotic attachments to the lid are higher, the levator muscle still typically functions normally. A normal levator function is 15 mm in adults. This is measured by assessing the excursion of the eyelid between downgaze and upgaze with the eyebrow fixed (Fig. 12.1). In addition to levator function and crease position, other standard lid parameters assessed should include the margin reflex distance 1 (MRD1), and the vertical palpebral fissure distance. The MRD1 is the distance between the corneal light reflex and the upper lid margin (Fig. 12.2). It is a true measure of eyelid ptosis as its reference point is the center of the pupil (light reflex). This measurement is not affected by lower lid position. The vertical palpebral fissure measures the

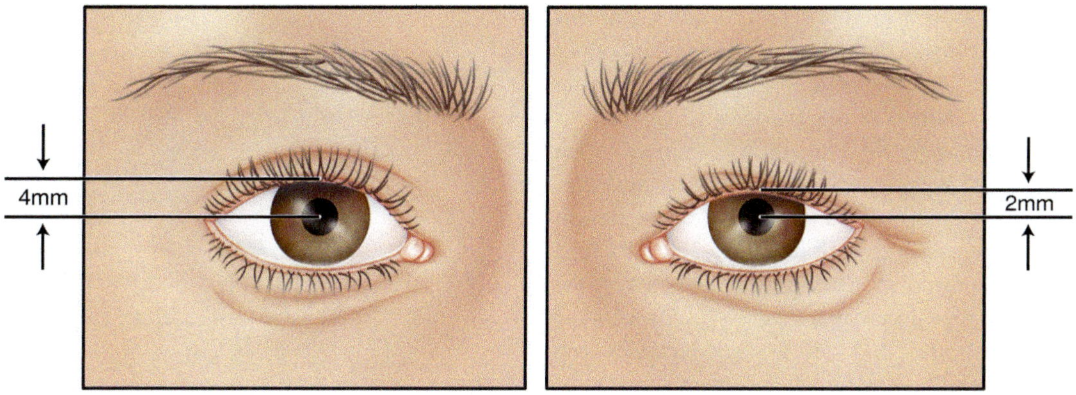

Fig. 12.2 The MRD1 is measured as the distance between the corneal light reflex and the upper lid margin. In this example, the MRD1 is 4 mm on the *right* and 2 mm on the left, representing 2 mm ptosis on the *left*

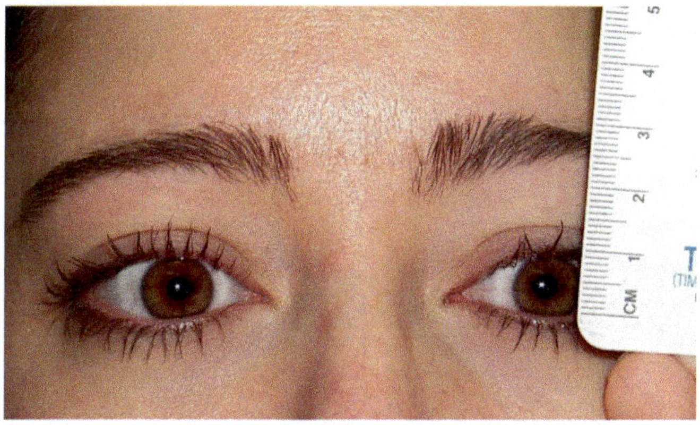

Fig. 12.3 The vertical palpebral fissure is determined by measuring, in millimeters, the distance between the upper and lower lid margin

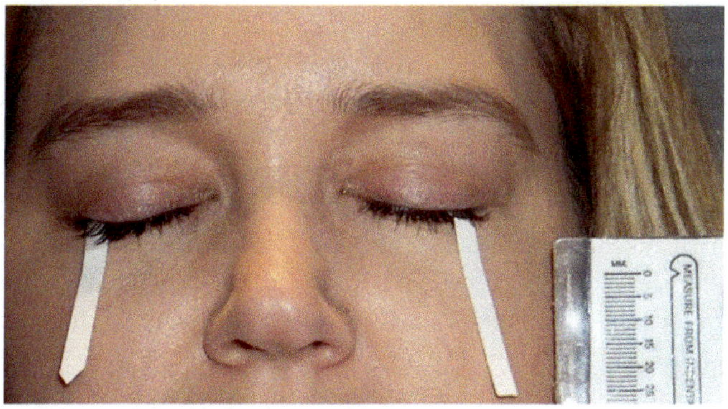

Fig. 12.4 After instillation of topical anesthetic, Schirmer strips are placed in the inferior fornix and measured after 5 min

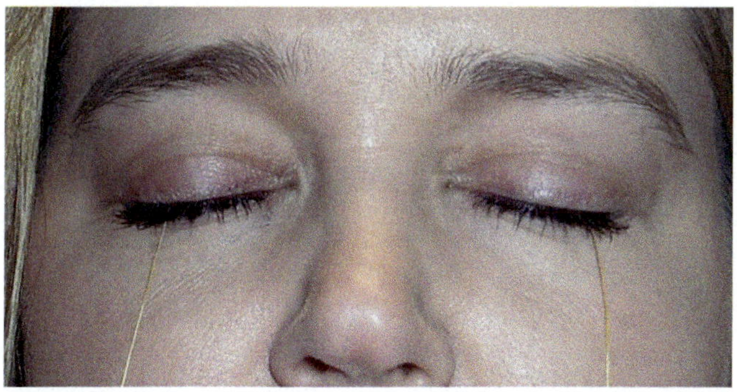

Fig. 12.5 The Zone-Quick can be performed in only 15 seconds without topical anesthesia

distance between the upper and lower lid margin (Fig. 12.3). It can be affected by both upper and lower lid position (i.e., lower lid retraction will increase this measurement) and thus is not the best measure of ptosis. A normal MRD1 is 3.5–4.5 mm. A normal adult vertical palpebral fissure is 10 mm.

An assessment of the Bell's phenomenon and orbicularis strength is important. The orbicularis strength is assessed by asking the patient to squeeze his or her lids tightly shut while the examiner attempts to pry them open. In a normal setting, it should be difficult to open the lids. To assess the Bell's phenomenon, ask the patient to relax the squeezing somewhat, manually open the lids, and check if the eye elevates under the upper lid. A normal response is elevation. When the Bell's mechanism and orbicularis strength is normal, the patient has inherent corneal protection from potential postoperative exposure symptoms. If either is reduced, there is a higher risk or corneal compromise. The same is true if preoperative lagophthalmos or lower lid retraction is present.

Examining the cornea is important with regard to dry eye symptoms. Any evidence of dry eye, corneal epithelial disease, or exposure may be a contraindication to surgery. Even with a normal-appearing cornea, the patient should be questioned about dry eye symptoms and whether or not artificial tear supplements are used. Schirmer testing, though not completely reliable, is still one objective way of measuring tear quantity and should be performed on every patient (Fig. 12.4) [8]. A strip of filter paper is placed in the lower conjunctival fornix of each eye for 5 min, and the amount of wetting of the filter paper is measured in millimeters. The Zone-Quick (Oasis, Glendora, CA) [9] technique can also be used. Fine cotton threads are placed in the inferior fornices of the eyelid for only 15 seconds (Fig. 12.5). When the threads become wet, they turn red. The amount of redness, again in millimeters, is measured. This test is quick and less irritating to the eyes. Finally, the presence of redundant upper eyelid tissue (skin, fat) should be determined so as to plan appropriately for the addition of blepharoplasty.

A final note on preoperative evaluation is that while the phenylephrine test is a necessary component of posterior ptosis surgery via conjunctival/Muller's muscle resection, it can also be helpful in levator resection patients [1]. If there is a positive response, it can demonstrate to the patient how the elevated eyelid may appear postoperatively [7]. Also, I have found that patients who respond well to phenylephrine drop testing also respond well to levator advancement surgery.

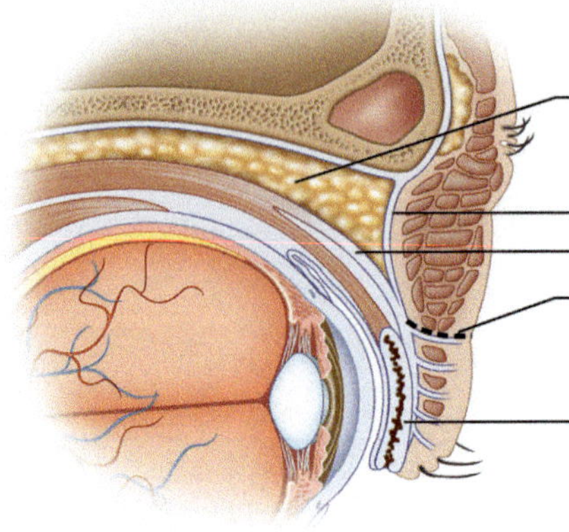

Fig. 12.6 An artist's rendition of the eyelid crease in Caucasians. The crease (*dotted line*) is formed by the superior aponeurotic attachments to the orbicularis muscle and eyelid skin

12.4 Anatomy

The eyelid is a dynamic structure which provides protection to the globe as well as conveys facial expression. Eyelid skin is the thinnest in the body with essentially no subcutaneous fat. The upper eyelid skin can be divided into two segments named for the underlying division of its associated orbicularis muscle counterpart. The pretarsal skin is below the eyelid crease and is firmly adhered to underlying tissue. The preseptal skin is above the eyelid crease, and is relatively mobile and lax allowing for eyelid movement.

The orbicularis oculi muscle, the sphincter (protractor) of the eyelid, consists of a palpebral (preseptal, pretarsal) and orbital component. The preseptal division overlies the orbital septum and the pretarasal segment the tarsus. The orbital division overlies the orbital rim and the corrugator muscle in the central lower forehead. As the orbicularis muscle is responsible for eyelid closure, it is recommended not to routinely debulk large amounts (especially with advancing age) of the muscle during surgery. Excessive muscle excision can leave the patient at risk for poor eyelid closure and exposure symptoms after surgery, even in the face of appropriate excision of skin. Also, maintaining the orbicularis muscle can enhance volume of the upper lid [10].

Beneath the skin and preseptal orbicularis muscle is the orbital septum. The septum is a dense connective tissue band which originates from the arcus marginalis of the superior orbital rim. The arcus marginalis is the fusion point of perisoteum overlying the orbit and frontal bone. In Caucasians, the septum inserts onto the levator aponeurosis several millimeters above the superior tarsal border. The eyelid crease is formed by the attachment of fibers of the distal levator aponeurosis to the orbicularis muscle and skin (Fig. 12.6). When the fusion of the septum to the aponeurosis occurs below the superior tarsal border, as in Asian individuals, it allows eyelid fat to lie more inferiorly, resulting in more fullness of the upper lid with blunting of the crease (Fig. 12.7).

The orbital septum is the anatomic landmark which separates the eyelid proper from the orbit [11]. Posterior to the septum are the eyelid fat pads, and below the fat is the levator aponeurosis. Identifying the aponeurosis, the critical structure for surgical repair, is the single most important step in surgery. The nasal fat pad is whiter in appearance and denser. The central fat pad, which lies on the levator, is yellow and more flaccid. There are only two fat pads in the upper lid (as opposed to the lower lid). Laterally, the upper lid may have a visible lacrimal gland (if it is prolapsed). Exercise caution when dissecting in this area so as not to inadvertently excise or damage the lacrimal gland. Care should also be taken not to overresect the central fat pad, as its natural tendency is to involute with age. This may lead to a hollowed upper sulcus postoperatively.

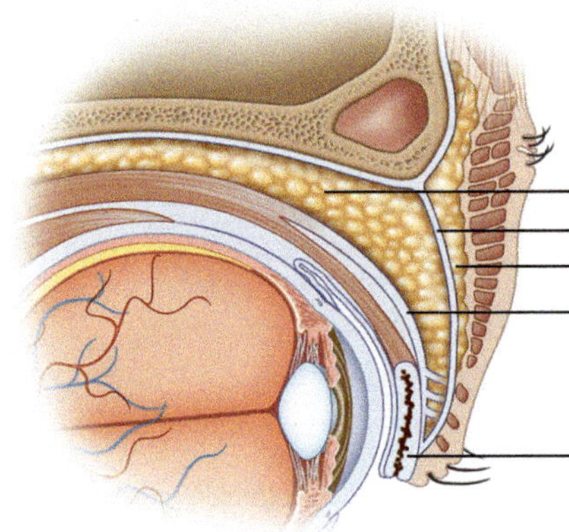

Fig. 12.7 In Asian patients, the crease is absent or indistinct. Note the lower attachment of the septum to the aponeurosis/tarsus, allowing fat to descend in the eyelid and blunt aponeurotic attachments to the skin

The levator aponeurosis, the tendon of the levator muscle (predominant retractor of the upper lid), lies just beneath the eyelid fat pad. The levator muscle originates from the posterior orbit at the lesser wing of sphenoid, extending anteriorly until approximately 15 mm from the superior tarsal border, where it becomes the fibrous aponeurosis. The muscle/aponeurosis transition occurs at Whitnall's ligament. The levator aponeurosis continues inferiorly until it attaches to

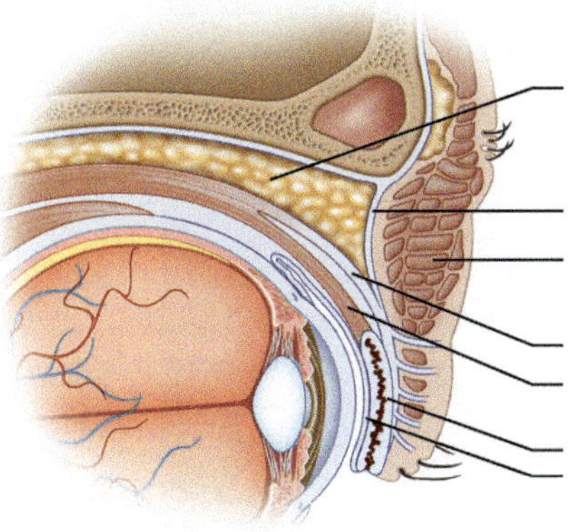

Fig. 12.8 A schematic of upper lid anatomy depicts all relevant anatomic structures

the anterior tarsal plate. Muller's muscle and conjunctiva are loosely adherent to the underside of the levator. During surgery, the levator can be gently dissected free from Muller's muscle for several millimeters superior to the tarsus. This allows isolation of the aponeurosis for resection/advancement. This should be done with care so as not to disturb the vascular arcades of the eyelid with resultant hematoma. Immediately posterior to the conjunctiva is the globe. It is recommended to place a corneal protector when dissecting in this area.

The tarsal plate lies posterior to the pretarsal orbicularis muscle. It is made up of dense connective tissue and provides the structural support to the lids. In the upper lid, the central tarsus is about 10 mm in vertical height [10, 11]. The tarsus is also an important landmark in levator ptosis surgery as it is the anchor point for levator reattachment during surgery.

Figure 12.8 depicts the relevant anatomic structures of the upper eyelid.

12.5 Procedure

A basic blepharoplasty tray is used for the procedure. The lid crease is marked with a fine-toothed marking pen. I prefer to use the patient's natural crease if it is present and favorably positioned. If the lid crease is significantly elevated, as in many patients with involutional ptosis, or if there is no visible crease, the incision is marked at approximately 10 mm from the central lid margin in women and at 8 mm in men. The crease is then tapered nasally and temporally to 5–6 mm from the margin to an endpoint of the puncta nasally and the canthus temporally. In Asians, the crease is drawn at a lower position as described in Chap. 14. When blepharoplasty is added, I demarcate an ellipse for skin excision. Even in isolated ptosis repair, I often excise mild amounts of skin, as the preoperative lid depression masks a degree of excess skin (latent dermatochalasis). That stated, it is important to note that caution must be taken when simultaneously lifting the lid and excising skin, to maintain

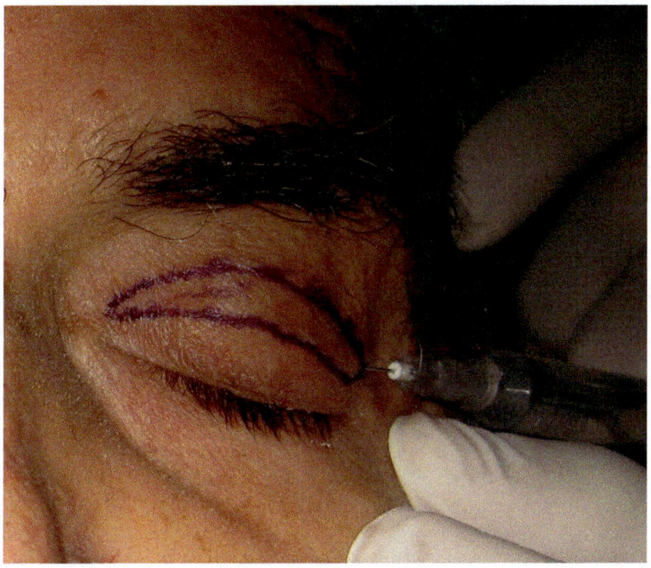

Fig. 12.9 After marking the lid, the local anesthetic mixture is infiltrated just beneath the skin, using minimal volume

postoperative lid dynamics (function, closure), and prevent exposure symptoms. An awareness of appropriate skin excision comes with surgical experience. In those cases when no skin excision is warranted, only the lid crease is demarcated [12, 13].

The eyelid skin is infiltrated with a 50:50 mixture of 2% lidocaine with 1:100:000 epinephrine and 0.5 or 0.75% bupivacaine. The solution may be buffered with sodium bicarbonate for pain control [14]. I do not add hyaluronidase to the mixture, as it may cause inadvertent spread of the anesthetic into the levator muscle, reducing native levator excursion and the surgeon's ability to accurately assess intraoperative lid position. The local anesthetic is infiltrated just beneath the skin (Fig. 12.9). It is important to use a minimal volume of anesthetic solution (1 cc or less, if possible), as the mechanical effect of volume can also cause spread of the solution to the levator muscle and reduce surgical accuracy. A small amount of local anesthetic is also injected subcutaneously over the central tarsus where the tarsal sutures will be passed. I avoid intramuscular infiltration to prevent hematoma formation and swelling. Intravenous sedation may be added, but with caution, as the patient must be fully cooperative during the lid adjustment phase of the surgery. I do not perform this procedure under general anesthesia as it is difficult to know how much to advance/resect the levator without patient cooperation. In the unusual circumstance where conditions dictate general anesthesia, a mild plication of the aponeurosis may be safest so as not to result in an overcorrection.

Following injection of anesthetic, topical anesthetic is instilled in the eyes, and the patient undergoes full face prep with a head drape and split sheet to leave the entire face exposed. Patients are more comfortable with the entire face left open,

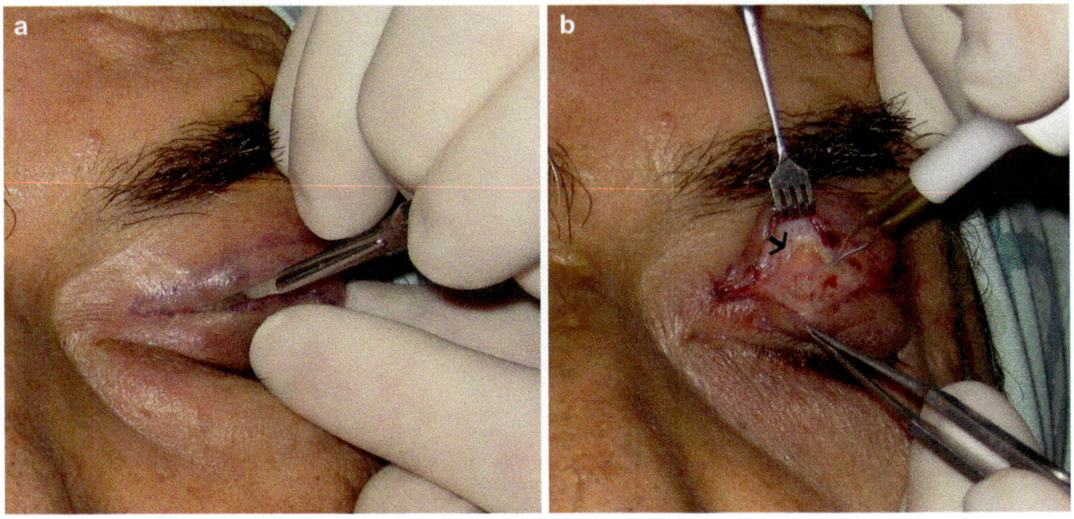

Fig. 12.10 (**a**) An incision is made through the skin, beginning with the inferior limb of the marking. A No. 15 blade, Colorado needle, or laser may be used. (**b**) Using a hand-held cautery, dissection is carried out superiorly to identify the orbital septum (*arrow*)

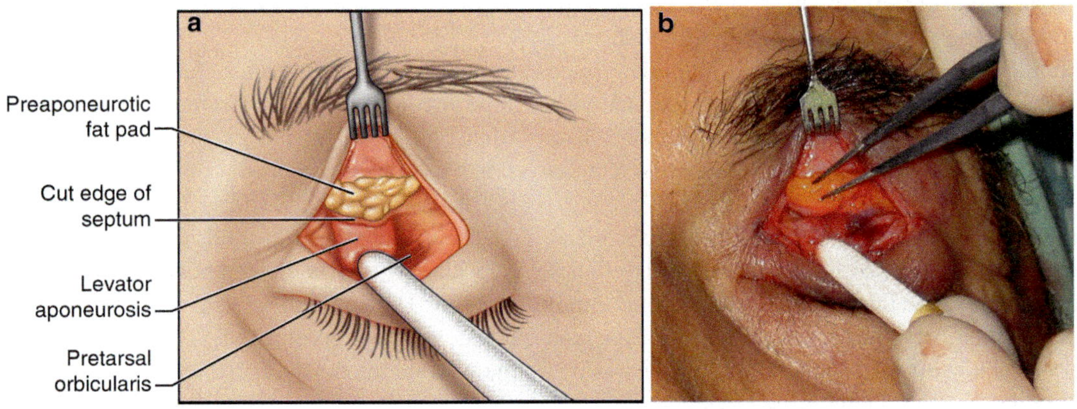

Fig. 12.11 (**a**) Artist's drawing (**b**) Surgical photo. Once the septum is opened, the preaponeurotic fat is identified (just below forceps) which lies just anterior to the levator. It may be shrunken with cautery or resected

and it allows both eyes to be compared during the procedure. A rigid corneal (or eye) shield is placed over the eye to protect the globe during the procedure.

The eyelid skin incision is made with a No. 15c blade along the demarcated line(s) (Fig. 12.10a). The skin is excised (if performed) with a Wescott scissors, Colorado needle, Ellman radiofrequency unit (Ellman International, Inc., Oceanside, NY), or CO_2 laser. Hemostasis is obtained with bipolar or monopolar cautery. With an assistant retracting the superior skin edge, the surgeon grasps the pretarsal orbicularis muscle inferiorly, and dissection is carried in a superior direction in the suborbicularis plane to identify the orbital septum (Fig. 12.10b). In older patients with a high lid crease (recessed levator) and in those with a deeper superior sulcus (recessed levator/septum with little or no preaponeurotic fat), it is especially important to dissect in a more superior direction to assure division of the septum. In these thin lids of older patients it is easy to mistaken tissue planes and inadvertently injure the levator aponeurosis when attempting to divide the orbital septum. Once the septum is identified and opened, the preaponeurotic fat prolapses into the field. As stated, identifying the fat is important as the levator aponeuriosis is just below it.

The preaponeurotic fat may be excised or contracted with cautery if desired (Fig. 12.11). Reduction of upper eyelid fat should proceed with caution so as not to create a hollow superior sulcus postoperatively. As discussed, there is no lateral fat pad in the upper lid. It is important not to confuse the lacrimal gland with eyelid fat pad. The lacrimal gland tends to be whiter in color and firmer in texture than fat. A dislocated lacrimal gland (Fig. 12.12a) can be repositioned but should not be excised.

Once the eyelid fat is reduced or brushed away, the levator aponeurosis is identified. In patients with involutional ptosis, there may be fatty infiltration of the levator muscle and/or attenuation of the aponeurosis. A frank disinsertion of the aponeurosis is less common. The assistant retracts the inferior skin edge of the wound and dissection is carried in a suborbicularis plane inferiorly to expose the tarsal plate (Fig. 12.12b).

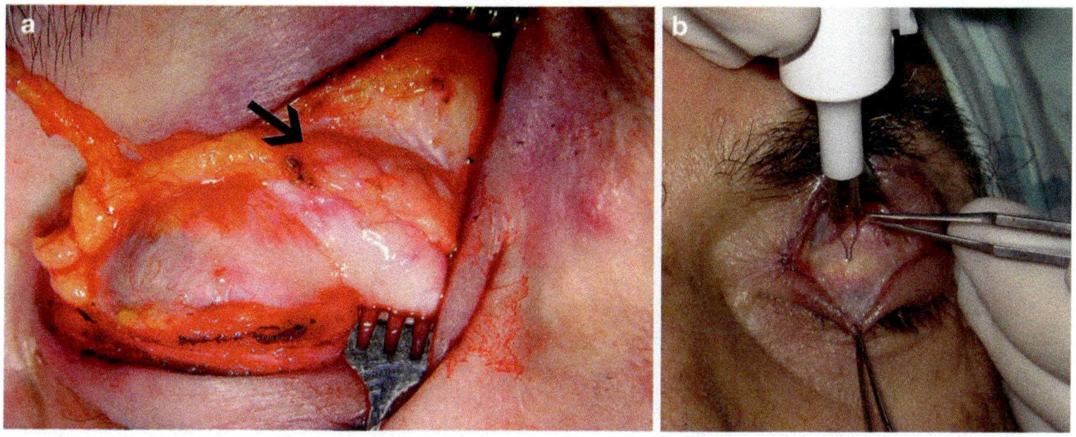

Fig. 12.12 (**a**) A dislocated lacrimal gland is noted intraoperatively (*arrow*). (Courtesy Guy G. Massry, MD). (**b**) Dissection is carried inferiorly through the pretarsal orbicularis muscle to expose the tarsal plate. The tip of the instrument is pointing to the tarsus

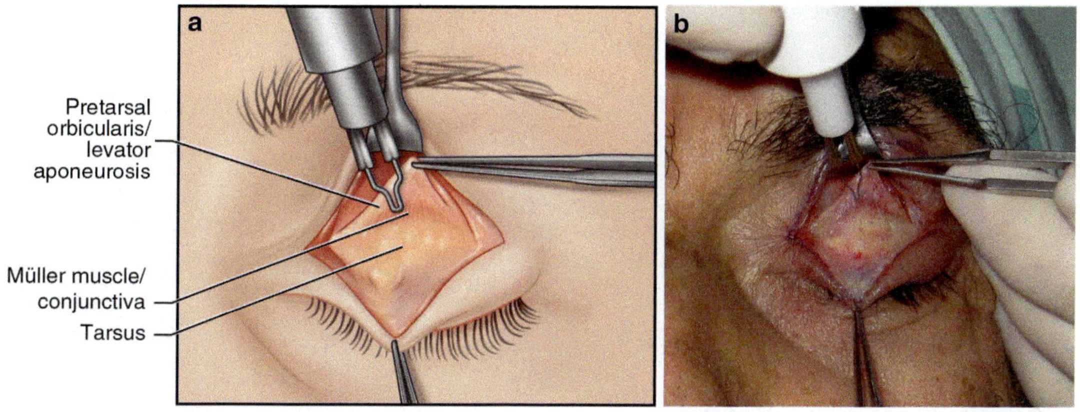

Fig. 12.13 (**a**) Artist's drawing (**b**) Surgical photo. Dissection is carried a few mm superiorly between Muller's muscle and the levator aponeurosis. The instrument is pointing to Muller's muscle

The aponeurosis is separated from the tarsal plate and from underlying Müller's muscle by dissecting superiorly in a graded fashion (Fig. 12.13). In appropriate patients, a strip of pretarsal orbicularis muscle can be excised to debulk the incisional portion of the eyelid and create a fresh edge of tissue which will adhere to the tarsus and help reform an eyelid crease (Fig. 12.14a).

The levator aponeurosis is isolated. Grasping the aponeurosis and asking the patient to look up will cause the muscle to retract into the orbit, and the surgeon will feel the pull as the muscle moves. This ensures that the tissue dissected free is the aponeurosis. The aponeurosis is now advanced to the tarsus. This can be done directly if there is a frank disinsertion. As stated previously, more often an aponeurotic attenuation is present. In this instance, the free edge of the aponeurosis is resected appropriately (to shorten and create a fresh edge) before advancement. A variety of sutures are used to secure the aponeurosis to the tarsus. These include both permanent and long-term absorbable sutures. I prefer a 5–0 absorbable polyglactin 910 or nonabsorbable 5–0 polypropylene suture. It is important to use a spatulated needle in order to pass the suture partial thickness through tarsus without cheese wiring the tissue. A double-armed suture is preferred, so that after the tarsal bite is placed, both ends can be passed through the aponeurosis for tying.

The suture is passed through partial-thickness tarsus, a few millimeters below its superior edge (Fig. 12.14b), in the central/medial region of the lid. I use a toothed forceps to engage the tarsus, elevate the lid, and evaluate contour, until I identify the best placement location. After passing the suture I evert the eyelid to ensure that the suture is not passed full-thickness, which may lead to corneal abrasion after surgery (Fig. 12.15a). Both needle ends are carried through the levator aponeurosis (Fig. 12.15b) and tied in a temporary slip knot (Fig. 12.16). If there is uncertainty as to what level of the levator to pass the suture, slightly below the muscle/aponeurotic border is a good place to start, however, the amount of ptosis and levator function should be taken into account. I have found that the greater the degree of ptosis, and the less the levator function, the higher the suture should be placed. However, I have been fooled.

Care should be taken when passing the levator suture to avoid inadvertent injury to the underlying Müller's

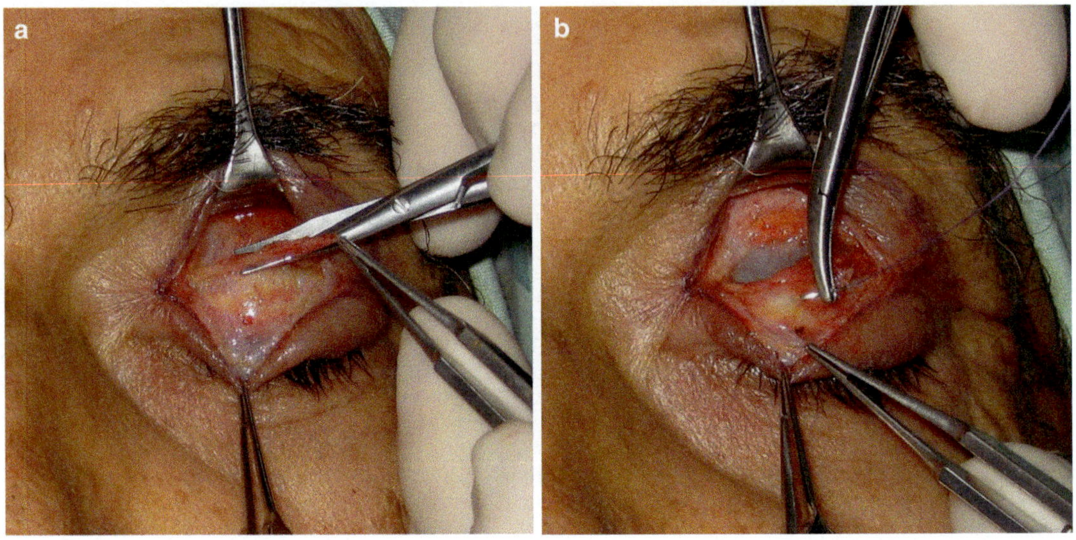

Fig. 12.14 (**a**) A strip of pretarsal orbicularis (in forceps) is excised. (**b**) Vicryl suture on a spatulated needle is passed partial-thickness through the anterior surface of the tarsus (*yellow tissue*)

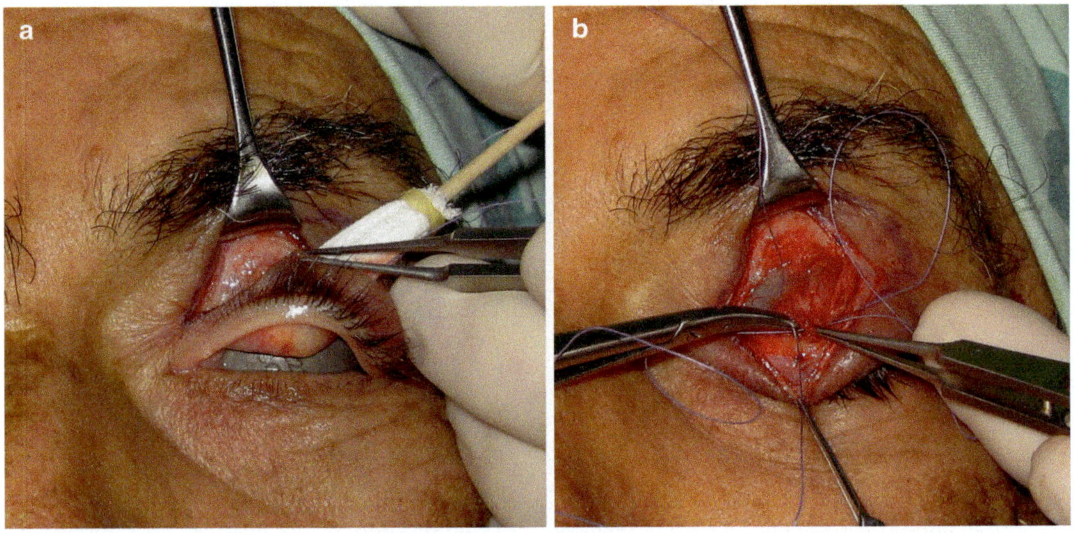

Fig. 12.15 (**a**) The lid is everted to ensure that the suture did not penetrate full-thickness through the tarsus where it could abrade the cornea. (**b**) One end of the 5–0 vicryl suture is passed through the levator aponeurosis (tissue adjacent to tip of forceps). The first arm of the suture has already been passed

muscle. An injury to Muller's muscle often results in a hemorrhage, making it more difficult to gauge eyelid position intraoperatively. After placement of the first levator suture, the eyelid is examined for height and contour**.** It is critical for the patient to be alert when examining lid position. If used, intravenous sedation (IV) is discontinued prior to evaluating eyelid position. The overhead lights are turned away from the patient's face and additional topical anesthetic can be given. I prefer to have the patient sit up intraoperatively as this provides a more physiologic assessment of the eyelid position and contour. This maneuver also helps to wake the patient in cases when IV sedation is used. The lid height should be set slightly above the desired level, allowing for normal postoperative drop. Tightening or loosening the suture can be accomplished in the sitting position until the desired lid height is achieved. When lid position is too high, or a central peak in contour is created, the suture can be loosened and allowed to hang back. This reduces the need to re-pass the suture. If the lid position is too low, the suture needs to be re-passed to a higher position on the aponeurosis. In this instance, the patient is returned to the supine position for suture adjustment.

Additional sutures are then placed just nasal and temporal to the central suture. The lid contour may appear appropriate intraoperatively with a single central suture. However, I have found that placement of additional nasal and temporal sutures helps to stabilize the eyelid contour postoperatively. This also helps take tension off of the central suture, reducing the chance of suture cheese wiring postoperatively. Once

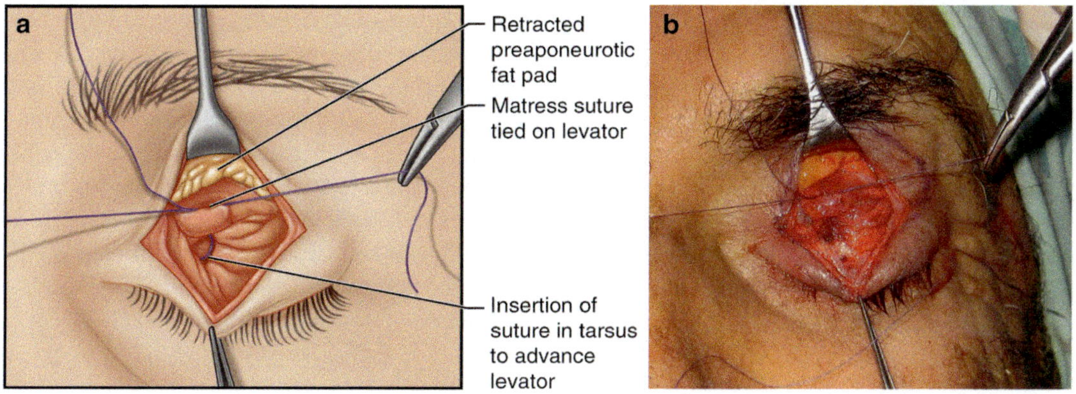

Fig. 12.16 (**a**) Artist's drawing (**b**) Surgical photo. Once both ends of the suture are passed, they are tied in a temporary slip-knot in order to evaluate the lid height intraoperatively

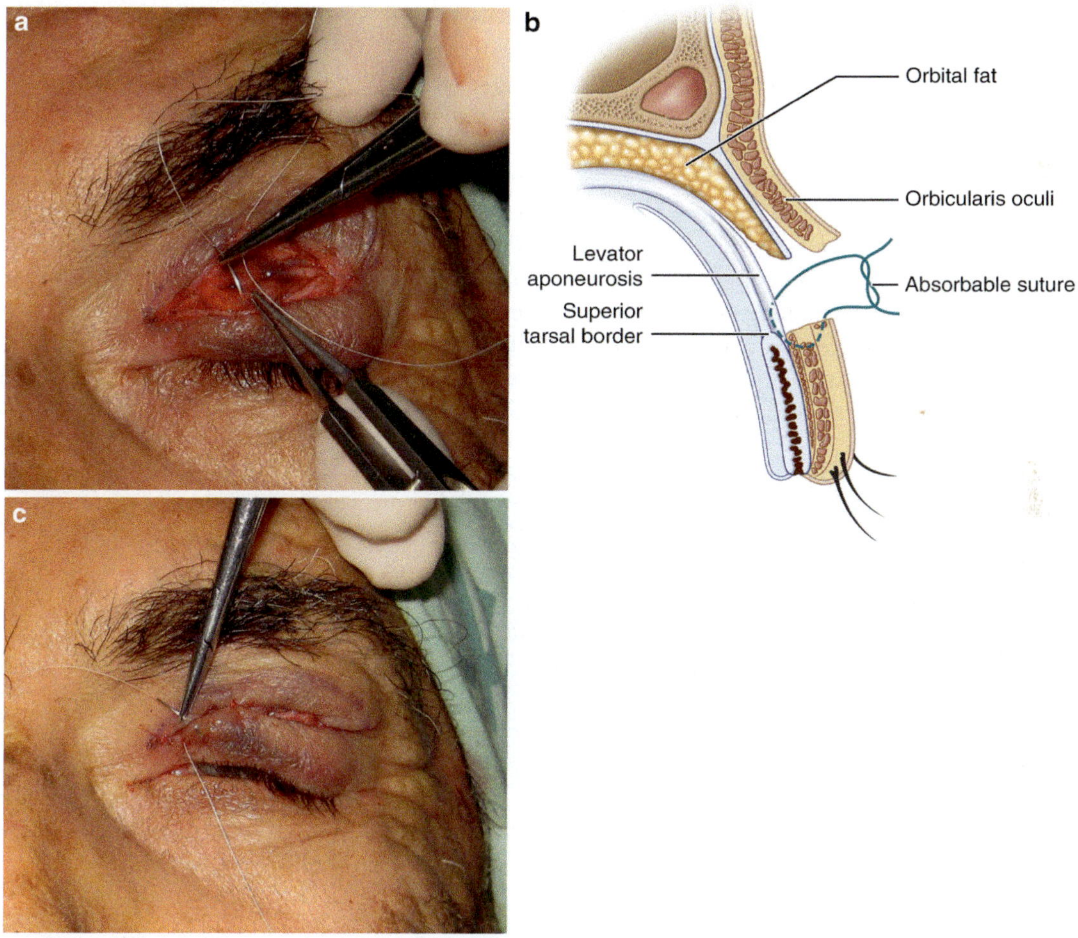

Fig. 12.17 (**a**) Once the aponeurosis has been resecured to tarsus, the lid crease may be reformed by passing an absorbable suture through one or both edges of the skin, or orbicularis muscle, while incorporating a bite of the edge of the levator aponeurosis (tip of needle in surgical photo). (**b**) Associated artist's rendition shows passage of suture. (**c**) The incision is closed with a running suture of 6–0 absorbable or nonabsorbable suture

the desired eyelid position and contour has been obtained, the sutures are tied and trimmed. The lid crease may be reformed, if desired, to more precisely define its location. This is accomplished by passing a few interrupted 6–0 absorbable sutures through one or both edges of the skin, or orbicularis muscle, while incorporating a bite of the edge of the levator aponeurosis (Fig. 12.17a,b). This supratarsal fixation creates a deep and well-defined crease. Alternatively, this step can be omitted, and a softer, less distinct, crease will form. The skin incision is closed with a running 6–0 plain gut or 6–0 Nylon or Polypropylene suture (Fig. 12.17c). Antibiotic ointment is applied to the wound.

Cold compresses are placed immediately after surgery. They are continued at frequent intervals for the next 48 h. The patient is advised to keep his/her head elevated, including sleeping on several pillows, in order to minimize postoperative edema. Antibiotic ointment is applied to the sutures 3 times daily for a week with artificial tear supplements used as needed. Patients are usually seen in the office at 5–7 days postoperatively, when nonabsorbable sutures are removed.

12.6 Complications

Mild lagophthalmos and exposure keratitis (dry eye) are probably the most common complications after surgery, and are typically self-limiting. Treatment for this problem includes the use of artificial tear supplements during the day and ointment before sleep for a short period postoperatively. The placement of punctal plugs can also be of benefit if symptoms persist. In addition, oral doxycycline may be helpful to correct meibomian gland dysfunction which can contribute to dry eye after surgery. In rare cases, corneal abrasion or ulcer may develop requiring the eyelids be closed temporarily with a tarsorrhaphy procedure [15, 16].

An over- or undercorrection of lid height can also occur. A small overcorrection may respond to gentle lid massage. Once the incision is sufficiently healed, the patient is instructed to use several fingers to hold the lid downward while simultaneously trying to open (creating countertraction) the lid for 5 min 4 times a day. If the overcorrection is more significant, a minor "in-office revision" is necessary. A small amount of local anesthetic is given (the incision site is typically partially denervated from the initial surgery), and the wound is partly opened by gently pulling apart the edges without re-incising. Sutures can then be adjusted to modify lid height and contour. If there is an obvious undercorrection, the same technique is used for revision. Conversely, if there is only mild undercorrection, it is best to wait until all the edema has subsided before considering revision [17].

12.7 Conclusion

Levator resection/advancement is a powerful technique for ptosis repair. Successful surgery requires a thorough appreciation of eyelid anatomy and experience with detailed dissection of the eyelid. In addition, comfort and familiarity with performing surgery on the awake patient and with intraoperative adjustment of lid height and contour are needed to attain consistent and reproducible surgical outcomes. Preoperative examination and counseling is essential in order to successfully identify and address both the ptosis and eyelid fullness (excess skin, herniated fat) components in cosmetic surgery patients (Figs. 12.18 and 12.19). In the appropriate setting, this surgery is an invaluable tool for the eyelid surgeon.

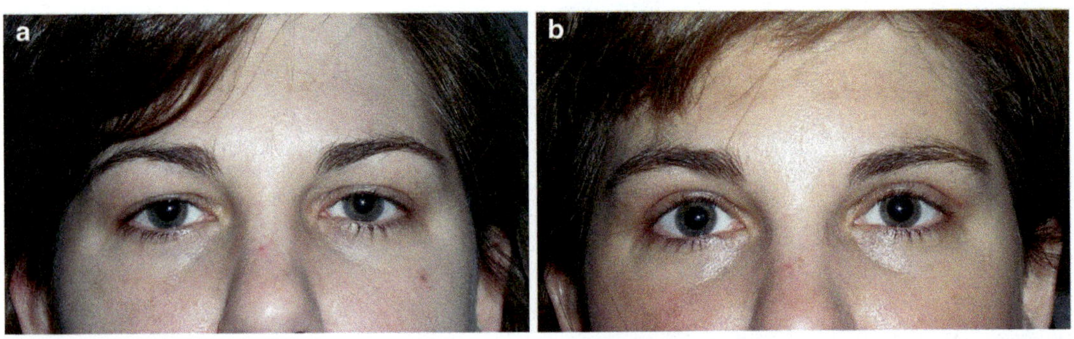

Fig. 12.18 (**a**) Preoperative and (**b**) postoperative photographs of a young patient who underwent upper blepharoplasty combined with minimal levator advancement to correct ptosis, more pronounced in the right eye

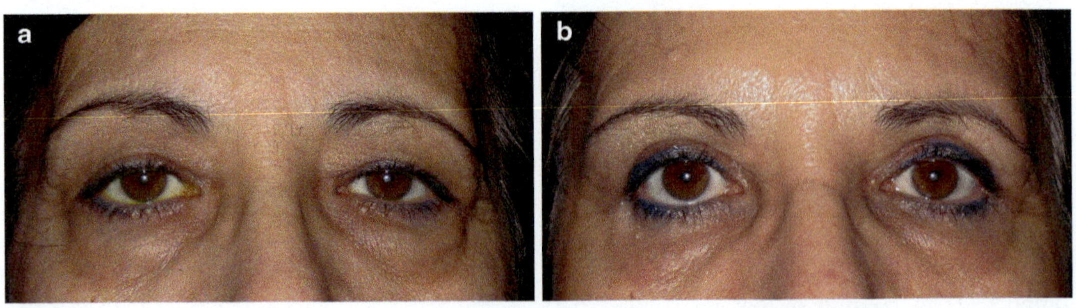

Fig. 12.19 (**a**) Preoperative and (**b**) postoperative photographs of middle-aged patient with significant dermatochalasis and ptosis. Both components were addressed surgically

References

1. Older JJ. Ptosis repair and blepharoplasty in the adult. Ophthalmic Surg. 1995;26(4):304–8. Review.
2. Beard C. Types of ptosis. In: Beard C, editor. Ptosis. 3rd ed. St. Louis: Mosby; 1981. p. 39–76.
3. Finsterer J. Ptosis: causes, presentation, and management. Aesthet Plast Surg. 2003;27(3):193–204.
4. Massry GG. Ptosis repair for the cosmetic surgeon. Facial Plast Surg Clin North Am. 2005;13(4):553–9.
5. Anderson RL, Dixon RS. Aponeurotic ptosis surgery. Arch Ophthalmol. 1979;97(6):1123–8.
6. Putterman AM, Urist MJ. Müller's muscle-conjunctival resection. Arch Ophthalmol. 1975;93(8):619–23.
7. Ben Simon GJ, Lee S, Schwarcz RM, et al. External levator advancement vs. Müller's muscle-conjunctival resection for correction of upper eyelid involutional ptosis. Am J Ophthalmol. 2005;140(3):426–32.
8. Lamberts DW, Foster CS, Perrry HD. Schirmer test after topical anesthesia and tear film meniscus height in normal eyes. Arch Ophthalmol. 1979;97(6):1082–5.
9. Mainnstone JC, Bruce AS, Golding TR. Tear meniscus measurements in the diagnosis of dry eye. Curr Eye Res. 1996;15:653–61.
10. Harris PA, Mendelson BC. Eyelid and midcheek anatomy. In: Fagien S, editor. Putterman's cosmetic oculoplastic surgery. 4th ed. Philadelphia: Elsevier; 2008. p. 45–62.
11. Patel BCK. Surgical eyelid and periorbital anatomy. Semin Ophthalmol. 1996;11:118–37.
12. Lucarelli MJ, Lemke BN. Small incision external levator repair: technique and early results. Am J Ophthalmol. 1999;127(6): 637–44.
13. Baroody M, Holds JB, Sakamoto DK, Vick VL, Hartstein ME. Small incision transcutaneous levator aponeurotic repair for blepharoptosis. Ann Plast Surg. 2004;52(6):558–61.
14. Moody BR, Holds JB. Anesthesia for office-based oculoplastic surgery. Dermatol Surg. 2005;31:766–9.
15. Pacella SJ, Codner MA. Minor complications after blepharoplasty: dry eyes, chemosis, granulomas, ptosis, and scleral show. Plast Reconstr Surg. 2010;125(2):709–18.
16. Hartstein ME, Kikkawa D. How to avoid blepharoplasty complications. Oral Maxillofac Surg Clin North Am. 2009;21(1): 31–41.
17. McCulley TJ, Kersten RC, Kulwin DR, Feuer WJ. Outcome and influencing factors of external levator palpebrae superioris aponeurosis advancement for blepharoptosis. Ophthal Plast Reconstr Surg. 2003;19(5):388–93.

Posterior Approach Ptosis Repair in the Aesthetic Patient With or Without Blepharoplasty

13

Kiran Sajja and Allen M. Putterman

Key Points

- The Müller's muscle-conjunctival resection procedure may be performed on ptotic patients with intact levator function and a response to the phenylephrine test.
- The advantage of this procedure over the levator aponeurosis advancement/resection procedure is a more predictable postoperative result decreasing the likelihood of reoperation.
- The advantage over the Fasanella–Servat procedure is preservation of the tarsus; allows for greater stability of the eyelid margin and less risk of suture keratopathy.
- The Müller's muscle-conjunctival resection procedure can be performed under local anesthesia with minimal discomfort. Alternatively, sedation or general anesthesia may be used without modifying the technique or decreasing the effectiveness/reliability of the technique.
- The most common complication from posterior eyelid ptosis repair is corneal irritation. Patients should be strongly encouraged to maintain an aggressive ocular lubrication regimen after surgery.

13.1 Introduction

Posterior eyelid ptosis repair via the Müller's muscle-conjunctival resection procedure with or without blepharoplasty is a valuable technique for periorbital rejuvenation in the aesthetic patient. The surgeon's ability to recognize eyelid ptosis, and comfort with performing posterior eyelid surgical procedures is paramount in successfully integrating this technique into surgical armamentarium.

A.M. Putterman (✉)
Professor, Department of Ophthalmology and Visual Sciences, Illinois Eye and Ear Infirmary, University of Illinois at Chicago, Chicago, IL, USA
e-mail: puttermanmd@hotmail.com

Age-related, or involutional, ptosis is common and must not be overlooked in the preoperative evaluation of an aesthetic patient. In our practice, patients often do not recognize the difference between upper eyelid ptosis and dermatochalasis. A detailed examination, including eyelid measurements and provocative testing, is important in determining the aesthetic and functional potential of eyelid ptosis repair with or without blepharoplasty.

Posterior eyelid surgical approaches may be daunting to the surgeon unfamiliar with surgical anatomy of the eyelid and orbit. In addition, the close proximity to the globe and potential for vision-threatening complications are variables that only clinical experience will alleviate. Appropriate selection of surgical candidates with realistic goals is vital in developing the skills necessary to feel at ease with posterior eyelid surgical approaches.

This chapter will detail the preoperative evaluation/planning, surgical technique, postoperative management, and potential complications of posterior eyelid ptosis repair via the Müller's muscle-conjunctival resection procedure with or without blepharoplasty.

13.2 Preoperative Evaluation

Before proceeding with any ptosis surgery, a detailed knowledge of eyelid anatomy and a thorough preoperative assessment of the suitability for ptosis surgery are necessary. These topics are discussed in detail in Chaps. 2 and 12. Please refer these chapters for reference.

13.2.1 Degree of Eyelid Ptosis

The margin-reflex distance 1 (MRD_1) measurement is used to assess the upper eyelid position (Fig. 13.1). The examiner holds a point light source at eye level directly in front of the patient and the patient is asked to gaze at the light. The distance from the corneal light reflex to the central upper eyelid

G.G. Massry et al. (eds.), *Master Techniques in Blepharoplasty and Periorbital Rejuvenation*,
DOI 10.1007/978-1-4614-0067-7_13, © Springer Science+Business Media, LLC 2011

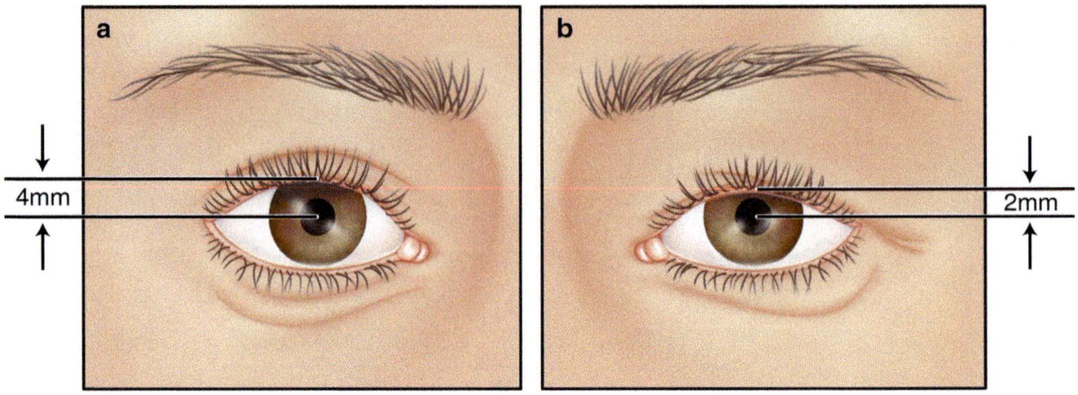

Fig. 13.1 Margin-reflex distance 1 (MRD_1): The distance from the corneal light reflex to the central upper eyelid margin. The MRD_1 is (a) +4 on the right and (b) +2 mm on the left upper eyelid

margin is the MRD_1. The MRD_1 is measured in positive millimeters if the eyelid is above the corneal light reflex and measured in negative millimeters if the eyelid obscures the corneal light reflex. In unilateral cases of upper eyelid ptosis, the difference in MRD_1 of the normal side and the ptotic side indicates the amount of ptosis. The normal MRD_1 is approximately 3.5–4.5 mm. This value may be used to determine the amount of ptosis in bilateral cases. The MRD_1 is a more valuable clinical measurement compared to the vertical palpebral fissure as it is independent of the lower eyelid position.

13.2.2 Levator Muscle Function

Levator function (LF) is used to assess the overall effectivity of the levator muscle/aponeurosis as an eyelid retractor. The levator muscle/aponeurosis is the principal eyelid retractor and decreased function may suggest dysgenesis of the levator muscle, abnormal innervation to the levator muscle, or traumatic disinsertion of the levator muscle/aponeurosis. The LF is measured as the excursion, in millimeters, of the upper eyelid from downgaze to upgaze with the frontalis muscle immobilized. The normal LF is approximately 15 mm. The frontalis muscle is an accessory eyelid retractor and if not immobilized will erroneously result in a higher LF measurement.

13.2.3 Phenylephrine Test

The Müller's muscle is a smooth muscle that is sympathetically innervated and involuntarily elevates the upper eyelid 2–3 mm [1]. Its origin extends from the posterior aspect of the levator muscle and inserts at the superior tarsal margin [2, 3]. The phenylephrine test uses an adrenergic agonist to stimulate the Müller's muscle and elevate the upper eyelid (Fig. 13.2).

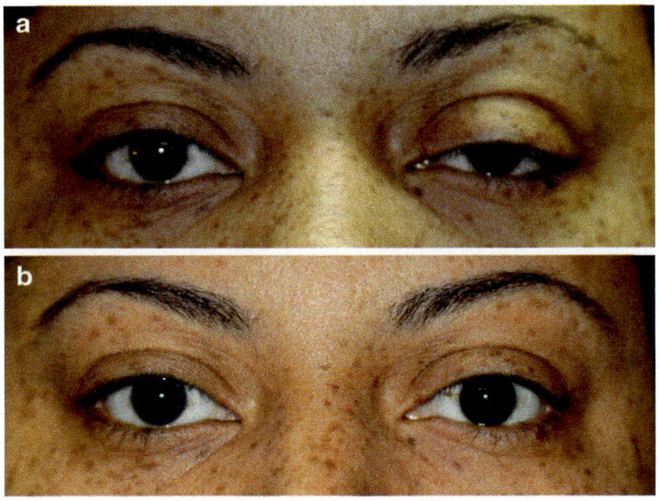

Fig. 13.2 A 37-year-old African-American woman presenting with left upper eyelid ptosis. (a) Prior to instillation of 2.5% phenylephrine drops. (b) Five minutes after instilling several drops of 2.5% phenylephrine onto the left superior fornix

The phenylephrine test is performed in three steps [4]. First, the MRD_1 is measured prior to instilling phenylephrine drops. Second, topical tetracaine drops are applied to the ocular surface and the patient's head is tilted backward, the upper eyelid is elevated, and the patient is asked to gaze downward. Several drops of 2.5–10% phenylephrine are instilled into the superior conjunctival fornix; this is repeated 2–3 additional times [5]. The patient is positioned in this manner to maximize effect on Müller's muscle and minimize ocular and systemic absorption. Finally, the MRD_1 is re-measured 3–5 min after instillation of the phenylephrine. The amount of upper eyelid elevation is used to determine the amount of Müller's muscle-conjunctival resection.

Prior to performing the phenylephrine test, the patient's clinical history should be thoroughly reviewed. Patients with a history of unstable or severe cardiac disease, hypertension, or angle-closure glaucoma should be excluded as systemic absorption of the phenylephrine may precipitate heart block, myocardial infarction, hypertensive crisis, or acute angle-closure glaucoma [5].

13.3 Anesthesia

The Müller's muscle-conjunctival resection ptosis procedure may be performed with minimal patient discomfort under local anesthesia consisting of 2% lidocaine with 1:100,000 units of epinephrine. In patients undergoing several concurrent periorbital rejuvenation procedures, oral/intravenous sedation or general anesthesia may be used without modifying the technique or decreasing the effectiveness or reliability of the postoperative result. This is not the case when performing an external levator advancement/resection ptosis repair as patients should be conscious to optimize intraoperative adjustments [6].

13.4 Surgical Technique

Once the preoperative evaluation is complete, it is vital to recruit the appropriate patients for posterior approach ptosis repair using the Müller's muscle-conjunctival resection procedure. Historically, patients with mild (≤2 mm) ptosis were considered appropriate, however, a recent study indicates that patients with moderate and moderate to severe ptosis may also be candidates. This suggests that patients with intact levator function (≥10 mm) and a response to the phenylephrine test are suitable for the Müller's muscle-conjunctival resection procedure.

In the initial report of the surgical technique [4], a response to the phenylephrine test in which the ptotic eyelid elevated to a normal level, 8.25 mm of Müller's muscle and conjunctiva, is excised. A 6.25–9.75 mm graded resection of Müller's muscle and conjunctiva is performed if the ptotic eyelid elevates slightly higher or lower than the normal eyelid or ideal eyelid position, respectively [7]. Several studies have attempted to develop an algorithm to determine the appropriate amount of Müller's muscle-conjunctival resection, however, results have been variable and no method has been universally accepted [8–12]. Clinical experience correlated with an individual surgeon's postoperative results is the most predictive factor in obtaining serial reliable operative results.

13.4.1 Step 1: Eyelid Marking for Upper Blepharoplasty

A sterile marking pen is used to mark the upper eyelid skin prior to injection of local anesthetic (Fig. 13.3a, b). The eyelid crease incision may be marked along the patient's natural eyelid crease; however, in patients with upper eyelid ptosis the eyelid crease may be displaced superiorly or poorly defined. This is often the case in patients with aponeurotic or involutional eyelid ptosis, the most common cause of eyelid ptosis in adults. Therefore, the crease may be measured and marked according to the patient/surgeon preference in regard to gender, ethnicity, anticipated prominence of the upper eyelid skin fold, and brow position.

The height of the eyelid crease above the eyelid margin may be marked at three positions (the upper punctum, the mid-pupil, and the lateral canthal angle) and connected in a curvilinear manner extending 1–1.5 cm temporally in a slightly upward direction. In men, the marks are usually 8 mm nasally, 10 mm centrally, and 9 mm temporally. In women, the marks are usually 9 mm nasally, 11 mm centrally, and 10 mm temporally [13].

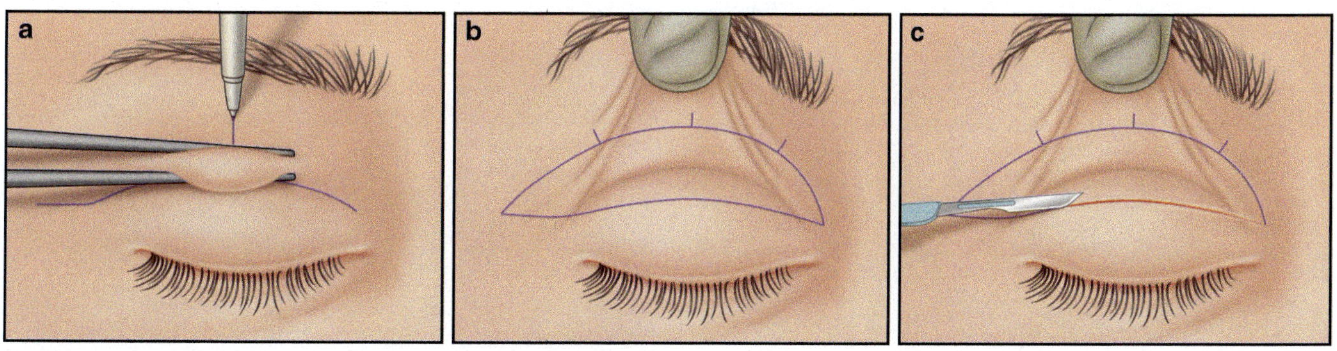

Fig. 13.3 (**a**) The upper eyelid crease is marked and the skin "pinch" technique is used to determine the amount of upper eyelid skin to be excised. (**b**) The upper eyelid markings designate an ellipse of tissue to be excised. Note the markings are positioned superior to the lateral canthus, mid-pupil, and upper punctum. (**c**) After a small amount of local anesthetic is injected below the skin, a surgical blade is used to make a superficial skin incision along the skin markings

A skin "pinch" technique may be employed to determine the amount of upper eyelid skin to be excised. A smooth forceps is used to grasp the eyelid skin at the mid-pupil crease mark and several millimeters above, in order to "pinch" the redundant eyelid skin and slightly evert the eyelashes without elevating the eyelid, and marked. This is repeated at the upper punctum and lateral canthal angle marks. The markings are connected in a curvilinear fashion and joined at the nasal and temporal ends to the eyelid crease marking.

See Chaps. 9 and 14 for further detail in surgical planning during upper blepharoplasty.

13.4.2 Step 2: Instilling Local Anesthetic for Upper Blepharoplasty

A small amount (0.5–1.0 mm) of local anesthetic is injected below the skin adjacent to the superficial skin markings. Overaggressive instillation of local anesthetic may cause inadvertent contraction of Müller's muscle in response to the epinephrine as well as making eyelid eversion more difficult. A surgical blade is used to make a superficial skin incision along the surgical markings (Fig. 13.3c).

13.4.3 Step 3: Performing the Frontal Block

A 23-gauge retrobulbar needle is used to perform a frontal nerve block (Fig. 13.4) [14]. This allows for sufficient anesthesia during the procedure without compromising normal eyelid architecture. One should palpate the supraorbital notch along the nasal aspect of the superior orbital rim to prevent inadvertent injury to the supraorbital neurovascular bundle. The retrobulbar needle is inserted into the superior orbit approximately 5–10 mm temporal to the supraorbital notch. The needle should hug the roof of the orbit during insertion and advanced to a depth of 4.0 cm; 1.5 mm of local anesthetic is injected. The needle should be withdrawn along the same path of insertion to avoid injury to the globe and orbital structures. Additional local anesthetic (0.25 mm) is injected subcutaneously over the center of the eyelid above the eyelid margin (Fig. 13.5a).

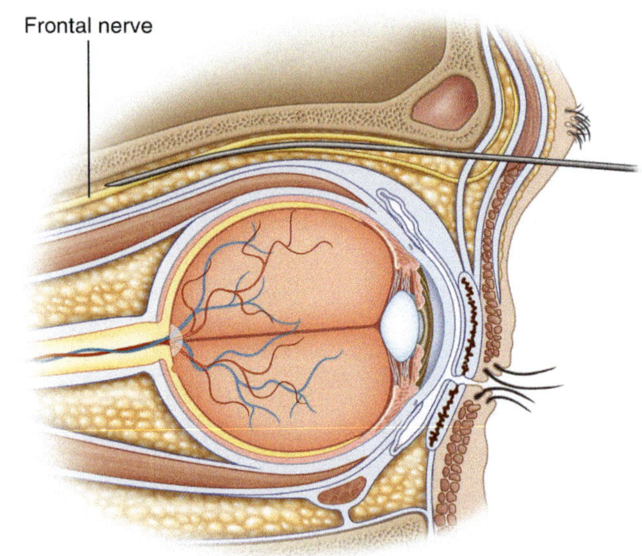

Fig. 13.4 Frontal nerve block: A sagittal view of the orbit detailing the path of the retrobulbar needle along the roof of the orbit

13.4.4 Step 4: Placement of the Traction Suture

A 4–0 silk traction suture is passed through skin, orbicularis muscle, and superficial tarsus 2 mm above the eyelid margin at the center of the eyelid (Fig. 13.5b). The silk traction suture is pulled superiorly and the eyelid is everted over a Desmarres retractor to expose the palpebral conjunctiva from the superior tarsal border to the conjunctival fornix. The size of the Desmarres retractor will depend on the laxity of the upper eyelid and the amount of conjunctiva-Müller's muscle to be excised; a medium and large-sized Desmarres retractor should be available. Several drops of topical tetracaine solution are irrigated over the globe and palpebral conjunctiva.

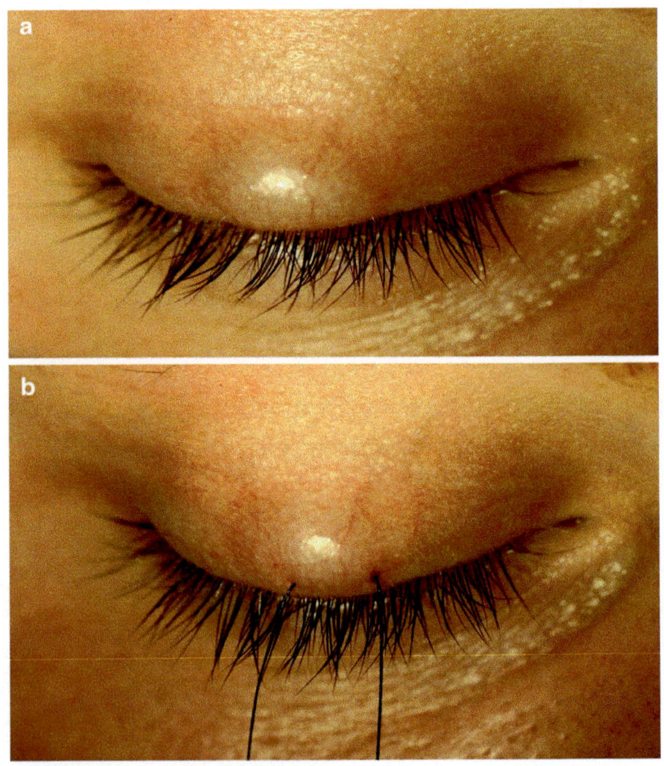

Fig. 13.5 Silk traction suture. (**a**) A small amount of local anesthetic is injected under the skin above the eyelashes at the central upper eyelid. (**b**) A 4–0 silk suture is passed through skin, orbicularis, and superficial tarsus approximately 2 mm above the eyelid margin

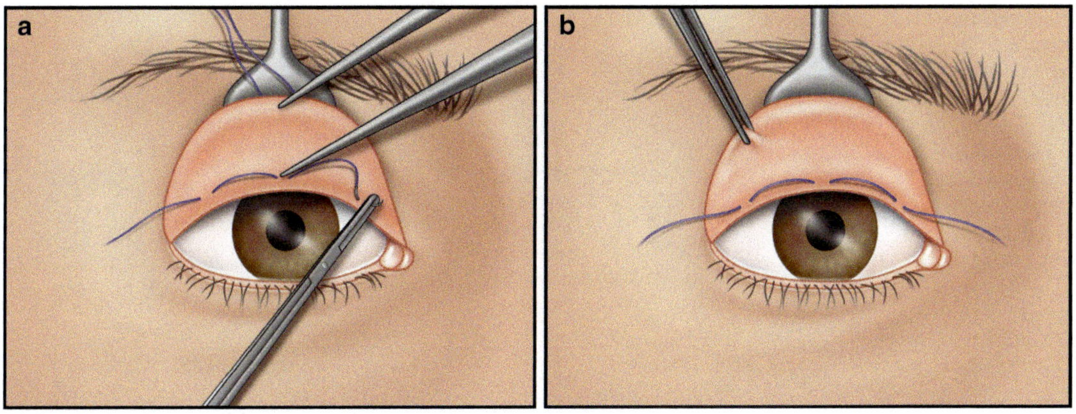

Fig. 13.6 (**a**) Silk marking suture: The upper eyelid is everted over a Desmarres retractor and a caliper is used to measure the distance above the superior tarsal margin. A 6–0 silk suture is passed through conjunctiva centrally and 7 mm nasally and temporally. (**b**) A toothed forceps is used to firmly grasp the conjunctiva and Müller's muscle between the superior tarsal border and the silk marking suture in order to separate Müller's muscle from the underlying levator aponeurosis

13.4.5 Step 5: Measuring Amount of Resection

A caliper is set at the amount of conjunctiva-Müller's muscle to be excised (Fig. 13.6a). One arm of the caliper is placed at the superior tarsal border and the other arm facilitates accurate placement of a 6–0 silk marking suture. The marking suture is passed through conjunctiva centrally and approximately 7 mm nasally and temporally. It is important to engage only conjunctiva during placement of the marking suture as inadvertent passage through Müller's muscle may result in subconjunctival hemorrhage.

13.4.6 Step 6: Separation of Conjunctiva and Müller's Muscle

A toothed forceps is used to firmly grasp the conjunctiva and Müller's muscle between the superior tarsal border and the silk marking suture in order to separate Müller's muscle from the underlying levator aponeurosis (Fig. 13.6b). This maneuver is possible because Müller's muscle is firmly attached to conjunctiva and only loosely adherent to the levator aponeurosis. Mild inferior rotation of the Desmarres retractor will decrease tension on the eyelid allowing for greater separation of the structures during this maneuver.

13.4.7 Step 7: Placement of the Ptosis Clamp

One blade of a specially designed clamp (Putterman Müller muscle-conjunctival resection clamp, Bausch & Lomb, Manchester, MO) is placed at the level of the silk marking suture (Fig. 13.7a, b). Each tooth of this blade engages the silk marking suture at its passage through the conjunctiva. The Desmarres retractor is slowly rotated from under the eyelid as the outer blade of the clamp engages the conjunctiva and Müller's muscle at the superior tarsal border. Any entrapped tarsus is pulled free from the clamp with the surgeon's thumb (Fig. 13.8a). The clamp is firmly compressed and the handle locked in position incorporating the palpebral conjunctiva and Müller's muscle between the superior tarsal border and the silk marking suture. It is important that the placement of the clamp should reflect the relative position of the tarsal plate. In elderly patients or patients with significant upper eyelid laxity, the tarsus is attenuated and, often, temporally displaced; the clamp should be adjusted temporally to avoid eyelid contour abnormalities.

13.4.8 Step 8: Preventing Inappropriate Ptosis Clamp Placement

The upper eyelid skin is pulled superiorly while the clamp is pulled in the opposite direction (Fig. 13.8b). If significant tension or a sense of attachment is noted between the skin and clamp during this maneuver, then the levator aponeurosis is likely incarcerated within the clamp; the clamp should be released and reapplied as instructed in Sect. 13.4.7. This maneuver is possible because the levator aponeurosis sends extensions to the orbicularis muscle and skin to form the eyelid crease.

13.4.9 Step 9: Passage of Suture

With the clamp held vertically, a double-armed 5–0 plain gut suture is run in a horizontal mattress fashion approximately 1.5 mm below the margin of the clamp along its entire width in

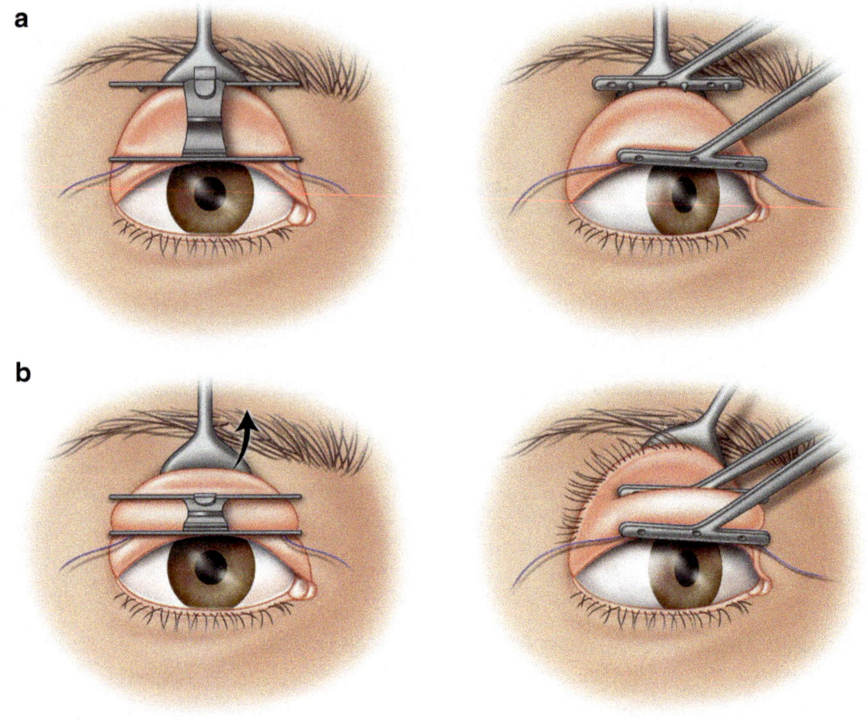

Fig. 13.7 Application of the Putterman Müller's muscle-conjunctival resection clamp. (**a**) The lower blade of the clamp is placed at the level of the silk marking suture. Each tooth of this blade engages the silk marking suture at its passage through the conjunctiva. (**b**) The Desmarres retractor is slowly rotated from under the eyelid as the outer blade of the clamp engages the conjunctiva and Müller's muscle at the superior tarsal border

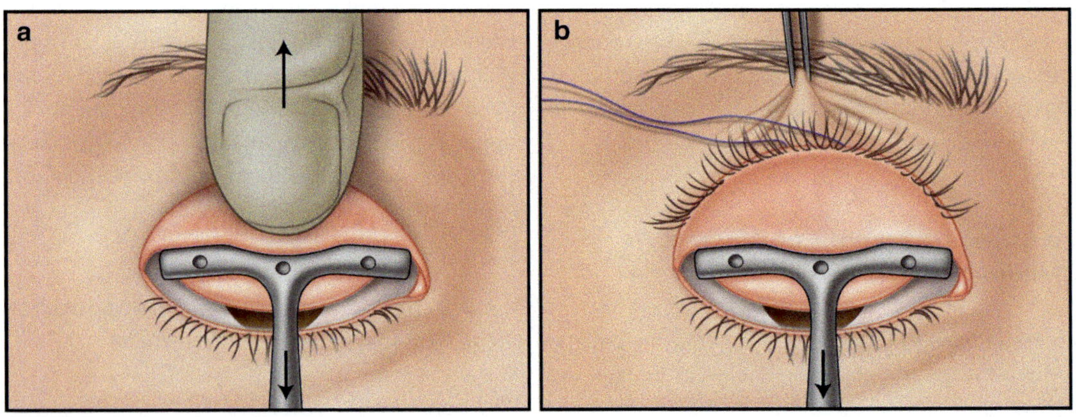

Fig. 13.8 (**a**) Any entrapped tarsus is pulled free from the clamp with the surgeon's thumb. (**b**) The upper eyelid skin is pulled superiorly while the clamp is pulled in the opposite direction. If significant tension or a sense of attachment is noted between the skin and clamp during this maneuver, then the levator aponeurosis is likely incarcerated within the clamp

a temporal to nasal fashion (Fig. 13.9a, b). The suture is passed through the conjunctiva and superior tarsal margin on one side of the clamp and conjunctiva and Müller's muscle on the opposite side of the clamp. In effect, the conjunctiva-Müller's muscle complex is advanced and reattached to the superior tarsal border. The suture passes are positioned adjacent to one another on the tarsal side and 2–3 mm apart on the opposite side of the clamp. This method decreases the corneal irritation and foreign body sensation experienced by the patient postoperatively.

13.4.10 Step 10: Excision of Conjunctiva and Müller's Muscle

A No. 15 surgical blade is used to excise the tissue within the clamp by cutting between the suture and the clamp (Fig. 13.10). The blade is beveled upward in direct contact with the clamp to prevent inadvertent lysis of the running suture. In addition, the surgeon must be careful not to cut the arms of the suture on either the nasal or temporal end of the clamp.

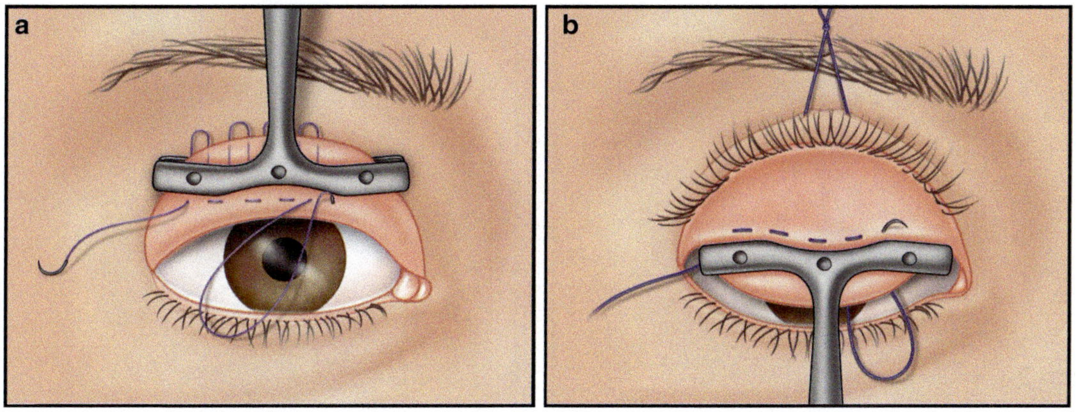

Fig. 13.9 Advancement of Müller's muscle and conjunctiva. (**a**) A double-armed 5–0 plain gut suture is run in a horizontal mattress fashion approximately 1.5 mm below the margin of the clamp along its entire width in a temporal to nasal fashion. View along the superior margin of resection adjacent to the superior conjunctival fornix. (**b**) View along the superior tarsal border

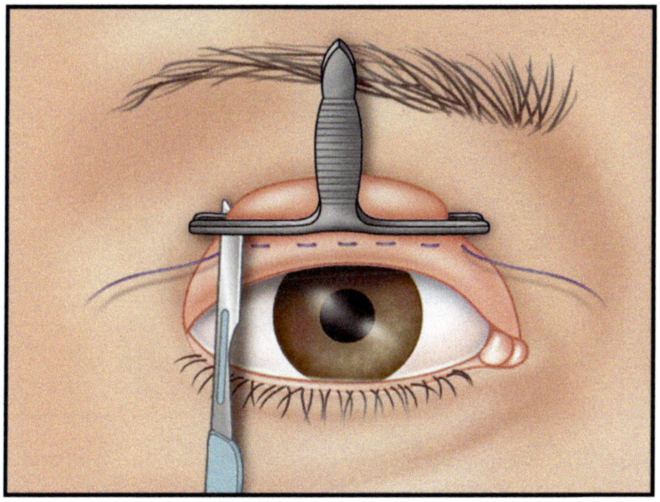

Fig. 13.10 Resection of Müller's muscle and conjunctiva: A No. 15 surgical blade is used to excise the tissue within the clamp by cutting between the suture and the clamp

13.4.11 Step 11: Closure of Conjunctival Wound

The Desmarres retractor is positioned to evert the eyelid while gentle traction is applied to the silk traction suture (Fig. 13.11a). The nasal arm of the plain gut suture is run in a continuous fashion in a temporal direction incorporating the superior tarsal border, Müller's muscle, and conjunctiva; each suture pass should be 2–3 mm apart. Great care must be taken to avoid cutting the original mattress suture with each pass; gentle suction and adequate hemostasis at the wound edges should be maintained. In addition, selection of a plain gut suture with a small, spatulated needle will help prevent inadvertent suture lysis.

13.4.12 Step 12: Burying the Suture Knot

Once the nasal arm of the plain gut suture reaches the temporal aspect of the wound, each arm of the suture is passed through conjunctiva and Müller's muscle into the wound (Fig. 13.11b). The arms of the suture are pulled from the interior of the wound and tied with a surgeon's knot. The ends of the suture are cut adjacent to the knot allowing the knot to retract into the subconjunctival space. This helps to prevent postoperative keratopathy and foreign body sensation. If the patient is undergoing concurrent upper blepharoplasty, the arms of the suture can be pulled from the interior of the wound and placed aside without tying the suture. The Desmarres retractor can be removed and the eyelid can be placed in its normal anatomic position. Once the eyelid skin or skin and orbicularis muscle has been excised and hemostasis maintained, the knot may be tied as previously instructed. Performing the excision of skin or skin/muscle and assuring hemostasis prior to tying the knot will prevent inadvertent suture lysis.

13.4.13 Step 13: Completion of Upper Blepharoplasty

The eyelid skin or skin/orbicularis muscle flap is excised using scissors or an electrocautery unit (Fig. 13.12a, b). Careful and aggressive hemostasis is maintained using unipolar/bipolar cautery. Orbital fat excision, lacrimal gland repositioning, and glabellar/brow procedures may be performed via the upper blepharoplasty incision. See Chaps. 9 and 10 for further discussion and surgical techniques. The eyelid crease is reconstructed by passing three 6–0 interrupted sutures through skin at the inferior wound edge, levator aponeurosis, and skin at the superior wound edge adjacent to the three eyelid crease markings. The wound is closed with a 6–0 running permanent suture.

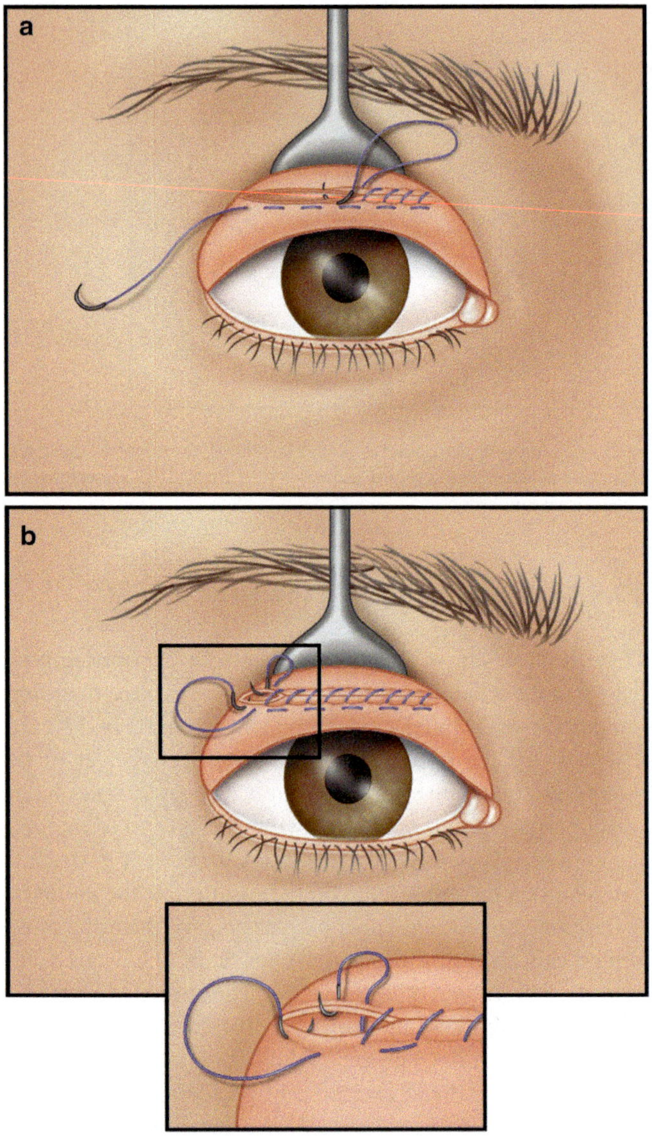

Fig. 13.11 Closure of conjunctival wound. (**a**) The nasal arm of the plain gut suture is run in a continuous fashion in a temporal direction incorporating the superior tarsal border, Müller's muscle, and conjunctiva; each suture pass should be 2–3 mm apart. (**b**) Once the nasal arm of the plain gut suture reaches the temporal aspect of the wound, each arm of the suture is passed through conjunctiva and Müller's muscle into the wound

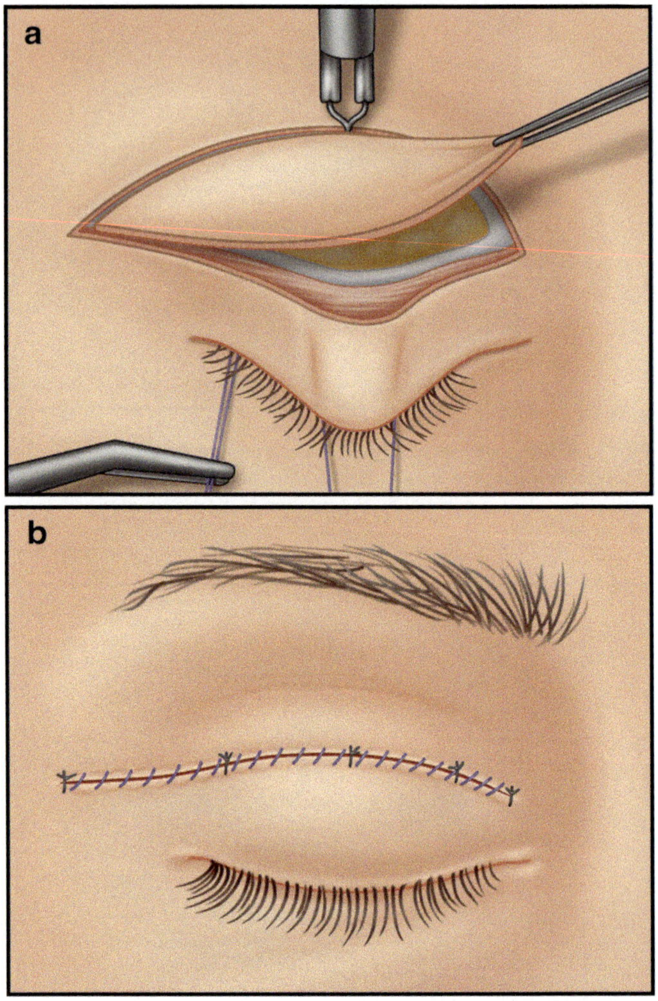

Fig. 13.12 Completion of upper blepharoplasty. (**a**) The eyelid skin or skin/orbicularis muscle flap is excised using scissors or an electrocautery knife. (**b**) Several 6–0 interrupted sutures reinforce eyelid crease reconstruction. The wound is closed with a 6–0 running permanent suture

13.5 Postoperative Management

A topical antibiotic ointment is generously applied over the surface of the eye at the completion of the procedure. The ointment should be applied 2–3 times daily for the first week and prior to bedtime for an additional week. A systemic antibiotic is not necessary following this procedure; however, if this procedure is combined with other periorbital rejuvenation procedures, prophylactic oral antibiotics may be added. Topical and/or systemic anti-inflammatory agents, such as steroids, are not necessary, but may be given as deemed appropriate in selected cases.

Cold compresses are applied over the eyelids for the first 24 h to help prevent postoperative edema and may be used thereafter for patient comfort. It is important that patients recognize that there may be continued sensory anesthesia to the eyelid 4–6 h after the procedure and that they should cycle the cold compresses to prevent superficial irritation.

Frequent use of ocular lubricants (drops and ointments) is important to prevent postoperative keratopathy and patient discomfort. Patients should be encouraged to use artificial tears throughout the day for suture- and exposure-associated symptoms.

Patients should be counseled on worsening eyelid swelling and ocular discomfort for the first 48–72 h following the

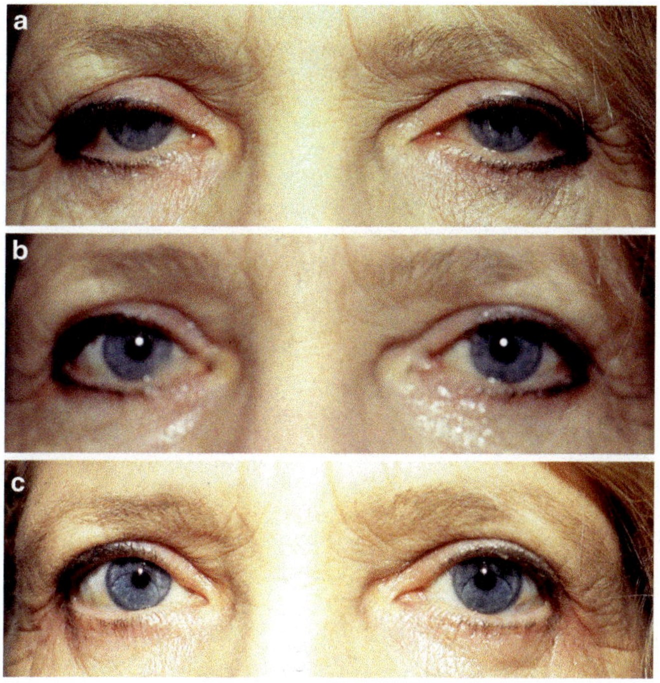

Fig. 13.13 A 56-year-old Caucasian woman presenting with bilateral upper eyelid ptosis. (**a**) Prior to instillation of 10% phenylephrine drops. (**b**) Five minutes after instilling several drops of 10% phenylephrine onto bilateral superior fornices. (**c**) Six weeks following bilateral Müller's muscle-conjunctival resection ptosis procedure combined with bilateral upper and lower blepharoplasty

procedure. Vision is often blurred and distorted secondary to uneven tear film and frequent ocular lubricant administration. As the eyelid swelling and ocular discomfort improves, the patient is instructed to use the artificial tears in lieu of the more viscous ocular lubricants. The eyelid usually attains its final level 3–6 weeks postoperatively (Fig. 13.13).

13.6 Complications

The most common complication from posterior eyelid ptosis repair is corneal irritation and/or abrasion [7]. The combination of exposed suture material, postoperative eyelid edema, and relative increase in exposed ocular surface area may contribute to corneal epithelial derangement. Patients with postoperative lagophthalmos are at particular risk of developing corneal abnormalities and should be strongly encouraged to maintain an aggressive ocular lubrication regimen. A bandage contact lens or collagen shield may be used in symptomatic patients. Rarely, a corneal abrasion may develop into a corneal ulcer. These patients should be referred for urgent ophthalmologic evaluation to prevent vision-threatening complications.

Over- or undercorrection of eyelid position is observed in approximately 3–5% of cases [13]. If a significant overcorrection occurs, downward massage of the eyelid while fixating the brow may be used in the early postoperative period. If the overcorrection persists, a levator recession procedure can be performed [13]. In cases of undercorrection, a repeat posterior eyelid ptosis procedure may be performed; however, results are frequently unpredictable; more often a levator advancement or resection ptosis procedure is employed.

In rare cases, persistent hemorrhage from the Müller's muscle may occur. The Müller's muscle is a highly vascularized structure and patients on anticoagulation therapy, or those who restart anticoagulation shortly after the procedure, are at increased risk. Firm pressure over the eyelid for approximately 5 min will often stop the hemorrhage; however, persistent hemorrhage may require exploration and cauterization.

13.7 Conclusion

Posterior eyelid ptosis repair via the Müller's muscle-conjunctival resection procedure is a safe and effective technique for periorbital rejuvenation in the aesthetic patient. Although posterior eyelid approach techniques can be daunting for the novice eyelid surgeon, with experience and patience this procedure is easily mastered. As opposed to levator advancement/resection ptosis repair, this surgery requires no patient cooperation, is quick, easier, and probably more appropriate for the surgeon not comfortable with advanced eyelid dissection techniques. Surgical outcomes are reliably consistent and reproducible, and typically yield high patient satisfaction.

References

1. Beard C. Müller's superior tarsal muscle: anatomy, physiology and clinical significance. Ann Plast Surg. 1985;14:324–33.
2. Müller H. Über glatte Muskeln an der Augenlidern des Menschen und der Säugetiere. Würzberg, Germany: Verhandl PMG; 1859; IX: 244. Cited by: Whitnall SE. The anatomy of the human orbit, 2nd ed. London: Oxford University Press; 1932. p. 145.
3. Dutton JJ. The eyelids and anterior orbit. In: Dutton JJ, editor. Atlas of clinical and surgical orbital anatomy. Philadelphia, PA: WB Saunders; 1994. p. 113–38.
4. Putterman AM, Urist MJ. Müller's muscle-conjunctival resection. Arch Ophthalmol. 1975;93(8):619–23.
5. Glatt HJ, Putterman AM, Fett DR. Comparison of 2.5% and 10% phenylephrine in the elevation of upper eyelids with ptosis. Ophthalmic Surg. 1990;21:114–22.
6. Ben Simon GJ, Lee S, Schwarcz RM, et al. External levator advancement vs. Müller's muscle-conjunctival resection for correction of upper eyelid involutional ptosis. Am J Ophthalmol. 2005; 140(3):426–32.

7. Putterman AM, Fett DR. Müller's muscle in the treatment of upper eyelid ptosis: a ten-year study. Ophthalmic Surg. 1986;17:354–60.
8. Mercandetti M, Putterman AM, Cohen ME, et al. Internal levator advancement by Müller's muscle-conjunctival resection: technique and review. Arch Facial Plast Surg. 2001;3:104–10.
9. Ben Simon GJ, Lee S, Schwarcz RM, et al. Müller's muscle-conjunctival resection for correction of upper eyelid ptosis: relationship between phenylephrine testing and the amount of tissue resected with final eyelid position. Arch Facial Plast Surg. 2007;9(6):413–7.
10. Ayala E, Galvez C, Gonzalez-Candial M, et al. Predictability of conjunctival-Müllerectomy for blepharoptosis repair. Orbit. 2007;26: 217–21.
11. Dresner SC. Further modifications of the Müller's muscle-conjunctival resection procedure for blepharoptosis. Ophthal Plast Reconstr Surg. 1991;7:114–22.
12. Perry JD, Kadakia A, Foster JA. A new algorithm for ptosis repair using conjunctival Müllerectomy with or without tarsectomy. Ophthal Plast Reconstr Surg. 2002;18(6):426–9.
13. Putterman AM, Fagien S. Müller's muscle-conjunctival resection ptosis procedure combined with upper blepharoplasty. In: Fagien S, editor. Putterman's cosmetic oculoplastic surgery. 4th ed. Philadelphia, PA: Saunders Elsevier; 2008. p. 123–33.
14. Hildreth HR, Silver B. Sensory block of the upper eyelid. Arch Ophthalmol. 1976;77:202–31.

14 Modern Advances in Asian Blepharoplasty

Kimberly J. Lee, Amir M. Karam, and Samuel M. Lam

Key Points

- The desires and expectations of Asian patients undergoing upper lid blepharoplasty are vastly different than those of Caucasian patients.
- It is critical to understand the ethnic characteristics of Asian eyelids before performing blepharoplasty on this group of patients.
- A lower attachment of the orbital septum on the levator aponeurosis with associated inferior fat displacement and crease attenuation; and the presence of a preseptal fat layer account for the anatomic differences of Asian upper lids from Caucasian upper lids.
- These anatomic differences cause Asian upper lids to be fuller than their Caucasian counterparts, and manifest a lower, indistinct, or fully absent crease.
- The presence or absence of a naturally occurring or previously created eyelid crease is essential to the preoperative assessment.
- The surgical plan should focus primarily on whether or not the patient desires a *single eyelid* (no crease), or a *double eyelid* (presence of a crease).
- Depending of preoperative findings and patient needs, surgery can involve one or all of the following: skin excision, fat excision, crease formation, or fat grafting.
- Conservative surgery is imperative.
- Westernization of eyelids should be avoided at all times.
- Revisional surgery in this patient population is very challenging.

14.1 Introduction

The pathogenesis of upper-eyelid aging involves degenerative changes in the skin, soft-tissue excess, and volume loss. The goal of facial rejuvenation is to restore a youthful look without altering appearance in an unnatural way. This is especially true in aesthetic rejuvenation of the Asian upper eyelid. This surgery can lead to loss of ethnic identity with resultant negative impression both from the patient, friends, and family. Successful upper eyelid rejuvenation in the Asian patient requires a thorough comprehension of the periorbital aging process specific to this population and a detailed understanding of the cultural nuances related to upper eyelid cosmetic surgery inherent to this group. What makes Asian blepharoplasty unique is the management of the eyelid crease. Although the presence of an eyelid crease can be a naturally occurring anatomic finding in the Asian population (double eyelid), individuals who lack this anatomic trait (single eyelid) will often seek "double eyelid" formation. The desire to have a double eyelid is largely cultural, as this feature is considered attractive. Consequently, it is necessary for the surgeon performing Asian blepharoplasty to have experience with upper eyelid crease formation, to meet patient needs.

There has been a paradigm shift away from Westernization of Asian upper lids. Traditionally, surgery has consisted of aggressive removal of skin, muscle, and fat. This has often led to a volume depleted upper lid with a deep sulcus and higher crease. The modern approach is aimed at restoring a more youthful and healthier appearing upper-eyelid region, which translates to performing conservative excision of skin, formal crease formation when necessary, coupled with some level of volume augmentation of the lateral eyebrow and infrabrow region. This approach is aimed at creating a less deflated and "fuller" eyelid, which will more accurately approximate the youthful Asian appearance. In this chapter, we will evaluate the aging process affecting the upper-eyelid region in the Asian patient, how to manage and treat the different anatomic types of the eyelid crease, how to perform an upper eyelid blepharoplasty in the Asian patient, and how to utilize complementary treatments to restore the youthful structure of this area.

S.M. Lam (✉)
Director, Willow Bend Wellness Center, Plano, TX, USA
e-mail: drlam@lamfacialplastics.com

G.G. Massry et al. (eds.), *Master Techniques in Blepharoplasty and Periorbital Rejuvenation*,
DOI 10.1007/978-1-4614-0067-7_14, © Springer Science+Business Media, LLC 2011

14.2 Anatomic Considerations of the Asian Upper Eyelid

The fundamental anatomic difference between Asian and Caucasian eyelid appearance pertains to the location of orbital septum insertion on to the levator aponeurosis. This attachment is lower in Asian eyes, even as low as the lower tarsal border. This lower point of insertion allows the preaponeurotic fat pad to descend lower on the aponeurosis, yielding a fuller eyelid appearance. In addition, the more inferior location of fat blunts the aponeurotic attachments to the orbicularis muscle. Clinically, these anatomic characteristics yield a puffy eyelid without, or with an indistinct crease. Consequently, approximately half of Asians do not have an upper eyelid crease while the remaining have some form of crease. Asians with a crease have a larger apparent palpebral fissure giving the appearance of a larger eye. The actual vertical palpebral fissure (upper to lower lid margin) does not change. However, an eyelid crease creates a tarsal platform (lid margin to upper lid skin fold). This additional pretarsal eyelid show makes the palpebral fissure appear larger. This feature is desirable aesthetically as it confers a more feminine appearance, and because it facilitates application of eye cosmetics.

Another anatomic difference between Asian and Caucasian eyelid anatomy helps account for increased fullness of the Asian upper eyelid. In Asians the brow fat pad has continuity into the post-orbicularis space of the eyelid proper. This preseptal (submuscular) fat can continue as low as the tarsus in many cases. In Caucasian eyelids the brow fat pad extension into the eyelid is an areolar connective tissue called the post-orbicularis fascia. The preseptal fat present in Asian eyelids adds to the more inferiorly displaced preaponeurotic fat (postseptal fat) to create a fuller Asian eyelid.

Figures 14.1 and 14.2 demonstrate the anatomic differences between Caucasian and Asian eyelids described above.

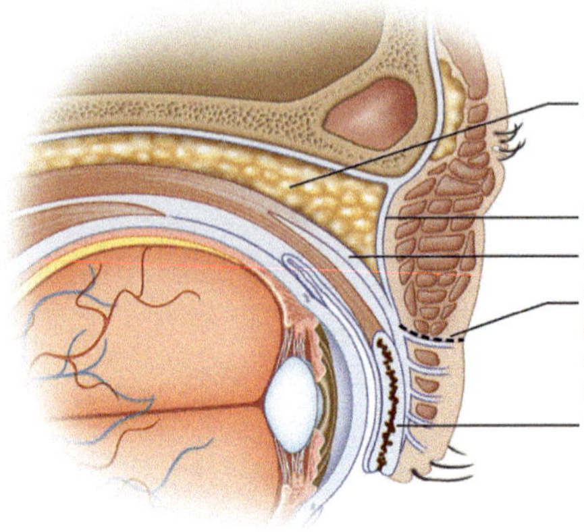

Fig. 14.1 Artist's drawing of Caucasian eyelid anatomy. Note the conjoined attachment of the orbital septum to the levator aponeurosis. This attachment point limits inferior displacement of eyelid fat. The levator sends fibers to the orbicularis and skin just below this attachment forming an eyelid crease (*dotted line*). Also note the absence of a preseptal fat layer (present in Asian eyelids). Instead there is an areolar connective tissue layer called the post-orbicularis fascia (not pictured)

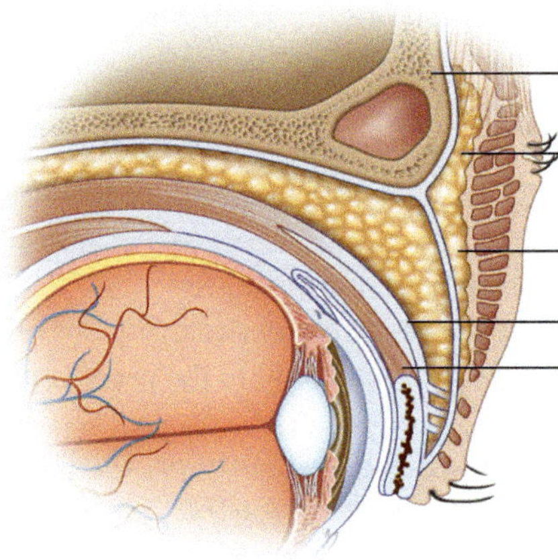

Fig. 14.2 Artist's drawing of Asian lid anatomy. Note the lower conjoined attachment of the orbital septum to the levator aponeurosis. This allows inferior displacement of eyelid fat and blunts levator attachments to the orbicularis and skin. The result is a fuller eyelid and variable crease formation. Also note the presence of a preseptal (submuscular) fat layer which is absent in Caucasian lids. This adds to the fullness of the Asian upper eyelid

14.2.1 Musculature

The orbicularis oculi muscle serves as the sphincter of the upper and lower eyelids and is innervated by the temporal, zygomatic, and buccal branches of the facial nerve. The transverse facial, supratrochlear, and supraorbital vessels supply the muscle. The muscle is divided into orbital and palpebral portions. The orbital portion is darker and thicker and is under voluntary control. It functions to close the eyelids, and secondary acts as a brow depressor. The palpebral portion acts involuntarily to close the eyelids or reflexively blink. The palpebral portion is thinner, lies directly over the eyelids, and is further subdivided into preseptal and pretarsal segments according to the anatomic structures they overlay [1–3].

14.2.2 Orbital Septum

The orbital septum lies beneath the preseptal division of orbicularis oculi muscle and is a continuation of the periorbita. The portion above the tarsus separates the muscular from the orbital fat compartment, while the inferior portion fuses with the anterior part of the tarsus [2]. The orbital septum is the anatomic separation of the eyelid from the orbit and segregates the fat. The upper eyelid crease is formed from the attachment of the levator fibers to the orbicularis muscle and eyelid skin.

In Asians, the orbital septum inserts approximately 3 mm from the base of the eyelid margin, while in non-Asians, it attaches at a higher position, 8–10 mm from the margin. The reason the crease is lower and indistinct in Asians is the levator fibers do not interdigitate as well with the orbicularis muscle and skin as the intervening fat prevents it from doing so.

14.2.3 Orbital Fat

Just posterior to the orbital septum are the fat pads of the upper eyelid. Unlike the lower eyelid, which has three fat pads, the upper eyelid has two fat compartments consisting of a medial and central compartment. The lacrimal gland may prolapse in the upper eyelid and should not be mistaken as a fat pad. Mistaken excision of the gland can lead to dry eye complications. Removal of the central fat pad is rarely required in surgery, as it can create an iatrogenic hollowing postoperatively (A-frame deformity). The medial fat pad is more commonly seen to have mild prolapse and is often conservatively excised in surgery.

14.2.4 Levator Palpebrae Superioris

The main muscle responsible for the eyelid opening is the levator palpebrae superioris muscle, which is innervated by the oculomotor nerve. Mueller's muscle, which lies posterior to the levator, anterior to the conjunctiva, and above the tarsus, is a smooth muscle responsible for 3–4 mm of eyelid opening. The levator muscle transitions to the aponeurosis at Whitnall's ligament. The levator aponeurosis sends attachments to the tarsus and to the orbicularis muscle and overlying skin to form the eyelid crease. As stated previously, specific to Asians is a lower attachment of the orbital septum to the aponeurosis. This causes the orbital fat to ride lower in the lid thereby making the eyelid fuller, blunting the attachment of the aponeurosis to the skin, and reducing the crease prominence.

14.3 Modern Management of the Upper Eyelid

Dermatochalasis is a significant contributor to the aging upper eyelid. The aged appearance is accentuated by volumetric depletion of fat and soft tissue beneath. In general, the trend in Asian upper blepharoplasty has moved away from the traditional aggressive removal of skin, fat, and muscle to a more conservative skin-only excision. The authors have also transitioned away from routine brow lifting. This is based on photo-documenting patients using current and past photographs. Often times, brows that appear to have fallen with age are noted to have the same or minimally changed position from youth. Accordingly, traditional eyelid and brow surgery performed in isolation can alter a person's identity in a fundamental and permanent way. Most young Asian women have a very low eyelid crease and relatively low brow position, but the shape and contour of that brow and eyelid are typically full. Traditional brow and eyelid surgical techniques rejuvenate the areas by extensive resection or lifting, which in turn ultimately increase the distance between the ciliary margin and the eyelid crease. Although a high and arched crease can exist naturally in the Caucasian race, it is generally quite rare to find in the Asian race. The authors believe that converting an Asian woman from a low crease to a high crease through browlift and subtractive eyelid surgery will alter the appearance in an unnatural way.

14.4 The Youthful Asian Upper Eyelid and its Age-Related Changes

The youthful Asian upper eyelid has minimal skin excess. The superior orbital rim and infrabrow region appear soft and full. A smooth layer of subcutaneous and submuscular fat exists over the contour of the bony orbital rim and the lateral aspect of the eyelid is free of hooding. In the Asian eyelid, there are three general configurations of eyelid crease. These are characterized by the following:

- Upper eyelids without a crease or fold.
- A naturally present crease, which typically lays 3–5 mm above the eyelid margin.
- A surgically created crease.

Postsurgical creases may be in a naturally occurring or elevated position. Management of each of these configurations needs to be considered by surgeons who perform Asian blepharoplasty.

During the aging process of Asian upper eyelids, volume depletion as well as progressive dermatochalasia can cause the skin to override the eyelid crease (if it exists). This process can shorten the pretarsal eyelid show (pretarsal skin or lid platform), or, in more severe cases, can lead to skin folding over the upper eyelid lash line. As the volume of the peribrow region diminishes, there is a descent of the lateral brow, further contributing to lateral hooding. The infrabrow volume loss results in skeletonization of the superior orbital rim. In certain cases, there may be mild prolapse of the medial fat pad.

14.5 Strategies for the Aging Asian Eyelid

The Asian upper eyelid is remarkably varied. As a result, several findings need to be identified and considered prior to performing these procedures. The essential questions are as follows:

- How does one manage an Asian patient with or without a natural crease who wants to have eyelid and brow rejuvenation?

- How does one manage an Asian patient who already had previous eyelid crease formation?

This section will elaborate a strategy that combines both cultural sensitivity and surgical judgment to approach an Asian patient for eyelid rejuvenation by classifying that individual into one of three categories: Asians with a natural eyelid crease, Asians without a crease, or Asians who have had an eyelid crease surgically fashioned in the past.

14.5.1 Asians with a Natural Crease

Although the surgical technique is exactly the same as that for a Caucasian patient, it should be noted that raising the visible eyelid crease height beyond 2–4 mm above the ciliary margin through reductive eyelid and brow surgery ultimately could render an Asian face unnatural in appearance. The "visible" eyelid crease is defined as the distance from the ciliary margin to the folded over upper-eyelid skin edge when the patient is viewed with open eyes and forward gaze. This typically corresponds to a height of 1–2 mm for a typical Asian eyelid. Conversely, the "surgical" eyelid crease refers to the point of fixation of the levator to the dermis, 5–6 mm from the ciliary margin. This will render a visible eyelid crease (after the skin eventually folds over the surgical crease) of 1–2 mm height above the lid margin. It is essential to maintain an eyelid crease position that is natural. This is the fundamental objective of every case. A strategy to maintain eyelid crease position is to avoid brow lifts in almost every case and to maintain or decrease eyelid position by using fat grafting in the upper eyelid and along the brow. Fat transfer to the upper eyelid/brow complex will reduce the height of the visible eyelid crease (causes skin fold to lower), as opposed to traditional excisional blepharoplasty, which often elevates the position.

If the eyelid skin rests along the ciliary margin, it is recommended to remove a small amount (2–3 mm) of skin (but typically no fat) from the upper eyelid, in conjunction with fat grafting (if necessary) to maintain an appropriate visible eyelid crease position. If the visible eyelid crease is 1 mm or greater above the ciliary margin, removal of skin is unnecessary (and counterproductive), and fat transfer alone is used. If the visible crease is higher than 1–2 mm, additional fat can be used to lower the crease further. Traditionally, 1–2 mL of fat is transferred to the brow and upper eyelid depending on the degree of brow and upper eyelid deflation as well as crease position. Looking at a patient's old photographs and discussing his or her desired changes should frame each aesthetic consultation.

14.5.2 Asians Without a Crease

Patients who do not have a natural crease present a much more complicated topic. Oftentimes, the absence of a fold already makes the eyes look narrower, so any brow and upper-eyelid deflation can lead to a worsening of the apparent palpebral fissure. Many surgeons simply decide on an arbitrary height at which to remove skin without reference to thinking about the crease. This is problematic for two reasons. First, arbitrary removal of skin without crease fixation can leave behind a visible scar (even if placed right above the ciliary margin) since there is no crease (with overhanging fold) to camouflage it. Second, the already narrow apparent palpebral fissure will not be significantly altered by skin removal without attention to the crease formation. Even if the patient has been accustomed to a narrow palpebral fissure throughout life, the patient expects a sufficient opening of the eyelid to have made the cosmetic endeavor worthwhile. This is difficult to achieve with simple skin removal. This is why fixating a crease is important. Often times, surgeons remove fat from the postseptal space, without crease fixation, with the thought that doing so will open the palpebral fissure. Although removal of eyelid fat without crease fixation can help debulk a prominent eyelid, it can be problematic. In this scenario, a lid crease can develop after surgery which is variable in position, complete or incomplete. This occurs because of unpredictable adhesion between the levator aponeurosis, muscle, and skin.

Two options should be presented to the patient when it comes to treating the Asian patient without a defined crease. One option is to create a crease. Making a crease opens up the eyelid shape enough to make an individual appear more "awake" or "open-eyed." The full-incision method (see below) is ideal, allowing the dermatochalasia to be directly addressed. Patients must, however, recognize that this procedure will change their "look" since the eyelid will appear rounder in configuration. Additionally, patients must be able to handle a longer healing process associated with a procedure in which a crease is formed.

If the patient does not want a surgically formed crease, then fat grafting to the upper eyelid and brow alone, without skin removal, can be an alternative way (option two) of improving the aesthetics without changing one's identity. Although the preseptal tissue is already full in both youth and adults in the Asian patient without a crease, converting an aging eyelid contour that is slightly concave to a more convex shape can bring back the look of a youthful eye. The patient must obviously understand the limitations in this approach.

14.5.3 Asians with Prior Surgery for Supratarsal Crease Formation

Asian patients who have a natural appearing but surgically created crease (not too high or overresected) can be treated with an approach similar to what has been described for individuals with a natural eyelid crease. Unfortunately, for many Asians who have undergone double eyelid procedures, their crease was surgically created during a time in which "Westernization" procedures were in vogue, i.e., overzealous fat and skin removal were in fashion along with very high crease formation. These patients offer a difficult situation to address. Removing additional skin or elevating their brows can make their crease appear even more unnatural and should be avoided.

Interestingly, 20 years following a Westernization procedure, the visible crease height can approximate a "normal" or low position of ~1 or 2 mm with ongoing brow and eyelid deflation. These individuals can be identified in that their visible crease appears to be of a normal, low height but there is something unmistakably unnatural appearing about their eyelids. The reason for this unnatural appearance is that the thick brow skin (all that remains after excessive eyelid skin removal) falls over the surgical eyelid crease and creates a thickened upper eyelid appearance. Removing more skin or lifting the brow can unmask a poor prior result, making the eyes appear more unnatural. If the surgeon is uncertain whether the previously created surgical crease is too high, he or she can simply lift the brow skin during the consultation. For these patients who have had a "Westernized" eyelid, adding fat along the brow and upper-eyelid complex may improve the overall aesthetic appearance. Even though a "thick" upper eyelid can appear unnatural, adding fat to the brow complex can actually improve the appearance as it converts a concave structure (which is unnatural) to a more convex structure thereby camouflaging the thick-skin appearance.

14.6 Eyelid Crease Formation

The primary goal of this technique is to create a natural appearing, eyelid crease. The desire to have a "double eyelid" is largely cultural, as this feature is considered attractive. To successfully perform this requires a comprehensive understanding of the natural eyelid crease shape as well as mastery of the surgical techniques required to fashion it.

Numerous techniques for Asian upper-eyelid blepharoplasty have been described in the literature, including suture ligation, external incision, and double suture twist (DST) methods [4, 5]. Mikamo [6] is thought to have published the first description of the suture ligation method in 1896. This was later elaborated on in a large series by Uchida [7]. The external incision method was described in 1929 when Maruo [8] reported both suture and incision techniques. It was not until 1961 that Pang [9] described what we now recognize as the partial-incision technique, with placement of full-thickness eyelid sutures to form an upper eyelid crease. It should be noted that during the era of Westernization upper blepharoplasty, the focus was on creating a high supratarsal crease found in Caucasian eyes. It was the evolution of results of this era that led to the current philosophy of preserving ethnic characteristics. The current techniques can be broadly categorized into suture-based, partial-incision, and full-incision techniques.

The suture ligation method is relatively noninvasive, with limited postoperative swelling and reversibility of the procedure by removing the sutures. However, crease asymmetry, cyst formation, and crease attenuation requiring full revision can occur. The disappearance of upper eyelid crease has been found to be higher in those with thicker skin of excess subcutaneous fat. The partial-incision method often requires multiple stab incision or needle passes through the skin to achieve the exposure and suture anchoring required to create an upper eyelid crease [5]. Again, crease attenuation can be problematic. The full-incision technique is favored because of its (1) relative permanent results compared with other methods, (2) independence from buried sutures to maintain the crease formation, (3) wide exposure to facilitate identification of structures, and (4) ability to manage dermatochalasis in the aging eyelid. The major disadvantage of the full-incision method is the 1–2-week recovery period and persistent swelling, which can remain for months if not a full year. Scarring has proven to be insignificant if the tissues near the epicanthus are avoided.

14.6.1 Preoperative Eye Evaluation and Crease Positioning

The patients' lids are evaluated for the presence or absence of a natural crease, and if asymmetries exist between the eyelids. How the fold terminates medially is then determined. Although several variations have been described, they essentially fall into one of two categories: inside fold or outside fold. This refers to the termination of the medial portion of the incision lateral to or medial to the epicanthus, respectively. The shape of the crease is then determined based on the preoperative consultation with the patient. The shape can be parallel to the normal anatomic shape of the eye (rounded) or slightly flared laterally (oval). The authors' preference is to pair an inside fold with a flared, oval configuration (Fig. 14.3).

14.6.2 Surgical Marking

The shape and configuration of the crease determined preoperatively are used as a guide to patient marking during surgery. The patient should be placed in a supine position, and the upper eyelid skin is held taut so that the eyelashes are slightly everted. Using calipers, the crease is demarcated

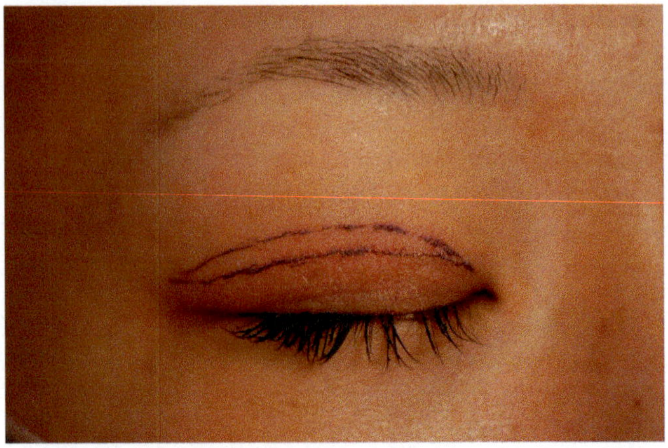

Fig. 14.3 Surgical marking illustrating the creation of an inside fold with a flared, oval configuration for the upper eyelid crease formation

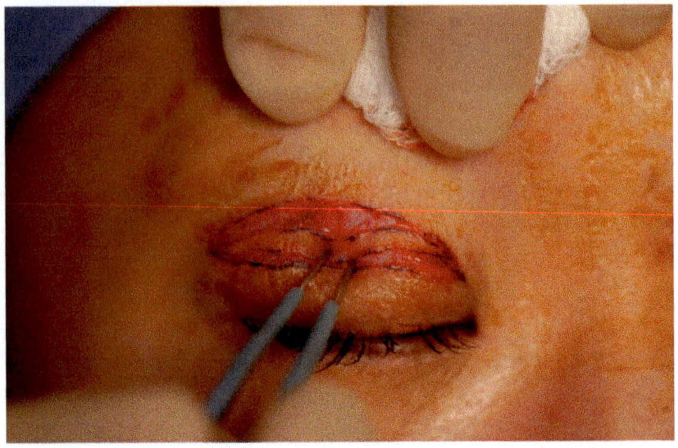

Fig. 14.5 Incision of the skin to the level of the orbicularis oculi muscle

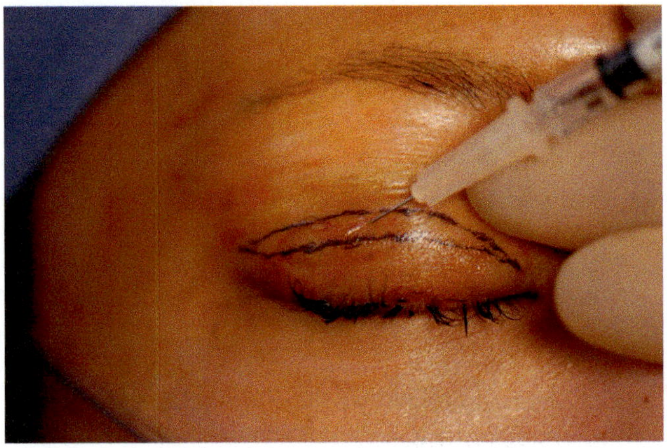

Fig. 14.4 Injection of local anesthetic to the upper eyelid via a 30-g needle

5–6 mm from the ciliary margin in order to create a natural appearing, low crease design. The degree of skin excision should allow approximately 3 mm between the upper and lower limbs of the incision, but should be tailored to each patient. It is recommended to err on the side of conservatism. Additionally, any preoperative asymmetry of skin excess must be compensated for during the skin marking.

14.6.3 Anesthesia

Some surgeons prefer patient cooperation throughout the procedure to help achieve symmetry, and avoid deep sedation if possible. Others prefer sedation or general anesthesia to facilitate patient comfort during the procedure. Local anesthetic, 0.5 cc of 1% lidocaine with 1:100,000 epinephrine mixed with 0.5 cc of 0.25% bupivacaine with 1:100,000 epinephrine, is infiltrated into the upper eyelid skin with a 30-g needle, by raising a subcutaneous wheal laterally which is then manually distributed along the entire length of the incision (Fig. 14.4). This method diminishes the likelihood of hematoma formation from multiple needle sticks.

14.6.4 Surgical Technique

The skin is incised to the level of the orbicularis oculi muscle with a scalpel blade (Fig. 14.5). The skin is excised with a scalpel, iris scissors, or electrocautery bovie unit. Meticulous hemostasis is achieved with cautery to maintain a bloodless, clear surgical field. The same steps are performed on the contralateral side and are continued in this alternating fashion to ensure symmetry.

If the patient does not have dry eye symptoms preoperatively, and the lid shows sufficient prominence, an iris scissors is used to excise a 1–2 mm strip of orbicularis muscle from the inferior edge of the wound (Fig. 14.6). Fibers of the underlying orbital septum are often times incorporated, to further decrease the fullness. This tissue "debulking" can enhance the final crease appearance.

The eyelid fat is addressed next. Balloting the eyeball can facilitate identification of the eyelid fat pads by forcing them forward for better identification. A small fenestration along the lateral extent of the wound edge just at the point where the strip of orbicularis was previously removed is made. With counter traction and balloting of the globe, dissection continues through the orbital septum until the preaponeurotic fat is identified (Fig. 14.7). This portion of the procedure requires meticulous attention to detail, to avoid injury to the levator aponeurosis. The fat pad identified is superficial to the levator aponeurosis and no deeper dissection is needed in blepharoplasty surgery. Once the fat is identified, the orbital septum can be opened to its full extent for exposure of the nasal and central fat pads (Fig. 14.8). A cotton-tipped applicator is used to bluntly dissect the preaponeurotic fat pad away from the underlying levator aponeurosis for exposure (Fig. 14.9).

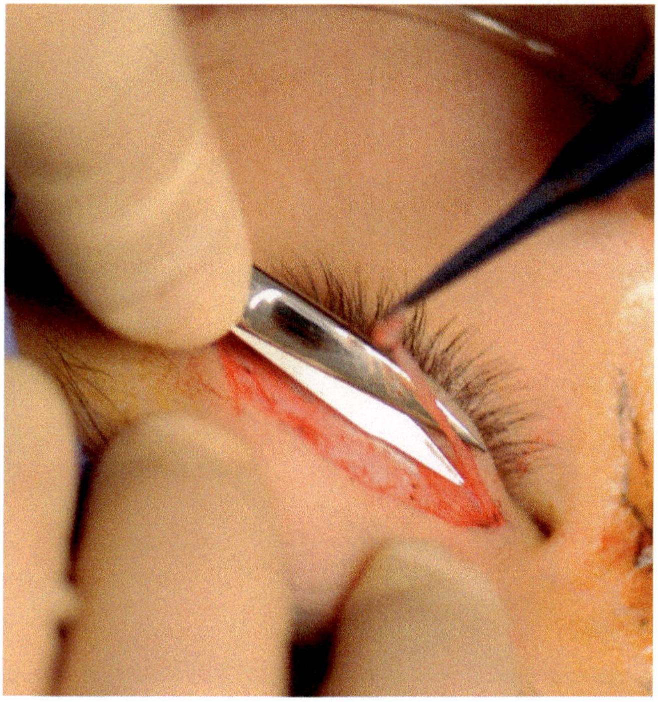

Fig. 14.6 Orbicularis muscle trim (excision) from inferior edge of the wound

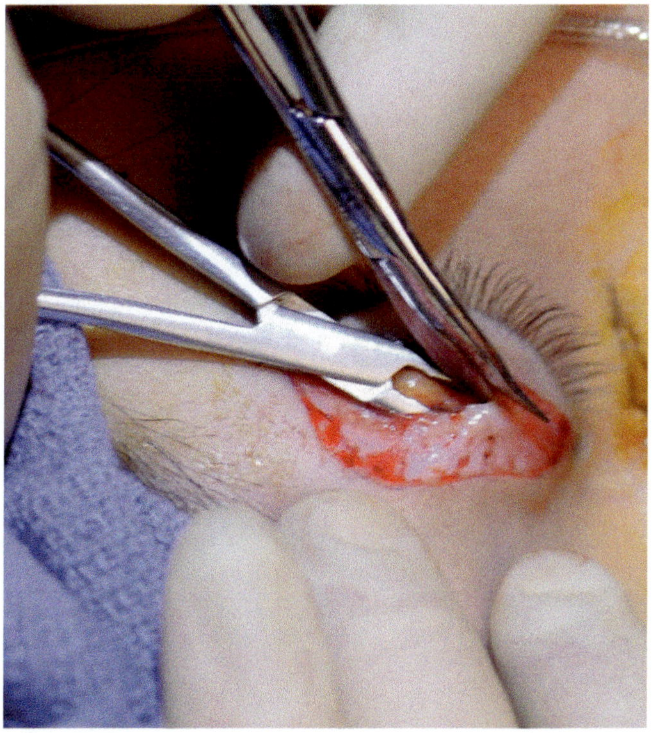

Fig. 14.8 Use of the mosquito clamp to elevate orbital septum/orbicularis layer from the levator aponeurosis, as these tissue planes are divided

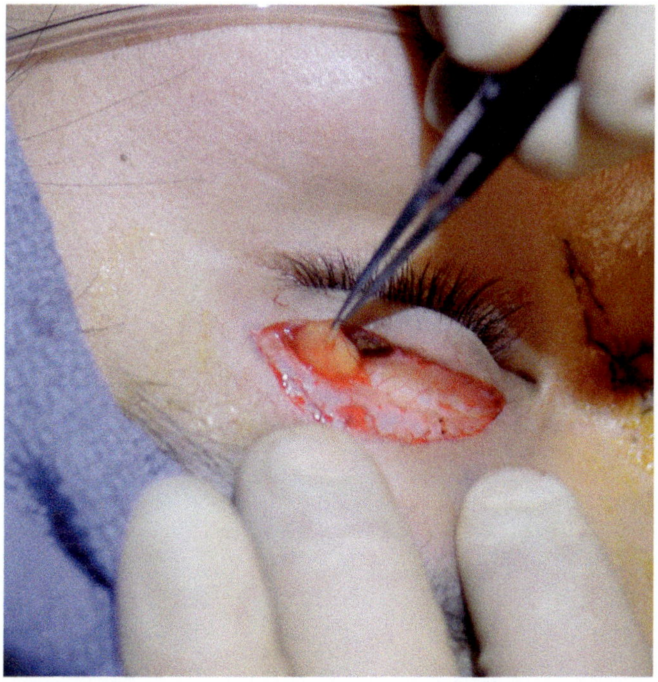

Fig. 14.7 Exposure of the preaponeurotic (postseptal) fat through an opening in the orbital septum

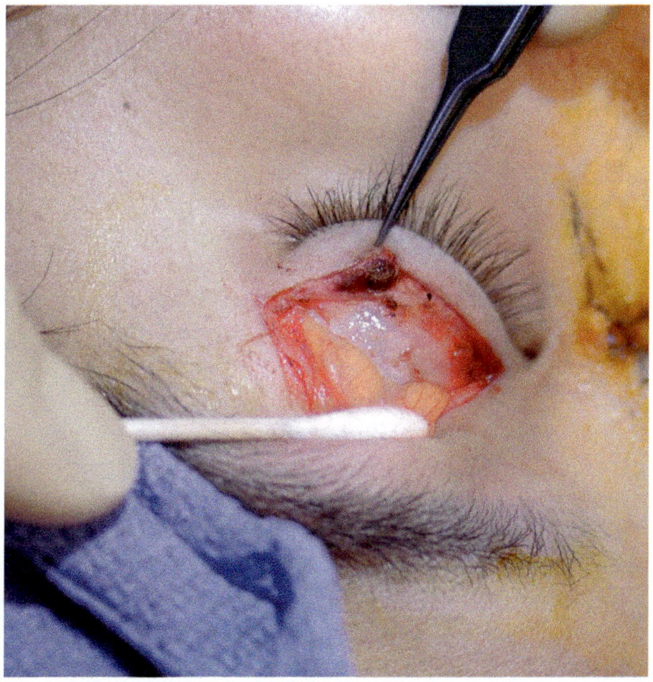

Fig. 14.9 Postseptal fat brushed away from fully exposed levator aponeurosis

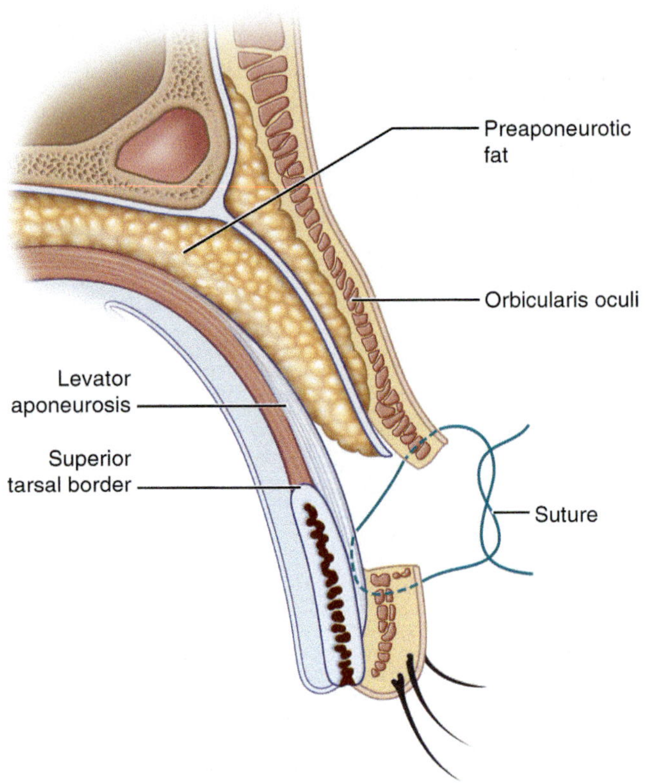

Fig. 14.10 Artist's drawing of crease fixation suture. A suture passes through the skin and orbicularis muscle at the superior margin of the wound, the levator aponeurosis, and through the skin and orbicularis muscle at the inferior margin of the wound. When tied, the suture creates a controlled adhesion of the levator to the orbicularis and skin. This creates a normal anatomic eyelid crease

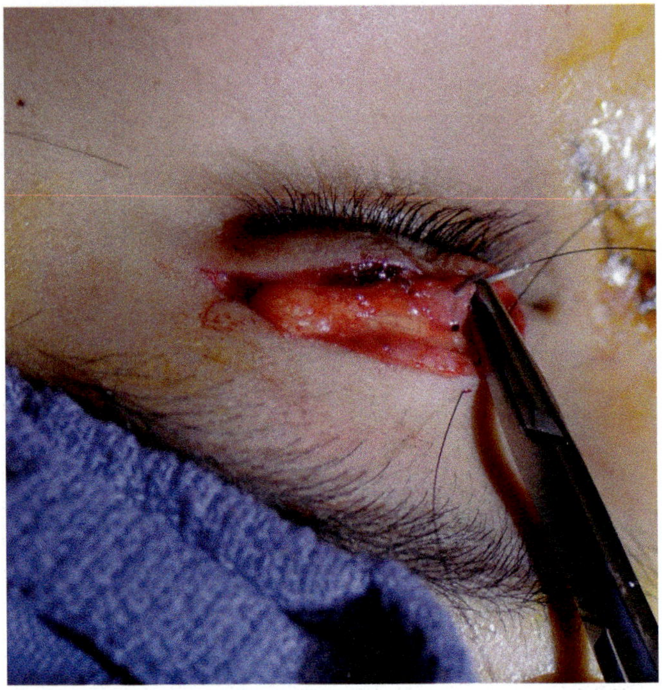

Fig. 14.11 A surgical photo demonstrating the placement of a 5–0 Nylon suture through the levator aponeurosis to set the height of the upper eyelid crease

14.6.4.1 Levator-to-Skin Fixation

To achieve a more open eyelid configuration, many surgeons remove excessive eyelid fat. However, in the authors' experiences, suture fixation of the levator aponeurosis to the eyelid skin is sufficient to achieve the desired open appearance of the palpebral aperture in 80% of cases. Therefore, excision of central preaponeurotic fat is rarely required. On occasion, nasal fat is conservatively sculpted.

The crease is now formed. The patient is asked to open his/her eyes to identify the mid-pupil location on forward gaze. A 6–0 nylon suture is placed through the upper skin edge at the mid-pupil line. The suture is then passed through the levator aponeurosis at its lower edge, and then through the lower skin edge at a corresponding point as the upper lid entry bite (Figs. 14.10 and 14.11). The patient is then asked to open his/her eyes after one suture is placed to determine proper crease depth, definition, and eyelash position (Fig. 14.12). The ideal suture will create a defined crease with slightly everted eyelashes. The eyelashes can be further everted with the aid of the electrocautery bovie applied to the orbicularis muscle just above the crease incision prior to suture placement. After suture placement, the crease height

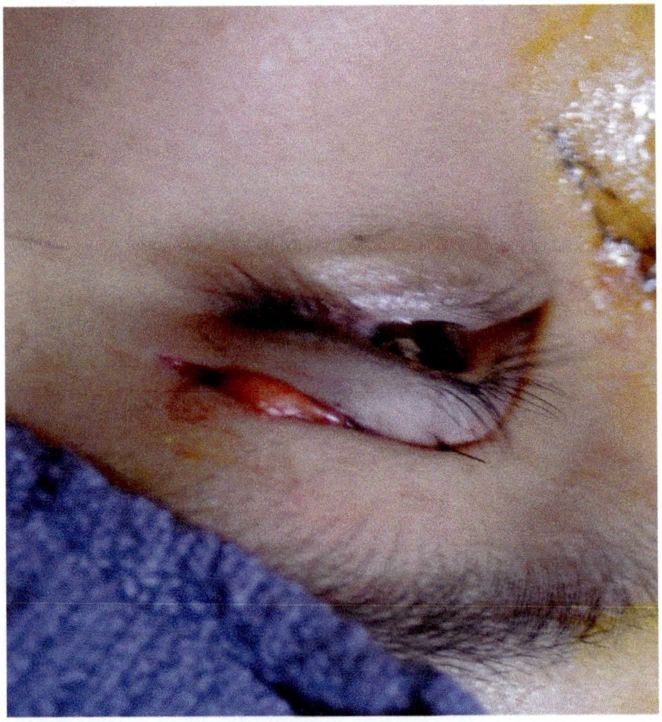

Fig. 14.12 A surgical photo corresponding to Fig. 14.10. The 5–0 Nylon crease fixation suture is placed. The patient is asked to open his/her eyes to assess positioning and symmetry

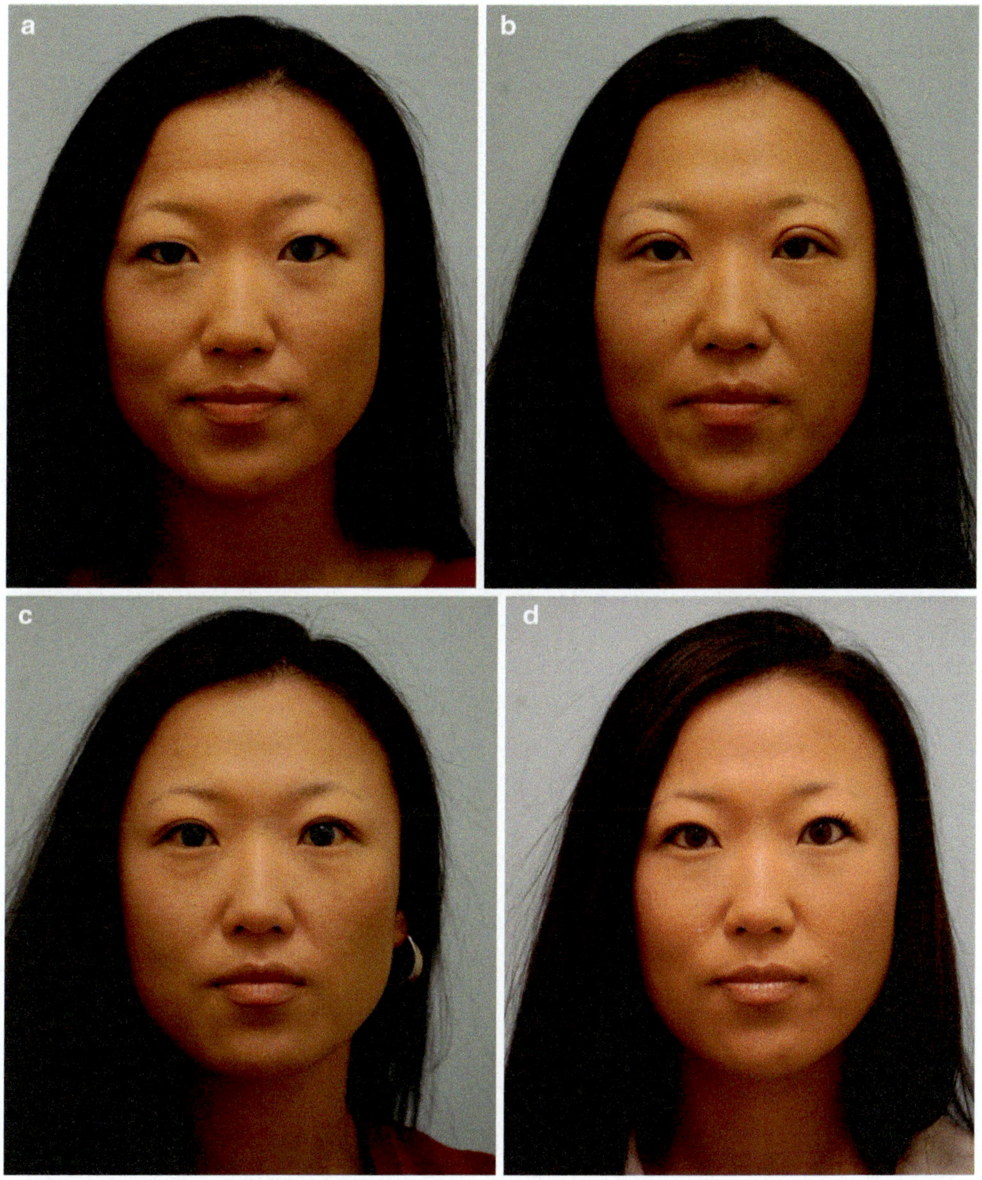

Fig. 14.13 (**a**) Preoperative photograph of an Asian woman with no upper eyelid crease. (**b**) Postoperative swelling in the upper eyelids at 1 week. (**c**) Gradual decrease in upper eyelid swelling after 3 months. (**d**) Final result 1 year out

will appear grossly elevated and should not be used as the desired goal (it will soften and descend with time). If the eyelash position as well as crease depth and position is deemed appropriate, the suture is secured with its ends left long enough for removal postoperatively. A higher crease can be created by placing a superiorly placed horizontal bite through the levator. Alternatively, a lower crease can be created by placing the suture more inferiorly along the levator. A second and third fixation sutures are aligned with the medial limbus and halfway between the lateral limbus and the lateral canthus, respectively. These fixation sutures can be adjusted intraoperatively if needed. The skin is then approximated with a loosely running, nonlocking 6–0 nylon suture. All sutures are removed a week after surgery. Figure 14.13 illustrates a patient before and 18 months after the described procedure.

14.6.5 Postoperative Care

Cold compresses are applied to the lids for the first 48–72 h to reduce edema. Ophthalmic antibiotic ointment is applied twice daily. The patient returns between the fifth and seventh postoperative day for suture removal. Occasionally, the patient may experience weakness in eye opening caused by eyelid edema or temporary levator aponeurosis dysfunction. This typically resolves within 1–2 months of surgery. Frank ptosis with poor lid excursion beyond the immediate postoperative period can signify levator injury requiring exploration. Pretarsal edema may persist for months and sometimes up to a year. This requires preoperative counseling and postoperative reassurance. Narrow, rectangular-shaped eyeglasses can camouflage some of the postoperative edema, which tends to lead to a noticeable high crease. The crease gradually lowers and softens over the course of the healing process. Female patients often use mascara to camouflage the height of the upper eyelid crease until the edema resolves.

14.7 Conclusion

Performing appropriate Asian upper eyelid blepharoplasty requires a detailed knowledge of Asian eyelid anatomy, an understanding of relevant periorbital aging changes and cultural preferences within this group, and experience with surgical crease formation. Traditional surgery tended to "Westernize" patients with creation of a high, arched crease. This result has fallen out of favor. Contemporary surgery focuses on volume preservation and restoration with less excision of tissue. A conservative excision of eyelid fat, with appropriate crease height, will contribute to ensuring a natural appearing result. The addition of fat grafting when appropriate can enhance outcome. With the full-incision method outlined in this chapter, the senior author (SML) has been able to achieve consistently excellent results with stable crease position over time.

References

1. Zide BM. Anatomy of the eyelids. Clin Plast Surg. 1981;8(4): 623–34.
2. Aguilar GL, Nelson C. Eyelid and anterior orbital anatomy. In: Hornblass A, editor. Oculoplastic, orbital and reconstructive surgery. Vol. 1: Eyelids. Baltimore: Williams & Wilkins; 1988.
3. Jones LT. New concepts of orbital anatomy. In: Tessier P, Callahan A, Mustarde JC, et al., editors. Symposium on plastic surgery in the orbital region. St. Louis: CV Mosby; 1976.
4. Kure K, Minami A. A simple and durable way to create a supratarsal fold (double eyelid) in Asian patients. Aesthet Surg J. 2001;21(3):227–32.
5. Chen WP. Suture ligation methods. In: Asian blepharoplasty and the eyelid crease. London: Elsevier; 1995. p. 39–50.
6. Mikamo K. A technique in the double eyelid operation. J Chugaishinpo. 1896.
7. Uchida K. The Uchida method for the double-eyelid operation in 1523 cases. Jpn J Ophthalmol. 1926;30:593.
8. Maruo M. Plastic construction of a 'double eyelid'. Jpn Rev Clin Ophthalmol. 1929;24:393–406.
9. Pang HG. Surgical formation of upper lid fold. Arch Ophthalmol. 1961;65:783–4.

Part IV

Lower Eyelid Rejuvenation

Transcutaneous Lower Eyelid Blepharoplasty

15

Stephen W. Perkins and Paul K. Holden

Key Points

- Properly executed and in the appropriate patient, transcutaneous lower eyelid blepharoplasty has minimal added risk of lower lid malposition as compared to other techniques.
- A complete ophthalmologic history, examination, and identification of the need for canthal suspension are critical to avoid potential adverse sequelae.
- Premorbid lower eyelid malposition and/or laxity must be identified before surgery and addressed during the procedure.
- Incisions placed 2–3 mm below the ciliary margin will preserve the pretarsal orbicularis oculi muscle, making the desired aesthetic and functional outcome more likely.
- It is important to redrape the skin–muscle flap in a superior-lateral direction and suspend the pretarsal orbicularis oculi muscle to the inner surface of the lateral orbit to prevent poor aesthetic and functional outcomes.
- When upper blepharoplasty is performed simultaneously, the lateral aspect of the upper eyelid incision should be closed first to prevent a visible incision.
- Overresection of fat must be avoided to prevent a sunken appearance after surgery.
- Fat transposition should be considered for effacement of the nasojugal groove ("tear trough" deformity).
- Festoons and orbicularis oculi muscle redundancy can be addressed with the malar extension technique.
- Aggressive ocular lubrication in the immediate postoperative period will reduce dry eye symptoms, speed recovery, and increase patient satisfaction.

P.K. Holden (✉)
Holden Facial Plastic Surgery, Scottsdale, AZ, USA
e-mail: holdenpk@gmail.com

15.1 Introduction

The transcutaneous approach to lower eyelid blepharoplasty is a commonly performed procedure and an important tool in the armamentarium of cosmetic surgeons. Although most consider it to be a relatively simple operation, proper patient selection and technique are crucial to achieve the best results while minimizing potentially vexing complications. The procedure best addresses true vertical excess of lower eyelid muscle and skin (dermatochalasis), offers ease of access to treat pseudoherniation of the orbital fat compartments, and is an ideal approach for adjunctive procedures such as malar extension, midface lift, lateral canthoplasty and fat transposition [1]. Additionally, the posterior lamella is preserved and the risk of corneal injury is minimized.

15.2 Patient Selection

Before proceeding with surgery, every patient should be carefully evaluated to determine the most appropriate procedure for rejuvenating the lower eyelid complex. Employing a standardized, logical approach to these patients will ensure optimal outcomes.

The evaluation begins with a complete ocular history including a review of prior surgeries and medical conditions which affect the eyes (such as glaucoma, diabetes, thyroid myxedema, dry eye syndrome, etc.). All of the patient's medications should be reviewed, especially those that may affect the eyes. For a patient without a history of ocular disease or complaints, and a normal examination, all that is required preoperatively is to perform a test of visual acuity and extraocular muscle movement. If a patient has any history of ocular problems or an examination that is unusual, then an evaluation by an ophthalmologist preoperatively is warranted. Common symptoms requiring referral include ocular pain, discomfort or irritation, a change in visual acuity, recurrent orbital edema, diplopia, dry eyes (especially in

G.G. Massry et al. (eds.), *Master Techniques in Blepharoplasty and Periorbital Rejuvenation*,
DOI 10.1007/978-1-4614-0067-7_15, © Springer Science+Business Media, LLC 2011

conjunction with xerostomia), chemosis, or epiphora. If there is a suspicion of a thyroid related orbital disorder, a thyroid panel is ordered.

In addition to an ocular assessment, surgical risk is evaluated. This includes identification of cardiopulmonary risk, the use of anticoagulation medications, as well as a history of diabetes, hypertension, and cancer. Prior surgical history, including response to anesthesia, should also be discussed.

Compared to transconjunctival surgery, the transcutaneous approach affords the ability to correct true vertical excess of lower lid skin and orbicularis oculi hypertrophy. However, there are specific indications for transconjunctival blepharoplasty. For example, young patients with excellent skin elasticity, presence of hereditary pseudoherniation of orbital fat, and no evidence of skin excess are ideally suited for the transconjunctival approach. Additionally, patients with Fitzpatrick skin types V–VI may benefit from transconjunctival blepharoplasty, as the scar from transcutaneous surgery may depigment and remain visible. Lastly, patients with residual fat herniation in an otherwise good result may be better suited for a transconjunctival revision.

15.3 Patient Examination

The initial examination of the eyes should include careful observation of extraocular movements, pupil and iris symmetry, evidence of prior surgery, skin quality, skin pigmentation, protrusion of the globe, pseudoherniation of fat, lower eyelid position/laxity, orbicularis oculi redundancy, depth of the nasojugal groove ("tear trough"), and position of the malar fat pad. This information will assist in surgical planning in order to avoid common pitfalls, and assure the best cosmetic result.

Skin quality varies according to age, ethnicity, smoking history, medical problems, sun exposure, genetics, and prior surgical or resurfacing history. In many cases, patients have structural signs of eyelid aging (pseudoherniation of fat, eyelid laxity) as well as pigmentary disturbances and telangiectasis of the skin (Fig. 15.1). Treatment of periorbital pigmentation and/or telangiectasis may require laser treatment, which can be performed at the same surgical setting as the lower lid blepharoplasty. These patients should be made aware of their skin changes in order to control expectations and plan for any additional procedures.

Lower eyelid skin redundancy is a major reason that patients seek surgical treatment. This is typically a consequence of age, sun exposure, and genetics, which all contribute to loss of skin elasticity and related changes (dermatochalasis). A simple skin pinch performed in the office can give the surgeon and patient an accurate assessment of the quantity of skin requiring excision. This is performed gently using blunt, flat forceps while the patient refrains from blinking. Skin that does not immediately recoil to its native position will likely require excision in order to provide optimal rejuvenation.

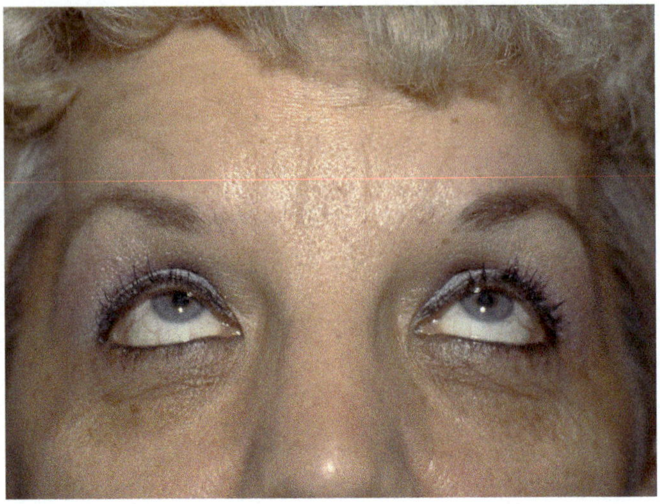

Fig. 15.1 A patient with lower eyelid hyperpigmentation. This can be improved with resurfacing, but not with blepharoplasty alone

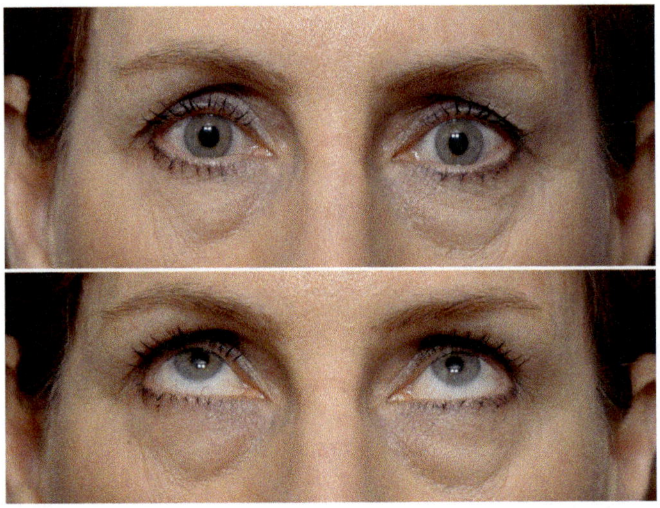

Fig. 15.2 A patient with pseudoherniation of periorbital fat, which is best demonstrated on upward gaze

Many patients complain of "bags" under their eyes that give a tired and aged look. This protrusion of the lower eyelid is usually a result of prolapsed orbital fat that becomes evident through an attenuated orbital septum. In addition to fat prolapse, the prominence may result from redundant, or lax, orbicularis oculi muscle, as well as midface volume loss and descent. Pseudoherniation of fat can be accentuated by having a patient look up during examination (Fig. 15.2). Gentle palpation of the globe during upward gaze can accentuate and better demonstrate the orbital fat components. In order to assess orbicularis oculi redundancy, patients are asked to squint or smile during forward gaze. As the muscle contracts, orbicularis redundancy will be apparent, especially in the pretarsal portion. In severe cases, the patient may have festoons, which are discussed below.

When patients report symptoms consistent with dry eyes, an objective test of tear film production may be beneficial to perform. The most common and reliable test for tear production is the Schirmer test, which is performed by the placement of a 35×5 mm size filter paper strip against the lateral fornix for 5 min. The resultant height of wetness of the paper is measured, and if it is less than 10–15 mm, the test is positive for dryness (with or without topical anesthetic). Xeropthalmia does not necessarily exclude patients from undergoing blepharoplasty, but usually requires more vigorous and prolonged attempts to maintain ocular lubrication during the recovery period.

15.4 Eyelid Position and Laxity

The position and tone (laxity) of the lower eyelid are considerations for surgery and must be addressed in order to avoid postoperative eyelid malposition such as retraction or ectropion. The lid distraction test and a snap test should be performed in order to assess the need for an eyelid tightening procedure (refer to Chap. 17 for detailed description of eyelid laxity and canthal suspension). The snap test is performed by gently pulling the lower eyelid inferiorly and laterally such that it pulls away from the eye (Fig. 15.3). The lid is then quickly released and should immediately return to its native position without blink. If this is not the case, lower eyelid tone is reduced, laxity is likely, and lid tightening should be performed via canthopexy or lateral canthoplasty [2].

The distraction test involves gently pulling the lower eyelid away from the eye and measuring the distance from the surface of the globe to the eyelid margin (Fig. 15.4). Distances greater than 10 mm are abnormal and indicate eyelid laxity. Lateral canthoplasty should be planned in these cases [2].

The lower eyelid should be at or above the inferior limbus. If below this level, eyelid retraction is present. The degree of retraction is measured as the distance between the lower eyelid margin and the inferior limbus (scleral show). Another measure of lower lid position is the margin–reflex distance-2 (MRD-2). This is the distance from the corneal light reflex to the lower eyelid margin, and should measure 5.5 mm or less. Distances greater than 5.5 mm are considered abnormal and likely secondary to lid retraction.

Relative lateral canthal position should also be assessed. Normally, the lateral canthus is positioned 1–2 mm superior to the medial canthus. If the lateral canthus is inferior to this level, laxity may be present, and canthal repositioning (via lateral canthopexy [3] or lateral canthoplasty [2]) should be considered for optimal outcome and to prevent lower eyelid malposition. In the most severe cases of eyelid laxity, horizontal lid shortening can be combined with lateral canthoplasty [2].

Protrusion of the globe will have a direct impact on the patient's recovery and the incidence of postoperative complications (see Chap. 26). Hertel exophthalmometry can be utilized to measure globe position relative to the orbital rim. Four classifications exist: Grade I: <15 mm protrusion (deep set eyes), Grade II: 15–17 mm, Grade III: 18–19 mm and Grade IV: >19 mm.[4] In Grade III–IV patients, globe prominence is present. In these cases, very conservative skin excision is performed in addition to modified lower lid support procedures, to prevent lid retraction, improve ocular lubrication, and enhance corneal protection. These include performing more superiorly directed lid suspension (above Whitnall tubercle), whether via canthoplasty or canthopexy, possible lid lengthening, and temporary placement of a support suture (Frost stitch, Fig. 15.5). An overcorrection of lid position is important, and care should be taken to avoid lid shortening lid procedures that can bowstring the globe [4].

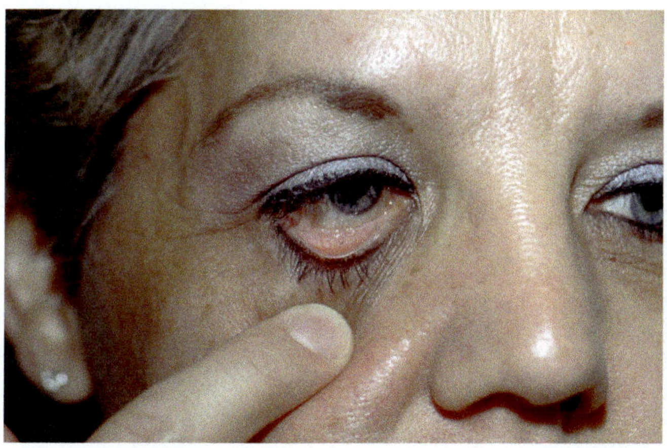

Fig. 15.3 The snap test is performed with inferolateral distraction of the eyelid with rapid release. Normally, immediate return of the eyelid to its native position occurs

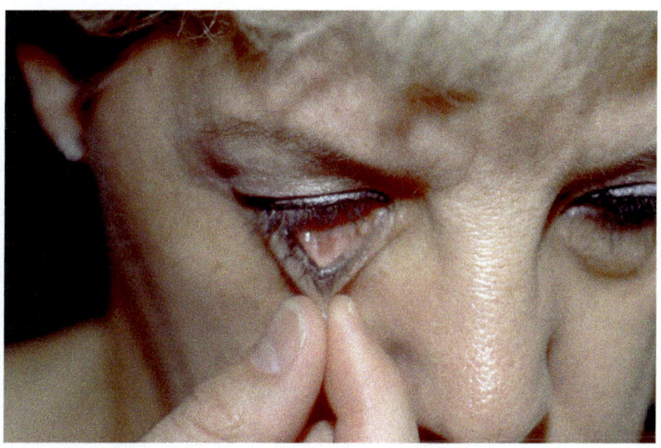

Fig. 15.4 The eyelid distraction test is performed by gently pulling the eyelid away from the globe and estimating the distance of distraction. Normal eyelid tone is present when distraction is 10 mm or less

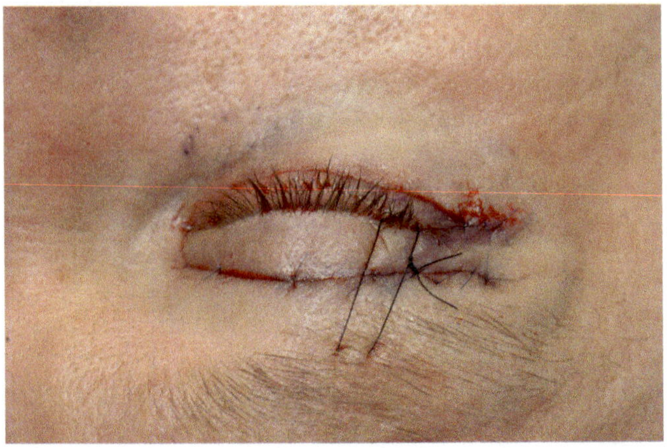

Fig. 15.5 A Frost suture is a horizontal mattress suture that suspends the lateral gray line of the lower eyelid to the midbrow. This suture is placed lateral to the cornea and usually left in place for 4–5 days

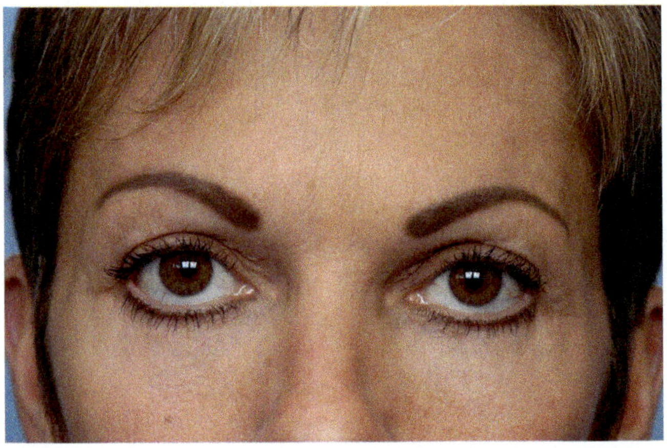

Fig. 15.6 Lateral lower eyelid rounding and scleral show is a preventable postoperative complication with proper suspension techniques

15.5 Revision Patients

Patients who have undergone previous eyelid surgery may have associated abnormalities of eyelid position and/or function. The examiner should take care to note lower eyelid deficiencies such as rounding (Fig. 15.6) or blunting of the lateral canthal angle, ectropion, entropion, skeletonization, malpositioned transposed fat, incorrectly placed incisions (visible scars), lower lid retraction with scleral show, and eyelid asymmetry [5].

Treatment of eyelid malposition is dependent on etiology. Mild cases of ectropion or lid retraction may only require canthal suspension, scar lysis and muscle plication. In more severe cases, middle lamella support with a spacer graft, such as hard palate mucosa, acellular dermis (Alloderm) or other spacing materials may be required. In severe cases, additional interventions such as transposition skin flaps from the upper lids or full thickness skin grafts may be necessary. Consideration should also be given to placement of a Frost suture and/or lateral tarsorrhaphy for corneal protection and temporary elevated support to the lower lid during the initial healing.

When entropion is present, release of the inner lamella with lid rotational techniques and potential spacer grafts, as previously mentioned, may be necessary.

15.6 Festoons and Malar Edema

Orbicularis hypertrophy can manifest as tissue excess that extends beyond the limits of the orbital fat. This tissue is thicker than skin alone. It can also extend below the orbital rim and to the malar eminence laterally (Fig. 15.7). The most severe manifestation of this are festoons. These are patulous

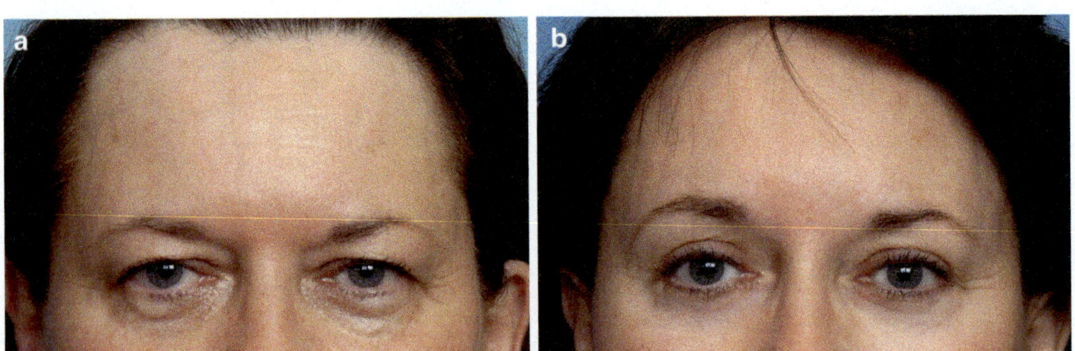

Fig. 15.7 Hypertrophy of the orbicularis oculi muscle is identified preoperatively and can be best improved using the transcutaneous skin muscle flap blepharoplasty technique. (**a**) Before and (**b**) after surgery

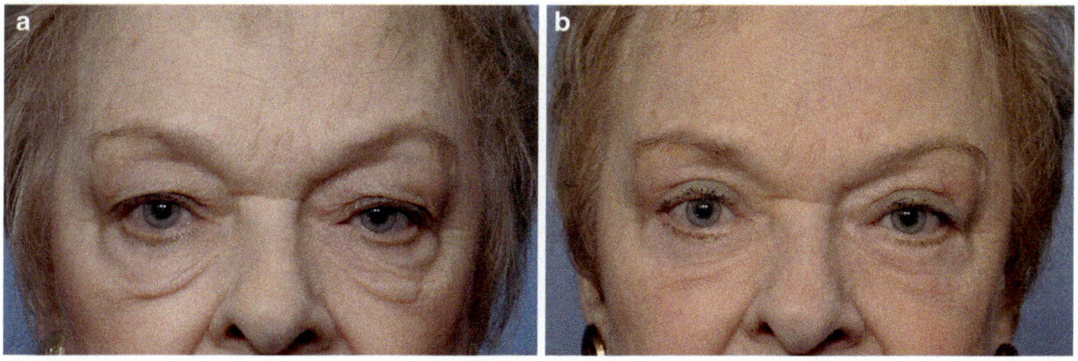

Fig. 15.8 Severe festoons often lead to ectropion, scleral show, and exposure keratitis. The technique of malar extension with lateral canthoplasty can give excellent improvement in these patients. (**a**) Before and (**b**) after surgery

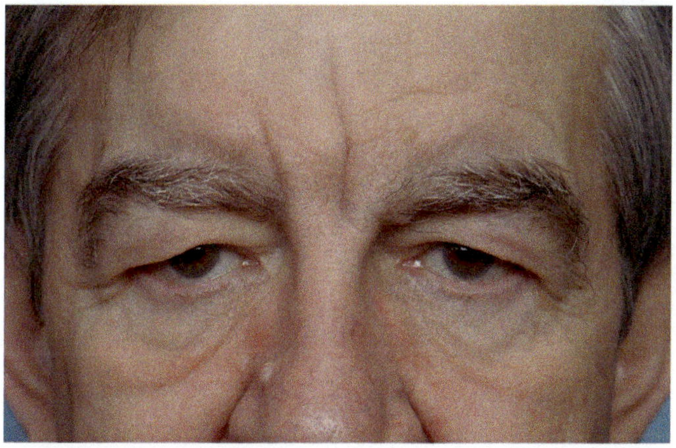

Fig. 15.9 Malar edema is visible during the preoperative examination. The patient should be advised that this condition might persist in the postoperative period for an extended period of time

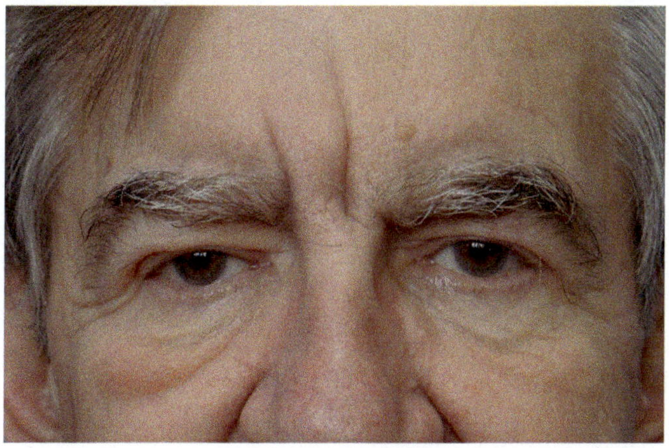

Fig. 15.10 Persistent malar edema following lower eyelid blepharoplasty

sacs of skin and muscle which appear to hang below the orbital rim from the medial to the lateral canthus in a hammock-like fashion (Fig. 15.8) [6, 7].

In these cases, extended transcutaneous lower eyelid blepharoplasty is an excellent treatment option [8]. Great care should be taken to document eyelid position and tension as the weight of festoons over time will often lead to severe laxity and malposition (Fig. 15.8).

Patients may also have malar edema (Fig. 15.9). This appears as subcutaneous fluid over the malar eminence, and usually follows minimal trauma or allergic response. Patients with a history of prolonged malar edema or those who manifest edema at the time of examination should be advised that lower eyelid blepharoplasty may trigger worsening edema after surgery, which may take months to resolve. Aggressive cold compresses, head elevation, and low-dose corticosteroids may be given at the time of surgery in order to minimize the severity of the problem. Patients should be counseled preoperatively of the possible postoperative course for this type of swelling (Fig. 15.10). Pressure taping of the lower lids with superolateral tension to the canthus and temple has been shown to be effective in reducing postoperative edema. Micropore tape (3M, St. Paul, MN) can be applied for 1 week.

15.7 Patient Expectations and Psychology

As with all cosmetic patients, psychology is an important factor in determining their suitability for surgery. During the consultation, the patients should be asked open-ended questions about their concerns while viewing themselves in a mirror. Allow the patients to verbalize their areas of concern and their expectations of surgery in their own words. Determine if the patients are reasonable and realistic in their expectations. Patients whose expectations can be easily directed with a little education are most appropriate.

Establish rapport with each patient and any family members or friends who accompany them. Listen carefully for warning signs, such as extrinsic motivation for surgery, overly inflated expectations, presence of emotional crisis, or a disapproving friend, spouse, or parent. In addition, be wary if there have been repeated prior procedures with another surgeon, especially if dissatisfaction over the prior results is present.

Patient and surgeon alike should be aware that transient depression after blepharoplasty is common and can exacerbate any preexisting depression. The inherent nature of the normal postoperative swelling, bruising, blurriness, and dry eye symptoms can create anxiety and depression until healing is more complete.

Ideally, patients should have intrinsic motivations, realistic expectations, and supportive family and friends. Furthermore, there should be an effortless development of a doctor–patient relationship. Any ongoing psychological conditions (if present) should have documented long-term stability with the patient's current regimen of treatment. In these instances, the success of surgery and patient satisfaction will be highest.

15.8 Important Surgical Anatomy

The lower eyelids consist of three lamellae. The anterior lamella consists of skin and orbicularis oculi muscle, and spans the full height of the lid. The orbicularis oculi muscle is further divided into a pretarsal, preseptal, and an orbital segment. Portions of the terminal pretarsal orbicularis muscle constitute a major component of both the medial and lateral canthal ligaments as they attach to the posterior lacrimal crest medially and the underside of Whitnall's tubercle laterally [9].

The middle lamella consists of the orbital septum, which is a connective tissue band originating from the periosteum of the inferior orbital rim (arcus marginalis) and fusing with the lower lid retractors 3–4 mm below the tarsal plate. A medial extension of the orbital septum called the orbitomalar ligament traverses the orbicularis muscle ending in cutaneous attachments and contributing to the nasojugal fold [10].

The posterior lamella consists of the tarsus and conjunctiva in the first 5 mm of the eyelid, and the capsulopalpebral fascia (lower eyelid retractors) and conjunctiva below the tarsus. The tarsus is the cartilaginous structure, which gives the lower eyelid support and is 4–5 mm in height, and 30 mm in width. The Meibomian glands lie within the tarsus, producing sebaceous secretions to the outer layer of the tear film, thereby preventing evaporation of tears.

The capsulopalpebral fascia originates from the inferior rectus muscle and, as stated above, fuses with the orbital septum before inserting to the inferior edge of the tarsus. This attachment is an important support structure of the lower eyelid. Disruption of this attachment may lead to entropion [10].

Orbital fat is located posterior to the orbital septum and anterior to the lower lid retractors. The lower orbital fat pads consist of three compartments: lateral, central, and medial pockets. The inferior oblique muscle divides the central fat pocket from the medial fat pocket, while the arcuate ligament separates the central from the lateral fat pad. The orbital fat gives volume to the inferior orbit and acts to cushion the eye and protect it from blunt trauma [11].

15.9 Operative Technique

The skin–muscle flap is the most commonly used transcutaneous technique by the senior author (SWP). The indications for this technique include true vertical excess of lower eyelid skin, orbicularis oculi muscle hypertrophy, and presence of pseudoherniation of orbital fat [12].

The incision is placed 2 mm inferior to the ciliary margin and extends from the lower punctum medially to a position 6 mm lateral to the lateral canthus following a natural skin crease (Fig. 15.11). Lateral extension of the incision to this position minimizes rounding of the canthal angle.

Following the skin incision, fine curved scissors are used to dissect through the orbicularis muscle at the lateral aspect of the incision (Fig. 15.12). A short separate skin flap is elevated

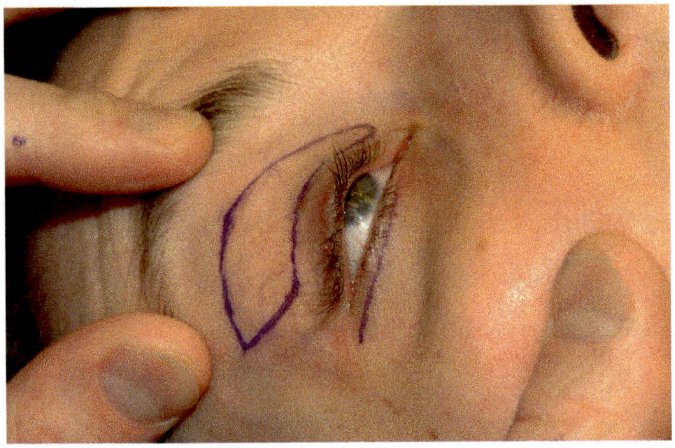

Fig. 15.11 Lower eyelid skin marking should be 2 mm below the lash line following a natural skin crease with extension from the punctum to approximately 6 mm lateral to the lateral canthus

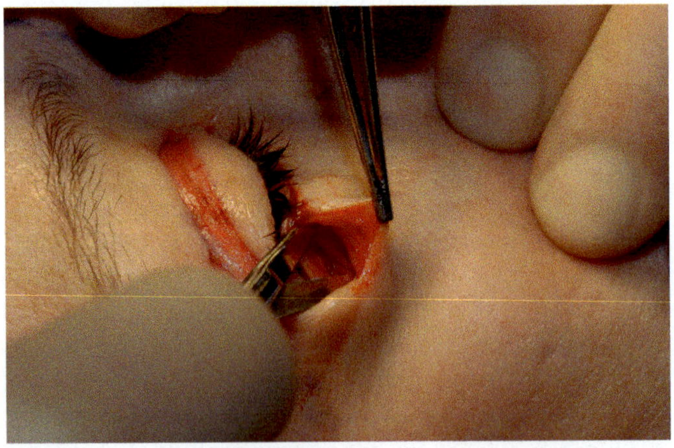

Fig. 15.12 Dissection through the lateral orbicularis oculi muscle to the level of the preseptal space

off the pretarsal orbicularis. Blunt scissors are then positioned posterior to the muscle at the lateral aspect of the incision and the skin–muscle flap is elevated off the orbital septum bluntly (spreading) along an avascular plane (Fig. 15.13). The subciliary incision is then completed using the scissors in a beveled manner to ensure the preservation of the pretarsal portion of the orbicularis oculi muscle, thus minimizing the risk of postoperative lower lid malposition.

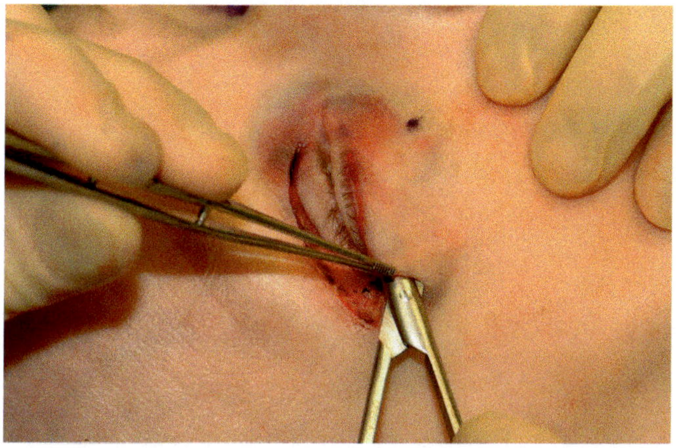

Fig. 15.13 Blunt elevation of the skin–muscle flap along an avascular plane should be free of resistance in nonrevision cases

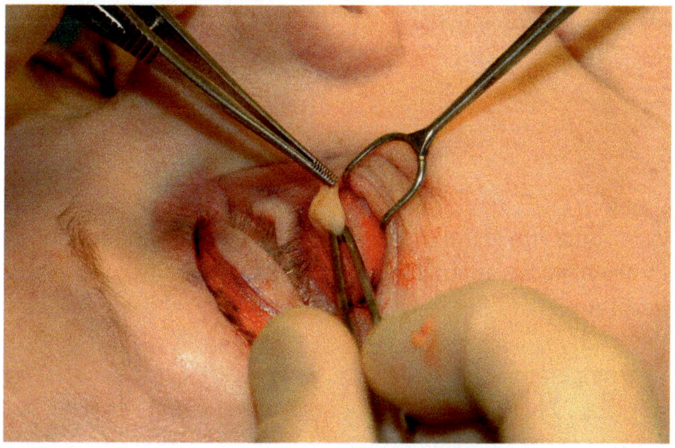

Fig. 15.14 Meticulous cauterization of fat with bipolar cautery prior to excision is crucial to the prevention of postoperative bleeding and retrobulbar hematoma

Small openings are made in the orbital septum to obtain access to the orbital fat compartments. Gentle palpation of the globe results in herniation of orbital fat through the aforementioned openings of the orbital septum. Herniated fat is gently grasped, and bipolar cautery is used to cauterize the base of each fat pad prior to excision (Fig. 15.14). Local anesthesia is infiltrated into the fat pocket to minimize pain. This maneuver is repeated for the lateral, central, and medial fat compartments. Gentle palpation of the globe following resection of orbital fat allows for reassessment of the remaining volume. A conservative approach to fat resection is maintained to avoid the creation of a sunken appearance after surgery [11]. In approximately 30–40% of cases, there is a preoperative physical finding of a nasal trough "deformity." In these cases fat transposition of the nasal, and occasionally middle fat pocket, is performed. The stalk of the visualized flap is positioned inferiorly beneath the orbicularis and sutured to the periosteum, 10–12 mm below the orbital rim.

The skin–muscle flap is now repositioned. If mildly sedated, the patient is asked to open the mouth and look up. This maneuver allows for maximal separation of wound edges and subsequent conservative resection of skin and muscle. On the other hand, if the patient is sedated, single-finger pressure at the inferomedial portion of the melolabial mound will create the same maximal stretch effect. During either maneuver, an inferiorly directed segmental cut is made at the lateral canthus to determine the amount of excess skin to excise (Fig. 15.15a). A tacking suture is placed to maintain the position of the skin–muscle flap (Fig. 15.15b). Eyelid scissors are then used to excise the overlapping skin (Fig. 15.15c). If orbicularis oculi muscle hypertrophy is evident, a 1- to 2-mm strip of muscle is resected to prevent overlapping of muscle and ridge formation with closure of the subciliary incision [13]. Conservative resection of both skin and muscle will decrease the incidence of postoperative lower eyelid malposition. If no additional procedures are planned, suspension of the orbicularis oculi muscle to the periosteum of the lateral

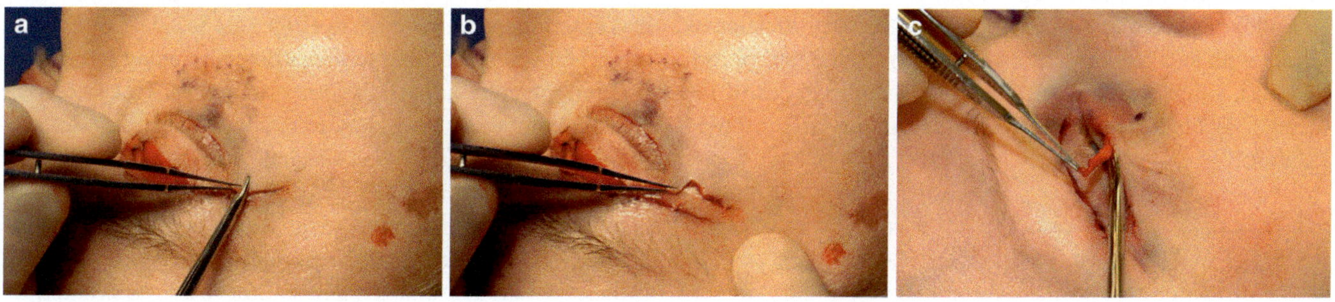

Fig. 15.15 Excess skin–muscle excision is first performed with a maximal stretch maneuver (as described) and (**a**) gentle overlay of excess laterally (**b**). A pair of fine skin scissors is then used to trim the redundant skin–muscle flap and it is tacked into position (**c**). Redundant skin and muscle can then be trimmed

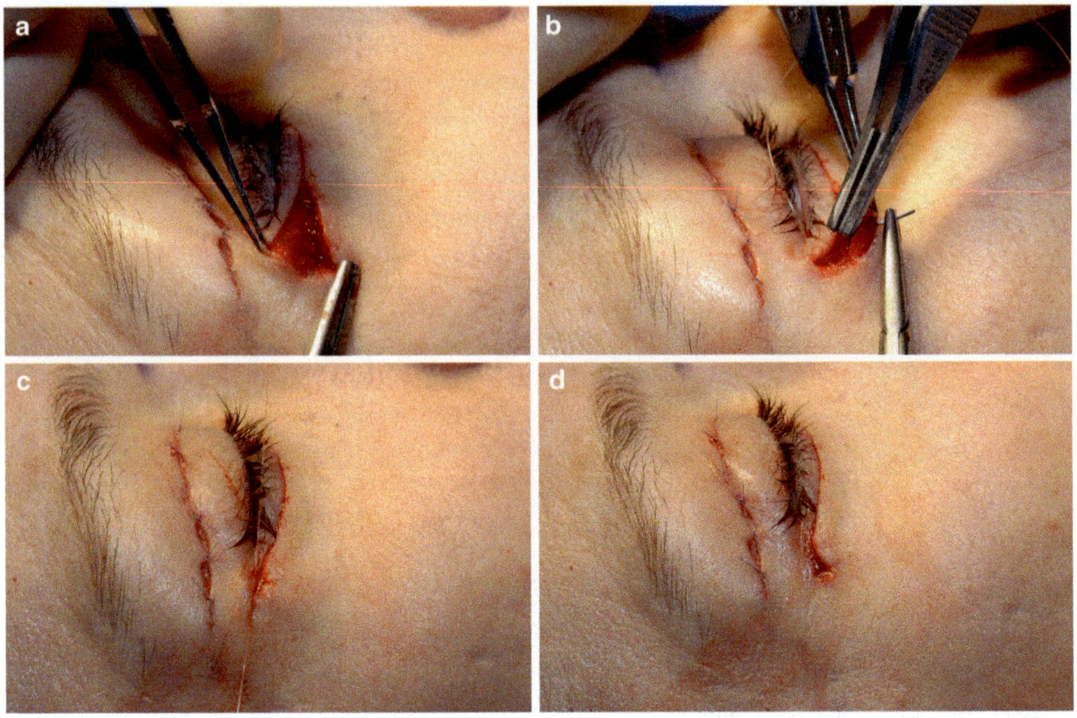

Fig. 15.16 The skin–muscle flap is suspended to the lateral orbital rim by (**a**) first passing the suture through the periosteum of the lateral orbital tubercle, (**b**) followed by the orbicularis oculi muscle. (**c**) Supporting sutures are then placed in buried interrupted fashion to further fasten the muscle in suspension (**d**) leaving minimal tension on the lower eyelid skin

orbital rim is performed using a 5–0 monocryl suture in buried fashion (Fig. 15.16a,b). Additional supporting sutures of the muscle flap are placed with one or two 5–0 vicryl sutures in a buried interrupted fashion (Fig. 15.16c,d).

If there is evidence of festoons or malar mounds, an extended lower lid blepharoplasty is performed inferior to the infraorbital rim [12]. The redundant orbicularis oculi muscle and/or malar mounds are addressed by first elevating and then advancing the entire skin-muscle flap and suborbicularis oculi fat (SOOF) unit superior-laterally (Fig. 15.17). Suspension of the skin–muscle flap is then performed in the same fashion.

Following muscle suspension, the subciliary incision is closed with 7–0 blue polypropylene suture at the lateral canthus in a simple, interrupted fashion. The remainder of the incision is closed with 6–0 plain gut suture in a running fashion.

15.10 Fat Transposition

Many methods have been described to efface the tear trough, including fat grafting[14], injectable fillers[15], alloplastic implants[16], and transposition of pedicled orbital fat over the orbital rim (fat transposition)[17]. Fat transposition via a transcutaneous approach in conjunction with lower lid blepharoplasty is our preferred method of addressing a tear trough deformity.

Preoperatively, the tear trough is carefully marked with a felt-tipped pen while the patient is sitting supine looking forward. Lower lid blepharoplasty with extension beyond the infraorbital rim is performed (Fig. 15.17). The orbital fat from the appropriate pocket(s) is isolated from the orbital septum. The fat is transposed over the orbital rim and positioned into a pocket posterior to the orbicularis oculi muscle and anterior to the periosteum (Fig. 15.18a). The transposed orbital fat is then secured to the periosteum using interrupted 6–0 polyglycolic acid (Polysorb)suture (Fig. 15.18b,c). The skin is redraped as necessary to evaluate tear trough effacement. The orbital fat is then softened with the use of bipolar cautery as needed (Fig. 15.18d,e). The medial fat compartment is most commonly transposed; however, the central and/or lateral fat compartments may also be repositioned if there is a greater quantity present, or if lid/cheek interface depression is present at a location more proximal to those compartments. The procedure is then completed as previously described.

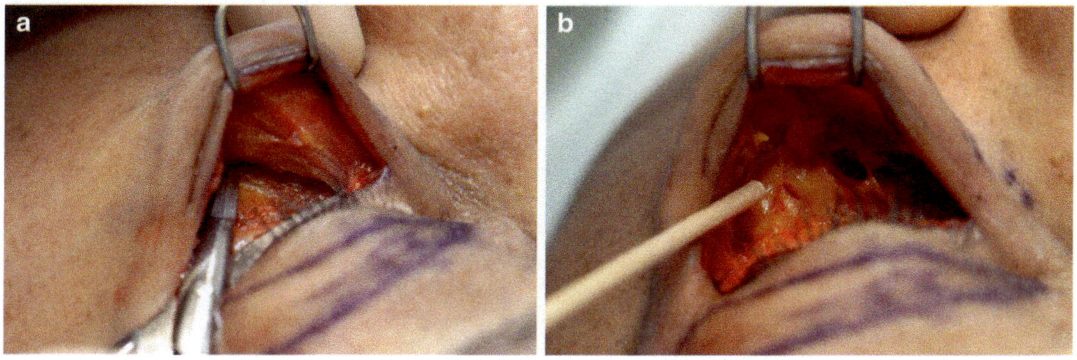

Fig. 15.17 Malar extension is performed by (**a**) dissecting between orbicularis oculi muscle and periosteum until (**b**) the SOOF and the skin–muscle flap are mobile as a single unit

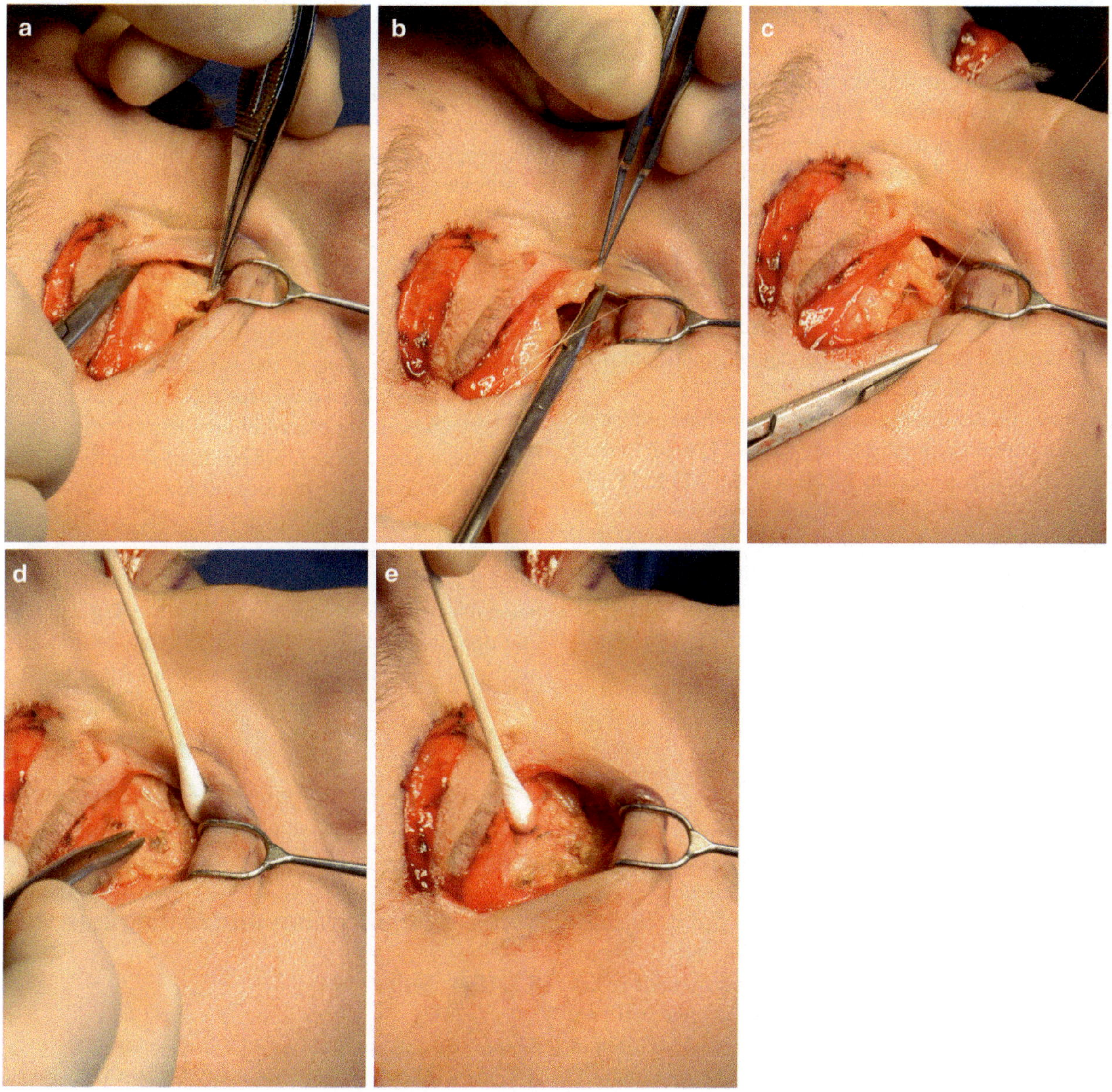

Fig. 15.18 Fat transposition is performed by (**a**) first advancing excess orbital fat through the septum and over the orbital rim. (**b**, **c**) Next, the fat is secured to the periosteum in the nasojugal groove. (**d**, **e**). Bipolar cautery is then used conservatively to contour the fat to avoid irregularities

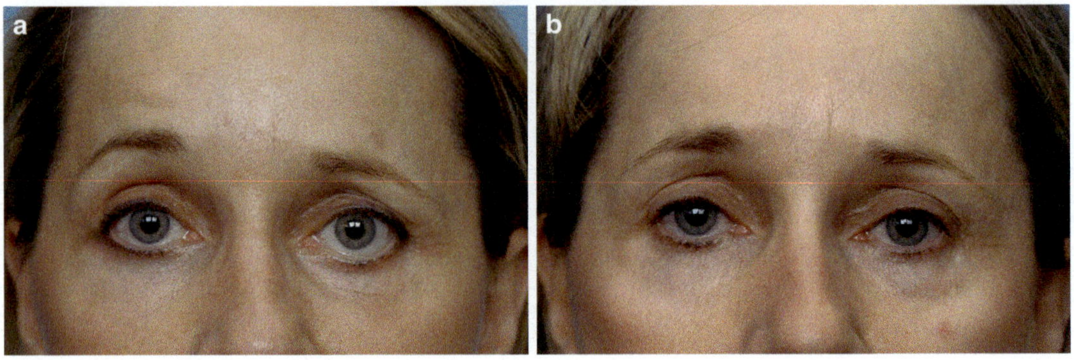

Fig. 15.19 (**a**) Lateral canthoplasty is indicated in patients with lower eyelid malposition preoperatively. (**b**) Improvement of lower eyelid position enhances the aesthetic and functional outcomes of surgery

15.11 Lower Eyelid Tightening

Several intraoperative maneuvers can help minimize postoperative lower lid malposition. These include preservation of the pretarsal orbicularis oculi muscle, conservative resection of skin and muscle, and suspension of the tarsus and/or pretarsal orbicularis oculi muscle to the periosteum of the lateral orbital rim.

For mild degrees of lower lid laxity, a canthopexy is performed prior to trimming the lower lid skin and muscle. A 5–0 monocryl suture is used to suspend and support the tarsus and pretarsal orbicularis to the medial superior periosteum of the superior orbital rim laterally.

If the lower lid demonstrates laxity or poor tone preoperatively, then a lateral canthoplasty (see Chap. 17) is performed in conjunction with lower lid blepharoplasty (Fig. 15.19). Following lateral canthotomy and inferior cantholysis, the terminal tarsus is dissected from the skin and muscle. The posterior surface of the tarsus is deepithelialized forming a tarsal strip. The appropriate amount of lower lid is excised. The tarsal strip is then secured to the inner aspect of the lateral orbital rim periosteum with a permanent suture in a posterosuperior vector.

15.12 Skin Resurfacing

Lower lid blepharoplasty cannot effectively address fine periorbital cutaneous rhytids. Therefore, chemical exfoliation or laser skin resurfacing can be performed in conjunction with surgery to improve skin quality. In the senior author's experience, the most effective and predictable resurfacing result is achieved using a phenol 88% chemical peel preferentially over CO_2 laser resurfacing. Ideal candidates for skin resurfacing of the lower eyelid include patients with Fitzpatrick skin types I–III. Blepharoplasty alone may result in vertical contracture of lower eyelid tissue. The addition of laser skin resurfacing will tighten lower lid skin, further shortening the anterior lamella. As such, it is essential to evaluate both lid position and support prior to performing skin resurfacing in conjunction with lower lid blepharoplasty. When appropriate, canthoplasty should be added to surgery to provide appropriate support

15.13 Postoperative Care

Immediately following surgery, ointment (antibiotic/steroid ophthalmic) is applied to the eye and the suture lines. This continues three times a day for the first week after surgery. Cold compresses are placed in the recovery room and for the first 2 days after surgery. Elevation of the head of the bed is important to minimize postoperative swelling.

Postoperative swelling may interfere with normal tear production and flow, leading to temporary epiphora and dry eyes. It is imperative to instruct the patient about the importance of artificial tear use throughout the day and nonantibiotic ophthalmic ointment placed onto the conjunctiva in the evenings. The patient is instructed to avoid physical activity for the first 48 h and heavy exertion (lifting, bending, or straining) for 2 weeks to minimize the risk of hematoma formation.

At 1 week postoperatively, the sutures are removed. Patients can then begin application of makeup.

15.14 Complications and Management

15.14.1 Milia

Milia are common findings after transcutaneous lower blepharoplasty. These are tiny, white keratin cysts found usually on or near the healed incision. The treatment is to first clean the area with rubbing alcohol and then extract the keratinaceous debris as a single unit with a 25 or 22g needle. A small dab of ointment is then placed over the excision site. Recurrence in the same location is very rare. In larger or recurrent milia, excision and closure with a simple interrupted 7–0 polypropylene suture is warranted.

15.14.2 Dry Eye/Chemosis

The signs and symptoms of dry eyes include a scratchy or foreign body sensation in the eye, epiphora, and presence of conjunctival edema (chemosis). If identified early and managed aggressively, more serious problem of exposure keratitis can be avoided. The patients should be educated with respect to dry eye, as they may find it difficult to comprehend that the eye is dry when they are experiencing copious amounts of tearing. Generous and frequent application of ophthalmic lubricant drops throughout the day and ointment in the evening is emphasized. A transition to a viscous artificial tear product is beneficial to those with chemosis [18]. If the chemosis is persistent and/or prominent, other maneuvers, such as placement of a Frost suture, lateral tarsorrhaphy, or, at the least, taping of the lower eyelid, are often beneficial both for symptomatic relief and accelerated recovery.

15.14.3 Hematoma

Hematomas after blepharoplasty range from a small self-limiting pool of blood under the suture line to an expanding collection that may extend into the retrobulbar space. The incidence of hematoma, in the senior author's experience, is extremely rare and is reduced by detailed history taking prior to surgery. A review of medications is essential. One must not only inquire about medications like aspirin and ibuprofen, but also herbal medications that may increase the risk of postoperative hemorrhage. Meticulous intraoperative hemostasis also greatly minimizes the risk of hematoma. Additional interventions include control of the blood pressure both intraoperatively and perioperatively, elevation of the head of the bed, application of cold compresses, and aggressive treatment of postoperative nausea with antiemetic medication.

While most small hematomas are benign and rare, their organization beneath the skin may result in an indurated mass which subsequently may lead to a thickened scar. Therefore, early treatment with steroid injection may be indicated.

Although extremely unlikely, a retrobulbar hemorrhage is a surgical emergency. There is a risk of blindness associated with increased orbital pressure which may result in either central retinal artery occlusion or ischemic optic neuropathy. A lateral canthotomy with inferior cantholysis performed immediately will alleviate the pressure. On rare occasions, an orbitotomy is needed. An ophthalmologic consultation should be urgently requested and the patient managed in an inpatient setting. In the senior author's experience of over 3,500 lower lid blepharoplasties, the incidence of acute retrobulbar hematoma is zero, in part due to meticulous bipolar cauterization of every fat stalk prior to excision.

15.14.4 Eyelid Malposition/Ectropion

Frequent patient follow-up in the initial 2–3 months after lower eyelid surgery can offer opportunities for intervention, which can prevent the need for further surgery. An important part of each examination is to look for and recognize early signs of lower eyelid malposition, such as increased scleral show, asymmetric positioning, decreased mobility, or early ectropion.

In most cases, gentle upward massage to release early scar formation and occasional corticosteroid injections will enable release of cicatrix and prevent the need for further intervention. In advanced cases, external superior traction with tape or placement of a Frost suture may be necessary. This is especially important when corneal protection is desired.

Revision surgery may be necessary after 6–8 weeks of conservative management if there is no improvement or the condition deteriorates. Earlier intervention is required when there is corneal exposure from rounding, scleral show, retraction, or ectropion. The cause of lid malposition should be determined. In cases of middle lamellar scarring, release of the middle lamella and resuspension of the skin–muscle flap may be all that is needed. Most often correction requires the performance of a lateral canthoplasty.

15.15 Conclusion

Transcutaneous lower eyelid blepharoplasty is an excellent and safe technique for lower lid rejuvenation. Figures 15.19–15.23 demonstrate preoperative and postoperative results of various patients who have undergone the surgery with and without the addition of adjunctive procedures. The skin–muscle flap method, when performed properly, carries minimal risk and yields natural and predictable results. Important considerations for surgery include proper patient selection,

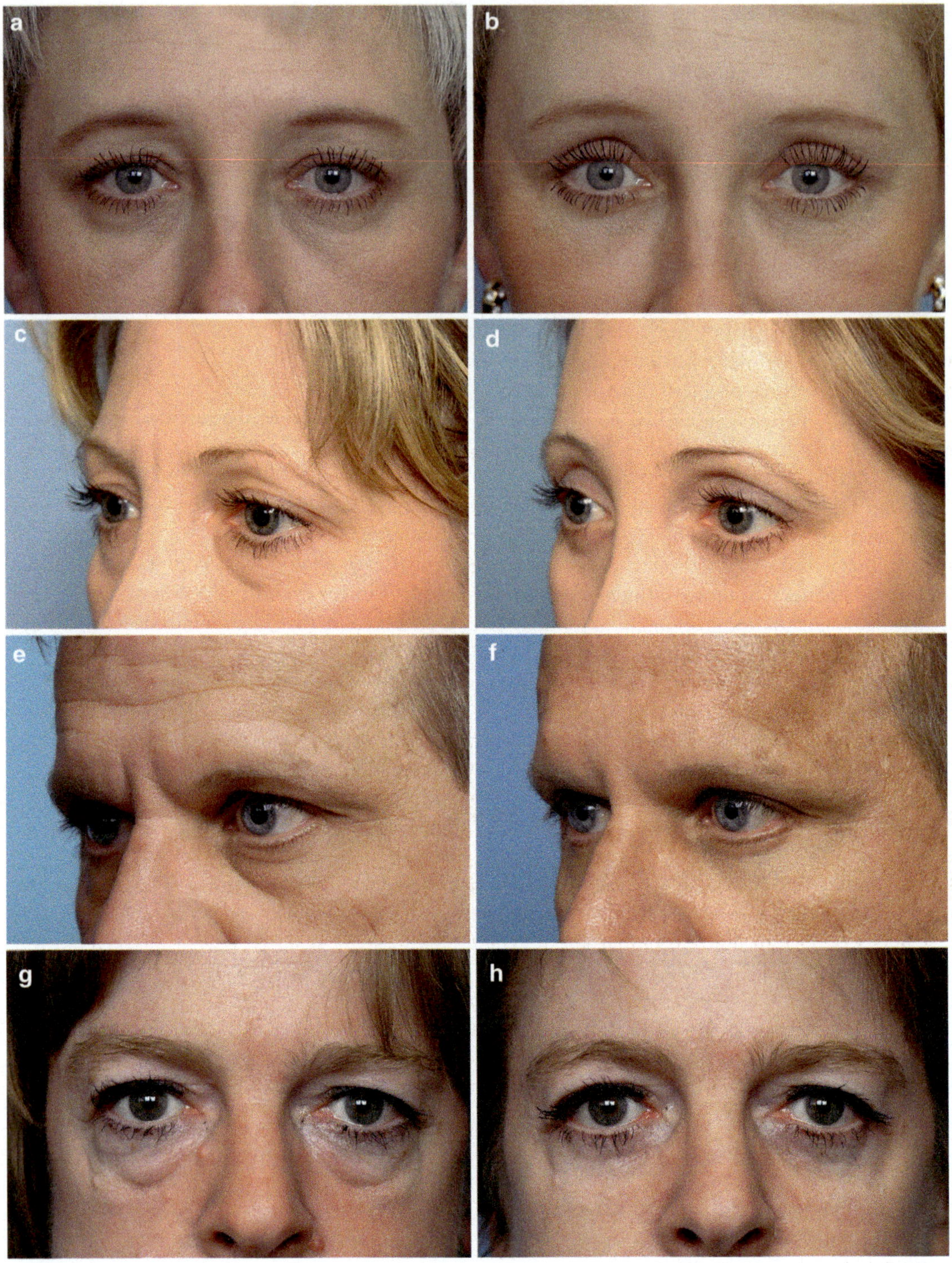

Fig. 15.20 Examples of preoperative and postoperative results in prototypical patients. Improvement is demonstrated in the (**a**, **b**) mild and (**c**, **d**) moderate cases of dermatochalasis with pseudoherniation of fat (**e**, **f**) Male patients and (**g**, **h**) cases of severe dermatochalasis can also achieve excellent results with proper technique

careful health history screening, and a thorough examination. This technique may be combined with lower eyelid resurfacing procedures, such as chemical peels or laser resurfacing, to improve skin texture and reduce wrinkling. Other adjunctive procedures such as malar extension, lower eyelid tightening, and fat transposition offer further refinement and versatility to the operation. Early and proper intervention of complications can greatly diminish the need for revision surgery.

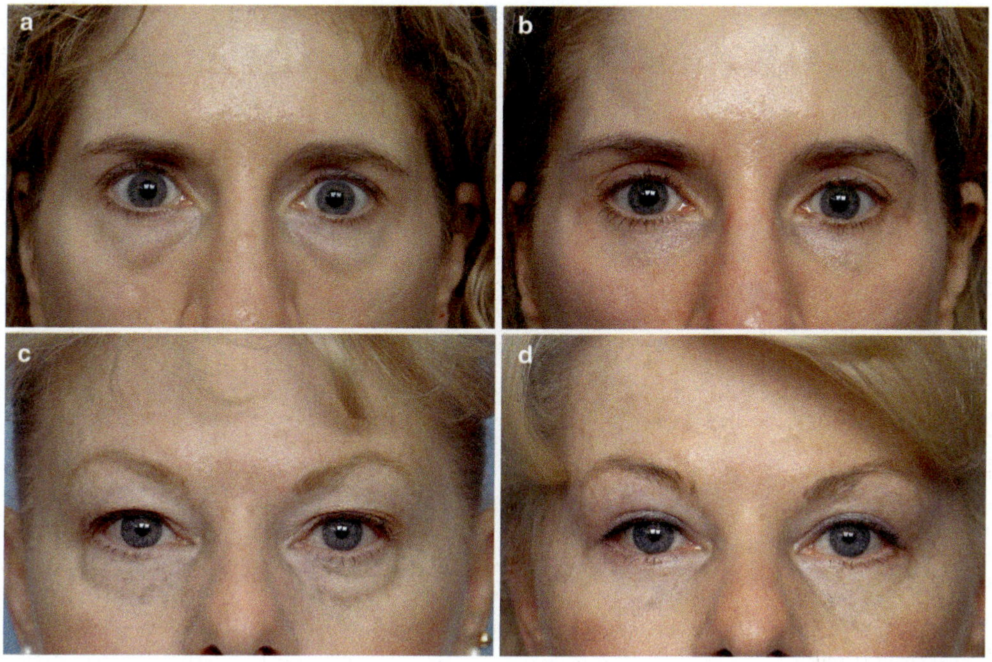

Fig. 15.21 Deep nasojugal grooves ("tear trough" deformity) are best addressed with fat transposition at the time of lower eyelid blepharoplasty. This can be addressed using the (**a**, **b**) medial (nasal) fat compartment but may also include the (**c**, **d**) central and lateral compartments depending on the patient's anatomy

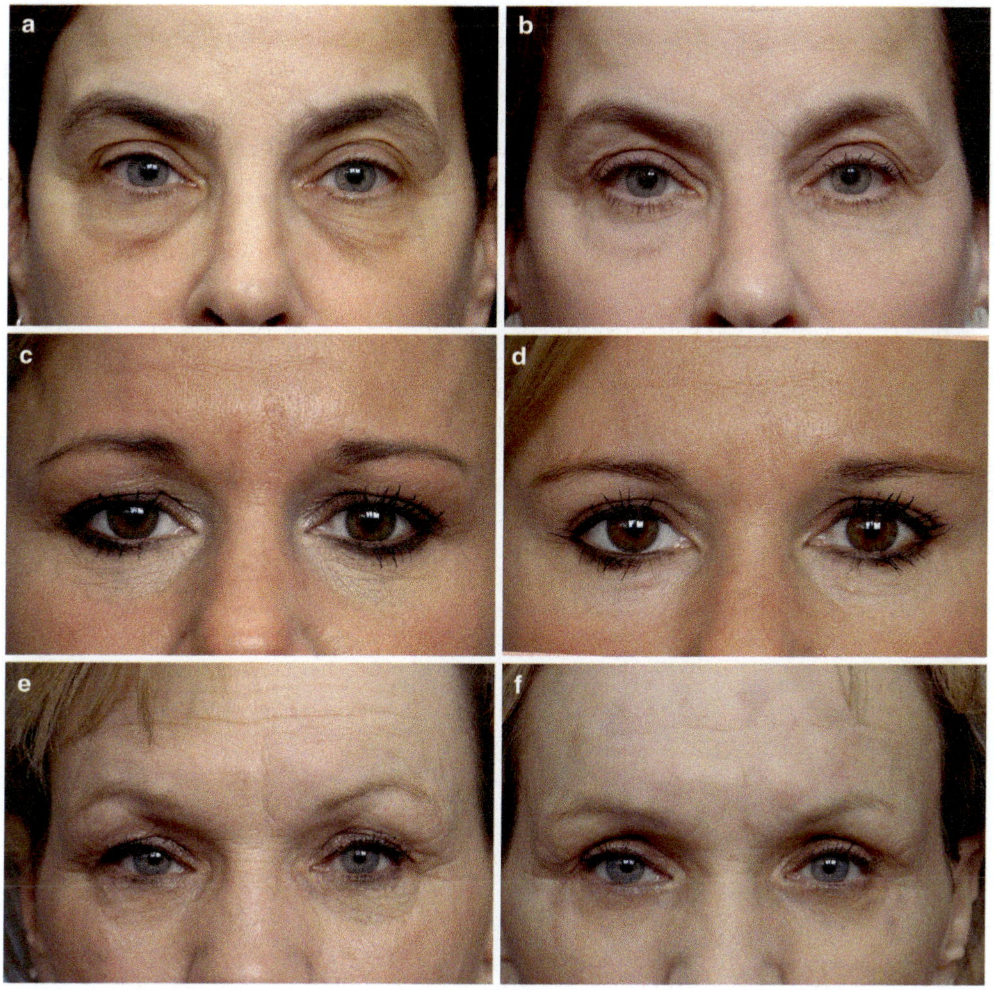

Fig. 15.22 Hyperpigmentation and persistent rhytids of the lower eyelid skin can be addressed at the time of lower eyelid blepharoplasty. In most cases, a chemical peel such as a (**a**, **b**) Baker's solution phenol chemical peel or even a (**c**, **d**) phenol 88% chemical peel can be employed. Alternately, (**e**, **f**) CO_2 laser resurfacing can also be employed

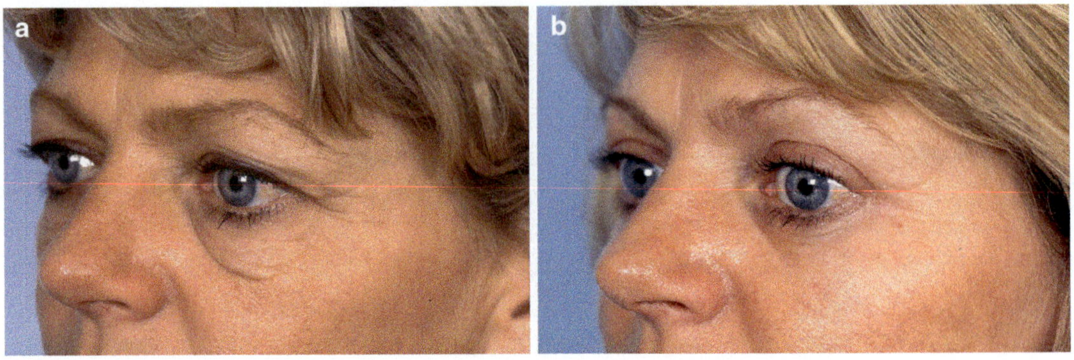

Fig. 15.23 (**a**, **b**) Malar extension with advancement and suspension of the SOOF and skin–muscle flap can give excellent improvement in festoons and orbicularis oculi redundancy

References

1. Honrado CP, Pastorek NJ. Long-term results of lower-lid suspension blepharoplasty: a 30-year experience. Arch Facial Plast Surg. 2004;6(3):150–4.
2. Rees TD. Prevention of ectropion by horizontal shortening of the lower lid during blepharoplasty. Ann Plast Surg. 1983;11(1):17–23.
3. Flowers RS. Canthopexy as a routine blepharoplasty component. Clin Plast Surg. 1993;20(2):351–65.
4. Hirmand H et al. Prominent eye: operative management in lower lid and midfacial rejuvenation and the morphologic classification system. Plast Reconstr Surg. 2002;110(2):620–8; discussion 629–34.
5. Patipa M. The evaluation and management of lower eyelid retraction following cosmetic surgery. Plast Reconstr Surg. 2000;106(2):438–53; discussion 454–9.
6. Furnas DW. Festoons of orbicularis muscle as a cause of baggy eyelids. Plast Reconstr Surg. 1978;61(4):540–6.
7. Furnas DW. Festoons, mounds, and bags of the eyelids and cheek. Clin Plast Surg. 1993;20(2):367–85.
8. Becker FF, Deutsch DB. Extended lower lid blepharoplasty. Facial Plast Surg Clin North Am. 1995;3:189–94.
9. Kikkawa DO, Lemke BN, Dortzbach RK. Relations of the superficial musculoaponeurotic system to the orbit and characterization of the orbitomalar ligament. Ophthal Plast Reconstr Surg. 1996;12(2):77–88.
10. Garcia RE, McCollough EG. Transcutaneous lower eyelid blepharoplasty with fat excision: a shift-resisting paradigm. Arch Facial Plast Surg. 2006;8(6):374–80.
11. Baker SR. Orbital fat preservation in lower-lid blepharoplasty. Arch Facial Plast Surg. 1999;1(1):33–7.
12. Papel ID. Muscle suspension blepharoplasty. Facial Plast Surg. 1994;10(2):147–9.
13. Bernardi C, Dura S, Amata PL. Treatment of orbicularis oculi muscle hypertrophy in lower lid blepharoplasty. Aesthetic Plast Surg. 1998;22(5):349–51.
14. Loeb R. Naso-jugal groove leveling with fat tissue. Clin Plast Surg. 1993;20(2):393–400; discussion 401.
15. Kane MA. Treatment of tear trough deformity and lower lid bowing with injectable hyaluronic acid. Aesthet Plast Surg. 2005;29(5):363–7.
16. Flowers RS. Tear trough implants for correction of tear trough deformity. Clin Plast Surg. 1993;20(2):403–15.
17. Kawamoto HK, Bradley JP. The tear "TROUF" procedure: transconjunctival repositioning of orbital unipedicled fat. Plast Reconstr Surg. 2003;112(7):1903–7; discussion 1908–9.
18. Enzer YR, Shorr N. Medical and surgical management of chemosis after blepharoplasty. Ophthal Plast Reconstr Surg. 1994;10(1):57–63.

16 Transconjunctival Lower Blepharoplasty: Fat Excision or Repositioning

Guy G. Massry and Paul S. Nassif

Key Points

- Transconjunctival lower blepharoplasty does not violate normal anatomic tissue planes (orbital septum and orbicualris muscle) as does its transcutaneous counterpart.
- The incidence of lower lid malposition and lateral canthal rounding is significantly less in transconjuncival vs transcutaneous surgery.
- Understanding lower lid anatomy and appropriate incision placement (4–5 mm below tarsus) is critical to attaining successful results.
- Fat can be excised or preserved (repositioned) depending on patient needs.
- Fat repositioning is an advanced technique, performed in a small surgical space.
- A variety of surgical nuances (traction suture, retracting the lower lid, retro-placing the globe) are used to improve exposure during surgery.
- The addition of various adjunctive procedures (canthoplasty, canthopexy, fat grafting, skin excision, etc.), when necessary, may enhance final results.
- An external skin excision or pinch allows fat and skin to be addressed simultaneously.
- When the surgical technique is mastered, patient satisfaction is high, and postoperative complications are infrequent and mostly self-limiting.

16.1 Introduction

Lower eyelid rejuvenation is a challenging aesthetic procedure. One of the key elements in lower blepharoplasty is the approach by which the orbital fat pads are identified. There are two standard ways to access the lower eyelid fat: transcutaneously (through the skin and muscle – see Chap. 15) and transconjunctivally (through the internal portion of the eyelid). Transcutaneous lower blepharoplasty is the more traditional approach to surgery [1, 2]. The skin, muscle, and fat are addressed through a single incision, thereby providing excellent anatomic exposure. However, the transcutaneous approach is fraught with a higher incidence of complications including lower eyelid retraction, ectropion and a rounded canthal angle [3–5]. This is primarily related to lack of eyelid support, overexcision of skin, and violation of the orbital septum (with subsequent scarring) and orbicularis muscle (with subsequent weakness) in accessing the fat pads.

Transconjunctival lower blephroplasty was first described by Bourguet in 1924 [6], but was not brought into mainstream modern cosmetic surgery until Baylis et al. re-introduced the technique in 1989 [7]. With this approach, orbital fat is addressed through an incision on the internal (conjunctival) surface of the eyelid, thereby preserving the integrity of the orbital septum and orbicularis muscle. These are essential steps in preventing lower eyelid malposition [8, 9] as there is less distortion of anatomy and postoperative cicatrization. For this reason, transconjunctival lower blepharoplasty has gained wide acceptance in cosmetic surgery across all subspecialties.

The transconjunctival procedure does not directly address excess skin or muscle or lid laxity when present. It requires additional procedures to do so. However, a simple skin excision, muscle placation, and lid tightening (see Chap. 17) can be added when necessary. We have found that the addition of these adjunctive procedures to transconjunctival surgery does not lead to the same incidence of the lid malposition complications seen with transcutaneous surgery. In the last decade, the advent of volume preservation/augmentation via fat redistribution or grafting has been an important addition to lower lid blepharoplasty and can be added to the surgery to enhance cosmetic results (see Chap. 22 for periorbital fat grafting technique).

In this chapter, transconjunctival lower blepharoplasty will be described in detail. Special attention will be given to the added technique of volume preservation via fat

G.G. Massry (✉)
Director, Ophthalmic Plastic Surgery, Spaulding Drive Cosmetic Surgery and Dermatology, Beverly Hills, CA, USA
e-mail: gmassry@aol.com

G.G. Massry et al. (eds.), *Master Techniques in Blepharoplasty and Periorbital Rejuvenation*,
DOI 10.1007/978-1-4614-0067-7_16, © Springer Science+Business Media, LLC 2011

repositioning. This is our preferred approach to lower lid surgery. An external skin excision and lid/muscle tightening is added when necessary. We have termed this sequence of fat reduction/preservation through a conjunctival incision, and an external skin-only excision the "bilamellar blepharoplasty." With this technique skin and fat are addressed, while the orbital septum and orbicularis muscle are left undisturbed. We feel this is a safer alternative to transcutaneous surgery when addressing skin and fat in the lower lid.

16.2 Lower Eyelid Anatomy

Transconjunctival lower blepharoplasty is performed from the inside of the eyelid. This can make anatomic orientation and surgical maneuvering difficult, as the surgical field is small and tight when compared to the open transcutaneous approach. For this reason, familiarization with lower lid anatomy (Chap. 2) is essential when performing this surgery.

The lower eyelid is divided into three layers or lamellae (Fig. 16.1). The outer or anterior lamella is comprised of the skin and orbicularis muscle. The middle lamella consists of the orbital septum. The posterior, or inner, lamella includes the tarsus and conjunctiva for the first 5 mm of the lid. Below the level of the tarsus, the posterior lamella continues as the lower eyelid retractors and conjunctiva. The tarsus forms the skeleton of the eyelid, giving it both support and flexibility. It is 4–5 mm in height, 30 mm in length, and 1 mm in thickness. It is bound by conjunctiva on its inner surface which abuts the globe, and by orbicularis muscle and skin on its outer surface.

Below the tarsus, the conjunctiva continues as the posterior extent of the lower eyelid to the inferior fornix. The lower eyelid retractors, also called the capsulopalpebral fascia, are just anterior to the conjunctiva and intimately associated with it. This sympathetically driven muscle (similar to Muller's muscle of the upper lid) originates from the tendon of the inferior rectus muscle and continues to fuse with the inferior border of the tarsus. Just anterior to the retractors are the fat pads. Anterior to the fat pads and limiting their forward extent is the orbital septum. This is a connective tissue layer originating from the periosteum at the orbital rim (arcus marginalis) and inserting on or fusing with the capsulopalpebral fascia 2–3 mm below the inferior tarsal boarder. A conjunctival incision just below the tarsus will divide the fused conjunctiva and lower lid retractors from the tarsus (Fig. 16.2). This plane is best suited for surgery desired in the postorbicularis fascial plane (avascular plane between the orbicularis muscle and orbital septum) such as addressing the orbital floor in fracture repair or for orbital volume augmentation. As dissection in this plane proceeds anterior to the septum, fat does not prolapse into the field. A transconjunctival incision below the fusion point of the orbital septum and lower eyelid retractors (4–5 mm below tarsus) is the entry point of choice for transconjunctival blepharoplasty as this is a direct route to the fat pads (Fig. 16.3).

There are three fat pads in the lower lid: nasal, central, and lateral. The nasal and central fat pads are divided by the inferior oblique muscle (Fig. 16.4). This muscle originates from the medial orbital floor and courses superolaterally to insert on the posterior globe. Careful attention must be given to avoid injury to this muscle. The central fat pad is separated from the lateral fat pad by the inferior arcuate ligament (Fig. 16.5).

The separation of the central and temporal fat pads by the arcuate ligament can often be seen clinically by asking a patient to look up. The same is typically not true of the nasal and central fat pads as they tend to override the inferior oblique muscle and blunt this separation (seen when performing surgery) (Fig. 16.6).

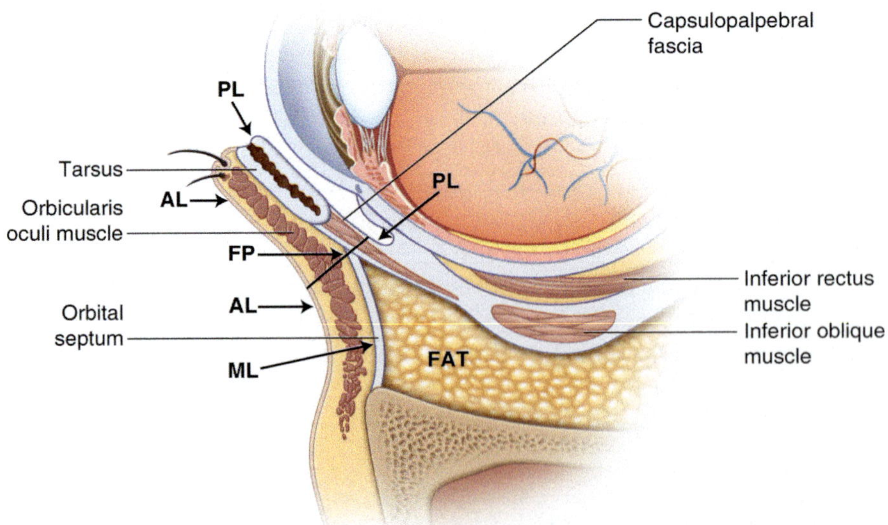

Fig. 16.1 Sagittal section of the lower eyelid demonstrating – (AL) the anterior lamella (skin/muscle), and (PL) posterior lamella above (tarsus/conjunctiva) and below (lower lid retractors/conjunctiva) the tarsus. The (FP) fusion point of the lower lid retractors and orbital septum, the (ML) middle lamella (orbital septum) and fat pads are also shown. The FP is critical for incision placement during surgery

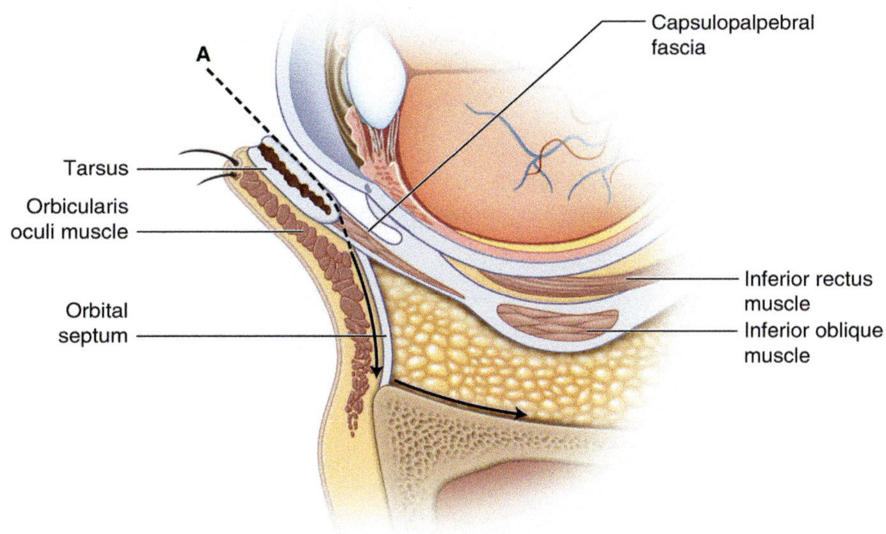

Fig. 16.2 Transconjunctival incision just below tarsus (dotted line) will lead to a preseptal dissection (between orbicularis muscle and orbital septum). This is the plane of dissection for accessing the orbital floor. To enter fat pads, the septum would be violated. This should be avoided in TCB

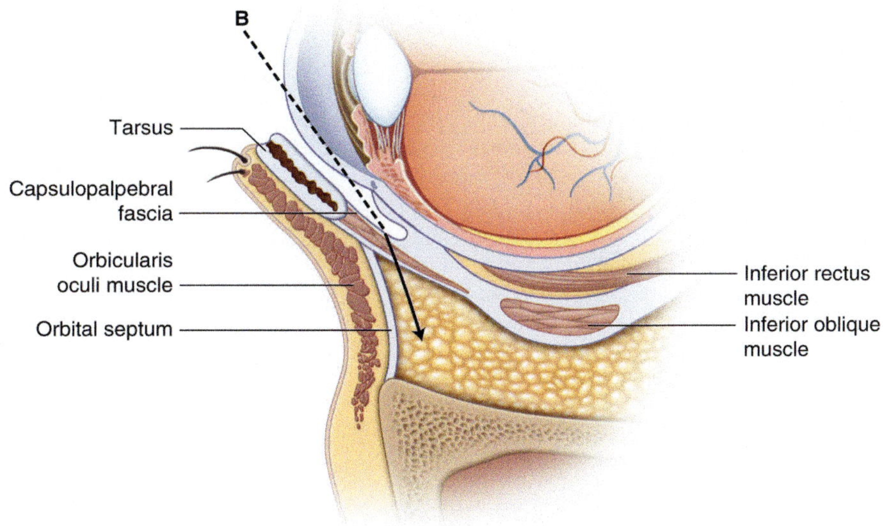

Fig. 16.3 Transconjunctival incision 4–5 mm below tarsus will lead to a postseptal or retroseptal dissection and direct entry into fat pads. This is the correct incision in TCB as it leaves the orbital septum intact

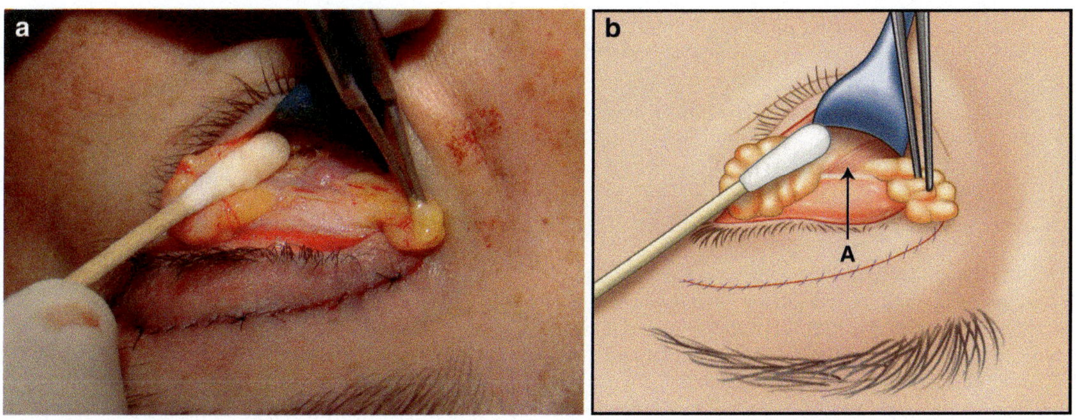

Fig. 16.4 (**a**) Surgical photograph with (**b**) accompanying illustration demonstrating the nasal and central fat pads divided by the inferior oblique muscle (**A**). This is an important surgical/anatomical landmark

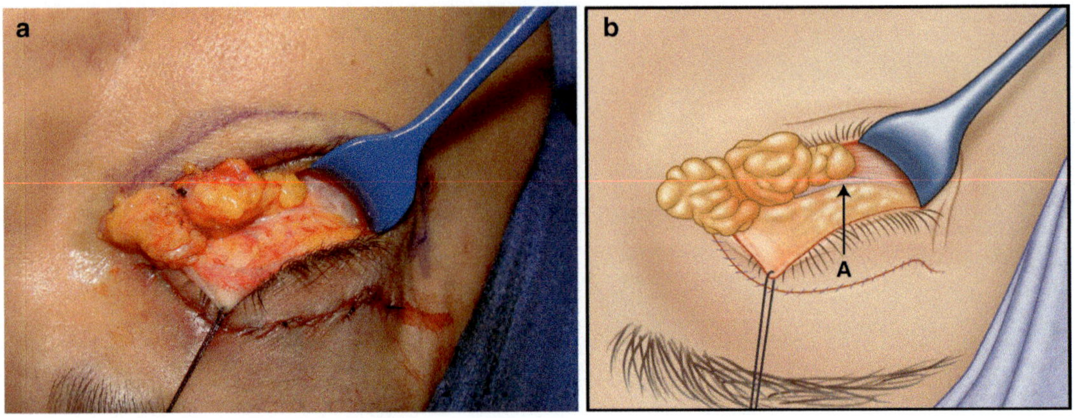

Fig. 16.5 (**a**) Surgical photograph with (**b**) accompanying illustration demonstrating the division of the central and temporal fat pads by the arcuate ligament (**A**)

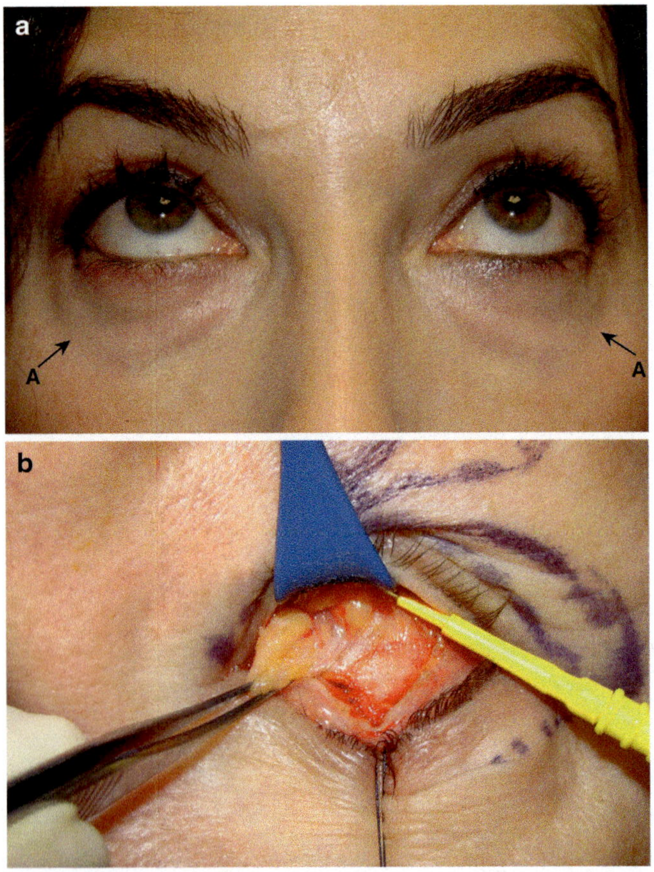

Fig. 16.6 (**a**) Patient photograph in upgaze demonstrating continuous nasal/central fat prominence, with an indentation (*arrows*) where the arcuate ligemant can be seen clinically to divide the central and temporal fat pad. (**b**) Surgical photograph demonstrating central fat pad overriding oblique muscle. This is why a clinical demarcation between the nasal and central fat pads (as opposed to the central and temporal fat pads) is typically not apparent

16.3 Eyelid Analysis/Preoperative Evaluation

As mentioned previously, to appropriately perform lower blepharoplasty, the surgeon may need to address excess or damaged skin, redundant and/or lax muscle, eyelid laxity, and displaced fat. In addition, volume deficits, involutional changes, and anatomic variations may also be present. The difficulty with surgery lies in correcting these deficiencies when support of the eyelid (including the effect of gravity) is typically against the surgeon. This is clearly not an easy task, and is the reason that surgeons have found lower blepharoplasty to be so challenging. As a result, it is important to understand the various factors which support and act against maintaining eyelid position (see below) [9]. This will provide a framework for planning appropriate surgery including the addition of adjunctive procedures necessary to attain the best possible outcomes.

The factors which support the lower lid (maintain height and position) include the following:

- Tendons: The medial and lateral canthal tendons act as a sling, maintaining lower lid height and keeping the lower lid abutted against the undersurface of the globe.
- Ligaments: There are retaining ligaments which fixate the eyelid and cheek soft tissue to the boney facial skeleton.
- Muscle: The orbicularis muscle which tonically elevates the lid with its sphincter action.
- Volume: Both soft tissue (fat) and hard tissue (bone) promote stabilization of facial structures including the lower eyelid.

The factors which reduce lower lid support (allow the lid to fall) include the following:

- The lower lid retractors, which like the orbicularis muscle, are in a tonic state of activity.

- Normal involutional changes. With age, canthal tendon and ligamentous laxity, loss of soft tissue and boney volume, and reduced muscular support all promote eyelid laxity and retraction
- Gravity: As lid support decreases with age, and gravity is constant, the equilibrium shifts to retraction.

The preoperative assessment should focus on the factors above. If only slight fat prominence is present (as with younger patients) a stand-alone transconjunctival blepharoplasty is appropriate. If, in addition, there is excess skin with good lid tone, a skin-only excision (or pinch) is added (bilamellar approach). If eyelid tendon laxity is present or muscle tone is reduced, a lid tightening procedure and/or muscle plication should be performed (Chap. 17). If significant volume deficit exists, fat preservation (see surgical section below), fat grafting (Chap. 22), or synthetic filler (Chap. 25) may be considered. If the midface retaining ligaments are deficient, re-suspension via midface lifting is added (Chap. 20).

16.4 Surgical Technique (With or Without Fat Preservation in the Subperiosteal Plane)

The eyelid is infiltrated transconjunctivally with 2 mL of 1% xylocaine with 1:100:000 epinephrine. If fat repositioning is planned, the tear trough (area to which fat will be repositioned) is marked preoperatively (Fig. 16.7). The tear trough is infiltrated with 1–2 mL of the same local anesthetic. We typically only reposition nasal and central fat. If there is a prominent lid/cheek junction depression lateral to this (orbitomalar groove), we prefer fat grafting (see Chap. 22) to this area. If the surgery is to be performed under local anesthesia only (no sedation), a cotton pledget (from cotton-tip applicator) soaked in Tetracaine is placed in the inferior fornix for 10 min prior to anesthetic injection. This maneuver usually renders the conjunctival injection of anesthetic solution painless.

After giving time for hemostasis and anesthesia to take place, the lower lid is displaced inferiorly with the index finger of your nondominant hand while the second finger of the same hand lightly retroplaces the globe. This maneuver elevates and exposes (balloons forward) the incisional site on the transconjunctival surface of the lid (Fig. 16.8). The free dominant hand is utilized to make an incision 5 mm below the tarsus to directly enter the fat compartment of the lower lid (Fig. 16.9). An electrocautery unit (Valleylab, Boulder, CO) with the Colorado tip microdissector (Kalamazoo, MI) or surgical scissors can be used to make this incision. As described in the section on eyelid anatomy, the orbital septum attaches to the capsulopalpebral fascia 2–3 mm below the tarsus. An incision above this area should be avoided as it enters the preseptal space. A dissection in this plane would require violating the orbital septum to identify

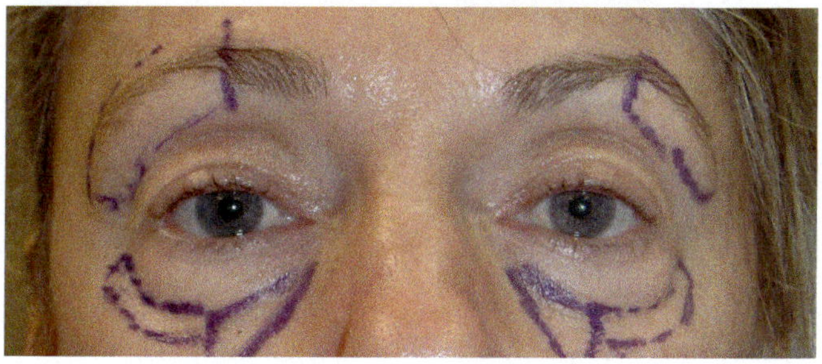

Fig. 16.7 The tear trough (nasojugal groove) is demarcated with a *solid line*. This area will undergo fat repositioning. The orbitomalar groove and lateral brows (demarcated with *dotted lines*) will undergo fat grafting

a

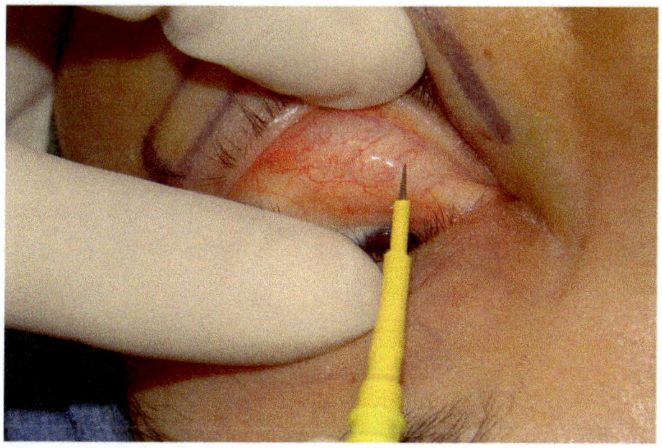

b

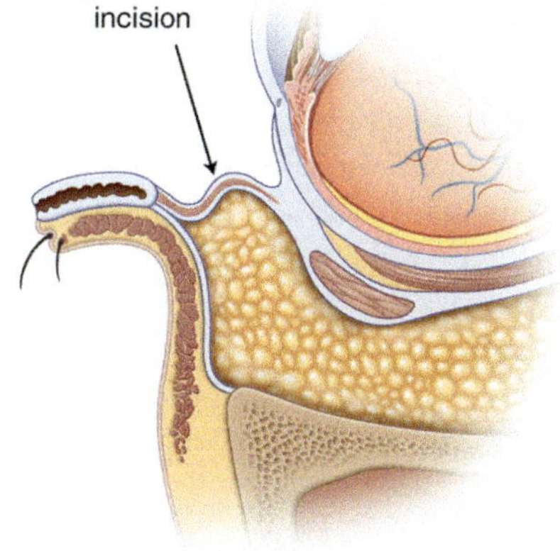

Fig. 16.8 (**a**) Retracting the lower eyelid while simultaneously depressing the globe increases the visible surface area of the conjunctiva, brings the fat forward and increases exposure of the surgical field. (**b**) The illustration demonstrates these changes and the location of the transconjunctival incision

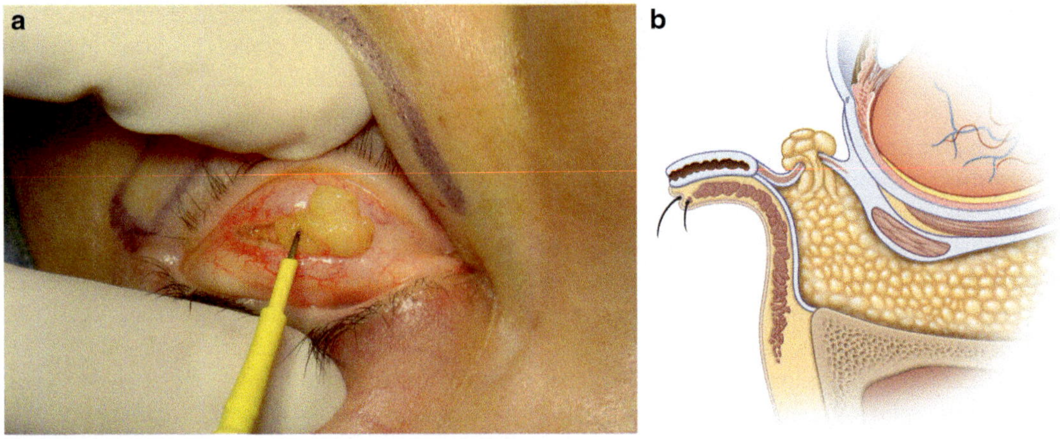

Fig. 16.9 (**a**) An incision 5 mm below the tarsus with the above maneuver provides direct entry into the fat pad. (**b**) This is seen clearly on the accompanying illustration

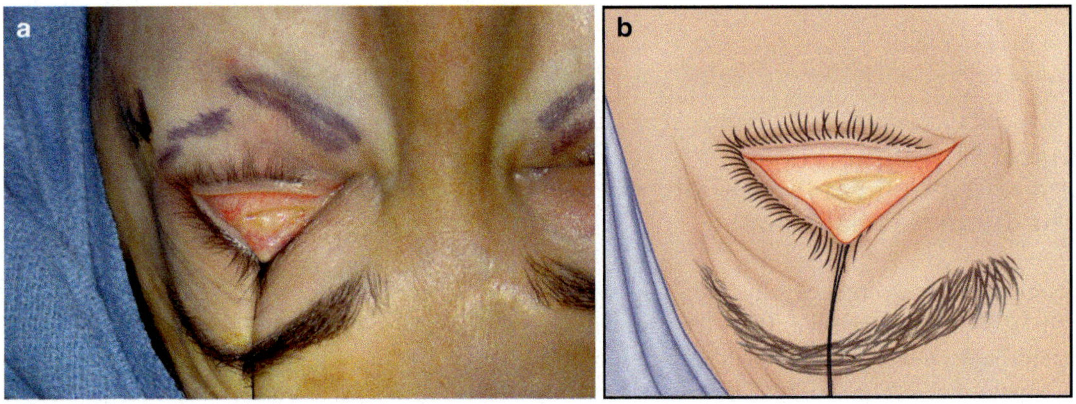

Fig. 16.10 (**a**) Surgical photo and (**b**) illustration of conjunctiva and retractors engaged with a 4–0 Silk traction suture which is secured to the head drape

and manipulate the fat pads. An incision below this attachment point will enter the postseptal or retroseptal space, provide direct access to the fat pads, and maintain the integrity of the orbital septum. This is a critical point as all attempts should be made to leave the orbital septum intact and avoid middle lamellar cicatrix.

The conjunctiva and retractors are then engaged with a 4–0 Silk suture which is secured to the head drape under tension (Fig. 16.10). This traction suture protects the globe, exposes the surgical field, and brings the fat pads forward (again via retroplacement of the globe). An insulated Desmarres retractor is used to retract the remainder of the lower eyelid (tarsus/orbicularis muscle and skin) inferiorly, further exposing the surgical field. It is important that the lip of the Desmarres retractor hits bone (orbital rim). If soft tissue (skin/muscle) gets trapped between the lip of the retractor and bone, it is possible to inadvertently lacerate this tissue and violate the skin.

By depressing the undersurface of the retractors, the fat pads balloon forward. In cases of fat excision only, all three fat pads are excised in a piecemeal fashion until they are flush with or just above the orbital rim (Fig. 16.11). In cases of fat preservation, the nasal fat pad is elevated with a small toothed forceps (0.5 mm Castroviejo). On occasion, it is necessary to amputate the tip of the fat pad to free it from overlying connective tissue elements Once the fat pad is identified, it is bluntly dissected free of surrounding attachments to the inferior oblique muscle, orbital rim, and the caruncle, to expose it in its entirety (Fig. 16.12). This may require some sharp dissection. We prefer the Colorado tip microdissection needle (Kalamazoo, MI) for dissection as it results in minimal bleeding, and obviates the need for clamping fat before cutting it which can be cumbersome and time consuming. Once the nasal fat pad is free, the Desmarres retractor is moved centrally to identify the central fat pad. Again blunt and sharp dissection is used to free the fat pad from the

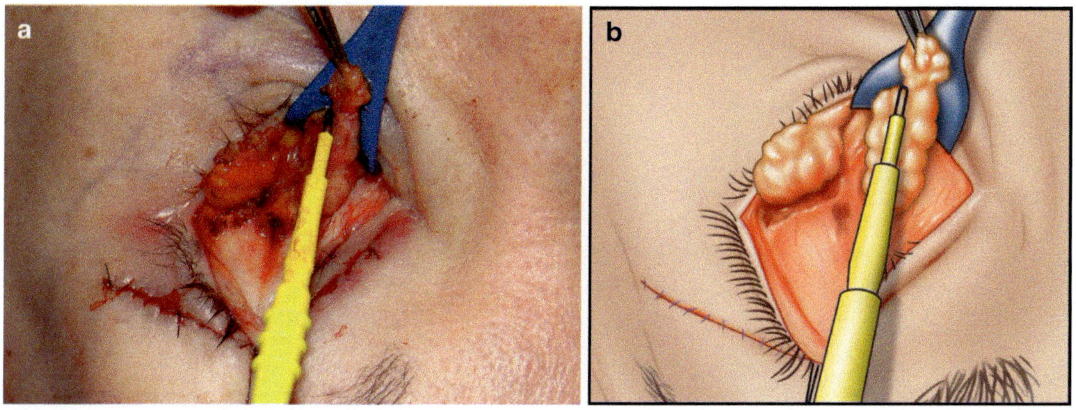

Fig. 16.11 (**a**) Surgical photo and (**b**) illustration of excision of fat pads

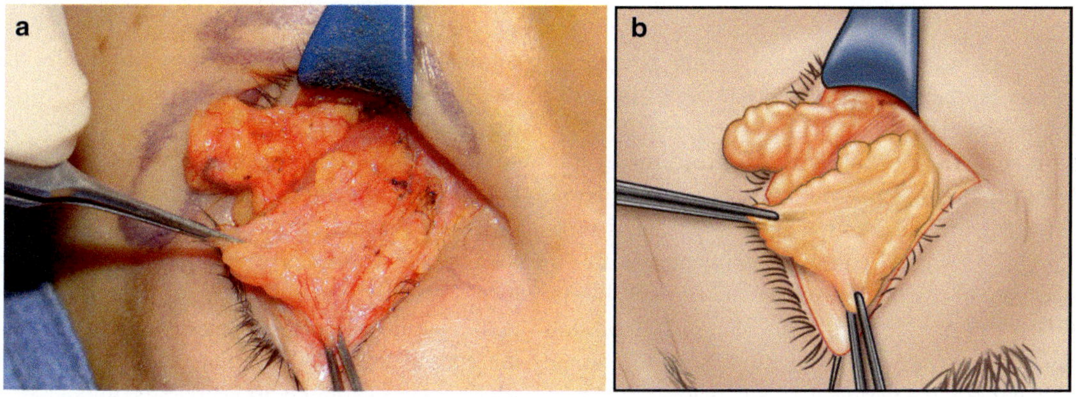

Fig. 16.12 (**a**) Surgical photo and (**b**) illustration of the creation of nasal fat pad pedicle

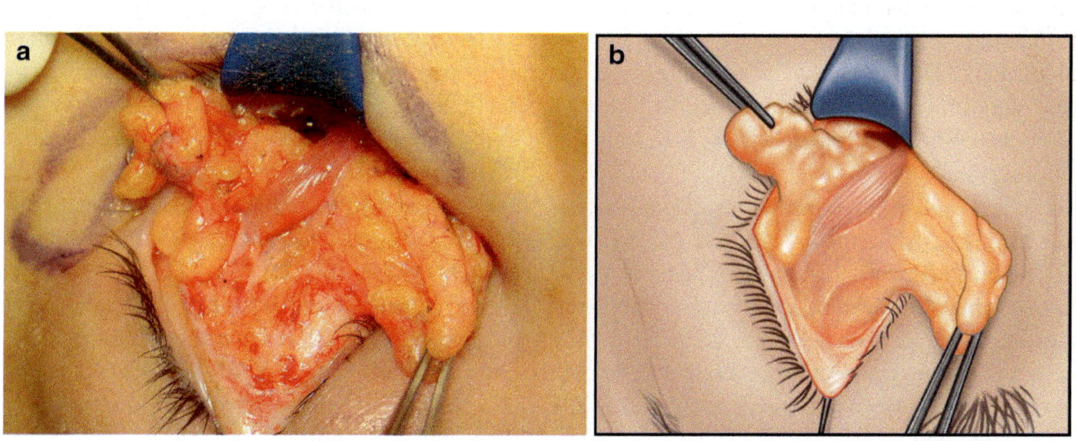

Fig. 16.13 (**a**) Surgical photo and (**b**) illustration of the free movement of nasal and central fat pad under inferior oblique muscle – "inverse shoe shine sign"

oblique muscle and orbital rim. When this is accomplished, it is critical to assure that there are no further attachments of fat to the muscle so that restriction of muscle movement is averted after the fat is repositioned. The nasal and central fat pad should be engaged with forceps and pulled in successive fashion to slide the fat freely under the muscle (Fig. 16.13). I call this the "inverse shoe shine sign" as it resembles shining a shoe in an inverted fashion. The lateral fat pad is conservatively excised or cauterized flush with the orbital rim as with standard fat excision blepharoplasty.

When the fat pedicles are free of all connective tissue attachments, they will move freely in all directions and are ready to be repositioned. The purpose of repositioning the fat is to fill (implant effect) the depression at the suborbital rim space (tear trough). If there is a long and thick pedicle, a portion may need to be trimmed and debulked to prevent overfilling

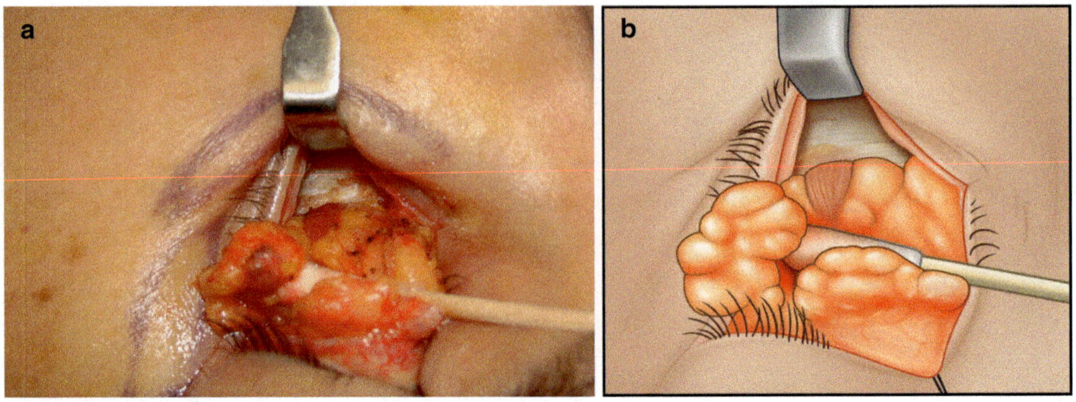

Fig. 16.14 (**a**) Surgical photo and (**b**) illustration of the subperiosteal dissection. Note the nasal and central fat pads separated by the inferior oblique muscle

and postoperative prominence. Conversely, if the pedicle is long and thin, the fat pad may be folded onto itself in order to increase the volume effect.

A Ragnell rake is used to inferiorly displace the eyelid from the orbital rim. This step is difficult with a Desmarres retractor as it is too wide and does not allow adequate visibility of the orbital rim. A blunt cotton-tip applicator and/or a Freer Elevator can be used to displace all suborbicularis oculi fat (SOOF) and muscle tissue elements off the orbital rim periosteum for approximately 3 mm below the arcus marginalis. I then incise the periosteum, just below the arcus, to bone (Fig. 16.14). The extent of the periosteal incision should match the area of the tear trough to be filled. It is imperative to maintain a blood-free field when creating the subperiosteal pockets. During this step, the edges of the attached periosteum limit elevation of tissue and visibility of the dissected pocket. With this reduced view, bleeding can severely limit progress.

A Freer Elevator is used to create the subperiosteal pockets. The dissection begins with the medial pocket whose lateral extent is the infraorbital neurovascular bundle. The nasal extent of the dissection is limited, as bleeding is typically encountered in this area. A second subperiosteal pocket (central) is then created lateral to the neurovascular bundle. Typically the central dissection dives down corresponding to a depression in the bone in that area. It is important to maintain this inferior plane of dissection, or more bleeding will occur. At this point, epinephrine soaked cotton pledgets (1:10,000 epinephrine) may be placed in the subperiosteal pockets for hemostasis. The traction suture is then released, and the transconjunctival incision on the opposite side is initiated. By the time the opposite side subperiosteal pockets are exposed, excellent hemostasis has been achieved on the initial side.

After the epinephrine-soaked pledgets are removed, the pockets are irrigated and a 4–0 prolene suture on a PS-2 (long) needle is passed through the inferior aspect of the tear trough transcutaneously and retrieved within the internal surgical space. The suture is passed to and fro through the fat pad (Fig. 16.15) and finally passed out from the internal wound to the outer skin. The prolene suture is tied over a cotton bolster. The knot should be taut but not too tight. The tighter it is, the more the fat may strangulate and lead to lymphedema and fat atrophy postoperatively. Also, for the fat to create its fullness over the bone, it should be allowed to recess slightly and fill the space in three dimensions. Too tight a suture will prevent this. The same step is repeated for the central fat pad. With the fat securely repositioned, the surgical view should demonstrate the implant effect of the fat, as it overrides the bone and possibly the inferior oblique muscle (Fig. 16.16).

The traction suture is released and the conjunctiva allowed to reoppose. Forced duction testing is performed. If forced ductions are not free, the wound is re-explored until all restriction is released. We now rarely perform forced ductions as we have found that appropriate lysis of connective tissue elements prevents restriction. At the conclusion of the case, the lid is in the appropriate position with the trough filled and the bolsters evident (Fig. 16.17).

Any adjunctive procedures (canthoplasty, fat grafting, etc. – refer to appropriate chapters) are now added if necessary. If excess skin exists, a pinch or simple excision is performed, and the wound is closed with a running 6–0 plain or fast-absorbing gut suture.

To reduce postoperative bruising and swelling, a pressure tape can be applied for the first week after surgery. I prefer 3M Microfoam tape (St. Paul, MN) applied over Mastisol (Ferndale Laboratories, Ferndale, MI) on the skin. The tape is secured from the lower lid angled towards the temple. When suture bolsters are present, a slit is cut on the tape to allow for the bolsters. This was suggested to me by Jonathan Hoenig, MD, and I have found it to significantly reduce healing time.

Figures 16.18–16.21 demonstrate examples of patient's appearance before and after surgery.

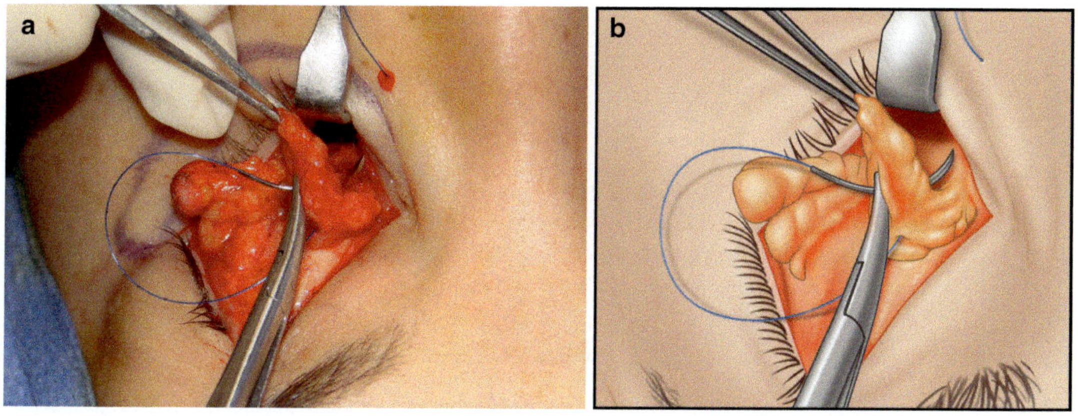

Fig. 16.15 (**a**) Surgical photo and (**b**) illustration of the prolene suture passed through fat pedicle

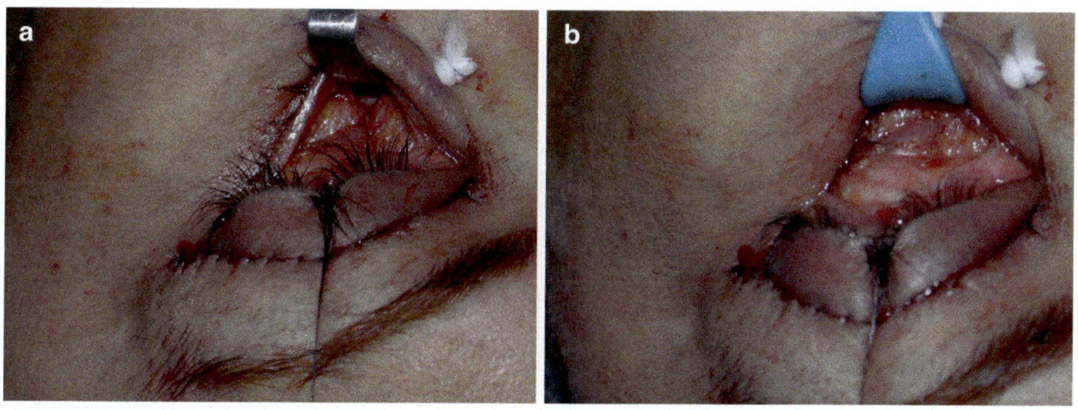

Fig. 16.16 Surgical view demonstrating (**a**) Ragnell retractor dividing repositioned fat pedicles, exposing bone and the inferior oblique muscle; (**b**) Desmarres retractor elevated from bone with fat pedicles filling space over bone and inferior oblique muscle (implant effect)

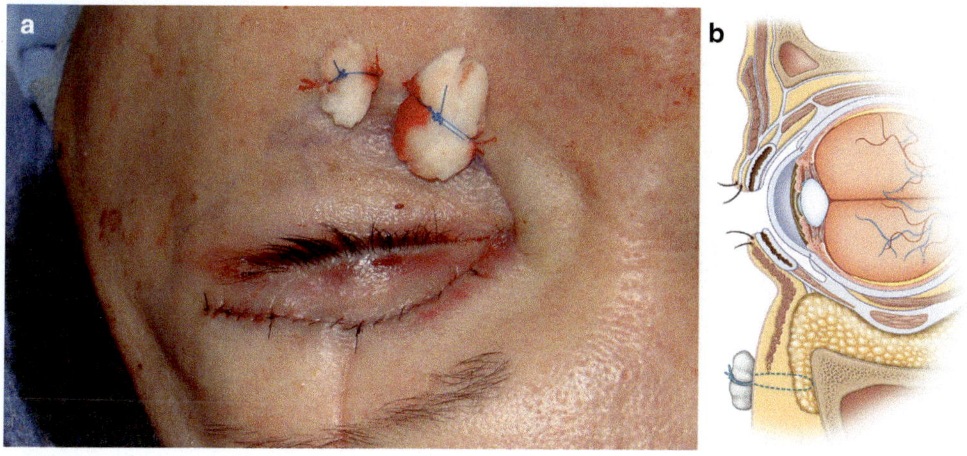

Fig. 16.17 (**a**) Final external appearance with bolster in place. (**b**) The illustration demonstrates repositioned fat pedicle secured in place with suture tied over bolster

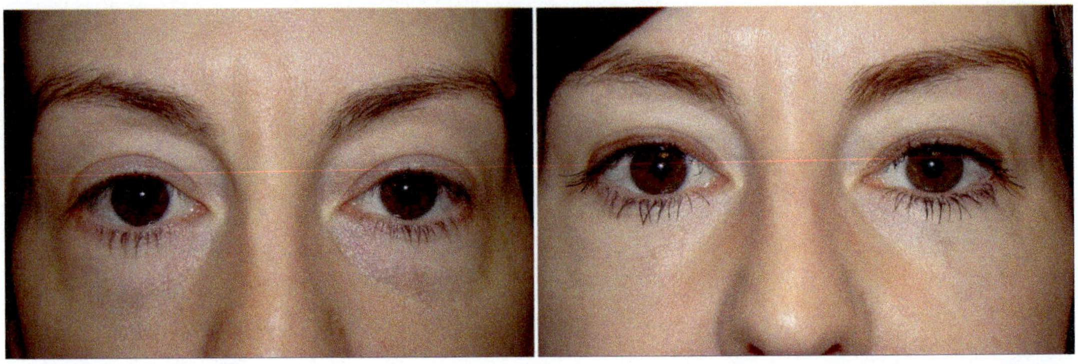

Fig. 16.18 A young woman who underwent transconjunctival lower lid blepharoplasty with fat repositioning only. (*left*) Before and (*right*) after surgery

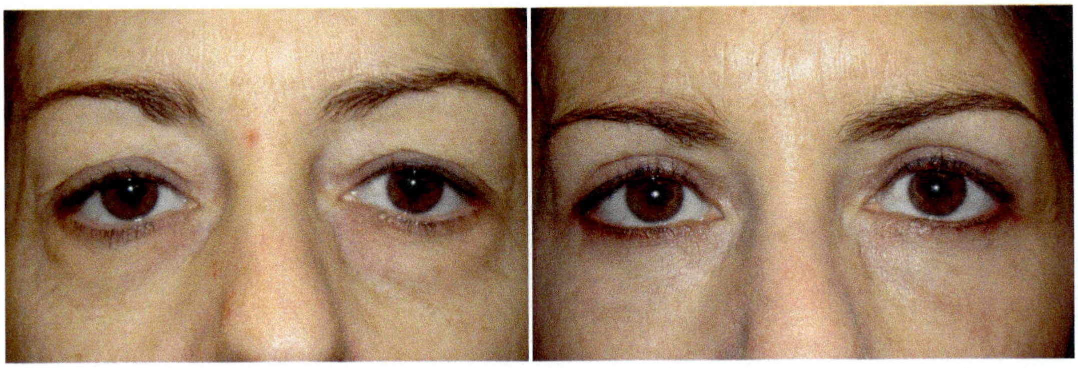

Fig. 16.19 Same procedure as Fig. 16.18 with the addition of fat grafting to the orbitomalar groove (lateral depression at lid/cheek junction). (*left*) Before and (*right*) after surgery

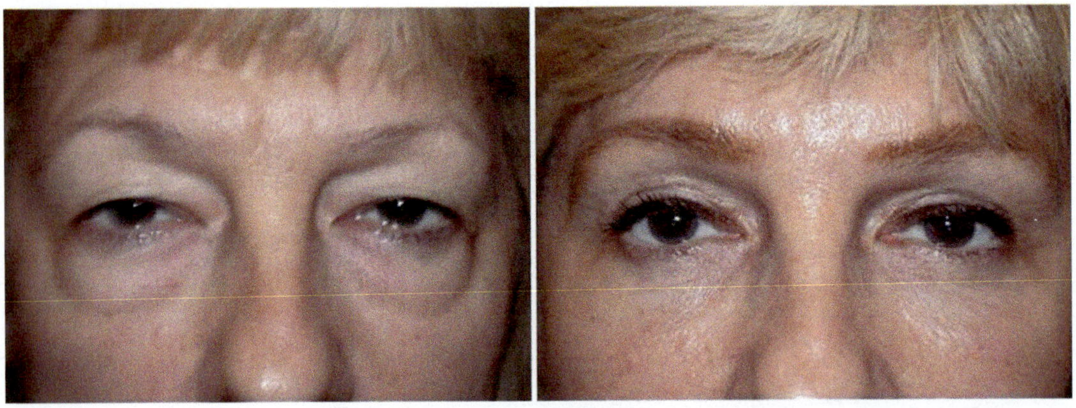

Fig. 16.20 Slightly older woman with same procedure as in Fig. 16.19. (*left*) Before and (*right*) after surgery

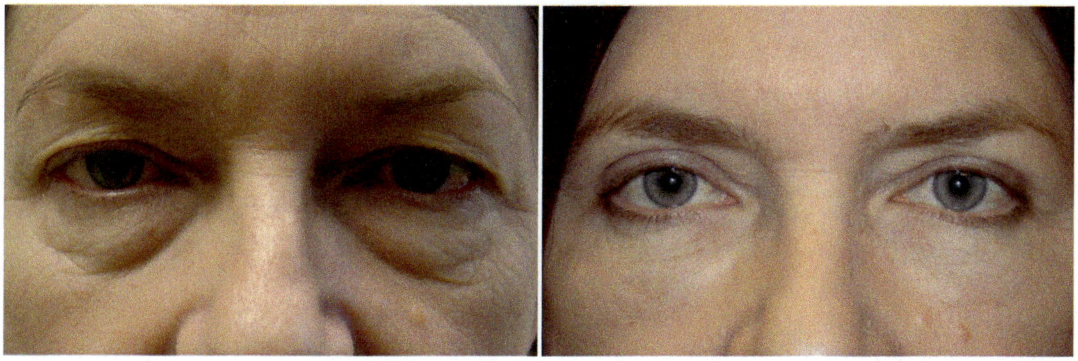

Fig. 16.21 Same procedure as in Fig. 16.20 with addition of canthoplasty, skin trim and orbicularis muscle plication. (*left*) Before and (*right*) after surgery

16.5 Postoperative Care

After surgery, patients are instructed to

1. Apply ice compresses ten minutes per hour while awake for 2 days after surgery.
2. Instill one drop of antibiotic/steroid combination eye drop (Tobradex, Alcon Laboratories, Irvine, CA) three times per day for the first week after surgery
3. Use a Medrol dose pack (Pfizer, Inc., New York, NY) if there are no contraindications.
4. Sleep with the head up (on two pillows) for the first week after surgery.
5. Avoid strenuous activity for the first 10 days after surgery.

The postoperative course typically involves normal bruising and swelling. We have not found postoperative pain to be a normal part of recovery, but blurred vision and tearing can be and usually resolve over the first week. If fat repositioning was performed, the Prolene bolster sutures are removed at day four. If Microfoam tape was applied, it is removed at 4–7 days after surgery.

16.6 Complications

Most of the surgical complications for fat excision and repositioning are similar. They typically include excessive bruising and swelling, chemosis, and subconjunctival hemorrhage. Excess swelling is best treated with reassurance. A higher dose of oral prednisone may be given if there are no medical contraindications. In cases of prolonged or refractory swelling, a history of excessive salt intake, leg swelling, or previous such history with other surgeries can sometimes be elicited. In these instances, a change in diet, compression, massage, and reassurance are often needed. When one side heals much different than the other, ask about sleeping on that side of the face and address the issue if needed.

Chemosis is subconjunctival edema which can occur with overzealous cautery, a low incision site, or when a canthal incision is added. There are various treatment modalities for chemosis depending on severity. Lubrication is important to prevent drying of the exposed conjunctiva. Topical and, especially, oral steroids can resolve the problem quickly. In persistent cases, temporary patching of the eye or an intermarginal suture can be of benefit by means of mechanical compression. On very rare instances, a conjunctival cutdown can be performed.

A subconjunctival hemorrhage can be very distressing to a patient. This is a bleed under the conjunctiva and typically reaches its maximum spread a few days after surgery and resolves in 1–2 weeks. Patient reassurance of the benign nature of the condition is important. If the patient describes conjunctival elevation of the hemorrhage, an evaluation is needed to rule out a more serious bleed.

An undercorrection or overcorrection of fat reduction can occur. This can lead to persistent fat prominence or hollowness. Undercorrections will require revision if the patient is bothered by the prominence. This is typically seen in the lateral fat pocket and a simple re-excision of fat can correct the issue. Overcorrections (hollows) can be problematic. This occurs less commonly with fat repositioning. This can be treated with a hyaluronic acid gel filler, or more permanently with autologous fat grafting.

An eyelid malposition is unusual with stand-alone transconjunctival surgery. Lower eyelid retraction is very rare without associated skin excision. Lower lid elevation can occur, most typically nasally, probably related to excessive or prolonged postoperative swelling which may gape the wound for an extended period of time. This usually resolves with reduction in swelling and time. If no resolution occurs, a resection and reattachment of the lower lid retractors is needed. An entropion can occur with a transconjunctival incision. It is typically spastic, cicatricial, or related to retractor disinsertion. The correction depends on the etiology as with standard entropion repair. A postoperative ectropion can rarely occur if severe preoperative eyelid laxity is not addressed. Finally, on rare occasions, postoperative trichiasis can develop. This is most likely related to damage to the eyelid blood supply and/or postsurgical scarring. Selective lash removal by electrolysis can provide a permanent solution.

When fat repositioning is performed, complications unique to this procedure can occur. These include diplopia (beyond the immediate postoperative period), fat granulomas, prolonged edema, tear trough irregularities, and cutaneous pigment changes at the bolster suture site. Diplopia is typically transient and related to anesthetic injection, edema, or inferior oblique trauma. This can be treated with higher dose oral steroids which should be tapered over a 10-day period. Most cases resolve over this time period. If permanent diplopia occurs, referral to a strabismus specialist is warranted. Fat granulomas are rare, and are treated with intralesional injections of low dose and concentration steroids (Kenalog 5 mg/mL, 0.1 cc). 5-Fluorouracil (5FU) can also be injected (Chap. 27). The granulomas usually resolve with 1–2 injections given 2–3 weeks apart. Surgical resection is rarely required. Prolonged edema is treated in a similar manner to diplopia with higher dose steroids. Tear trough irregularities are typically due to fat granulomas and resolve with intralesional steroid (or 5 FU) injections. Transient hyperpigmentation can occur at the exit site of the cutaneous prolene suture. Topical bleaching preparations may be necessary if the hyperpigmentation does not spontaneously resolve.

16.7 Conclusion

Transconjunctival lower blepharoplasty is an excellent procedure to address lower eyelid fat prominence. When an adjacent tear trough is present, fat repositioning is added to efface the depression. While the learning curve for surgery is steep, the procedure can be mastered with appropriate knowledge, guidance, and experience. When necessary, adjunctive techniques such as canthopexy, canthoplasty, skin excision, and fat grafting can be added to enhance the final outcome. This surgery maintains normal anatomy to a greater extent than does the traditional transcutaneous approach. This in turn leads to less postoperative cicatrization of tissue planes and potential lower eyelid malposition. In the hands of an experienced surgeon, postoperative complications are infrequent, generally self-limiting, and patient satisfaction is high.

References

1. Katzen LB. The history of cosmetic blepharoplasty. Adv Ophthal Plast Reconstr Surg. 1986;5:89.
2. Reidy JP. Swelling of eyelids. Br J Plast Surg. 1960;13:256.
3. Neuhaus R, Baylis H. Complications of lower eyelid blepharoplasty. In: Putterman AM, editor. Cosmetic oculoplastic surgery. New York, NY: GrundStratton; 1982.
4. McGraw BL, Adamson PA. Postblepharoplasty ectropion. Arch Otolaryngol Head Neck Surg. 1991;117:852–6.
5. Taban M, Douglas R, Li T, et al. Efficacy of "thick" acellular human dermis (alloderm) for lower eyelid retraction. Arch Facial Plast Surg. 2005;7:38–44.
6. Bourguet J. Les hernies graisseuses de l'orbite. Notre treitement chirugical. Bull Acad Med (Paris). 1924;92(3 ser):1270.
7. Baylis HI, Long JA, Groth MJ. Transconjunctival lower lid blepharoplasty. Technique and complications. Ophthalmology. 1989; 96(7):1027.
8. Mullins JB, Holds JB, Branham GH, et al. Complications of the transconjunctival approach: a review of 400 cases. Arch Otolaryngol Head Neck Surg. 1997;123:385–8.
9. Massry GG. Comprehensive lower eyelid rejuvenation. Facial Plast Surg. 2010;26(3):209–21.

17 Managing the Lateral Canthus in the Aesthetic Patient

Guy G. Massry

Key Points

- Canthal suspension is an integral part of lower blepharoplasty surgery.
- The incidence of postoperative lower lid malposition is reduced when the eyelid is properly secured.
- Aesthetic canthoplasty/canthopexy should be approached differently than traditional reconstructive canthoplasty.
- Familiarization with canthal anatomy and a thorough preoperative evaluation (eyelid laxity, globe prominence) are critical to attain appropriate outcomes.
- Become comfortable with operating on the canthus and understand the important points of surgery:
  - In most aesthetic cases, avoid lid shortening and disrupting the deep attachments of the lower eyelid to the orbital rim.
  - Reattach the lower lid to the inner orbital rim (to conform to globe).
  - Realign the canthal angle.
- Canthoplasty/canthopexy surgery has a unique set of potential complications which can be very bothersome to patients. It is important to familiarize oneself with these problems and know how to best manage them.
- Avoid high risk patients. Patients unhappy with this form of surgery are often the most difficult to manage.

17.1 Introduction

One of the major complications of lower blepharoplasty (especially with transcutaneous surgery), has been postoperative eyelid malposition, primarily lower lid retraction, or ectropion [1–7]. This is a result of excessive skin excision, weakening of the orbicularis muscle, scarring of the orbital septum, and not addressing pre-existing eyelid laxity. Lower eyelid tightening at the lateral canthus has significantly reduced the incidence of lower lid malposition after surgery [8, 9]. Consequently, canthal surgery has become an essential adjunct for the lower blepahroplasty surgeon, with numerous variations having been described [10–13].

Unfortunately, canthal surgery (canthoplasty, canthopexy) can be an area of difficulty and confusion for the cosmetic surgeon, especially if there is a lack of familiarity with surgery in this area. A change in canthal height, lower eyelid slope and curvature, a squinty or "cat eye" appearance, a smaller appearing eye, canthal rounding, and canthal pain, tenderness, scarring, and webs can occur. This has made canthal surgery intimidating. It has been hard to identify the best canthal support procedure. The simpler procedures provide less support of the lower lid, while the more significant techniques carry higher risks of the canthal distortion.

My goal in this chapter is threefold. I will provide a thorough understanding of lateral canthal anatomy, emphasize the essential factors which should run through the surgeon's mind when planning surgery, and review various canthal procedures. Hopefully, this will simplify an area of surgery which has, at times, been a challenge to many aesthetic surgeons.

17.2 Canthal Anatomy

To understand the lateral canthus, some basic tenets of lower eyelid anatomy must be outlined. The horizontal palpebral fissure measures 30 mm in an adult. It terminates where the upper and lower lids fuse laterally. The angle formed by this union is known as the lateral canthus, while the point of fusion is termed the lateral commissure. The lateral canthus maintains its position and stability by a deeper (subcutaneous) connection to bone. This connection is called the lateral canthal tendon (LCT). I prefer the term lateral palpebral ligament (LPL) as this fibrous structure integrates dense connective tissue (the tarsus) to bone (Whitnall's tubercle) (Fig. 17.1).

G.G. Massry (✉)
Director, Ophthalmic Plastic Surgery,
Spaulding Drive Cosmetic Surgery and Dermatology,
Beverly Hills, CA, USA
e-mail: gmassry@aol.com

G.G. Massry et al. (eds.), *Master Techniques in Blepharoplasty and Periorbital Rejuvenation*,
DOI 10.1007/978-1-4614-0067-7_17, © Springer Science+Business Media, LLC 2011

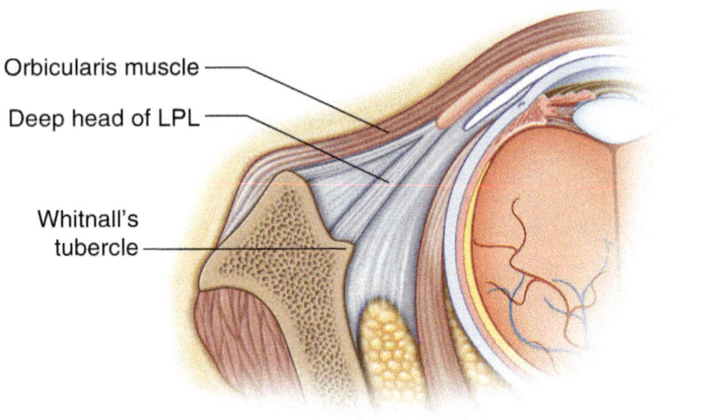

Fig. 17.1 Axial section of the lower lid and lateral orbital rim demonstrating the LPL (lateral palpebral ligament) with its posterior attachment to Whitnall's tubercle

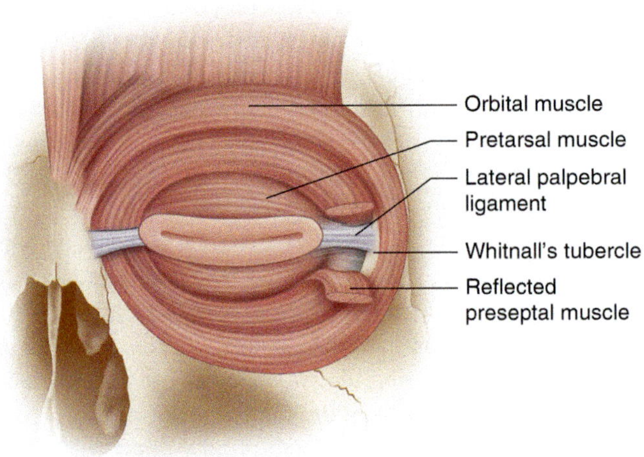

Fig. 17.2 Upper and lower lid orbicularis muscle (orbital, preseptal, and pretarsal) relationship to LPL

The eyelids are composed of both anterior and posterior lamella with components of both contributing to the formation and integrity of the LPL. The orbicularis oculi muscle is the protractor of the eyelids, comprises part of the anterior lamella, and is divided into an oribital and palpebral portion. This division of the orbicularis is anatomic and functional in nature [14]. The palpebral portion of the orbicularis muscle is further divided into a preseptal and pretarsal segment. The pretarsal portion overlies the tarsus. At the termination of the tarsus, it continues as a superficial and deep connective tissue band which forms the LPL. The deep head attaches to the lateral orbital tubercle (Whitnall's tubercle), a boney prominence 3 mm posterior to the lateral orbital rim. This is the critical attachment of the LPL as it maintains the lid's apposition to the globe (Fig. 17.2). Also of note is that the attachments of the LPL maintain the lateral canthus slightly higher than the medial canthus.

17.3 Patient Evaluation for Canthal Surgery

The goal of aesthetic canthal surgery is to provide support and stability for the lower eyelid, while preserving the position and appearance of the lateral canthus. To do this correctly, the anatomic attachments of the LCT must be recreated and maintained in both an antero-posterior and supero-inferior dimension. The preoperative evaluation is critical in determining the most appropriate way to accomplish this.

The presence of lower eyelid laxity must be identified on all patients. Eyelid laxity, a measure of the integrity of the canthal tendons and orbicularis tone, is determined in two standard ways. The first is the lower lid distraction test. The lower lid is pulled away from the globe (Fig. 17.3). Clinically significant laxity (poor canthal tendon support) is present if the lower lid can be pulled more than 8 mm from the globe. In addition, a snap-back or snap test can be performed. The lower lid is manually displaced inferiorly, and its ability to snap back into normal position, without blink, is assessed (Fig. 17.4). If the lower lid does not return to normal position without blink quickly, the eyelid tone is reduced. While the lower eyelid distraction test and snap test may primarily assess different parameters of lower lid support, the results are typically the same as both canthal tendon integrity and orbicularis tone are needed to properly support the lower eyelid.

The preoperative examination modalities reviewed above were initially described to assess eyelid laxity in the setting of eyelid malposition (ectropion, lid retraction, etc.). They measure gross eyelid deficiencies but may miss subtle changes. When performing blepharoplasty, subtle changes are important as preserving lid position; not treating eyelid malposition is the objective. This is particularly true with trancutaneous lower blepharoplasty. In this setting, when even small amounts of eyelid laxity are present, and/or tone is reduced,

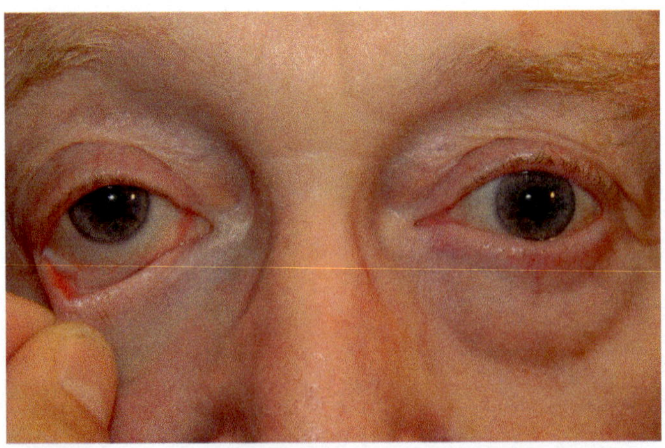

Fig. 17.3 Lower lid distraction test

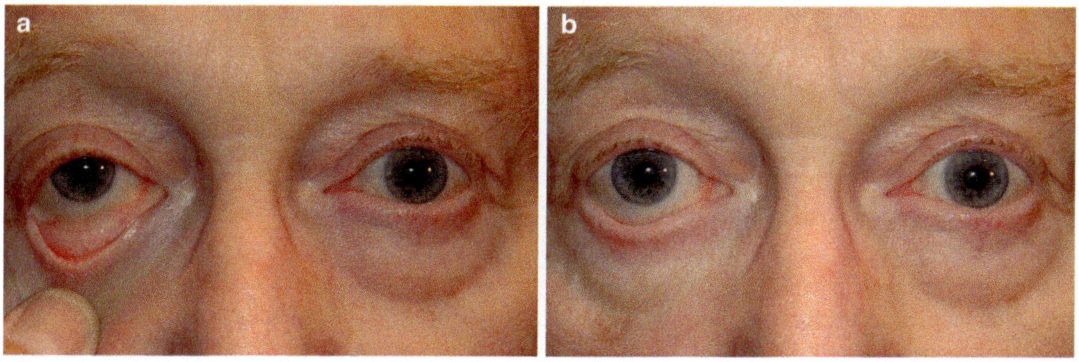

Fig. 17.4 Lower lid snapback test. (**a**) Lid pulled inferiorly; (**b**) lid returns without blink. Note that the lower lid demonstrates laxity (decreased tone) as it does not return to normal position (compare to opposite side)

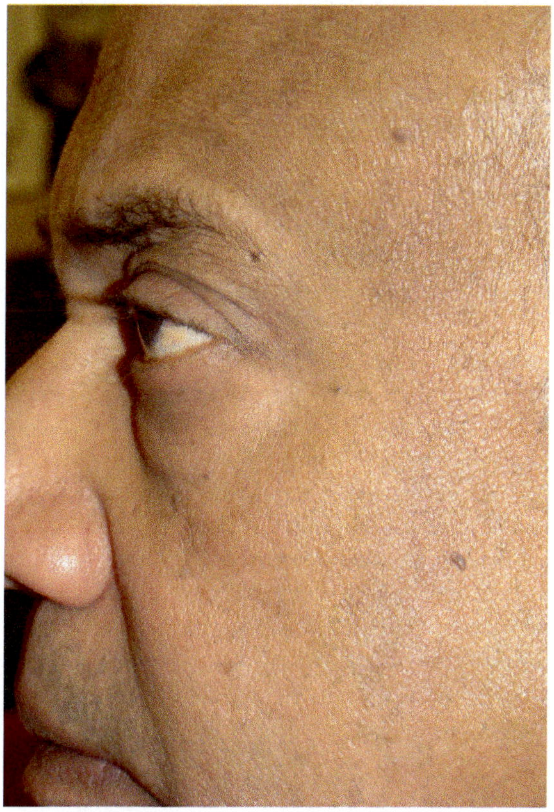

Fig. 17.5 Side view of a patient revealing negative vector eyelid as the globe protrudes further than the suborbital rim tissue

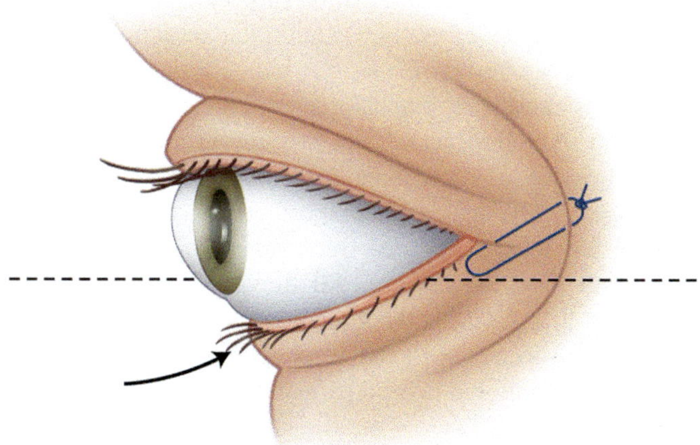

Fig. 17.6 Illustration of canthal suspension in a prominent globe. Note "bowstringing of the globe." with increased sclera show (*dotted line* to *arrow*)

lid tightening is always warranted. An omission of this step will most assuredly lead to lower eyelid malposition. In transconjunctival surgery, the lower lid is at less risk of lid retraction or ectropion, and lid tightening is needed only if the degree of laxity is more significant or if a separate skin excision is to be performed.

It is also important to evaluate globe prominence when considering lid tightening. When the anterior projection of the globe protrudes further than the midface, a negative vector eyelid is present (Fig. 17.5). This can occur as a result of relative globe prominence (large eye, shallow orbit, etc.) or midface (bone/soft tissue or both) recession. When the lower lid is tightened in this scenario, it can bowstring the globe, increase or create scleral show (true or pseudo-lid retraction), and make the eye (globe) appear more prominent (Fig. 17.6). There are techniques to reduce these complications (see surgical technique section below and Chap. 26). However, in this setting, it may be prudent to forgo the blepharoplasty altogether.

17.4 Surgical Techniques

As previously mentioned, it is important to differentiate reconstructive canthal surgery from the aesthetic procedure. The traditional canthoplasty was described for the reconstructive patient with significant eyelid laxity and malposition [15, 16]. This surgery involves complete disinsertion of the lower eyelid from its attachment to the lateral orbital rim (canthotomy and cantholysis). The terminal eyelid is then shortened and resecured to the bone via a tarsal tongue. This *lateral tarsal strip* technique is the classic canthoplasty procedure [17]. While the surgery is not overly complex in the hands of an experienced surgeon, it does involve significant anatomical distortion. In the best of hands, this surgery can lead to small degrees of canthal malalignment and changes in the canthal angle. This is well-tolerated by the older reconstructive patient with involutional eyelid changes. The procedure is not appropriate for the typical cosmetic eyelid patient where complete surgical eyelid disinsertion and lid shortening is rarely needed. In cosmetic surgery, a tarsal strip is typically reserved for patients who are older with more severe lid changes (excess skin, rhytids, laxity, etc.). In this small sub-group of aesthetic patients, the overall improvement in appearance after surgery is so significant that a discrepancy of the two canthi after surgery is usually not a significant concern.

In most aesthetic blepharoplasty patients who require lower lid tightening, two other procedures will likely provide a better overall outcome: a modified canthoplasty or a canthopexy. The incidence of postoperative canthal angle changes or discrepancies between sides is much less common with these procedures. All three procedures will be described below. These three techniques will allow the surgeon a full spectrum of canthal suspension surgical options which can be tailored to each patient depending of preoperative findings.

17.4.1 Canthoplasty (Lateral Tarsal Strip)

The canthus is anesthetized transcutaneously to the lateral orbital rim periosteum and transconjnuncitvally with Xylocaine 1% with 1:100:000 epinephrine. A 7–8 mm canthotomy is performed (Fig. 17.7). An incision is made through orbicularis muscle to the orbital rim periosteum. Blunt dissection with a cotton-tipped applicator is useful for freeing tissue off the periosteum. It is not uncommon to identify a small fat pad (Eilser's fat) during this step. This fat pad should be left undisturbed if possible. The terminal eyelid is grasped with a toothed forceps and a Wescott scissors or an electrical cutting device is used to engage the inferior crus of the LCT (feels like a dense band). This attachment is lysed with a resultant dynamic release of the eyelid (Fig. 17.8). The amount of lid shortening is then determined by bringing the lid to the inner orbital rim and approximating the excess. The tarsus is released from the conjunctiva and retractors below (Fig. 17.9). The corresponding amount of lid margin is then trimmed (Fig. 17.10), and the anterior and posterior lamellae are split (Fig. 17.11). The excess skin is excised (Fig. 17.12) and the tarsal tongue is now formed. The tarsus is then de-epithelialized with a scalpel or light cautery. The tarsus is shortened as needed and engaged with a suture for reattachment (Fig. 17.13). A 4–0 Vicryl suture on a half-circle needle (P2 or S2) is utilized for the suspension. Vicryl suture works well as it is reactive (induces scar) and absorbs after 3 months, thus avoiding suture spitting which can occur with permanent sutures. The tarsus is secured to the inner periosteum of the lateral orbital rim (Fig. 17.14a) at the level of Whitnall's tubercle. After the periosteal bite is completed, the suture can be passed through the superior limb of the LPL. This maneuver aids in formation of the canthal angle. The suture is approximated without tying in order to assess the lid position. I prefer a slight (2 mm) over-correction in anticipation of postoperative drop. If lid position is appropriate, the suture is tied (Fig. 17.14b). The canthal angle is then reformed with a grey line–grey line suture (see detailed description in modified canthoplasty section). The canthus is closed with either absorbable (6–0 chromic) or permanent (6–0 silk) suture (Fig. 17.15). The permanent sutures are removed in 1 week.

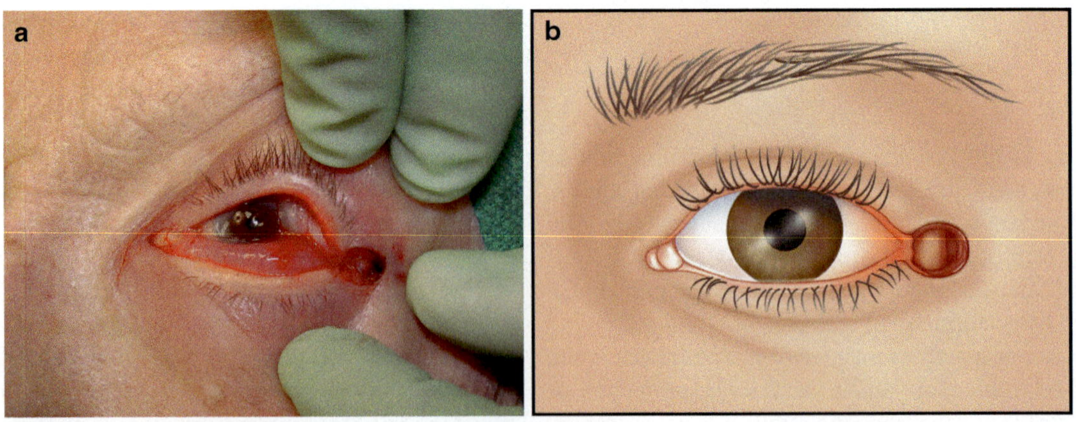

Fig. 17.7 A canthotomy initiates the procedure (**a**) Surgical photo and (**b**) illustration

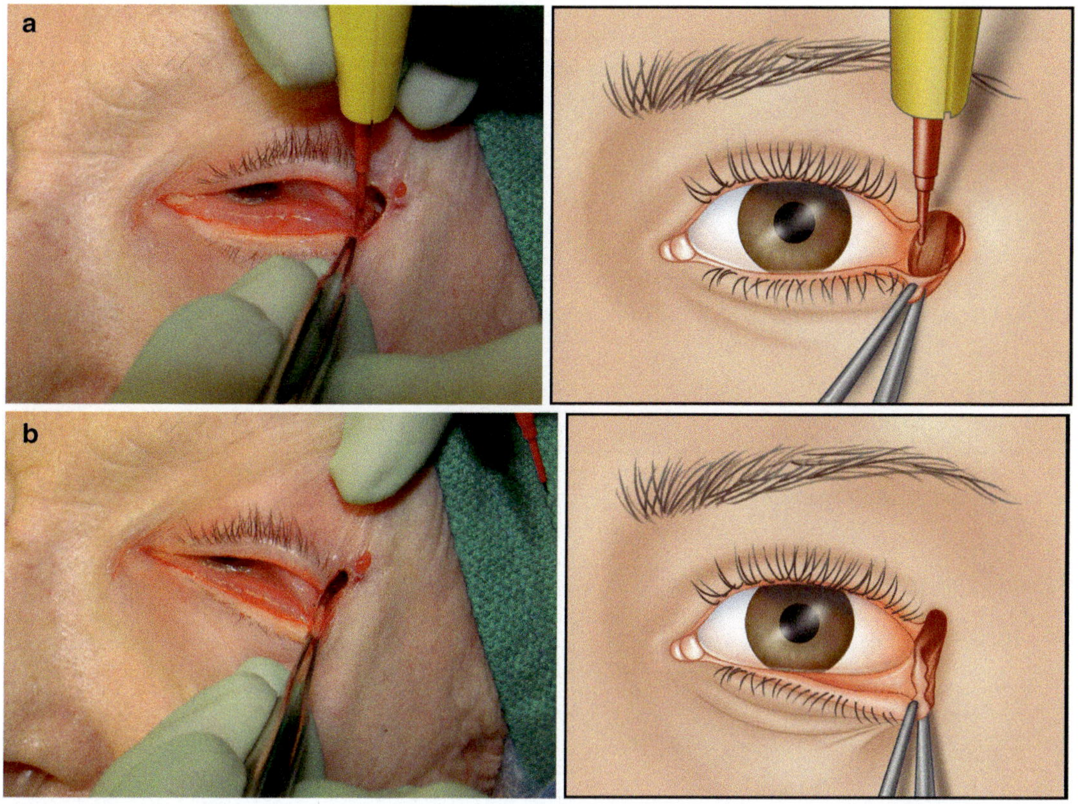

Fig. 17.8 (**a**) The inferior crus (attachment) of the LPL is lysed (cantholysis) with (**b**) dynamic release of the lower lid. Note surgical photo and accompanying illustration for both

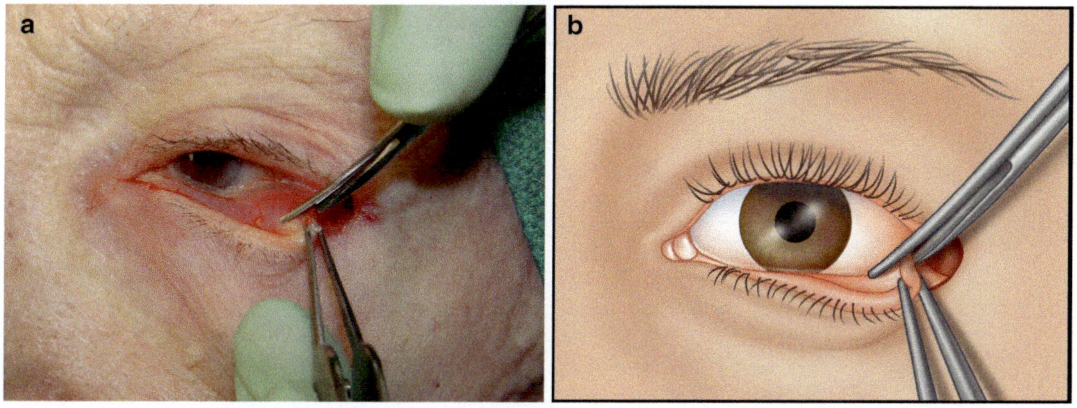

Fig. 17.9 Separation of conjunctiva from tarsus in preparation for formation of tarsal strip (**a**) Surgical photo and (**b**) illustration

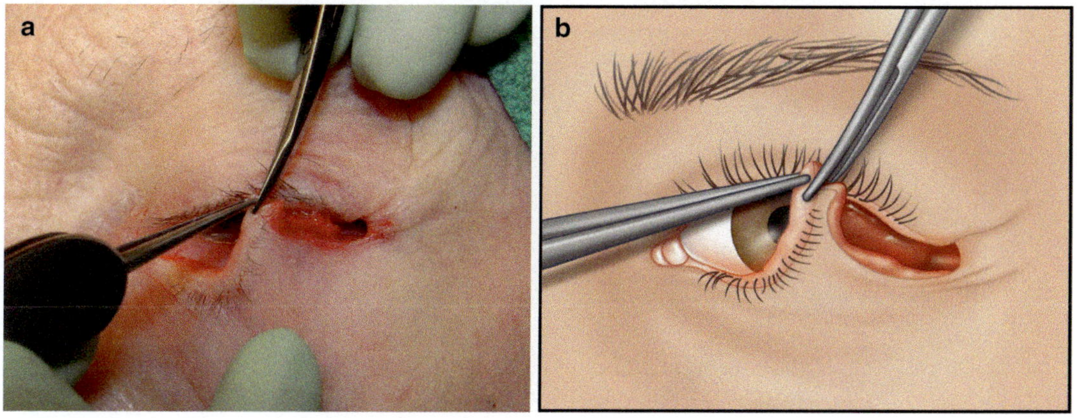

Fig. 17.10 The lid margin (muco-cutaneous junction) is trimmed (**a**) Surgical photo and (**b**) illustration

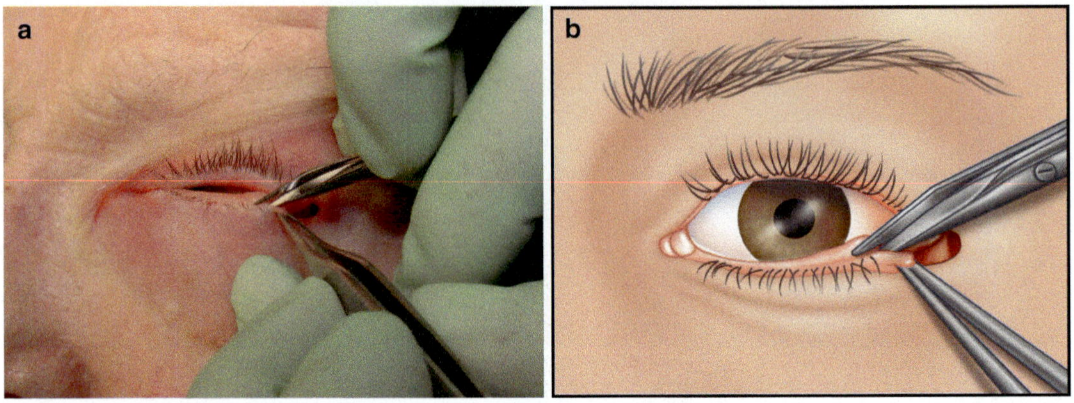

Fig. 17.11 The anterior and posterior lamellae are split (a) Surgical photo and (b) illustration

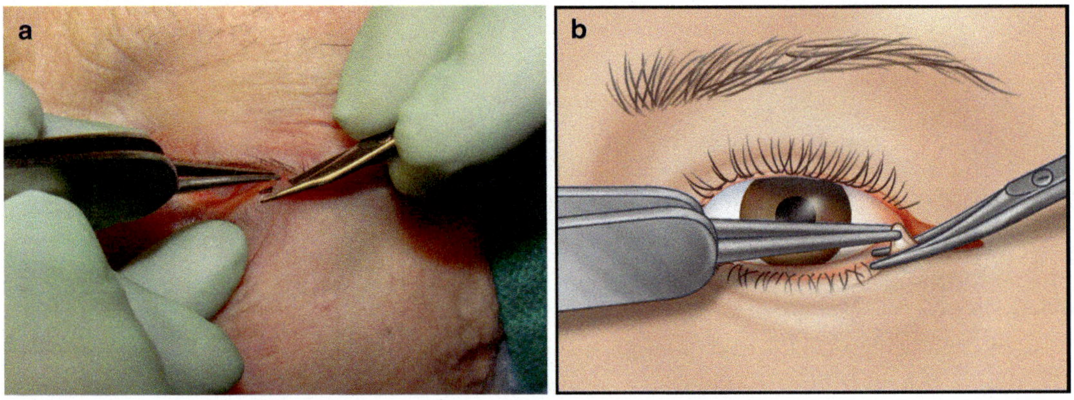

Fig. 17.12 Excess skin is trimmed (a) Surgical photo and (b) illustration

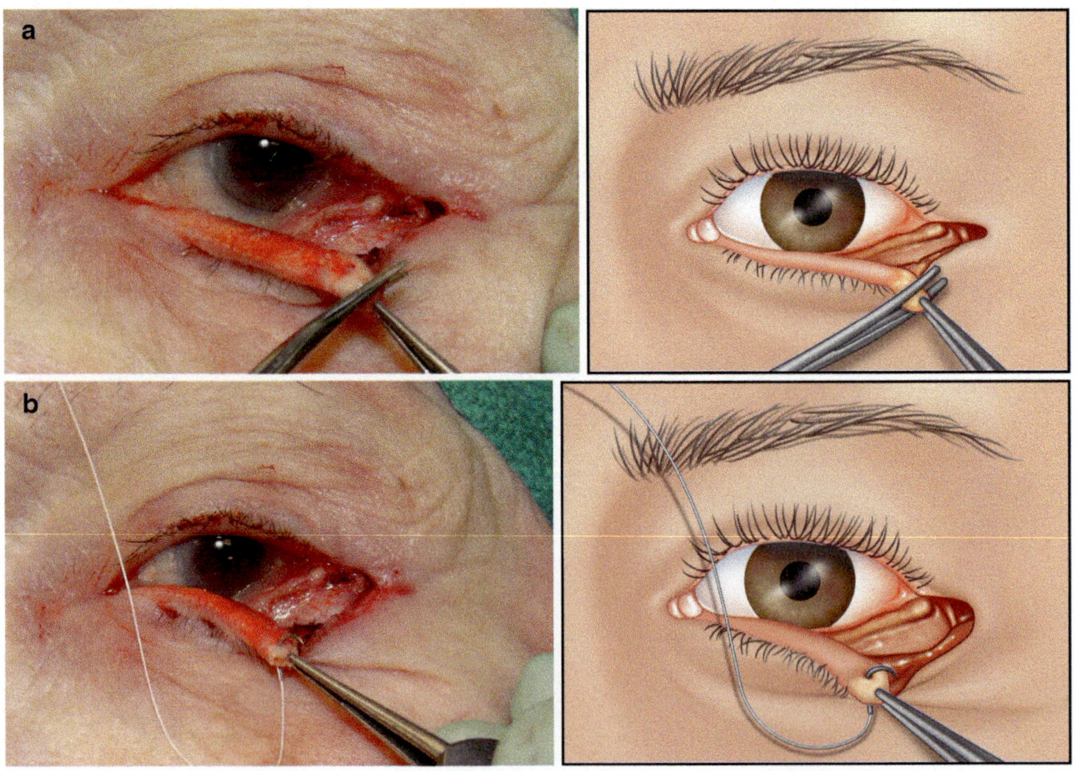

Fig. 17.13 (a) The tarsus is shortened and (b) engaged with a suture for reattachment to the orbital rim. Note surgical photo and accompanying illustration for both

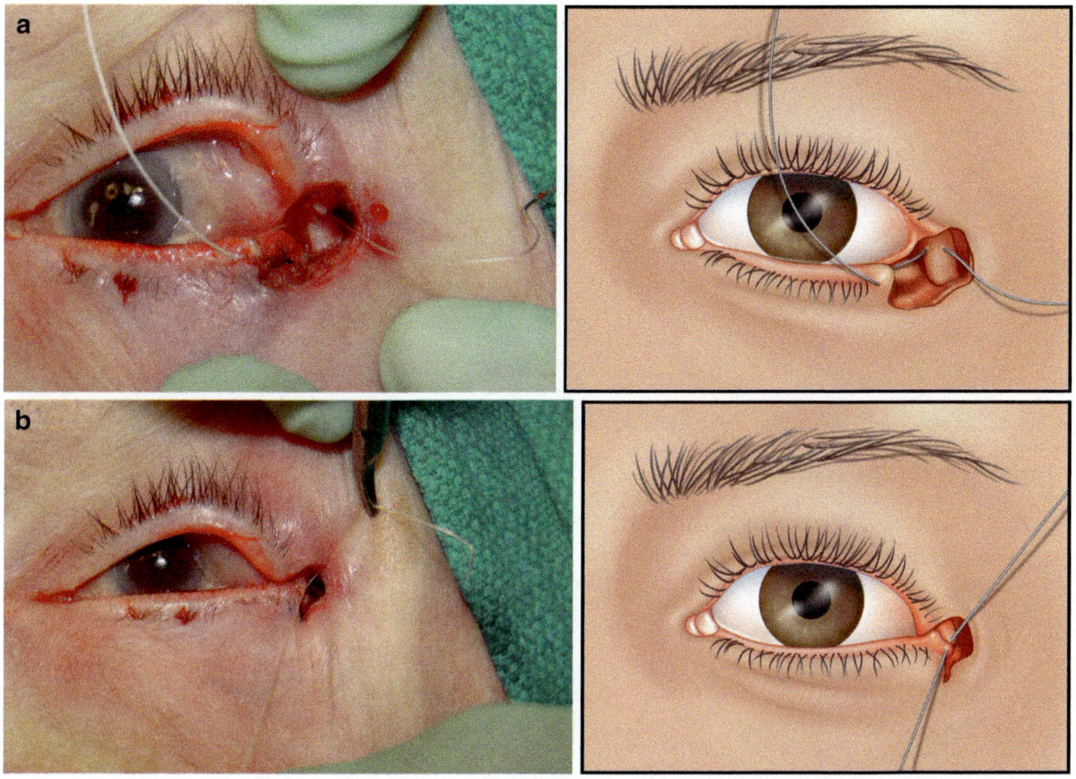

Fig. 17.14 (**a**) The tarsal tongue is sutured to the inner orbital rim periosteum and (**b**) secured. Note surgical photo and accompanying illustration for both

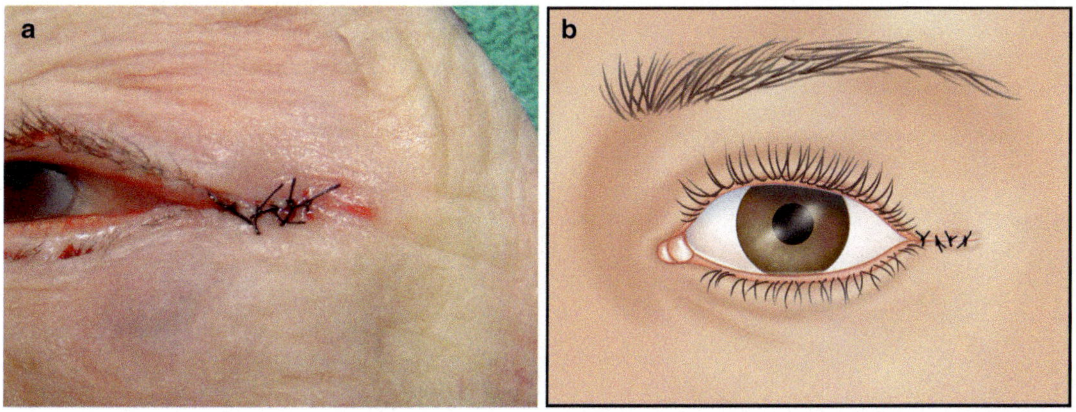

Fig. 17.15 The canthus is closed (**a**) Surgical photo and (**b**) illustration

17.4.2 Modified Canthoplasty

A canthotomy and dissection to the orbital rim is performed as described above. No cantholysis or lid shortening ensues; however, the canthal angle is split (upper from lower lid). As stated previously, complete lid disinsertion and shortening is rarely needed in cosmetic eyelid surgery. The goal in this procedure is to secure the lid laterally with less distortion of canthal anatomy as is inherent to the more powerful tarsal strip procedure. The terminal eyelid is grasped (Fig. 17.16). A small separation of skin/muscle from underlying tissue (tarsus or LPL) is created. The terminal tarsus or ligament is engaged with a 4–0 Vicryl suture in a similar fashion as with the tarsal strip procedure (Fig. 17.17). The suture is secured to the inner orbital rim periosteum and checked for position (Fig. 17.18). When appropriate, the knot is tied. The canthal angle is then recreated with a grey line–grey line suture (6–0 chromic or 6–0 silk) (Fig. 17.19). The grey line is the terminal

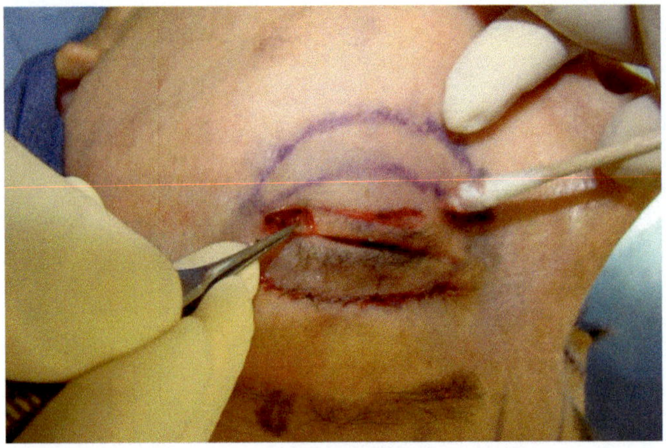

Fig. 17.16 The terminal eyelid is grasped

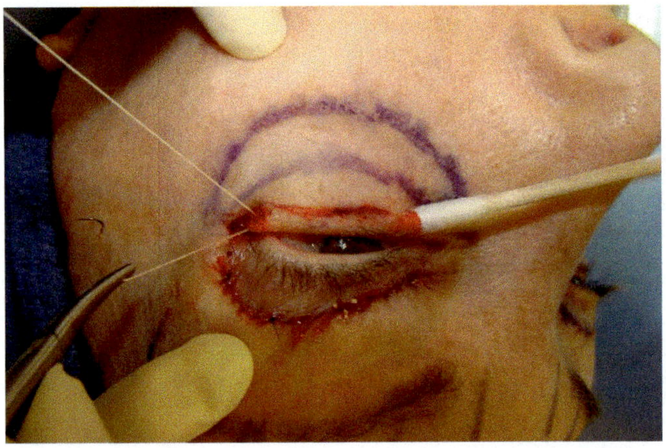

Fig. 17.17 The tarsus/LPL is engaged with suture for fixation

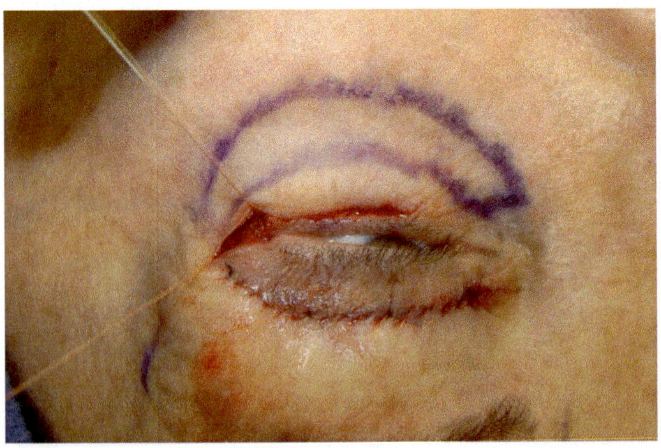

Fig. 17.18 The lid is secured to orbital rim

fibers of the pretarsal orbicularis muscle (muscle of Riolan). It is just anterior to the openings of the meibomian glands. The suture is passed through the grey line of the terminal upper and lower eyelid. Engaging the periosteum with suture between the grey line bites may be performed to further enhance the canthal angle before securing this suture. When tying this suture, special attention is given to make sure the upper and lower lid meet equally at the canthal angle. This will prevent one lid from over-riding the other, and a blunted or irregular appearance to the canthal angle after surgery. The canthus is then closed as with the tarsal strip surgery.

17.4.3 Canthopexy (Muscle suspension)

In this procedure, the canthotomy is through skin and muscle only. It is not necessary to split the canthal angle. A subcutaneous dissection of skin from preseptal orbicularis muscle is performed. If there is associated skin excision, an infracilliary incision is made continuous with the canthotomy and an open exposure of the orbicularis is created. The terminal orbicularis is engaged with a 5–0 Prolene or Vicryl suture and secured to orbital rim periosteum for fixation. In isolated lower blepharoplasty surgery, the suture is secured to the orbital rim periosteum through the canthotomy incision (Fig. 17.20). When performed in conjunction with upper eyelid blepharoplasty, the suture may be secured to the periosteum of the orbital rim at a higher position through a temporal upper eyelid crease incision (Fig. 17.21). This is performed by tunneling a connection between the upper lid crease incision and the canthotomy incision. This technique often provides more support to the eyelid. If folds or puckers are created in the lower lid skin when the suture is tied, further subcutaneous dissection is necessary. The canthus is closed with 6–0 chromic or Nylon suture (Fig. 17.22). A grey line suture is not needed as the canthal angle is not disrupted.

17.4.4 The Prominent Globe

Patients with negative vector eyelids (prominent globes) present a special challenge when lid tightening is performed. Whichever procedure is selected can lead to "bowstringing" of the globe by the lid. This occurs because the length of lid needed to overcome the additional globe surface area (from globe prominence/projection) is lacking. When a relatively short lid is secured to the lateral orbital rim, it rides down the globe. In this setting, the globe will appear to protrude further and the lower lid will retract. This is discussed in detail in Chap. 26.

A surgical modification which may avert this problem is to hang back the canthal support suture. When the lower lid is secured to the lateral orbital rim, the suture can be left loose. This anteriorizes the attachment site of the lid and may prevent bowstringing as the lid is psudo-lengthened by the suture. The suture tying can be graded to select the best lid position. In addition, the suture can be secured to a higher

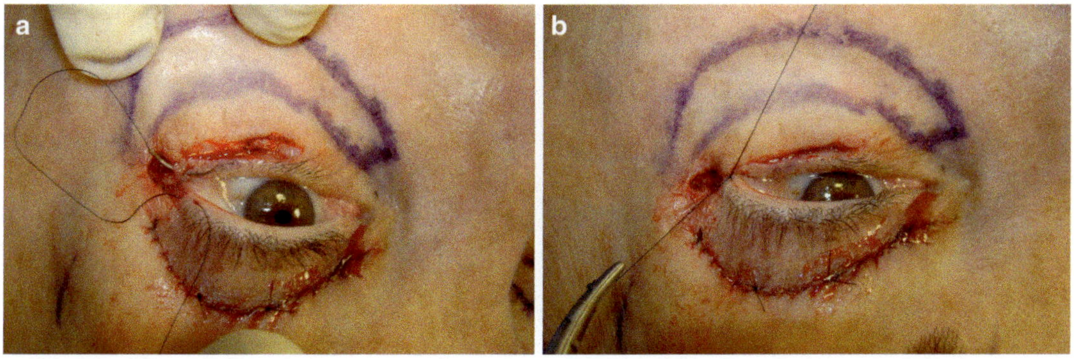

Fig. 17.19 Canthal angle reformed with (**a**) *grey line*–grey line suture from upper to lower lid and (**b**) securing of suture

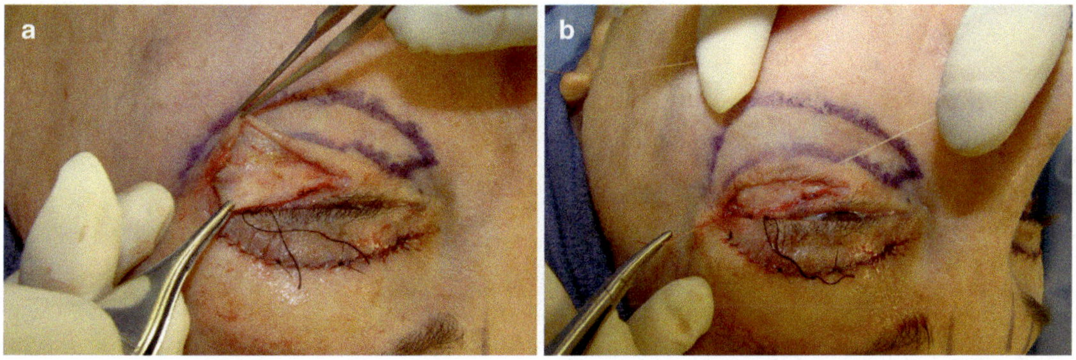

Fig. 17.20 Through an infracilliary incision, the terminal orbicularis muscle is (**a**) grasped and (**b**) secured to periosteum at the lateral orbital rim

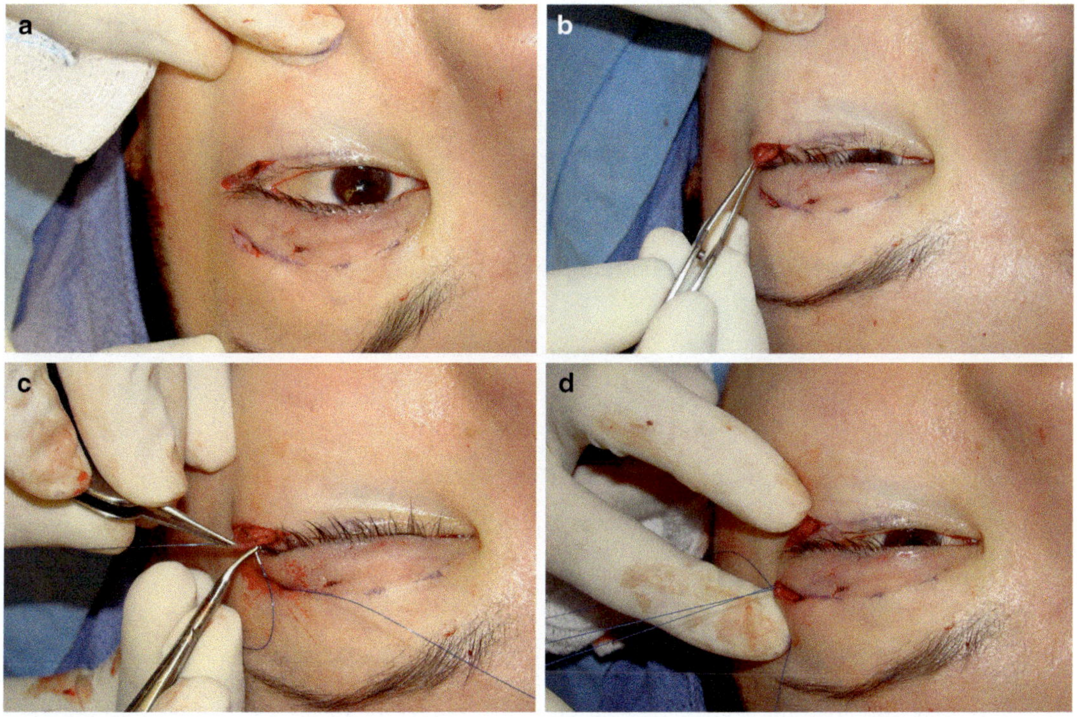

Fig. 17.21 (**a**) A temporal lid crease and canthal incision is made. (**b**) The orbicularis is undermined and grasped, (**c**) engaged with a suture, and (**d**) tunneled from the canthal to lid crease incision and secured to periosteum at the supero-lateral orbital rim

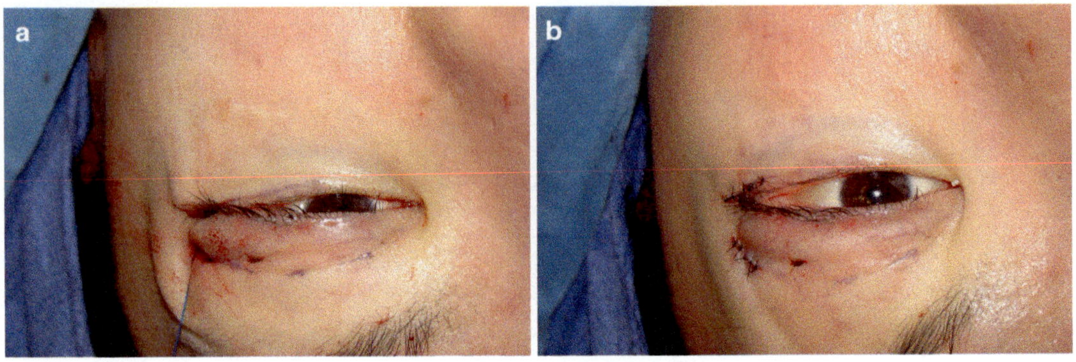

Fig. 17.22 (**a**) Skin puckering after tying suture. (**b**) The puckers resolve with undermining of the skin, and the incisions are closed

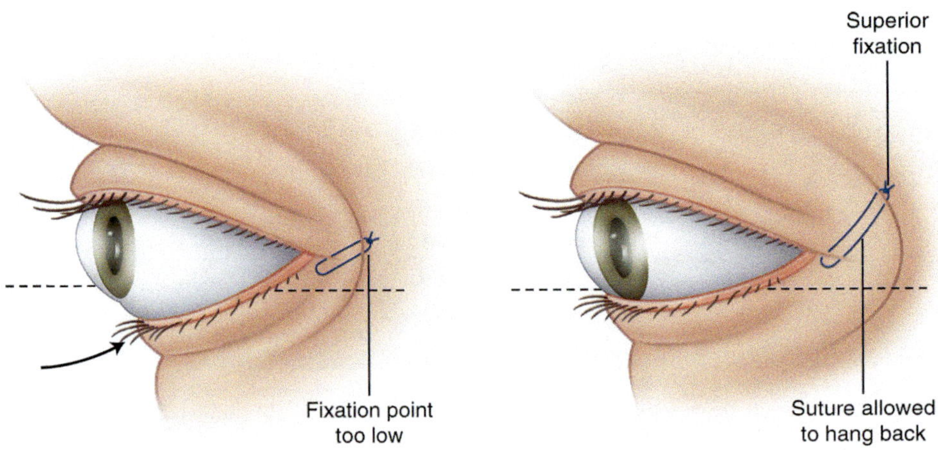

Fig. 17.23 Artist's illustration of (*left*) bowstringing of a prominent eye with lid tightening as is shown in Fig. 17.6. Note scleral show and lid retraction (*arrow*) created by lid tightening. (*Right*) Modification of canthoplasty by hang-back and supra-placement of eyelid fixation suture. This prevents the "bowstringing" effect. Note elevation of lower lid and reduction of scleral show

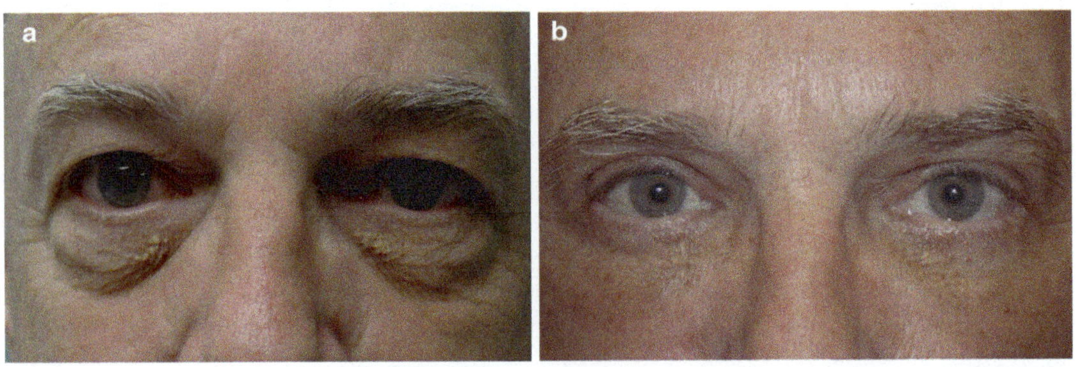

Fig. 17.24 This man underwent canthoplasty, skin trim, and orbicularis suspension in addition to lower lid transconjunctival blepharoplasty with fat repositioning to the nasojugal groove (tear trough) and fat grafting to the orbito-malar groove (temporal lid/cheek junction depression). (**a**) Pre- and (**b**) postoperative frontal views

point on the lateral orbital rim providing a greater elevating effect. These two modifications can help in preventing lid/globe deficiencies (Fig. 17.23).

Figures 17.24–17.28 demonstrate representative outcomes of patients who underwent aesthetic canthal surgery.

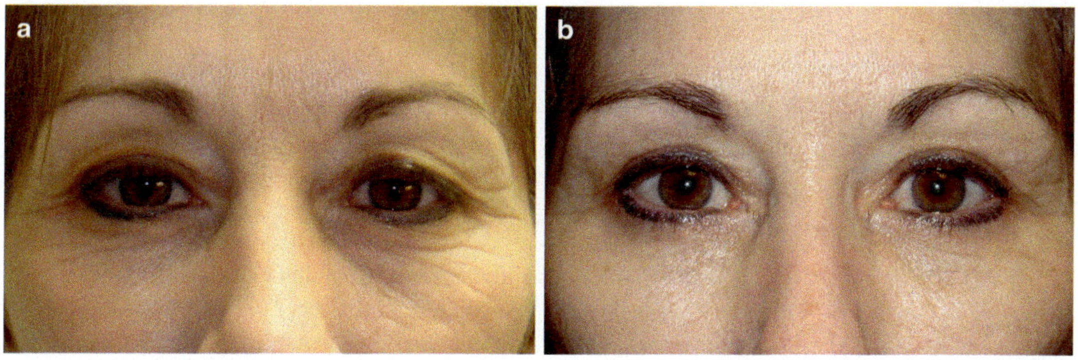

Fig. 17.25 (**a**) Pre- and (**b**) postoperative views of a woman who underwent canthoplasty, orbicularis suspension, skin trim, fat grafting to the tear trough, and mild lower lid postoperative Botox. Note *slight lid margin* eversion temporally on the *left* after surgery. The patient was not bothered by this

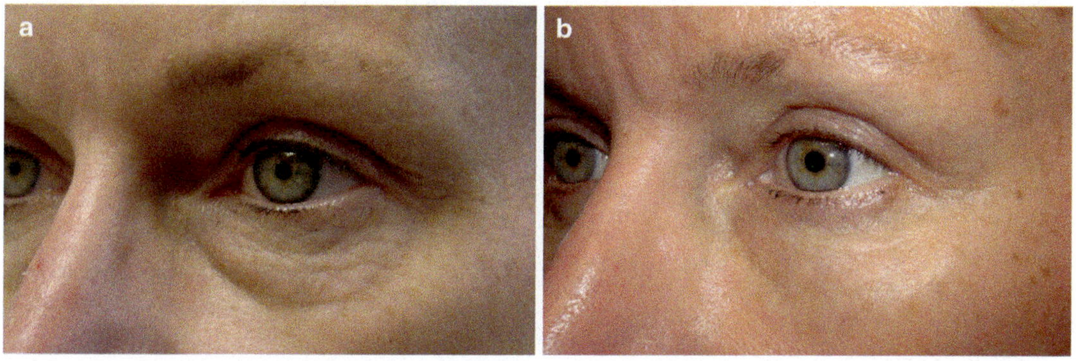

Fig. 17.26 (**a**) Pre- and (**b**) postoperative oblique views of a woman who underwent canthoplasty, skin trim, and orbicularis suspension, in addition to transconjunctival lower lid blepharoplasty with fat repositioning

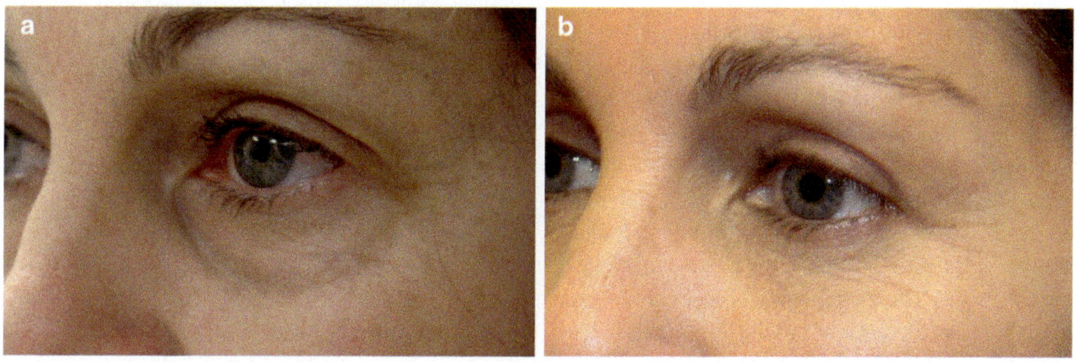

Fig. 17.27 Same procedure as patient in Fig. 17.26. Note the canthal angle is unchanged after surgery. (**a**) Before and (**b**) after surgery

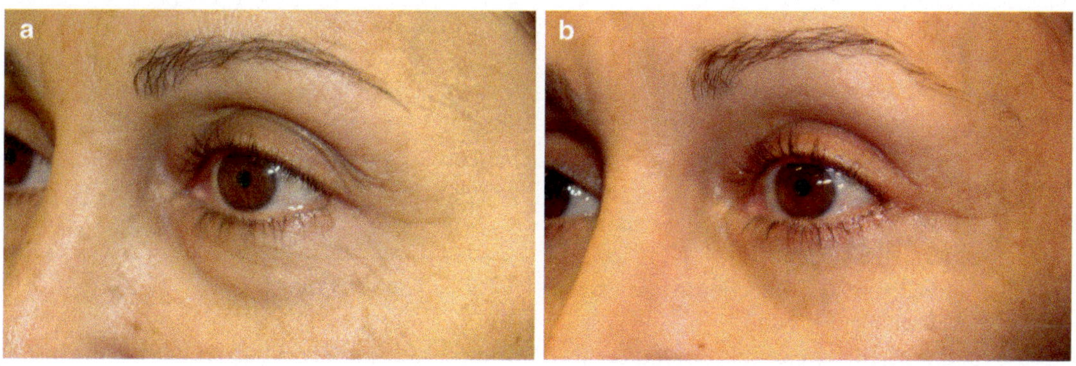

Fig. 17.28 Identical procedure as patient in Fig. 17.27 (**a**) Before and (**b**) after surgery. There was minimal effacement of the tear trough (little fat to reposition), but the canthal angle maintained its normal appearance. Her infracilliary scar is slightly apparent. She did not complain of this

17.5 Postoperative Care

Patients are instructed to perform the following:

1. Apply an antibiotic ointment to the sutures three times a day for the first week after surgery.
2. Instill a combination antibiotic–steroid drop to the eye three times a day for the first week after surgery.
3. Apply ice compresses 10 min per hour while awake for the first 48 h after surgery.
4. Sleep with the head elevated (few pillows) for the first week after surgery.
5. Avoid exercise and more than light physical activity for the first week after surgery.

Patients are seen at 1 week after surgery for suture removal if non-absorbable sutures are used. The grey line canthal angle suture is typically kept in place longer (10 days) in order to ensure that the angle remains anatomically intact. In the immediate postoperative period, patients typically have an over-correction of lower lid height with exaggerated slant, pain, and tenderness at the canthal angle, a degree of chemosis near the angle, and a feeling of tightness. These issues typically resolve within the first month after surgery.

17.6 Complications

Surgery on the lateral canthus can lead to number of complications which are mostly benign in nature and short-lived, but often a nuisance to patients. Some of these problems require further intervention, and may persist indefinitely. As surgery secures the lower eyelid, patients may complain of a tight feeling. Patients have a difficult time describing the complaint, as it is an obscure sensation. This tightness usually subsides within the first month after surgery, but may rarely last for a year or more. The patient needs to be reassured that this is a normal part of surgical healing. In the rare case when this is prolonged, injections of low dose steroid (0.2 cc Kenalogue 5 mg/mL) or 5-flourouracil (5FU see Chap. 27) or a combination of the two solutions, mechanical massage, stretching, and botulinum toxin-A injections may be of benefit. I have not found a consistent correlation of releasing the canthus surgically with resolution of this symptom.

Pain and tenderness, without signs of cellulitis, abscess, or granuloma, at the canthus is another cumbersome complaint. This follows the same course and recovery as lid tightness described above. This is likely related to periosteal manipulation/disruption, nerve entrapment/injury, or low lying inflammation at the surgical site. Steroid/5FU injections as described previously may help in resolving this issue.

Suture abscesses and granulomas can also occur after surgery. They typically present a few weeks after surgery. Warm compresses and antibiotic treatment (oral and topical) may help in a small percentage of abscesses (the abscess can self-express). If this does not lead to resolution, a canthal cutting down with suture removal in the office, under local anesthesia, should help resolve the abscess. In cases of granuloma, steroid/5FU injections as described previously are given. On occasion excision is needed.

Chemosis is usually treated with topical and oral steroid preparations. Rebound chemosis can occur, so a slow taper is warranted. In the more recalcitrant cases, pressure patching, a temporary tarsorrhaphy, and a conjunctuval cut-down can be considered depending on the mind-set of the patient.

Canthal angle discrepancies and changes from preoperative shape and position are especially troublesome, as they often require a surgical revision. The canthus is such a delicate structure and has such a great effect on lid appearance that even subtle changes can bother the patient significantly. The best way to handle this is preparedness (explain the possibility to the patient in the preoperative discussion), avoidance (manipulate the canthus as little as possible whenever possible), and readiness (become comfortable with surgery and revision). I have found canthal angle distortion is rarely a problem when the deeper attachments of the LPL are left undisturbed and no lid shortening is performed (as with most aesthetic procedures). If surgery is warranted, I like to wait 6 months to a year prior to intervening.

Canthal webs can occur, especially when upper blepharoplasty is simultaneously performed and there was insufficient distance between the upper lid incision and the canthotomy. The webs result from a relative shortage of skin in the vertical dimension compared to the horizontal plane, and can be addressed with various combinations of mini-flaps (Y-V and Z-plasties). Surgical revision should be performed no earlier than 6 months after the initial procedure. In the interim, the area can be injected with steroid–5FU combinations as previously described. The surgical revision can enhance outcome; however, scarring, wound contracture, and only partial improvement can occur.

An elevation of the canthus/lower lid with elevation of the brow is another rare but troublesome complication. This is typically seen in the setting of simultaneous upper eyelid blepharoplasty. This complication is likely a result of cicatrix at the junction of upper eyelid, lower eyelid, and canthus. This is a difficult problem to correct as patients often look great without brow animation. Early steroid/5FU injections and massage may help, but the issue typically persists. Patients usually acclimate to the problem with time if the aesthetic result is otherwise good.

17.7 Conclusion

There are a variety of procedures which can be used to suspend and reinforce the lower lid via the lateral canthus during blepharoplasty. These procedures have improved surgical outcomes and reduced postoperative complications significantly. Understanding the anatomy of the canthus, indentifying preoperative deficiencies that may lead to canthal/eyelid malposition, minimizing canthal disruption, and understanding the nuances of reconstructing the canthus correctly is critical to attaining these results. When these concepts are kept in mind, canthal suspension can be performed safely and reproducibly in aesthetic lower lid surgery.

References

1. Edergton Jr MT. Causes and prevention of lower lid ectropion following blepharoplasty. Plast Reconstr Surg. 1972;49(4):367.
2. Rees TD. Correction of ectropion resulting from blepharoplasty. Plast Reconstr Surg. 1972;50(1):1.
3. Levine MR, Boynton J, Tenzel RR, et al. Complications of blepahroplasty. Ophthalmic Surg. 1975;6(2):53.
4. Tenzel RR. Surgical treatment of complications of cosmetic blepharoplasty. Clin Plast Surg. 1978;5(4):517.
5. Neuhaus R, Baylis H. Complications of lower eyelid blepharoplasty. In: Putterman AM, editor. Cosmetic oculoplastic surgery. New York, NY: Grund Stratton; 1982.
6. McGraw BL, Adamson PA. Postblepharoplasty ectropion. Arch Otolaryngol Head Neck Surg. 1991;117:852–6.
7. Taban M, Douglas R, Li T. Efficacy of "thick" acellular human dermis (alloderm) for lower eyelid retraction. Arch Facial Plast Surg. 2005;7:38–44.
8. Nowitzki T, Anderson RL. Advances in eyelid malposition. Ophthal Plast Reconstr Surg. 1985;1:145.
9. Carraway JH, Mellow CG. The prevention and treatment of lower lid ectropion following blepharoplasty. Plast Reconstr Surg. 1990;85(6):971.
10. Shorr N, Goldberg R, Eshagian B, Cook T. Lateral canthoplasty. Ophthal Plast Reconstr Surg. 2003;19(5):345.
11. Fagien S. Algorithim for canthoplasty: the lateral retinacular suspension: a simplified suture canthoexy. Plast Reconstr Surg. 1999;103:2042–53; discussion 2054–2058.
12. Chong KK, Goldberg RA. Lateral canthal surgery. Facial Plast Surg. 2010;26(3):193–200.
13. Massry GG. Comprehensive lower eyelid rejuvenation. Facial Plast Surg. 2010;26(3):209–21.
14. Shovlin JP, Lemke B. Clinical eyelid anatomy. In: Bosniak S, editor. Principals and practice of ophthalmic plastic and reconstructive surgery. Philadelphia, PA: WB Saunders; 1996. p. 261–80.
15. Converse JM, Smith B. Canthoplasty and dacryocystorhinostomy. Am J Ophthalmol. 1952;35(8):1103.
16. Beard C. Canthoplasty and brow elevation for facial palsy. Arch Ophthalmol. 1964;71:386.
17. Anderson RL, Gordy DD. The tarsal strip procedure. Arch Ophthalmol. 1979;97:2192.

Management of the Post-lower Eyelid Blepharoplasty Retracted Eyelid

18

Dan Georgescu, Geeta Belsare, John D. McCann, and Richard L. Anderson

Key Points

- Lower eyelid retraction after blepharoplasty surgery is perhaps the single most difficult challenge in aesthetic reconstructive surgery.
- The mechanism of eyelid retraction following surgery can be related to eyelid laxity, weakness of the orbicularis oculi muscle, inadequate anterior lamella, scarring of the middle lamella and/or posterior lamella, or any combination of these deficits.
- Common sequelae of lower eyelid retraction include exposure keratopathy, irritated eyes, blurry vision, lateral canthal dystopia, a round eye, and sclera show.
- The incidence of eyelid retraction can be reduced if the surgeon carefully evaluates the anatomical changes that prompted the patient to seek surgical treatment. Most patients have very little excess skin or muscle in the lower eyelids and removing these tissues is one of the most common causes of eyelid retraction after blepharoplasty.
- There are patients that respond well to removal of tissue, such as the young patient with a familial tendency towards excess fat in the lower eyelid and the older patient who truly has excess skin in the lower eyelids. In these patients, the appropriate layer of tissue can be conservatively removed.
- The blepharoplasty surgeon must recognize that some very common conditions, such as altered texture of the lower eyelid skin and fluid retention over the malar eminence, are not improved by removal of tissue from the lower eyelid.
- Understanding the mechanism of eyelid retraction preoperatively is crucial for selecting the proper reconstructive technique to achieving the desired, long lasting result.
- Disrupting the orbicularis oculi muscle, with or without excision of tissue, can result in lower eyelid retraction related to paralysis or weakness of the muscle. This common cause of lower lid retraction is often reversible over a period of several months without surgical intervention.
- Cosmetic patients chose to have surgery for appearance, so they will rarely accept reconstructive techniques that negatively impact on cosmesis, such as full-thickness skin grafting. In many patients with lower eyelid retraction and anterior lamellar insufficiency, skin grafting can be avoided with midface elevation that recruits skin and muscle into the lower eyelid.
- Middle and posterior lamellar deficiency are best treated with lysis of the scar tissue and placement of a spacer graft.

18.1 Introduction

Lower eyelid blepharoplasty is an operation that should aim first to maintain or regain proper eyelid function and structure and second to remove or reposition muscle, skin, and fat to give the patient a more youthful appearance. Unfortunately, even the most skilled surgeons will sometimes have a patient that develops postblepharoplasty round eyes and sclera show. Lateral canthal dystopia and lower eyelid retraction predictably occur in a small number of patients that underwent transcutaneous lower eyelid blepharoplasty by even the most experienced surgeons, sometimes years after surgery (Fig. 18.1) [1, 2]. In many cases, the eyelid retraction or laxity is the result of continued facial aging and sagging combined with the postoperative changes that occurred in eyelid structure. However, the most common scenario is when a "skin-focused" young surgeon removes too much anterior lamellar tissue at the time of surgery, which results in eyelid

D. Georgescu (✉)
Clinical Assistant Professor, Wilmer Eye Institute, Johns Hopkins Medical Center, Baltimore, MD, USA
e-mail: dan.oculoplastics@gmail.com

G.G. Massry et al. (eds.), *Master Techniques in Blepharoplasty and Periorbital Rejuvenation*,
DOI 10.1007/978-1-4614-0067-7_18, © Springer Science+Business Media, LLC 2011

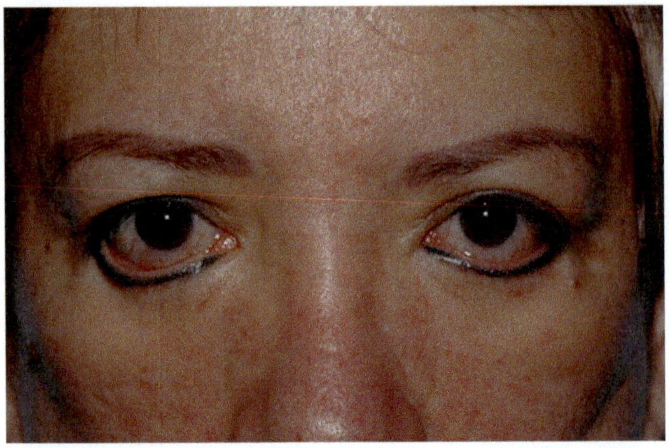

Fig. 18.1 Clinical photograph showing severe lower eyelid retraction 5 years after skin and muscle flap lower eyelid blepharoplasty in a middle-aged patient

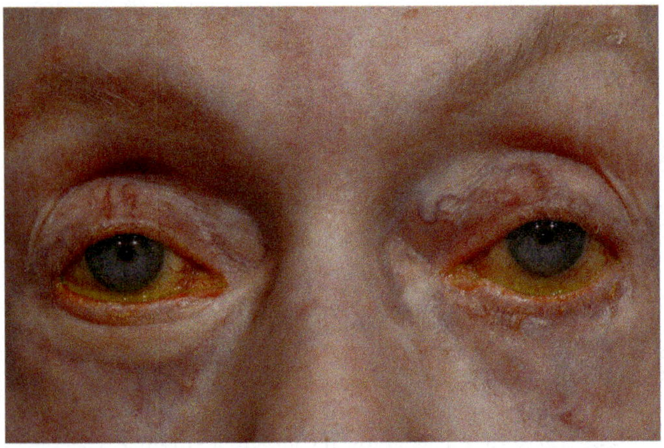

Fig. 18.2 Clinical photograph of a patient who underwent retroauricular skin grafting in the right lower eyelid for the correction of severe eyelid retraction after bilateral skin and muscle flap blepharoplasty. Note the color difference with the "stuck on" appearance of the graft, which made the patient very unhappy with the cosmetic result despite the relative improvement in lower eyelid position on the right side compared to the left

retraction and ectropion. This same surgeon will then believe that the only cause for this complication is the removal of too much skin and will try to correct it by performing a full-thickness skin graft which is very likely to make the unhappy patient unhappier, because of skin color and texture differences (Fig. 18.2).

The postblepharoplasty patient with eyelid retraction was motivated to have the original surgery for cosmetic considerations and will rarely be satisfied with an excellent anatomic reconstitution in the presence of an even faintly visible skin graft. Only a minority of these patients will accept to trade appearance for function, in order to alleviate the severe ocular complications of eyelid retraction. Most patients with eyelid laxity or retraction present with symptoms of exposure keratopathy such as ocular irritation, photophobia, and blurry vision [2, 3]. In addition, some patients present with tearing, typically related to reflex secretion from exposure keratopathy or to stenosis of the lacrimal puncta from keratinization of the lid margin and medial ectropion. Tearing can also functional naso-lacrimal duct obstruction, from altered eyelid mechanics and weakness of the orbicularis oculi muscle with malfunction of the lacrimal pump.

18.2 Anatomy of the Eyelid and Cheek

The normal position of the lower eyelid margin is tangential to the inferior limbus while the lateral canthal angle should rest approximately 2 mm above the position of the medial canthus [3, 4]. After successful blepharoplasty, the lateral canthus should continue to sit 2 mm above the medial canthus. If the lateral canthal angle is inferiorly displaced, a round eye will result, which is cosmetically undesirable (Fig. 18.3). If the lower eyelid margin is inferiorly displaced, even if the position of the lateral canthus is adequate, the patient will present with eyelid retraction and scleral show, both of which cause cosmetic and functional deficit (Fig. 18.4) [3, 5, 6].

Anatomically, the lower lid is composed of three lamellae (Fig. 18.5) [3, 4, 7]. The anterior lamella consists of skin and the orbicularis oculi muscle and may be thought of as a continuum from the corner of the mouth to the lower eyelid

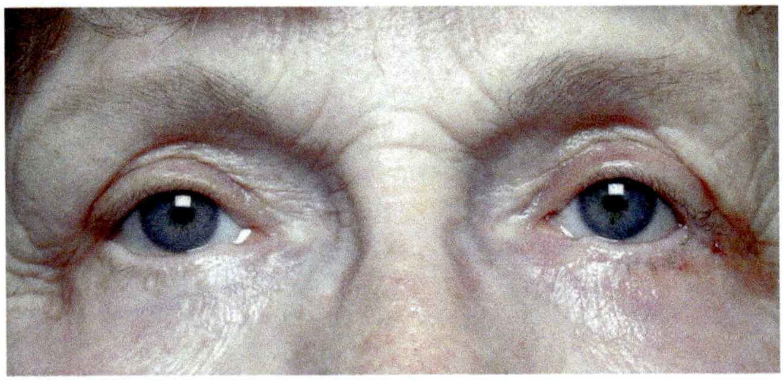

Fig. 18.3 Clinical photograph showing marked rounding of lateral canthi and shortening of the horizontal palpebral aperture in a patient who underwent skin and muscle flap lower eyelid blepharoplasty 6 years ago

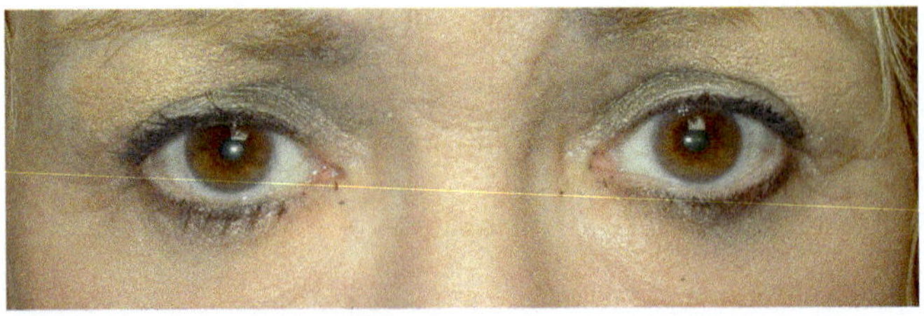

Fig. 18.4 Clinical photograph showing eyelid retraction, after skin and muscle flap lower eyelid blepharoplasty, despite normal position of the lateral canthi

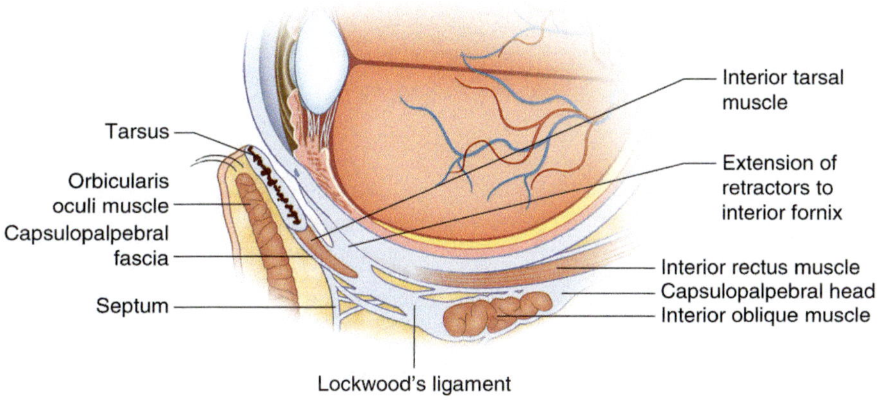

Fig. 18.5 Lower eyelid anatomy in sagital section. The anterior lamella is composed of skin and orbicularis oculi muscle. The middle lamella is composed of the septum. The posterior lamella is composed of tarsus and conjunctiva superiorly and lower lid retractors (inferior tarsal muscle and Lockwood's ligament) and conjunctiva inferiorly

margin. The middle lamella consists of the orbital septum, which originates from the arcus marginalis at the inferior orbital rim and inserts on the inferior tarsal margin. In the unoperated state, the septum is distensible (stretchable) but becomes rigid if scarring occurs secondary to surgery or trauma. The posterior lamella is composed of conjunctiva and either tarsus (superiorly) or lower eyelid retractors (inferiorly). The eyelid fat lies between the orbital septum and the eyelid retractors, similar to the preaponeurotic fat in the upper eyelid.

The orbicularis oculi is a circular sphincter muscle with three parts: the pretarsal orbicularis oculi, which lies anterior to the tarsus; the preseptal orbicularis oculi, which overlies the orbital septum and the orbital orbicularis oculi, the part that overlies the bone surrounding the orbit (Fig. 18.6). The tissue layers just below the inferior orbital rim, from anterior to posterior are skin, orbital orbicularis oculi muscle, suborbicularis oculi fat (SOOF), periosteum, and bone. The SOOF is continuous inferiorly with the cheek fat pad (Fig. 18.7). After the fourth decade, the orbital orbicularis oculi muscle, the SOOF, and the cheek fat pad start to descend [8]. Thus, when reconstructing the lower eyelid, the mobilization and elevation of the SOOF, either in a pre- or a subperiosteal plane, will elevate the overlying orbital orbicularis oculi muscle and the skin. Midface advancement recruits skin for the eyelid and helps avoid skin grafting.

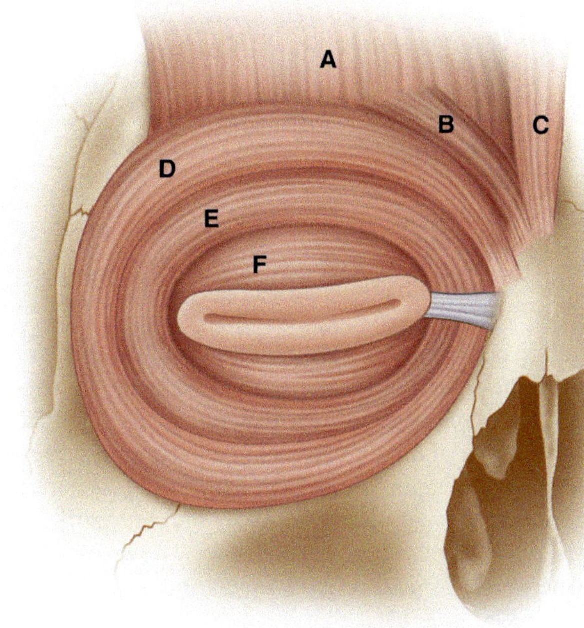

Fig. 18.6 Anatomy of the orbicularis oculi (upper and lower lid) and adjacent muscles. (**A**) Frontalis muscle; (**B**) corrugator muscle; (**C**) procerus muscle; (**D**) orbital portion of the orbicularis oculi muscle; (**E**) preseptal portion of the orbicularis oculi muscle; (**F**) pretarsal portion of the orbicularis oculi muscle

18.3 Pathophysiology of Postblepharoplasty Lower Eyelid Retraction

After blepharoplasty, the structure and the position of the eyelid should be preserved. The lateral canthus should continue to be 2 mm superior to the medial canthus and the lower eyelid margin should still lie tangential to the inferior limbus. Consequently, each of the three lamellae should have adequate vertical height. There are five possible causes of postblepharoplasty lower eyelid retraction: untreated horizontal eyelid laxity, vertical inadequacy of the anterior lamella, vertical inadequacy of the middle lamella, vertical inadequacy of the posterior lamella, and weakening or paralysis of the orbicularis oculi muscle. Eyelid malposition after surgery can result in ectropion, if the anterior lamella is vertically shortened; entropion, if the posterior lamella is vertically shortened; or retraction, if the middle lamella is vertically shortened [1–14].

The incidence of postblepharoplasty lower lid retraction is also influenced by the prominence of the globe relative to the anterior projection of the inferior orbital rim (see chap. 26),

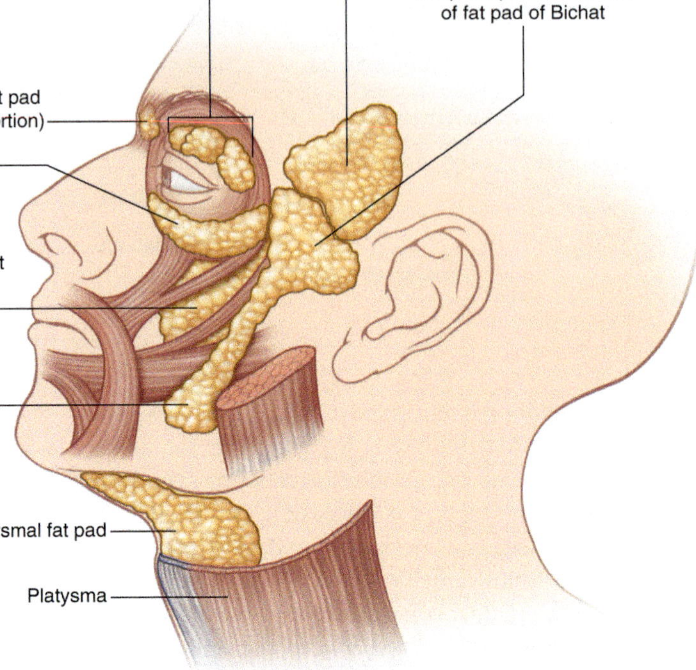

Fig. 18.7 Anatomy of periocular fat pads. *SOOF* suborbicularis oculi fat

by intra and postoperative bleeding, and by the degree of disruption of the orbital septum which results in inflammation and subsequent scarring [12–14]. The wound healing process also plays a role in the development of lower eyelid retraction. Hematoma within the surgical planes induces contraction during the healing process. An eyelid with horizontal laxity or even a normal eyelid may be pulled down by gravity under the weight of postoperative edema and heal in an inferior position [10, 12, 13].

The most common surgical error that causes eyelid retraction is the excessive removal of skin and muscle from the lower eyelids. Removing anterior lamellar tissue in the face of uncorrected lower lid laxity further increases then incidence ectropion and/or lower eyelid retraction.

18.4 Presentation

The unhappy post-lower eyelid blepharoplasty patients usually complain of the loss of the almond shaped of their eyes, pulled down lower lids, and a tired or fatigued appearance. Frequently, they also have functional concerns such as blurry vision, red eyes, ocular discomfort, irritation, and tearing [1, 3, 5, 6]. Even though these patients have inadequate vertical lower eyelid skin, they often complain of excess lower eyelid tissue, especially when they smile. The apparent excess skin in the lower eyelids after blepharoplasty is due in part to the loss of skin elasticity and cannot be corrected by further removal of skin.

18.5 Preoperative Evaluation

The evaluation of patients with lower eyelid retraction starts with measuring the lateral canthal position relative to the medial canthus and the margin-reflex distance 2 (MRD2) which is the distance from the pupillary light reflex to the lower eyelid margin. The “distraction” and “snap” tests are then performed to assess for horizontal lower eyelid laxity and elasticity, respectively. Vertical adequacy or inadequacy of the lower eyelid is determined next and is an essential part of the evaluation. Asking the patient to squint and smile helps determine if the eyelid can rise without restriction. The patient is then asked to close the eyelids gently and raise the eyebrows and any degree of lagophthalmos should be measured. It is also important to note if the lower eyelid moves upward and the punctum moves medially, with lid closure. Failure of the eyelid to move in and upward with closure is suggestive of paralysis of the orbicularis oculi muscle. The lower eyelid is then pushed superiorly with one or two fingers to determine whether there is any tethering to the inferior orbital rim. The patient is asked to open the mouth to see if stretching the anterior lamella pulls the eyelid inferiorly. The relative degree of proptosis is measured with the Hertel exophthalmometer. The degree of globe prominence relative to the cheeks and inferior orbital rim is probably even more important, as this dictates whether the lower eyelid needs to be horizontally shortened or vertically elevated. The shortest distance between two points is a straight line. However, as the eyelids travel on the meridian of the globe, for prominent globes the distance from the medial canthus around the globe to the lateral canthus is greater. The "procedure surgeon" who plans to horizontally tighten the lower eyelid in the face of a prominent globe in hopes of vertically elevating the lid will find that horizontal eyelid tightening over a prominent globe results in lowering of eyelid position.

18.6 SurgicalP rocedures

There are two groups of surgical interventions that are necessary for the correction of postblepharoplasty lower eyelid retraction in the cosmetic patient. The first group of procedures, called "lateral canthal resuspension," is aimed at horizontally tightening the lower eyelid and can be either a canthopexy or a canthoplasty [1–10]. A canthopexy involves tightening the lateral canthal tendon without opening the canthal angle. In contrast, a canthoplasty implies performing a canthotomy/cantholysis before resuspending the lower eyelid to the lateral orbital rim periosteum. The lateral tarsal strip (LTS), first introduced in 1979, remains one of the most common canthoplasty procedures performed today [6, 15–17]. LTS is a powerful technique, very useful in cases of profound eyelid laxity or ectropion where horizontal eyelid shortening is necessary to achieve adequate eyelid tightening. Unfortunately, this can also lead to shortening of the horizontal palpebral aperture, which is cosmetically undesirable, and patients will complain about it [18]. It seems that nobody wants a smaller appearing eye. Another unwanted effect of the tarsal strip procedure is the imbrication of the upper and lower eyelids laterally from supraplacement and shortening of the lower eyelid with preservation of the upper eyelid length [18, 19]. A modified LTS procedure that addresses this issue in patients with severe eyelid laxity, as seen in the floppy eyelid syndrome, has recently been described [20].

For less severe eyelid laxity, a canthopexy can be performed through either an upper or a lower eyelid incision, where the suture is passed under the skin without externalization through the lateral canthal angle [6, 21, 22]. A modified canthopexy technique where the suture is passed ab externo through a small incision in the lateral canthal angle has also been described [23–25]. With this technique, a double armed suture is buried in the lateral canthus and looped around the lateral canthal tendon. An upper eyelid incision is used to retrieve the suture and to attach it to the lateral orbital rim. Although horizontal palpebral aperture shortening is usually not an issue with canthopexy techniques, eyelid imbriction can be seen if the inferior crus of the lateral canthal tendon is preferentially tightened or supraplaced.

We use a modified lateral canthal resuspension technique that tightens the upper and lower eyelids simultaneously without imbricating the eyelids and without shortening the palpebral aperture. This technique also obviates the need for performing a canthotomy and is done through an upper eyelid incision for which reason we called it "the lateral canthal resuspension-sine canthotomy" (LCR-SC, in press). One must realize that canthoplasties and canthopexies can only correct for horizontal eyelid laxity. If the lower eyelid is vertically inadequate, performing only a canthoplasty or a canthopexy procedure will not correct the problem.

The second group of procedures is of those that correct for the vertical inadequacy of the lower eyelid [4, 5, 8, 10, 11, 26–47]. The more prominent the globe, the less likely horizontal tightening will improve the final eyelid position. The standard horizontal eyelid tightening procedures can be anticipated to fail in patients with vertical inadequacy and to worsen the final lower eyelid position in patients with vertical inadequacy as well as relative prominence of the globe. After lysing the entire eyelid cicatrix that inhibits upward movement by tethering the eyelid to the inferior orbital rim, each individual layer is vertically augmented, as necessary. The anterior lamella is lengthened by performing a midface lift in which the entire cheek, which is continuous with the eyelid, is advanced and supported superiorly by suturing the orbital orbicularis oculi muscle and the SOOF, or the undermined cheek periosteum in subperiosteal midface elevation, to the orbital rim periosteum or temporalis fascia [5, 9, 10, 21, 23, 24]. To correct for middle lamella inadequacy, the vertically tethering middle lamella is horizontally divided from the inferior tarsal margin and all the scar tissue is lysed. A graft, the dimensions of which are calculated during the preoperative evaluation of the lower eyelid position, is then placed in the posterior lower eyelid to act as a spacer and prevent middle and posterior lamellar contraction during healing [4, 5, 8, 10, 11, 26–35, 40–47]. The posterior lamella is reconstructed by the same spacer graft placement between the inferior tarsal margin and the recessed conjunctiva and lower eyelid retractors. The graft becomes an inferior vertical extension of the existing tarsal plate and acts not only as a spacer but also as a buttress to support the lower eyelid. This buttress support for the lower eyelid is particularly useful and important in helping maintain a superior position of the reconstructed eyelid in the presence of a prominent globe.

In this manner, a total lower eyelid reconstruction, using a layer-by-layer independent reconstruction technique is performed. The anterior lamella is reconstructed with the mid-face lift, by recruiting both skin and muscle. The middle lamella is reconstructed by separation and scar lysis.

The posterior lamella is reconstructed by vertically augmenting the mucosal surface with the spacer graft.

Different materials have been used as spacer grafts throughout time. Desirable qualities of a spacer graft include easy accessibility and storage, affordability, short preparation time, and good handling properties allowing intraoperative manipulation, sizing, shaping, placement, and fixation. The graft should also induce minimal inflammation after implantation and permit native tissue ingrowth without shrinkage. With time, the implant should become virtually incorporated in the native tissues and provide long lasting support. For the purpose of eyelid reconstruction, the ideal material should mimic a tarso-conjunctival composite in thickness, surface quality, and resilience. Many different materials have been used, including autogenous, allogenic, and synthetic grafts. Commonly used autogenous grafts are hard palate, ear cartilage, temporalis fascia, fascia lata, buccal mucosa, nasal septal cartilage, tarsus, and periosteum [4, 5, 8, 10, 11, 29–39]. Allogenic donor sclera and, more recently, bioengineered grafts such as Alloderm (LifeCell, Branchburg, NJ), tarSys (IOP, Costa Mesa, CA), Enduragen (Porex, Newnan, GA), and DermaMatrix (Synthese, West Chester, PA) have also been used [40–47]. Although promising results with the use of each one of these grafts have been reported, none of them is perfect. Scleral grafts are not permanent and tend to be degraded by the body, resulting in graft shrinkage over time [40]. Temporalis fascia grafts do not replace the conjunctiva, which can lead to ocular irritation initially and contraction of the graft later on [32]. Auricular cartilage grafts, on the other hand, are much stiffer than the tarsus and do not replace the conjunctiva [31, 34]. Composite grafts such as the palate and nasal septum have the distinct advantage of replacing both tarsus and conjunctiva. Unfortunately, some of these techniques have the inconvenience of poor access, limited tissue availability, and donor site morbidity.

The gold standard spacer for lower eyelid reconstruction remains, however, the hard palate graft, which is harvested from an area between the gingiva and the palatine raphe. The use of hard palate mucosal grafts in lower eyelid reconstruction was first described by Siegel in 1985 for repair after tumor excision [35]. Its use as a spacer graft was subsequently reported for patients with cicatricial entropion, eyelid retraction secondary to thyroid eye disease, postblepharoplasty lower eyelid retraction, lagophthalmos after surgery for paralytic ptosis, and contracted socket [4, 5, 8, 10, 11, 29, 35, 39]. Hard palate mucosa serves as an ideal material for posterior lamella replacement for many reasons. It is a composite tissue that provides both structural support and mucous membrane replacement. Its mucosal surface nicely replaces conjunctiva, whereas its stiff structure provides eyelid support similar to that of tarsus. The dense concentration of collagen fibers in the lamina propria of the hard palate gives this tissue its stability and firmness, but at the same time it has enough flexibility to allow it to maintain its contour and act as a tarsal replacement with excellent eyelid appearance and function, unlike ear or nasal cartilage. Acting as an internal splint, the palate mucosal graft also prevents shifting of the overlying layers. The eyelid remains stable, and therefore comfortable, for many years. In addition, hard palate mucosa is abundant, easily obtained, easy to handle, and it takes reliably with minimal shrinkage following grafting because of quick vascularization. Furthermore, being an autograft, it is not at risk for rejection. The rule of thumb for determining the vertical height of the spacer graft is to add one millimeter to the amount of vertical inadequacy between the existing and the desired eyelid margin positions. In the more proptotic patient, an additional 1 or even 2 mm of vertical height may be added to compensate for the inferior force exerted by the globe and for the anticipated loss of support due to the lesser horizontal tension that must be used when the globe is prominent.

Hard palate grafts have unfortunately their own disadvantages, including donor site morbidity (postoperative discomfort or bleeding, oral candidiasis, and oronasal fistula), increased operating time for graft harvesting, and occasional keratinization of the mucosal surface with potential ocular surface irritation [4, 5, 8, 11, 29].

The authors commonly use the DermaMatrix allograft, a non-crosslinked acellular human dermis that is processed to allow for fast vascular and cellular ingrowth. We have found that DermaMatrix becomes covered with conjunctiva within several weeks after implantation. Although not a rigid composite graft like the hard palate, DermaMatrix obviates the problems related to donor site morbidity, limited tissue availability, and prolonged operative time. DermaMatrix also comes in a thin and a thick version, with the thick version giving more support when placed in the lower eyelid.

A critical step in the reconstruction process of any retracted lower eyelid is vertical eyelid splinting at the end of surgery using a Frost type suspension suture. This allows the three reconstructed layers of the lower eyelid to fuse in the desired configuration and preserves the vertical dimension of the spacer graft in the early postoperative period.

18.7 Surgical Technique

18.7.1 Scar Lysis and Mobilization

Before making the incision, the lower eyelid margin is grasped with a forceps and pulled superiorly to determine the amount of restriction to superior movement. In the case of scarring of the middle or posterior lamella, this test will be positive. This superior traction test is repeated frequently throughout the procedure. An incision is made centrally through the conjunctiva and lower eyelid retractors at the inferior tarsal margin with Stevens scissors. The incision is extended medially and laterally all the way to the caruncle and the lateral canthus, respectively. Care is taken to avoid damaging the inferior canaliculus and the semilunar fold medially. Injury to the canaliculus may result in epiphora, and injury to the semilunar fold may result in diplopia. Superiorly directed lower eyelid traction is again performed. If scarring is present, this usually shows persistent restriction, because only the posterior lamellar attachments to the inferior tarsal margin have been divided. Now, the posterior lamella (conjunctiva and lower lid retractors) is grasped at its leading edge and pulled superiorly to assess its vertical adequacy. A 4.0 silk traction suture passed through the conjunctiva and lower lid retractors can be used to put superior tension on the posterior lamella. At this point, the posterior lamella should be entirely free and should stretch superiorly without restriction. If it does not, the surgeon will find a cicatrix between the lower lid retractors and inferior orbital rim. Dissection is continued in the preseptal plane as far inferiorly as the arcus marginalis at the inferior orbital rim. At this point, superior traction is limited by middle lamellar tether, anterior lamellar inadequacy, or both. To further determine the cause of restriction, the cheek (anterior lamella) is digitally pushed superiorly. If this fully relieves the retraction, then the restriction is in the anterior lamella. In contrast, if the eyelid is still tethered, then most likely the restriction is midlamellar in which case the cicatrix in the plane of the septum that tethers the lower eyelid retractors to the inferior orbital rim has to be lysed. The conjunctiva and lower lid retractors are then pulled superiorly again. If the procedure did not fully release the entire middle lamellar cicatrix, the septum can be dissected free from the arcus marginalis along the inferior orbital rim to provide further release.

The orbitomalar ligament is then incised sharply with Stevens scissors and the orbicularis oculi muscle is elevated from the orbital rim, in a preperiosteal plane, using a vertical spreading technique with Stevens scissors followed by a Sayre elevator. The orbitomalar ligament is released all across the inferior and infero-lateral orbital rim to allow for superior mobilization of the orbicularis oculi muscle, in preparation for the midface lift.

18.7.2 Midface Elevation

The authors' current thinking on midface elevation focuses less on SOOF lifting and more on repositioning of the orbicularis oculi muscle. In our hands, a preperiosteal midface elevation technique performed through an upper eyelid blepharoplasty or lateral skin crease incision is the procedure of choice. A large preperiosteal myocutaneous flap is created first that extends all the way from the brow to the cheek. Dissection initiates in the lateral brow area, where an incision is made with Stevens scissor through the posterior leaf of the deep galea to elevate the brow fat pad from the periosteum (Fig. 18.8). To mobilize the brow, dissection continues for 2 cm above the superior-lateral orbital rim, between the posterior leaf of the deep galea and the periosteum, using a vertical spreading technique. To break into the midface and the lower eyelid, a sharp incision is made with Stevens scissors at the supero-lateral orbital rim beneath the orbicularis oculi muscle to expose the preperiosteal plane. The orbicularis oculi is elevated by releasing the orbitomalar and the zygomaticomalar ligaments using a vertical spreading technique with Stevens scissors (Fig. 18.9). The lateral raphae and the

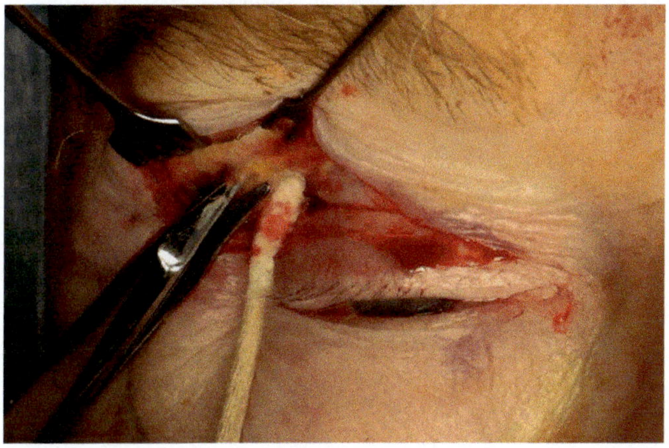

Fig. 18.8 Intraoperative clinical photograph showing the release of deep galea from the arcus marginalis at the superior orbital rim with Stevens scissors. A plane is created between deep galea and periosteum to elevate and mobilize the brow fat pad

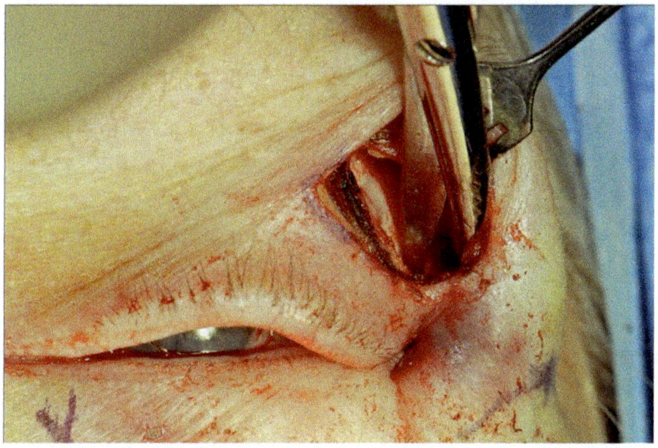

Fig. 18.9 Intraoperative clinical photograph showing elevation of orbicularis oculi muscle at the lateral orbital rim using a vertical spreading technique with Stevens scissors in the preperiosteal plane. The orbitomalar and the zygomaticomalar ligaments are released to create a large myocutaneous flap and mobilize the brow, the lateral canthus, and the cheek as one unit

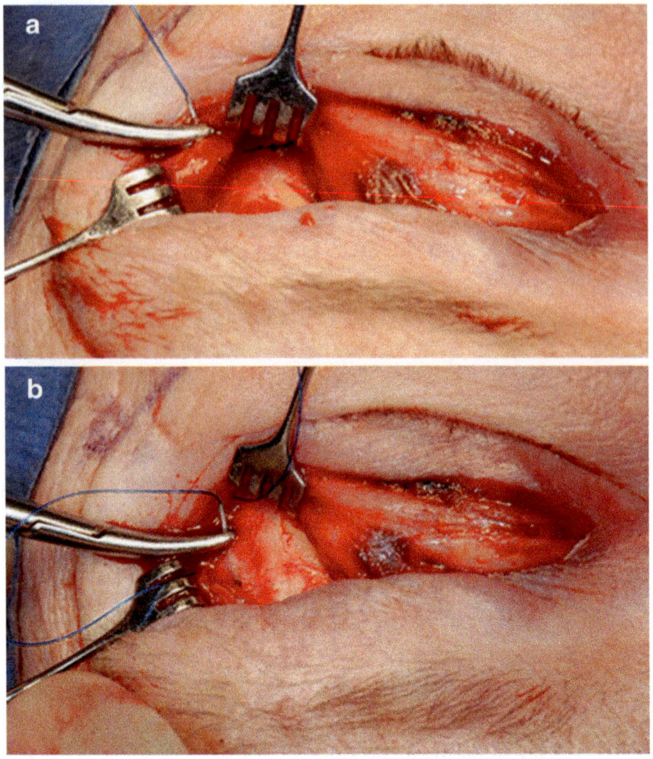

Fig. 18.10 Intraoperative clinical photograph of preperiosteal midface elevation where the (**a**) lateral orbicularis oculi muscle and the fibrous suborbicularis oculi fat (SOOF) (tissues engaged with suture) are (**b**) resuspended to the periosteum overlying the lateral orbital rim with 6.0 Prolene sutures

lateral orbital thickening (LOT) are elevated from the periosteum. However, the posterior limb of the lateral canthal tendon is left attached to the Witnall's tubercle. The dissection is then extended downwards in a plane between the zygomaticus muscles and the SOOF. The planes of dissection created via the transconjunctival lower eyelid incision and the upper lid blepharoplasty incision are united. The midface is then resuspended with one or two 4.0 Prolene sutures. The sutures are passed through the infero-lateral portion of the orbital orbicularis oculi muscle and the fibrous SOOF and attached to the dense periosteum overlying the lateral orbital rim. This creates an orbicularis oculi muscle sling that lifts the cheek superiorly (Fig. 18.10).

18.7.3 Graft Placement

The chosen spacer graft is cut to fit the horizontal lower eyelid defect. As mentioned previously, we use roughly a 1:1 ratio plus 1–2 mm for the vertical dimension, especially with the hard palate mucosal grafts or the rigid synthetic grafts such as tarSys or thick Alloderm. The graft is sutured to the lower border of the tarsal plate with a running 6.0 chromic suture with the knots externalized to the skin. The lower border of the spacer graft is usually left unattached although it can be sutured to the conjunctiva inferiorly with a running 6.0 chromic suture.

18.7.4 Lateral Canthal Resuspension

In our hands, the LCR-SC is the procedure of choice for the majority of patients. To resuspend the lower eyelid, a 4.0 Prolene suture on a P3 needle is passed through the upper eyelid blepharoplasty incision, beneath the orbicularis oculi muscle but above the lateral canthal tendon, and externalized through the apex of the lateral canthal angle at the muco-cutaneous junction (Fig. 18.11a). The suture is then passed back through the same hole in the canthal angle created by the forward pass, but this time inferior and deep to the lateral canthal tendon, and externalized through the blepharoplasty incision (Fig. 18.11b). The suture is then secured to periosteum just inside the lateral orbital rim at the desired height (Fig. 18.11c). This procedure combined with a midface lift can be the only intervention necessary in patients that present with lower lid laxity without vertical shortening of the eyelid. However, in patients with vertical eyelid insufficiency, the LCR-SC and the mid-face lift performed through an upper eyelid incision can lead to complete restoration of the eyelid anatomy only when combined with a lower eyelid transconjunctival scar lysis and spacer graft placement. On occasion, an LTS canthoplasy-type procedure is required to correct an advanced lower lid laxity [15–17].

18.7.5 Eyelid Splinting and Casting

In patients with vertical eyelid insufficiency, to ensure adequate anatomical fixation of the reconstructed lower eyelid and to prevent reattachment of the middle lamella to the periosteum and the inferior orbital rim, the eyelid is placed on upward traction for a couple of days. After a bandage contact lens is placed in the eye, a 6.0 Prolene horizontal mattress Frost-type suture is passed vertically through the brow and upper eyelid tarsus and then horizontally through the lower eyelid tarsus and back the same route to the brow. The suture is tied above the brow to place the lower eyelid on an upward stretch. Either one single central suture or two sutures, one medial and one lateral, are placed in this fashion. A tight patch is then placed over the eye using Mastisol® liquid adhesive (Eloquest Healthcare, Ferndale, MI) to act as a cast and prevent postoperative hematoma formation and movement between the lower eyelid lamellae. The patch and the Frost suture are left in place for 3–5 days.

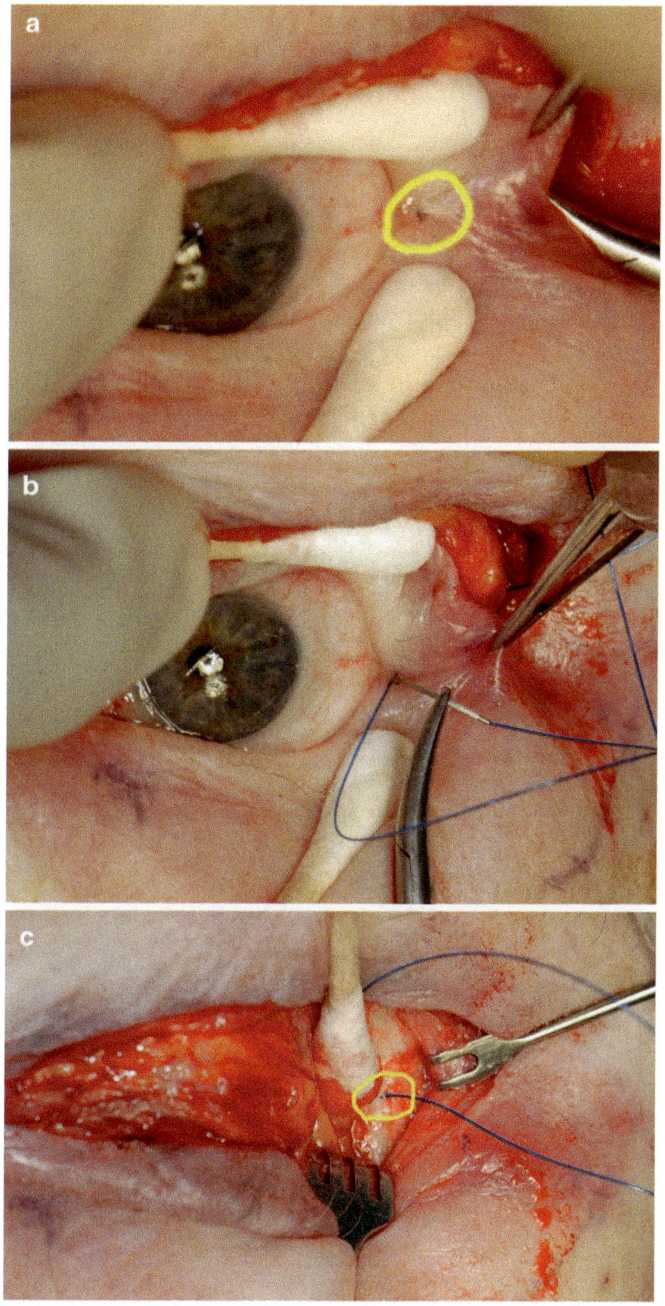

Fig. 18.11 Intraoperative clinical montage showing the three critical steps of the lateral canthal resuspension sine canthotomy technique (LCR-SC). (**a**) Forward pass of a single-armed 6.0 Prolene suture on a P3 needle through the upper eyelid blepharoplasty incision, under the orbicularis oculi muscle but above the lateral canthal tendon, and externalization through the apex of the lateral canthal angle at the mucocutaneous junction (*yellow circle*). (**b**) The suture is passed backwards through the same hole but this time under the lateral canthal tendon and externalized through the blepharoplasty incision. (**c**) The suture is anchored to the periosteum inside the lateral orbital rim (*yellow circle*)

18.8 Conclusion

Lower eyelid retraction remains one of the most dreaded complications of eyelid surgery and occurs in as many as 20% of patients undergoing skin and muscle flap lower eyelid blepharoplasy [1, 2]. Even the most experienced surgeons will occasionally encounter a post-lower eyelid blepharoplasty patient with rounded lateral canthi and retracted lower eyelids. However, the vast majority of cases are the result of skin-focused blepharoplasty procedures and surgical techniques that alter important eyelid structures, such as the orbicularis oculi muscle and the orbital septum, which leads to postoperative eyelid weakening and scarring.

Some techniques that have been proposed for avoiding this complication are proper wound closure to avoid tether of the orbital septum in the operative site, a tight pressure dressing immediately following surgery to prevent hematoma formation, a Frost suture to apply upward traction on the lower eyelid during the early postoperative period, and a transconjunctival approach to fat to avoid violation of the septum and reduce the risk of scar formation [3, 6, 12–14, 48–50].

A thorough preoperative evaluation is essential for determining the pathophysiologic mechanism of eyelid retraction and deciding on the appropriate combination of surgical procedures needed to address the problem. Therefore, a lower eyelid "snap" test, a vertical traction test, and an evaluation for malar descent should be done at a minimum to assess for the contributing factors.

Many different procedures have been proposed for the correction of lower eyelid retraction. Inferior retractor weakening by releasing the sympathetically innervated lower tarsal muscle, recession of the capsulopalpebral fascia, and various horizontal shortening procedures have been used successfully to treat mild cases of eyelid retraction or laxity. For patients presenting with horizontal laxity of the lower eyelid only, without middle lamella scarring and malar descent, studies have shown that a lateral canthoplasty or canthopexy procedure can usually correct the problem [22–25, 51]. However, these lateral canthal resuspension procedures are usually ineffective when used alone in the presence of vertical inadequacy of the lower eyelid [4, 5, 8, 10, 11, 26–35, 40–47]. These patients require correction of the vertical inadequacy by reconstructing all eyelid lamellae involved, in addition to horizontal lower eyelid tightening. We found that, in the majority of patients with severe lower lid retraction, all three factors (lateral canthal tendon laxity, vertical eyelid shortening, and midface descent) are contributing to some extent to the eyelid malposition. For this reason, approaching the problem with any one surgical technique alone is unlikely to lead to optimal correction. Instead, we treat all three components as a functional and cosmetic unit by performing a combined lateral canthopexy, spacer graft placement, and midface elevation. For the rare case where midface lifting is insufficient for reconstruction of a very short anterior lamella, surgeons may have to place a full-thickness skin graft, albeit at an aesthetic expense. This procedure has very low acceptance among cosmetic patients and should be used only as a last resort.

Although the middle and posterior lamellae are more difficult to reconstruct because of the lack of an ideal and readily available graft material, the cosmetic result is more acceptable to the patient. Thus, conjunctiva and tarsus are often supplemented by "spacers," which are free grafts of "substitute" tissue that have physical and histologic properties that make them suitable to support eyelid structures and protect the globe [4, 5, 8, 10, 11, 26–35, 40–47]. The required "spacers" provide augmentation by lengthening the lower eyelid retractors and giving vertical height and stiffness to support the lower eyelid following release of the cicatrix.

Commonly used spacers include autogenous tissue (e.g., hard palate, ear cartilage, nasal septal cartilage, tarsus, periosteum, temporalis fascia, fascia lata, and sclera) as well as alloplastic implants, such as AlloDerm (LifeCell Corp., Branchburg, NJ), Mersilene mesh (Ethicon, Johnson & Johnson, Piscataway, NJ), Enduragen (Porex, Newnan, GA), and DermaMatrix (Synthese, West Chester, PA). AlloDerm has compared unfavorably to palatal grafts in lower eyelid reconstructive surgery. In one series, the use of acellular dermis grafts was associated with a 57% contraction rate as compared with a 16% rate observed with hard palate mucosal grafts [42]. A more recent study using thick AlloDerm grafts showed results comparable to those obtained with hard palate grafts and superior to those obtained with thin AlloDerm grafts [52]. Donor sclera was at one time a popular method; however, it suffers from a number of disadvantages, including postoperative shrinkage and folding, unpredictable final lid position, erythema, bulkiness, and the lack of a mucosal surface. Ear cartilage is also a popular choice but, despite being easy to harvest, it tends to be thicker and stiffer than natural tarsus, resulting in a relatively immobile lower eyelid. Because cartilage is difficult to contour, it can also result in a noticeable bump in the lower eyelid. Furthermore, re-epithelialization is unpredictable over cartilage grafts. Free tarsal grafts are certainly ideal but necessitate surgery on the upper lid tarsus, risking possible untoward changes in the normal upper eyelid contour and height. However, this technique is useful in the rare instance when an upper eyelid tarsectomy is performed for the correction of concurrent upper lid ptosis.

The hard palate graft remains the gold standard because it most closely resembles tarsus in terms of consistency and stiffness, and provides a mucosal surface and good ocular comfort. Moreover, as these patients present after previously unsatisfactory or unsuccessful aesthetic surgery, a graft that provides predictable results is critical. The use of hard palate grafts for the correction of lower eyelid retraction was first described by Kersten et al. in patients with thyroid orbitopathy, with good vertical eyelid splinting achieved even in the setting of advanced proptosis [4]. Cohen and Shorr subsequently reported good results with hard palate grafting for postblepharoplasty lower lid retraction [8]. The dense collagen matrix gives the palatal mucosa a firm consistency to provide adequate support without significant shrinkage.

A variety of approaches to midface elevation have been described in the literature [53–58]. These include upper and lower blepharoplasty incisions, a lateral canthotomy incision, and preauricular techniques. With the aim of maximal superolateral pull, we prefer the upper blepharoplasty approach when combined with a lateral canthopexy and placement of a spacer graft. This allows for well-hidden scars with adequate access to the malar fat pad. Although a subperiosteal malar elevation has been reported to be effective for recruiting skin to the lower eyelid, we have found the preperiosteal dissection quite satisfactory. If the anterior lamellar deficiency cannot be compensated by midface elevation because of the lack of recruitable skin, the patient may require skin grafting to provide adequate external coverage to the eyelid.

While each component of the tripartite procedure can be performed using various techniques described in the literature, we have chosen and modified certain procedures that we feel are most suitable for this patient population. For addressing the lateral canthal laxity, we find our LCR-SC to be an adequate technique for the vast majority of cases. The LCR-SC, a canthopexy-type procedure, is performed through an upper eyelid incision and avoids three common complications seen with the canthoplasy procedures: imbrication of the upper and lower eyelids, postoperative chemosis, and shortening of the horizontal palpebral aperture. In postsurgical patients, avoiding further shortening of the lower eyelid and scarring in the lateral canthal angle is desirable and better achieved with a canthopexy rather than a canthoplasty-type procedure. In addition, our technique is very useful because the same upper eyelid incision is used to perform a midface lift. However, there are certainly cases where a traditional LTS-type procedure is necessary to correct the horizontal lower eyelid laxity by shortening the tarsal plate laterally. Thorough preoperative evaluation should be done to determine the best procedure for each individual patient.

In conclusion, by combining the individual techniques of lateral canthopexy, spacer grafting, and midface suspension into a single tripartite procedure, the moderate to severe lower eyelid retraction found in some post-lower eyelid blepharoplasty patients can be effectively corrected. This approach leads to predictable anatomic results and has a high rate of patient satisfaction.

References

1. Neuhaus R, Baylis H. Complications of lower eyelid blepharoplasty. In: Putterman AM, editor. Cosmetic oculoplastic surgery. New York, NY: Grune & Stratton; 1982.
2. McGraw BL, Adamson PA. Postblepharoplasty ectropion. Arch Otolaryngol Head Neck Surg. 1991;117:852.
3. Patipa M. The evaluation and management of lower eyelid retraction following cosmetic surgery. Plast Reconstr Surg. 2000;106:438.
4. Kersten RC, Kulwin DR, Levartovsky S, et al. Management of lower-lid retraction with hard-palate mucosa grafting. Arch Ophthalmol. 1990;108:1339.
5. Shorr N, Fallor MK. "Madame Butterfly" procedure: combined cheek and lateral canthal suspension procedure for post-blepharoplasty, round eye, and lower eyelid retraction. Ophthal Plast Reconstr Surg. 1985;1:229.
6. Jordan DR, Anderson RL. The tarsal tuck procedure: avoiding eyelid retraction after lower blepharoplasty. Plast Reconstr Surg. 1990;85:22.
7. Wolff E. Anatomy of the Eye and Orbit. 7th ed. Philadelphia, PA: Saunders; 1976.
8. Cohen MS, Shorr N. Eyelid reconstruction with hard palate mucosa graft. Ophthal Plast Reconstr Surg. 1992;8:183–95.
9. McCord Jr CD, Ellis DS. The correction of lower lid malposition following lower lid blepharoplasty. Plast Reconstr Surg. 1993;92:1068.
10. Shorr N. Madame Butterfly procedure with hard palate graft: management of post-blepharoplasty round eye and scleral show. Facial Plast Surg. 1994;10:90.
11. Patel BC, Patipa M, Anderson RL, McLeish W. Management of post-blepharoplasty lower eyelid retraction with hard palate grafts and lateral tarsal strip. Plast Reconstr Surg. 1997;99:1251.
12. McCord Jr CD, Shore JW. Avoidance of complications in lower lid blepharoplasty. Ophthalmology. 1983;90:1039.
13. Edgerton Jr MT. Causes and prevention of lower eyelid ectropion following blepharoplasty. Plast Reconstr Surg. 1972;49:367.
14. Tenzel RR. Complications of blepharoplasty, orbital hematoma, ectropion and scleral show. Clin Plast Surg. 1981;8:797.
15. Anderson RL, Gordy DD. The tarsal strip procedure. Arch Ophthalmol. 1979;97(11):2192–6.
16. Anderson RL. Tarsal strip procedure for correction of eyelid laxity and canthal malposition in the anophthalmic socket. Ophthalmology. 1981;88(9):895–903.
17. Jordan DR, Anderson RL. The lateral tarsal strip revisited. Arch Ophthalmol. 1989;107(4):604–6.
18. Karesh JW, Nirankari VS, Hameroff SB. Eyelid imbrication. An unrecognized cause of chronic ocular irritation. Ophthalmology. 1993;100(6):883–9.
19. Donnenfeld ED, Perry HD, Schrier A, Zagelbaum B, Rodgers R. Lid imbrication syndrome. Diagnosis with rose bengal staining. Ophthalmology. 1994;101(4):763–6.
20. Vagefi MR, Anderson RL. The lateral tarsal strip mini-tarsorrhaphy procedure. Arch Facial Plast Surg. 2009;11(2):136–9.
21. Webster RC, Davidson TM, Reardon EJ, Smith RC. Suspending sutures in blepharoplasty. Arch Otolaryngol. 1979;105(10):601–4.
22. Whitaker LA. Selective alteration of palpebral fissure form by lateral canthopexy. Plast Reconstr Surg. 1984;74(5):611–9.
23. Hamra ST. The role of the septal reset in creating a youthful eyelid-cheek complex in facial rejuvenation. Plast Reconstr Surg. 2004;113(7):2124–41; discussion 2142–4.
24. Hamra ST. The zygorbicular dissection in composite rhytidectomy: an ideal midface plane. Plast Reconstr Surg. 1998;102(5):1646–57.
25. Rizvi M, Lypka M, Gaon M, Kovacev T, Eisemann B, Eisemann MJ. Minimally invasive lateral canthopexy (MILC). J Plast Reconstr Aesthet Surg. 2010;63(9):1434–6.
26. Shorr N, Perry JD, Goldberg RA, et al. The safety and applications of acellular human dermal allograft in ophthalmic plastic and reconstructive surgery. Ophthal Plast Reconstr Surg. 2000; 16:223.
27. Rubin PA, Fay AM, Remulla HD, Maus M. Ophthalmic plastic applications of acellular dermal allografts. Ophthalmology. 1999;106:2091.
28. Fay AM, Pieroth L, Rubin PAD. An animal model of lower eyelid spacer grafting with acellular dermis. Ophthal Plast Reconstr Surg. 2001;17:270.
29. Patipa M, Patel BC, McLeish W, Anderson RL. Use of palate grafts for treatment of post-surgical lower eyelid retraction: a technical review. J Craniomaxillofac Trauma. 1996;2:18.
30. van der Meulen JC. The use of mucosa-lined flaps in eyelid reconstruction: a new approach. Plast Reconstr Surg. 1982;70:139.
31. Marks MW, Argenta LC, Friedman RJJ, Hall JD. Conchal cartilage and composite grafts for correction of lower lid retraction. Plast Reconstr Surg. 1989;83:629.
32. Holt JE, Holt GR, Van Kirk M. Use of temporalis fascia in eyelid reconstruction. Ophthalmology. 1984;91:89.
33. Obear MF, Smith B. Tarsal grafting to elevate the lower lid margin. Am J Ophthalmol. 1965;59:1088.
34. Baylis HI, Rosen N, Neuhaus RW. Obtaining auricular cartilage for reconstructive surgery. Am J Ophthalmol. 1982;93:709.
35. Siegel RJ. Palatal grafts for eyelid reconstruction. Plast Reconstr Surg. 1985;76:411.
36. Vecchione TR. Palatal grafts for lip reconstruction. Ann Plast Surg. 1983;10:301.
37. Yoshimura Y, Nakajima T. Tracheoplasty with palatal mucoperiosteal graft. Plast Reconstr Surg. 1990;86:558.
38. Hall HD, O'Steen AN. Free grafts of palatal mucosa in mandibular vestibuloplasty. J Oral Surg. 1970;28:565.
39. Holck DE, Foster JA, Dutton JJ, Dillon HD. Hard palate mucosal grafts in the treatment of the contracted socket. Ophthal Plast Reconstr Surg. 1999;15:202.
40. Doxanas MT, Dryden RM. The use of sclera in the treatment of dysthyroid eyelid retraction. Ophthalmology. 1981;88:887.
41. Karesh JW, Fabrega MA, Rodrigues MM, Glaros DS. Poly tetrafluoroethylene as an interpositional graft material for the correction of lower eyelid retraction. Ophthalmology. 1989;96:419.
42. Sullivan SA, Dailey RA. Graft contraction: a comparison of acellular dermis versus hard palate mucosa in lower eyelid surgery. Ophthal Plast Reconstr Surg. 2003;19:14.
43. Wainwright DJ. Use of an acellular allograft dermal matrix (AlloDerm) in the management of full-thickness burns. Burns. 1995;21:243.
44. Tobin HA, Karas ND. Lip augmentation using an AlloDerm graft. J Oral Maxillofac Surg. 1998;56:722.
45. Kridel RW, Foda H, Lunke KC. Septal perforation repair with acellular human dermal allograft. Arch Otolaryngol Head Neck Surg. 1998;124:73.
46. Jones FR, Schwartz BM, Silverstein P. Use of a nonimmunogenic acellular dermal allograft for soft tissue augmentation. Aesthet Surg Q. 1996;16:196–201.
47. Patrinely JR. Application of acellular dermal allografts. Ophthalmology. 2000;107:1966.
48. Zarem HA, Resnick JI. Expanded applications for transconjunctival lower lid blepharoplasty. Plast Reconstr Surg. 1991;88:215.
49. Kim JW, Ellis DS, Stewart WB. Correction of lower eyelid retraction by transconjunctival retractor excision and lateral eyelid suspension. Ophthal Plast Reconstr Surg. 1999;15:341.
50. Goldberg RA, Lessner AM, Shorr N, Baylis HI. The transconjunctival approach to the orbital floor and orbital fat: a retrospective study. Ophthal Plast Reconstr Surg. 1990;6:241.
51. Baylis HI, Nelson ER, Goldberg RA. Lower eyelid retraction following blepharoplasty. Ophthal Plast Reconstr Surg. 1992; 8:170.

52. Taban M, Douglas R, Li T, Goldberg RA, Shorr N. Efficacy of "thick" acellular human dermis (AlloDerm) for lower eyelid reconstruction: comparison with hard palate and thin AlloDerm grafts. Arch Facial Plast Surg. 2005;7(1):38–44.
53. Spinelli HM. Atlas of aesthetic eyelid and periocular surgery. Philadelphia: Saunders; 2004. p. 23–57, 120–35, 163.
54. Anderson RDA, Lo MW. Endoscopic malar/midface suspension procedure. Plast Reconstr Surg. 1998;102:2196.
55. Hinderer UT. Vertical preperiosteal rejuvenation of the frame of the eyelids and midface. Plast Reconstr Surg. 1999;104:1482.
56. Hester TR, Codner MA, McCord CD. The "centrofacial" approach for correction of facial ageing using the transblepharoplasty subperiosteal cheek lift. Aesthet Surg Q. 1996;16:51.
57. Edelstein C, Balch K, Shorr N, Goldberg RA. The transeyelid subperiosteal midface-lift in the unhappy postblepharoplasty patient. Semin Ophthalmol. 1998;13(3):107–14. Review.
58. Patel MP, Shapiro MD, Spinelli HM. Combined hard palate spacer graft, midface suspension, and lateral canthoplasty for lower eyelid retraction: a tripartite approach. Plast Reconstr Surg. 2005;115(7):2105–14; discussion 2115–7.

19 Laser Management of Festoons

Adam J. Scheiner and Sterling S. Baker

Key Points

- Correcting lower eyelid festoons adds greatly to overall rejuvenation of the lower eyelid–cheek complex.
- Traditional incisional techniques to correct festoons are often time intensive and yield suboptimal results.
- Festoons have been reported to result from damage to the skin, and potentially to oppositional underlying muscular forces in the tissue deep to the festoons. Our experience and results have substantiated the skin as a primary etiologic factor.
- Both CO_2 and certain Er:Yag lasers can be used to treat lower eyelid skin folds and festoons effectively.
- It is important to distinguish between the relatively thin skin above the orbital rim and the relatively thick skin below the orbital rim when treating festoons with laser skin resurfacing.
- The lower eyelid skin should be treated more conservatively above the orbital rim and more aggressively below the rim.
- The end point for laser treatment of lower eyelid festoons is no further tissue shrinkage with the last laser application.
- It is important to create a transition zone with lighter laser ablations around the border of the more aggressively treated skin to avoid creating a demarcation line from the treated region to the untreated surrounding skin.
- Application of laser safety principles is critical when using lasers to improve festoons.
- Knowledge of postoperative laser skin healing care and possible complications is critical to the clinical and aesthetic outcome.

S.S. Baker (✉)
Assistant Clinical Professor, Departments of Ophthalmology and Dermatology, University of Oklahoma College of Medicine, Oklahoma City, OK, USA
e-mail: sbaker@baker-holloman.com

19.1 Introduction

Skin folds that may occur at the junction of the lower eyelid and cheek are known as festoons [1]. They are a difficult finding to treat in rejuvenation of the lower eyelid–cheek complex. While skin excision, muscle plication, canthal suspension, and judicious removal or translocation of orbital fat can improve the contour of the lower lid and midface, the quality of the overlying skin can often dramatically affect the final cosmetic outcome.

Clinically, festoons appear in the inferior area of the lower eyelid where the thin eyelid skin transitions into the thicker facial skin of the cheek. While festoons are often seen with prolapsed orbital fat, their distinguishing feature is redundant or ballotable skin caudal to this area of transition. Festoons can vary in severity from localized folds of skin in the inferior lower lid to protuberances on the cheek (Fig. 19.1). Furnas and others have suggested that laxity in the orbicularis oculi muscle of the lower eyelids is implicated as an etiology based largely on their intraoperative observations. This explanation seems counter-intuitive when considering the movement of the muscle itself.

The facial muscles of the lower eyelid and cheek are the orbicularis oculi muscles above and the upper lip elevators below. The skin and subcuticular tissues in this region are secured to deep structures by orbitomalar retaining ligaments which were demonstrated in convincing microscopic detail by Kikkawa et al. [2]. In their paper, Mendelson et al. [3] further expanded the anatomic definition of this area by describing a prezygomatic area bounded by the lower eyelid above, the lower temple superolaterally, the cheek laterally, and the infrazygomatic cheek below. Their cadaver studies led them to conclude that the zygomatico-cutaneous ligaments at the inferior border of the area are stronger than the orbicularis retaining ligaments at the superior border of this region. On the basis of these observations, we can surmise that festoons may form as a consequence of this comparative

G.G. Massry et al. (eds.), *Master Techniques in Blepharoplasty and Periorbital Rejuvenation*,
DOI 10.1007/978-1-4614-0067-7_19, © Springer Science+Business Media, LLC 2011

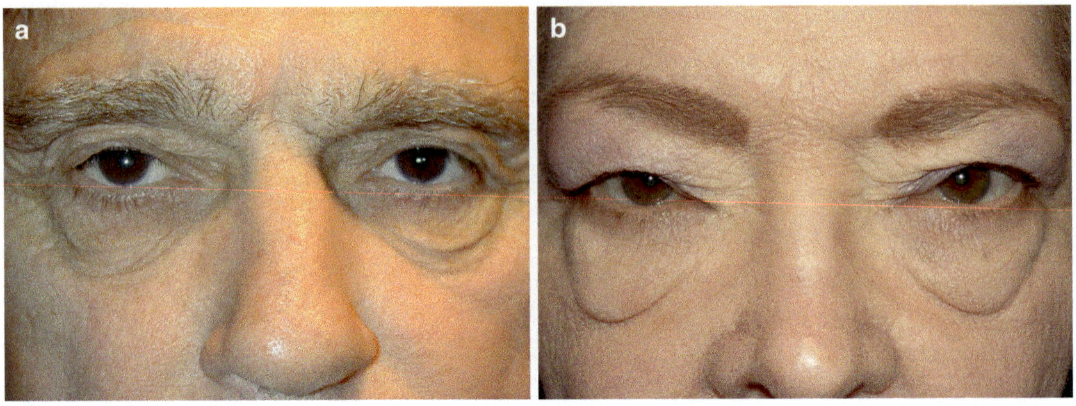

Fig. 19.1 (**a**) Sixty-six-year old man with festoons of the lower lid; (**b**) 67-year-old woman with festoons of the upper cheek

weakness in the superior orbicularis retaining ligament, allowing the overlying lax skin to slide caudally over the relatively stronger support of the zygomatico-cutaneous ligament.

Festoons are predominantly found as a condition of aging. However, other factors such as solar elastosis, tobacco abuse, or other environmental factors contribute to skin laxity and festoon formation. Another possible explanation may be muscular in origin. Festoons tend to occur at the level of the junction of the orbital orbicularis oculi muscle, which contracts in a horizontal direction, and the upper lip elevators, which contract in a vertical direction. These two muscle groups act at approximate right angles to each other, which could damage intrinsic skin elasticity as well as stretch the deeper retaining ligaments.

Festoons may occur as a familial trait and can be exacerbated by allergies. Goldberg et al. [4] proposed that loss of skin elasticity in the malar eminence leads to festoon formation. While festoons are most often cosmetic concerns, they can rarely be significant enough to produce functional defects by compromising the inferior visual field. Esmaeli et al. described such a case of lower lid festoons, which occurred during treatment of chronic myelogenous leukemia [5].

Medical treatment of festoons with oral diuretics or steroid injections may produce minimal improvement, which is usually transient. Superficial skin procedures such as chemical peels can improve rhytids but are largely ineffective for festoons. Surgical treatment by creating large lower lid skin or skin muscle flaps has been described as being effective [1]. These flaps involve relatively extensive dissections that risk iatrogenic ectropion formation. In addition, they are often suboptimal in their results. Another surgical alternative is the direct resection of the festoon itself, but this surgery is seldom used because it has the potential to create a visible scar on the midface [6]. Laser resurfacing is a relatively simple and effective alternative to these surgical flaps. One of us (SSB) initially presented and published the technique in the mid 1990 [7].

19.2 Laser Tissue Interactions

Patel developed the CO_2 laser [8], which emits at 10,600 nm. The concept of selective photothermolysis explains the tissue effect produced by lasers [9]. The chromophore or target in tissue for both the CO_2 and Er:Yag lasers [9, 10] is water. Early incisional applications of the CO_2 laser were developed chiefly by gynecologists and otolaryngologists. In 1984, the first extensive periorbital CO_2 laser application was reported in as a series of blepharoplasties [11]. In1988, laser techniques were developed for tranconjunctival lower lid blepharoplasty [12]. In 1985, initial laser resurfacing techniques for facial lesions were reported for the treatment of actinic cheilitis [13]. Further uses of topical laser therapy were developed as resurfacing applications to treat periorbital facial rhytides [14]. Newer, pulsed, and high energy CO_2 and Er:Yag lasers (emitting at 2,940 nm) have extended precision and predictability to laser skin resurfacing of the face by producing dermal changes in a controlled fashion [10, 15–21].

CO_2 and Er:Yag lasers produce skin changes by vaporizing water in the skin. Skin, which is damaged to less than full thickness, will heal by forming new elastin and new more tightly cross-linked collagen. In their clinical applications, these lasers differ in their coefficient of absorption with the Er:Yag being more efficiently absorbed by water than the CO_2 laser. Vaporization of water in the skin requires a fluence of 4.5–5.0 J/cm^2 at the wavelength emitted by the CO_2 laser while ablation from the Er:Yag laser requires approximately 1.0 J/cm^2. In terms of clinical relevancy, this means that more of a given ablative pulse of CO_2 energy remains at the site of application in the form of sub-ablative thermal energy than an equivalent pulse of energy emitted by an Er:Yag laser. The duration of the laser pulse also determines how much thermal energy is conducted to adjacent tissue from the site of application. The thermal relaxation time of skin is about 800 μs. If ablation occurs in less than that time interval, most of the thermal energy produced during vaporization will not be conducted to adjacent tissue. The most reliable way to achieve that objective is to deliver the laser energy in the form of an ablative pulse of less duration than the thermal relaxation time of skin. The Er:Yag laser energy is emitted from a doped crystal, which is limited by its design to a pulsed emission of about 250 μs. CO_2 lasers are gas lasers which emit in a continuous fashion. To generate time limited exposure to tissue, CO_2 lasers must be rapidly swept across the target tissue or gated in some fashion to be effective at limiting thermal damage. Even in the limited exposure mode though, they still impart a moderate amount of thermal damage to the tissue adjacent to the wound because of their relatively less efficient coefficient of absorption. This factor can be used to the practitioner's advantage in achieving festoon reduction. The same clinical result can be achieved from the Er:Yag laser by combining two pulses in rapid succession. The first pulse emits at a fluence higher than the ablative threshold while the second pulse emits at a sub-ablative fluence. This second pulse imparts thermal energy in a tunable fashion [10, 19–27].

Residual thermal energy at the site of the laser application accomplishes two objectives. First, bleeding from superficial vessels in the upper dermis is controlled by the cautery effect of that residual thermal energy. This control is necessary because the water in blood on the surface of the treated skin becomes the chromophore for successive passes of the laser, thereby limiting the effect of the laser to the surface of the target tissue. Second, thermal energy in skin produces relatively deep collagen fiber devitalization, and most importantly collagen contraction [22]. This becomes the framework for the new collagen formation in the healing skin.

19.3 Preoperative Evaluation and Patient Selection

Laser skin resurfacing is an excellent treatment option for festoons. However, it is an elective procedure requiring an interval of time for healing, with potential postoperative morbidity. As such, it is important to evaluate patients thoroughly and confirm that they have realistic expectations, and understand potential complications about the procedure. The areas of the face to be treated with the laser should be confirmed, and patients should be educated about the course and importance of their postoperative care.

Patients are informed of the traditional indications for laser skin resurfacing including improvement of sun damaged skin, including actinic keratoses and seborrheic keratoses; facial rhytids; dyschromia; and scar revision. They are then told how the laser can also be used to reduce, or eliminate, the prominence of their festoons.

Any suspicious skin lesions must be biopsied and treated appropriately before undergoing treatment with the laser. If either a frank or latent ectropion is noted on exam, plans should be made to correct that condition at the time of surgery. Patients should be shown photos of the actual daily healing progress of previous patients. This can be helpful in preparing the patient for what can be a challenging postoperative recovery.

The patient should be educated on all the possible complications and their treatment.

Photography of the treatment areas is critical and can be valuable in discussing the patient's expectations. The goal is to improve facial rhytids and festoons. It is not appropriate to guarantee that these conditions can be fully resolved. The strategy of under promising and over delivering can serve the practitioner well.

Medical and dermatologic histories should be obtained. The pigmentation skin type should be noted. Fitzpatrick Class III skin types or darker have an increased risk of pigmentation change after the procedure. The healing of the skin after laser skin resurfacing depends on the density of the pilosebaceous appendages in the treatment area. Any factors which may affect the pilosebaceous glands such as previous facial radiation or use of oral retinoids for 1 year prior can put the patient at risk for poor healing after laser treatment. Active acne should be treated prior to resurfacing. Tobacco use can delay healing and should be avoided. Any interruption in healing can result in scarring. Other contraindications include active skin infections, vitiligo, pregnancy, and a history of keloids or hypertrophic scars.

Anti-virals should be started one day preoperatively and continued until full re-epithelialization occurs. Medications given before laser skin resurfacing to reduce the incidence of hyperpigmentation include topical retinoids and hydroquinones. Their use is stopped after the procedure, and can be restarted after full re-epithelialization has been achieved. Patients should expect relatively long healing times (typically about 14–16 days to re-epithelialization) and persistent postoperative erythema when treating to the depth necessary to reduce festoons. Preoperative consultation with informed consent reviewing potential complications is crucial to the examination process. All potential anesthesia-related complications should be discussed as well.

19.4 Treatment Protocols

Anesthesia is typically achieved with a mixture of 2% lidocaine with 1:100,000 epinephrine (AstraZeneca, LP) mixed in a 1:1 ratio with 0.75% bupivacaine (Hospira, Inc.). Two to four milliliters of this mixture is injected as a bolus transorally to block the infraorbital nerve. An additional 1–2 mL boluses are injected transcutaneously at the lateral orbital rim to block the zygomaticotemporal and the zygomaticofacial nerves. The patient is prepped with non-flammable solutions and draped with non-flammable drapes. Standard laser safety protocol is observed. Laser safe eye shields are placed to protect the eyes during the application of the laser.

When resurfacing the lower lid, it is useful to divide this area into two zones roughly demarcated by the inferior orbital rim. The upper zone (lid margin to orbital rim) includes the thin eyelid skin, which has relatively sparse subcutaneous tissue between the deep dermis and the orbicularis muscle. There is a risk of producing a cicatricial ectropion from overly aggressive treatment in this region. Therefore, resurfacing should be performed conservatively in this upper zone.

The second treatment zone extends from the inferior orbital rim caudally to the junction of the lid skin with the cheek skin overlying the malar eminence. Festoons lie within this lower zone. This lower zone is treated aggressively with multiple passes of ablative laser energy. For example, when using the Sciton Contour Er:Yag laser (Sciton, Inc.), multiple passes are made at an ablative fluence of 10–15 J/cm^2 with 50–100 μm of nonablative coagulation. Table 19.1 shows representative laser settings for a few common lasers in use today. Between passes, the desiccated tissue residue can be removed by gentle debridement using saline soaked gauze. However, mechanical removal of this residue is not a necessary component to achieve festoon resolution. Typically, the first two passes of laser ablation remove epidermis and most of the papillary dermis. These passes also substantially alter the water content of the remaining dermis. Subsequent passes do not produce much additional desiccated tissue debris but do continue to produce shrinkage of the residual reticular dermis. The laser passes are continued over the area of the festoon until the last application of laser energy no longer produces visible shrinkage of the festoon. The total number of passes typically ranges from seven to 10. The margins adjacent to the main treatment area should be lasered in a "feathering" fashion with declining fluences to avoid demarcation lines by blending the treated area with the untreated area.

Postoperative wound care is a critical factor in achieving the clinical results from this procedure. Many approaches to treating a second degree burn, which characterizes this postoperative wound, have been reported. Our preferred approach includes an oral antiviral medication (e.g., Valtrex®, GlaxoSmithKline) (500 mg po BID) to prevent the herpes simplex virus from interfering with wound healing. This is begun the day before and continued throughout the postoperative healing regimen. Immediately following the procedure, bio-occlusive topical wound dressings (e.g., Flexzan®, Advanced Medical Solutions Limited) are applied for 1–3 days. During this time, the areas of treated skin not covered by the bio-occlusive dressing are coated with a topical lubricant (e.g., Aquaphor®, Beiersdorf Inc.) (Figs. 19.2 and 19.3).

The Flexzan® bandages are removed by gentle soaking during a shower on the second post op day (Fig. 19.4).

The patient is followed closely with multiple postoperative clinic visits in order to help guide patient compliance with the healing regimen and observe for signs of compli-

Table 19.1 Laser settings for laser festoon reduction

Passes	Area	Settings	
Sciton Contour Erbium:Yag laser			
1st	Upper and lower zone	10–20 J/cm^2	No coagulation
2nd	Lower zone	10–20 J/cm^2	25–50 μm coagulation
3rd–10th	Lower zone	10–20 J/cm^2	25–100 μm coagulation
Last	Wound margins	5–15 J/cm^2	No coagulation
Coherent Ultrapulse CO_2 laser			
1st	Upper and lower zone	Pattern 4, size 5–7, density 3 × 300 mJ and 60 W	
2nd–10th	Lower zone	Pattern 3, size 5–7, density 5 × 300 mJ and 60 W	
Last	Wound margins	Pattern 4, size 5–7, density 3 × 300 mJ and 60 W	
Nidek Unipulse 1040 CO_2 with Fastscan CPG			
1st	Upper and lower zone	10 W, spot size 1.02 mm, 30% overlap, laser off time 0.4 s	
2nd-10th	Lower zone	18 W, spot size 1.02 mm, 30% overlap, laser off time 0.4 s	
Last	Wound margins	10 W, spot size 1.02 mm, 30% overlap, laser off time 0.4 s	

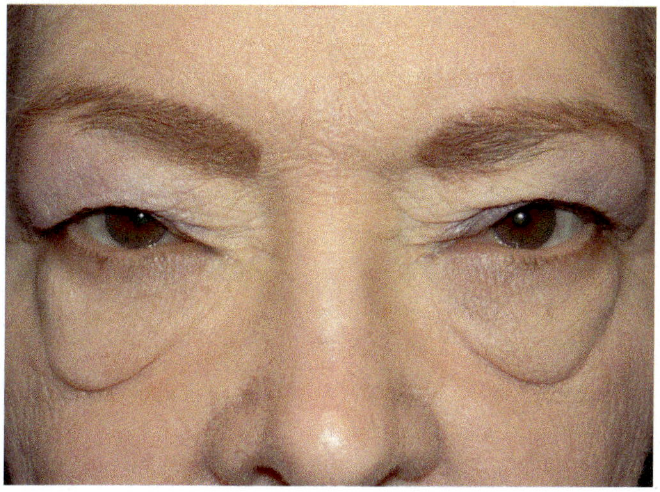

Fig. 19.2 Sixty-seven-year old woman before surgery

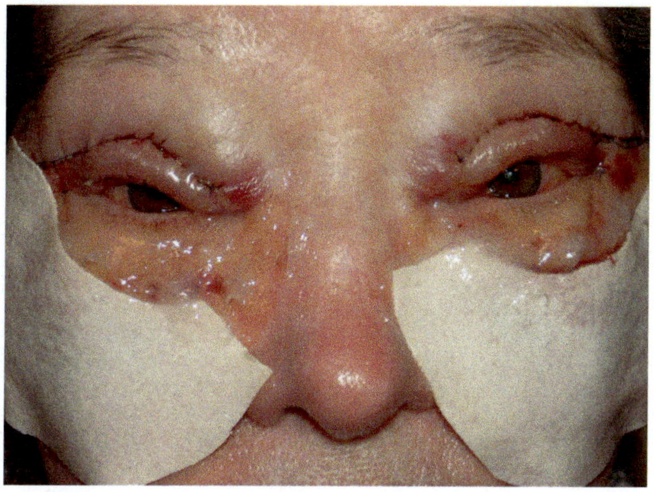

Fig. 19.3 One day following levator advancement, upper lid blepharoplasty, modified tarsal strip, transconjunctival lower lid blepharoplasty, and lower lid erbium laser skin resurfacing

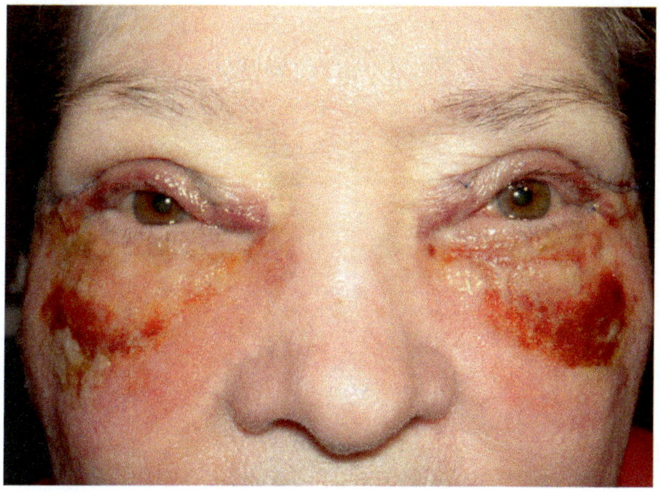

Fig. 19.4 Three days post op

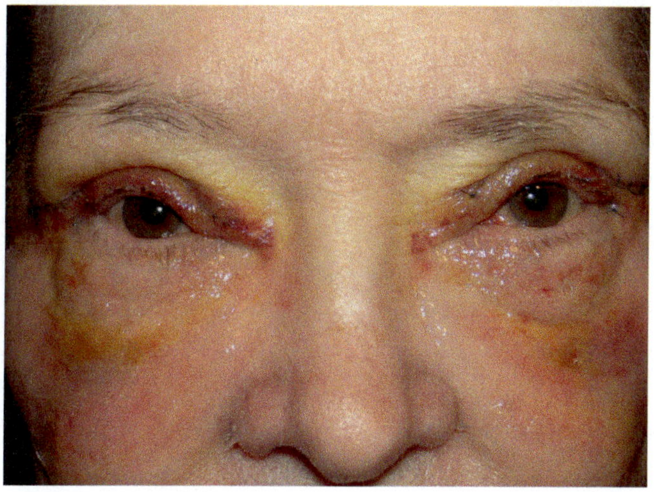

Fig. 19.5 Five days post op

cations. The healing regimen includes soaking the skin with a dilute solution of acetic acid (e.g., vinegar water) at the concentration of 1 teaspoon – 1 tablespoon per cup of water. Clean cloths are soaked in this solution and applied sopping wet to the healing skin for a half hour per application. The cloth can be resaturated during this half hour soak. The acetic acid facilitates the debridement of the thermally devitalized tissue and creates an acidic environment. The acidic washes reduce the growth of bacterial and fungal elements, which is why antibiotics or antifungals are rarely needed during the healing process. After soaking, the skin is coated with a topical lubricant (e.g., Aquaphor®) to prevent tissue desiccation and encourage epidermal healing until the next vinegar water application. These cycles of vinegar water soaks followed by the application of healing ointments are constant throughout the healing process. The patient is encouraged to do the vinegar soaks 6–10 times per day. The authors tend to see the patient every 2–4 days until the skin is fully epithelialized (Figs. 19.5–19.10).

This frequency of follow-up allows observation of the wounds and early detection of wound healing problems. If herpes simplex virus is suspected to be interfering with wound healing, the dose of the antiviral can be increased to fight such an infection. Likewise, if bacterial or fungal infections are suspected, appropriate medications should be used. The treated area re-epithelializes generally in 14–16 days. Once the target area has fully epithelialized, the frequency of post

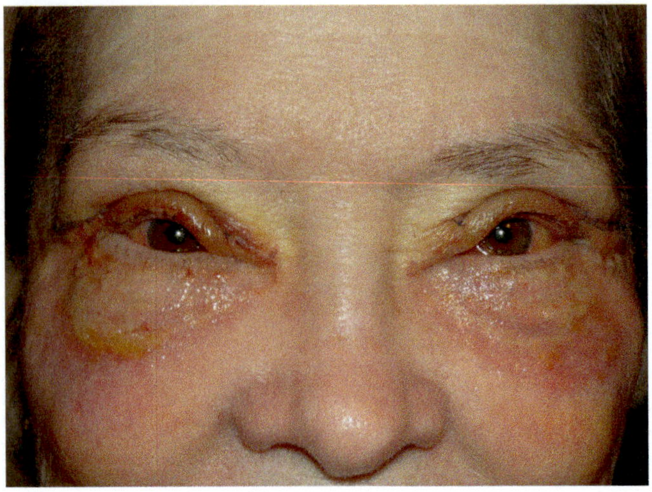

Fig. 19.6 Seven days post op

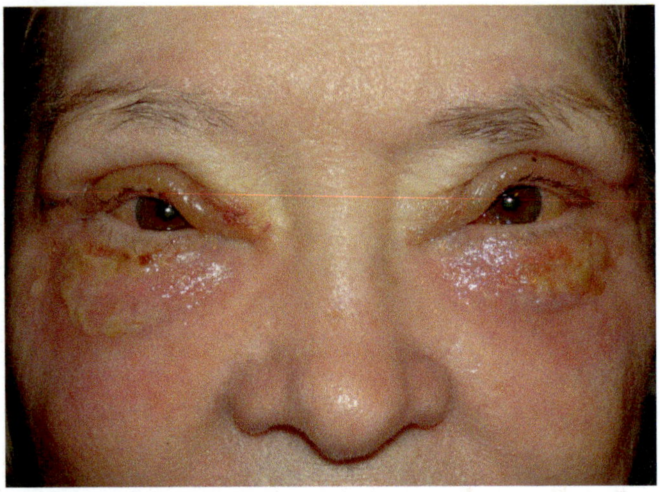

Fig. 19.7 Nine days post op

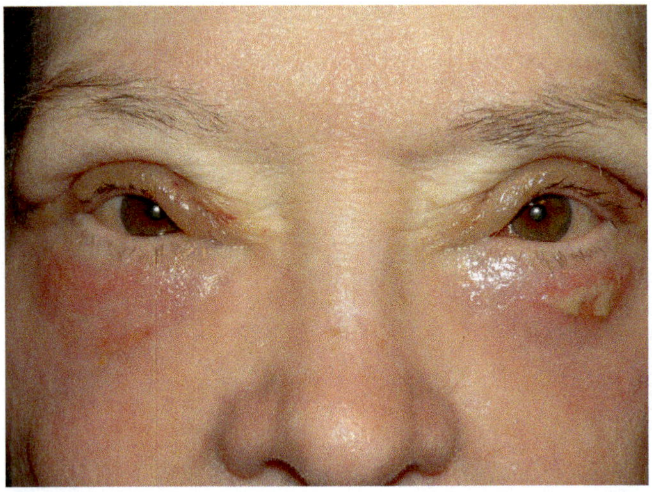

Fig. 19.8 Eleven days post op

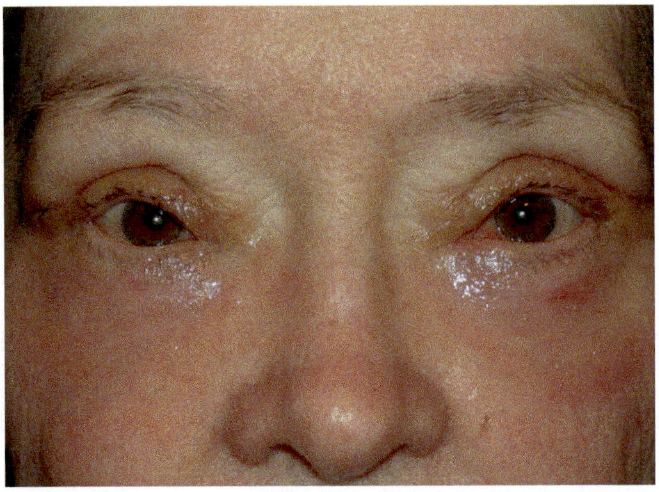

Fig. 19.9 Fourteen days post op

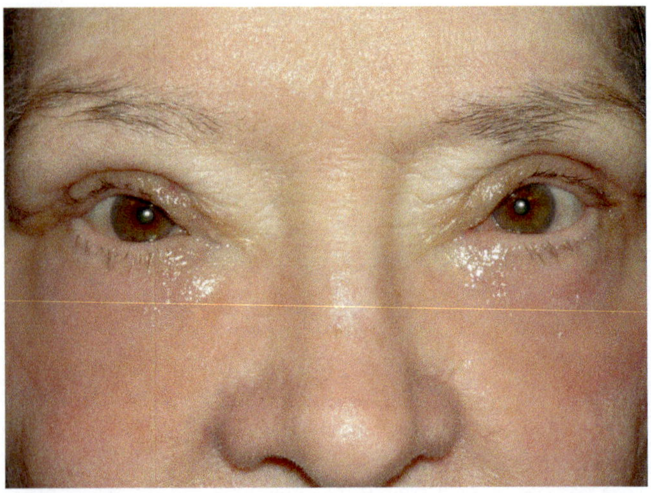

Fig. 19.10 Sixteen days post op

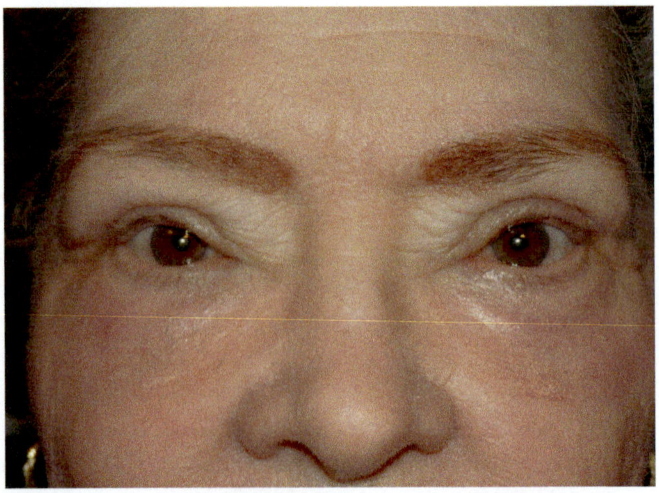

Fig. 19.11 Thirty days post op

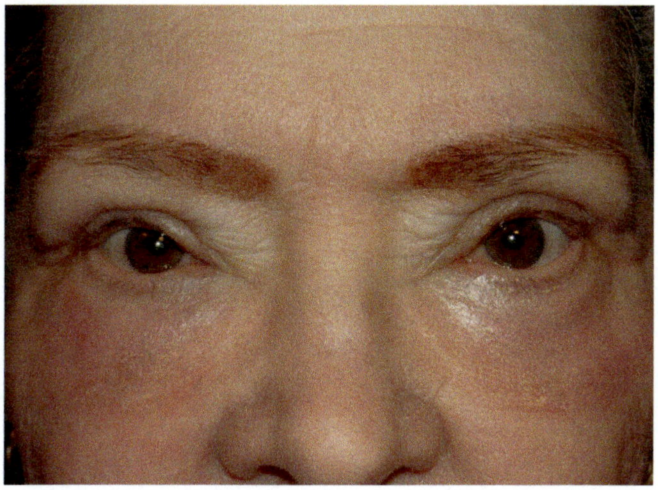

Fig. 19.12 Forty-two days post op

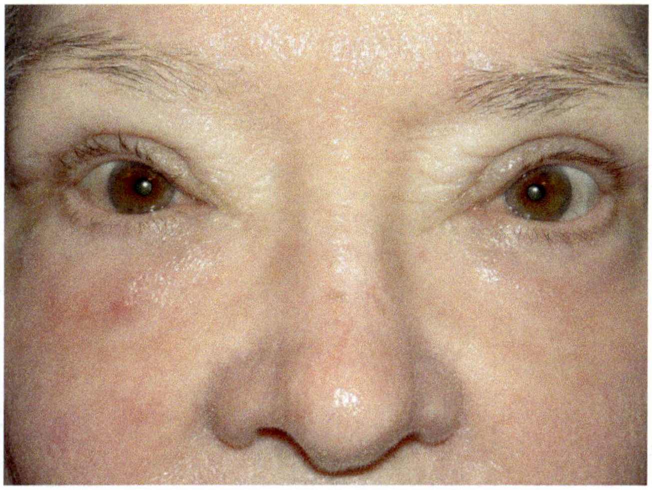

Fig. 19.13 Seventy-three days post op

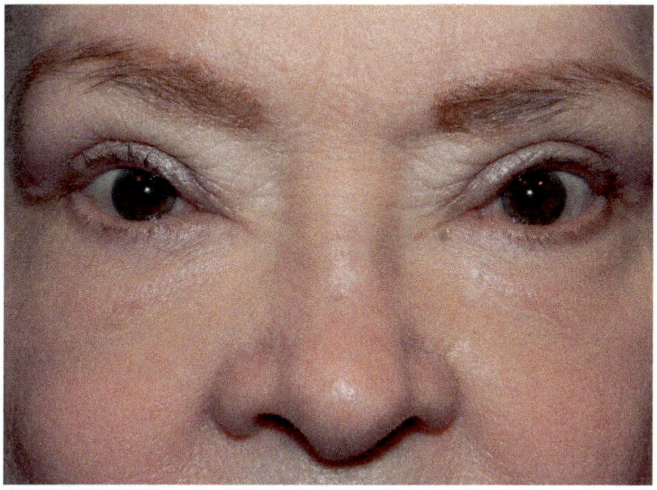

Fig. 19.14 One-hundred and eight days post op

op appointments is reduced (Figs. 19.11–19.14), daily sunblock is used, and camouflage makeup can be applied as needed to conceal postoperative color variations.

19.5 Complications

The most difficult aspect of laser skin resurfacing is the postoperative care and recognizing the signs of complications. For the surgeon beginning laser skin resurfacing, a preceptorship or formal partnership with an experienced surgeon is invaluable. Avoiding complications is the goal, but complications do occur and can be managed successfully with proper treatment and patience.

A herpes simplex infection is a potentially serious complication which can arise during the first 2 weeks of postoperative healing. This can be challenging to identify during the early stages of healing because these infections usually present with epithelial changes, and the epithelium is absent during this stage.

In the following photos, the evolution and treatment of a herpetic infection can be seen (Figs. 19.15–19.21). This patient was treated with a relatively light skin laser ablation to improve the skin quality of the lower lid and reduce periocular rhytids. Healing typically occurs relatively quickly, with re-epithelialization at 7–10 days. At 3 days, the wound looked appropriate (Figs. 19.15 and 19.16).

But at 7 days after laser skin resurfacing (Fig. 19.17), the lack of healing indicated a problem. The patient was instructed to increase the concentration of the vinegar in her soaks to help with the removal of the exudate on the lower lid. The patient was seen daily at this point and on postoperative day 13 (Fig. 19.18), the presence of only a border of healed epithelium (suboptimal epithelialization) gave the indication of a secondary factor influencing wound healing. The wound was cultured for bacterial and fungal elements, but the strong suspicion was for a herpetic infection, and the dose of Valtrex® was doubled from 1 g per day to 2 g per day.

The patient was followed up daily. The preliminary microbiologic cultures came back without growth, and the dose of Valtrex® was again increased to 3 g per day. At this point, the wound started to improve slowly (Fig. 19.19). By day 22, the wound was healing nicely (Fig. 19.20).

As the wound continued to heal, it was confirmed that the poor healing was due to the herpes simplex virus. The patient was continued on 3 g of Valtrex® until the skin was fully epithelialized and was then tapered off over 2 weeks. The patient healed well without scar formation (Fig. 19.21).

Other possible infections which occur in the first 1–2 weeks following laser treatment include a bacterial cellulitis and fungal infection. Bacterial infections typically present

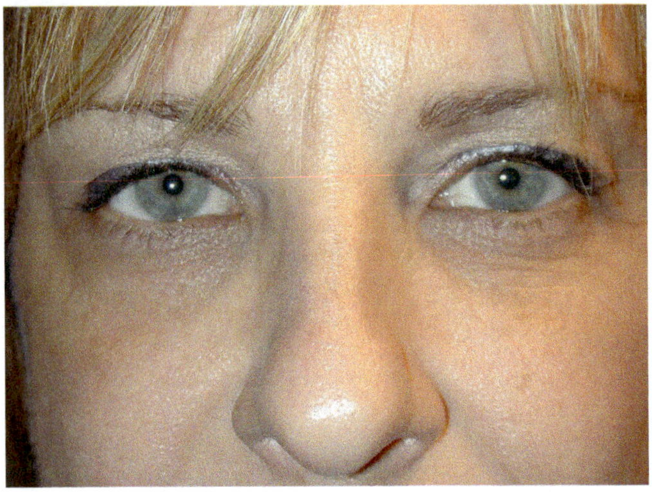

Fig. 19.15 Forty-seven-year-old woman before surgery

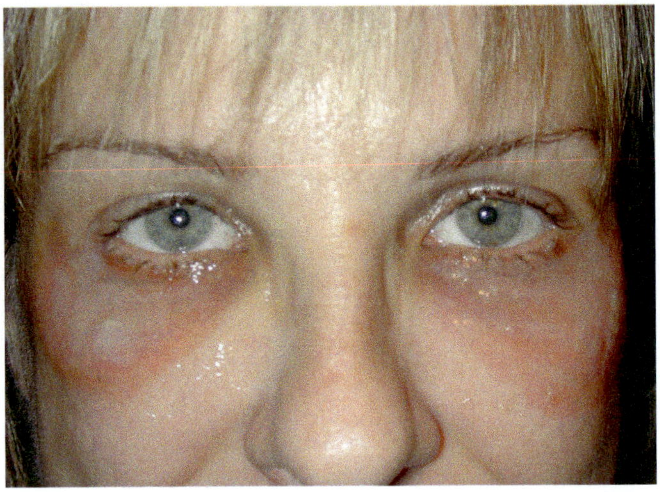

Fig. 19.16 Three days following transconjunctival lower lid blepharoplasty and lower lid erbium laser skin resurfacing

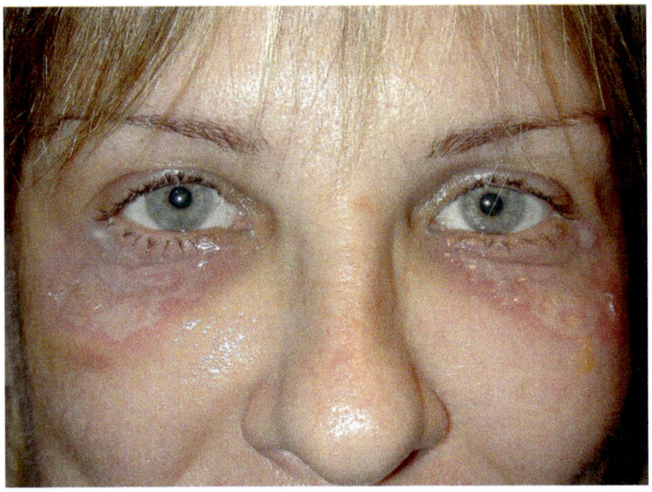

Fig. 19.17 Seven days post op

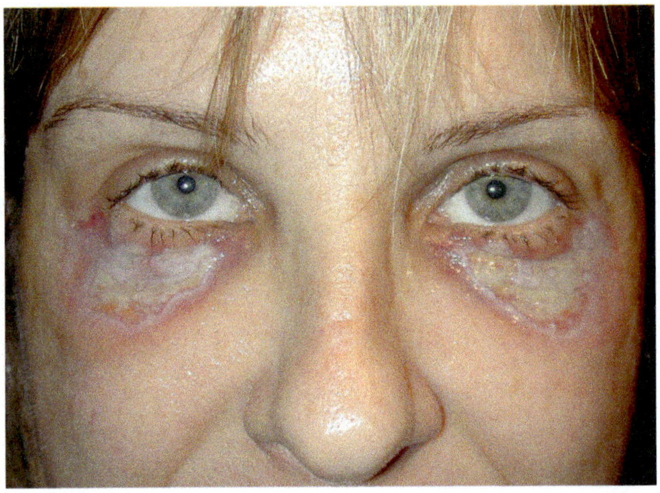

Fig. 19.18 Thirteen days post op

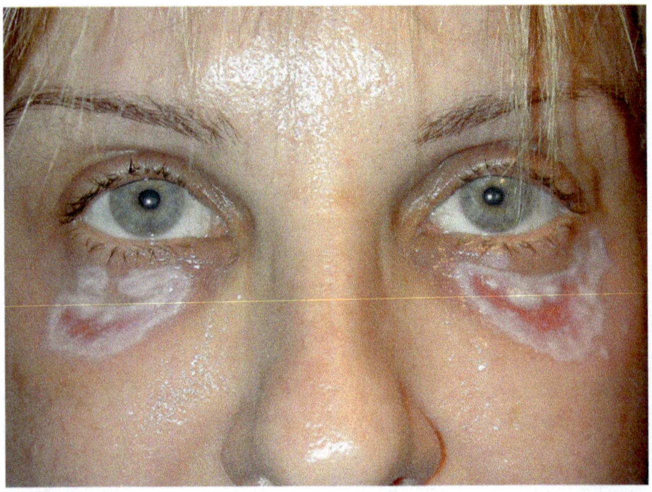

Fig. 19.19 Seventeen days post op

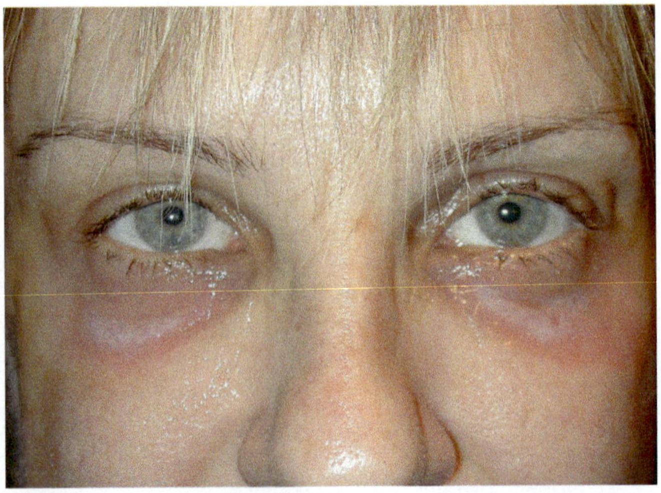

Fig. 19.20 Twenty-two days post op

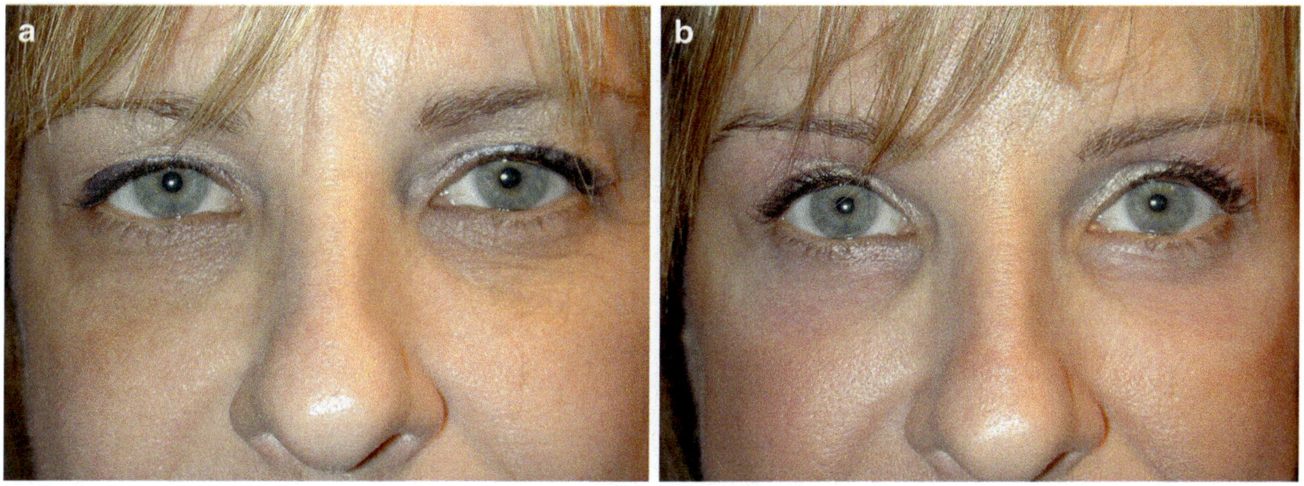

Fig. 19.21 (**a**) Presurgery; (**b**) 60 days post op

with redness, pain, exudates, and foul odors. Culturing these wounds is paramount. Antibiotics including intravenous administration, should it be warranted, may be given depending on the severity of the infection. When infections do occur, a polymicrobial nature can be seen. Some typical pathogens include pseudomonas, staphylococcus, and streptococcus. Some surgeons propose prophylaxis with antibiotics to aid in prevention of these infections.

Fungal infections, such as Candida, usually appear as soft white plaques on an erythematous base. Satellite lesions can be seen and diagnosis with a KOH preparation can help identify and differentiate these infections. Some surgeons treat with antifungal medications as prophylaxis against these infections as well.

Acne eruptions are possible after resurfacing and can be treated with an oral tetracycline. Milia can present in the first month and may be treated with glycolic acid peels and low dose retinoic acid.

Pigmentary changes can occur after laser treatment. Postinflammatory hyperpigmentation typically presents in the first month. It is more likely to occur in those patients with Fitzpatrick skin types III–VI. Treatment options include observation as many resolve over 4–6 months, topical bleaching with hydroquinones, topical retinoids, topical steroids, and the use of sun avoidance and sunblock. If a patient is in the skin types at risk, some surgeons pre- and posttreat with topical hydroquinones and retinoids.

Hypopigmentation is less commonly seen. When present, it is typically a pseudo-hypopigmentation. This laser procedure causes a relative reduction in the normal age related pigment deposition in the skin. This would normally lead to a transition zone of relatively lighter (treated) skin to darker (untreated) skin. However, this finding is diminished by the use of decreasing laser energies in the border region around the heavily treated skin. Decreasing the level of ablation in a graded fashion around the central treatment area creates a transition zone which blends the clinical effect and pigment changes between the treated and adjacent untreated skin.

Absolute hypogimentation is rare. When present, this may be due to thermal injury to the deep melanocystes of the skin. Excimer lasers have been used to stimulate the melanocytes in these cases and have been helpful, but a more simple treatment involves the use of camouflage makeup.

Erythema is normally seen during the first 12 weeks after treatment and then decreases over time. If erythema persists, mild topical steroids can be helpful. Makeup can be used to camouflage the erythema.

Scarring and ectropion are rare complications after laser skin resurfacing, and are usually preventable with proper intraoperative technique and postoperative care. In the treatment of festoons described in this chapter, the authors have not experienced scarring or ectropion in over 15 years of experience. Subdividing the lower lid into a more superficially treated zone from the eyelid margin to the orbital rim and a more aggressively treated zone adjacent and distal to this area probably mitigates these complications.

As described in this chapter, to treat festoons, multiple laser applications are needed. Treating other portions of the face with this approach is aggressive, may lead to scar formation, and is not recommended. If scars from laser skin resurfacing do form, the surgeon must recognize and treat them with steroids, anti-metabolites, and/or vascular lasers. In certain stable scars, surgical excision may be indicated. Careful patient selection, safe laser technique, and attentive postoperative management mitigate the risk of scars after surgery.

As mentioned above, we have not seen ectropion after laser application. This is most likely related to our laser application technique (graded zoned treatment), and a thorough preoperative evaluation identifying patients with eyelid

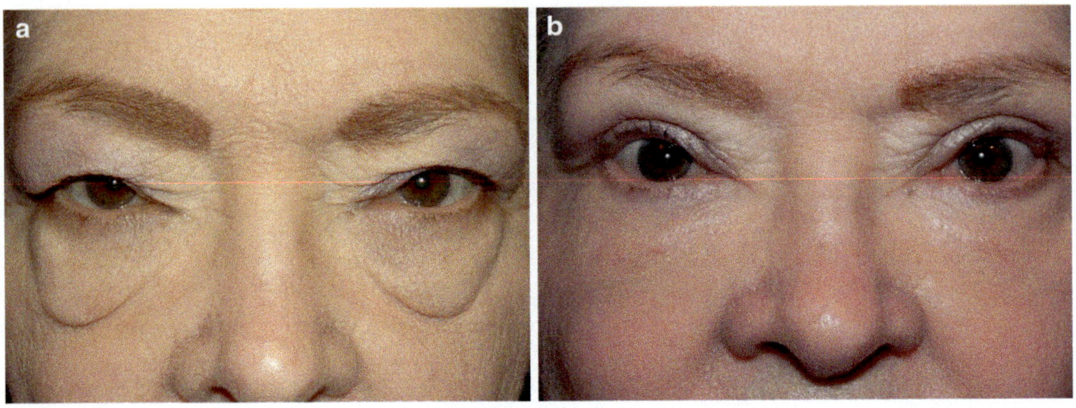

Fig. 19.22 Sixty-seven-year-old woman from Fig. 2 (**a**) before and (**b**) 108 days after levator advancement, upper lid blepharoplasty, modified tarsal strip, transconjunctival lower lid blepharoplasty, and lower eyelid erbium laser skin resurfacing to treat lower eyelid festoons

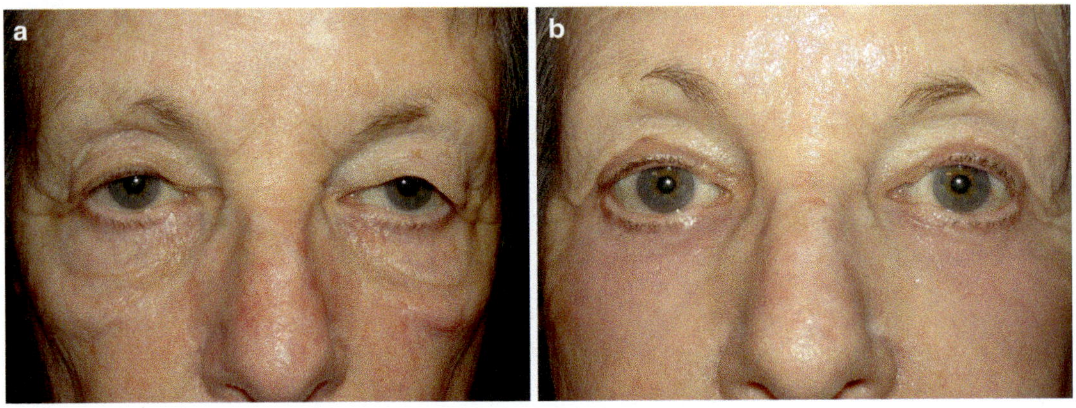

Fig. 19.23 Seventy-three-year-old woman (**a**) before and (**b**) 77 days after upper lid blepharoplasty, modified tarsal strip, transconjunctival lower lid blepharoplasty, and lower eyelid erbium laser skin resurfacing to treat lower eyelid festoons

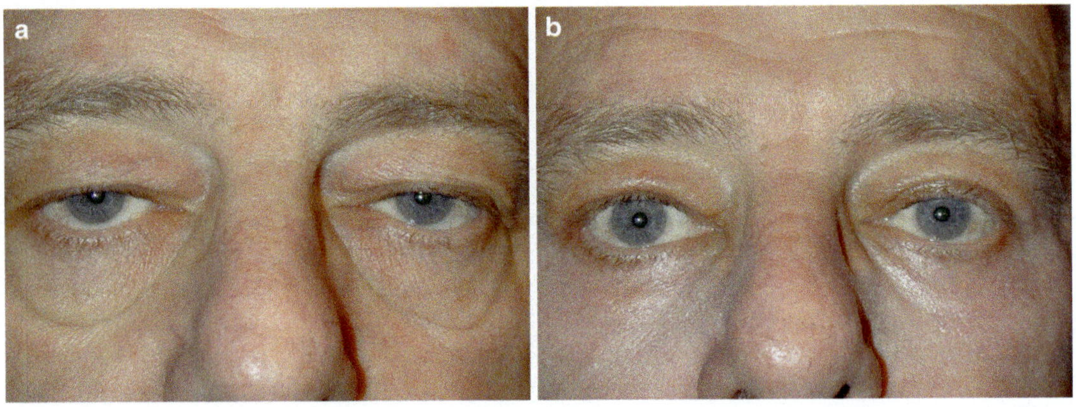

Fig. 19.24 Sixty-five-year-old man (**a**) before and (**b**) 6 weeks after levator advancement, upper lid blepharoplasty, modified tarsal strip, transconjunctival lower lid blepharoplasty, and lower eyelid erbium laser skin resurfacing to treat lower eyelid festoons

laxity who are at risk of post-laser eyelid malposition. If permanent post-laser ectropion were to develop, appropriate surgical management is needed.

Performing laser treatment of festoons, its postoperative care, and the management of possible postoperative complications can seem daunting. However, with proper adherence to the technique described in this chapter practitioners can perform the procedure safely and effectively.

Pre- and postoperative results of our technique can be seen in Figs. 19.22–19.24.

19.6 Conclusion

We have had tremendous success using laser skin resurfacing techniques to treat festoons. We believe this suggests that festoons are primarily a cutaneous rather than muscular pathologic entity. As previously stated, the clinical endpoint of laser skin resurfacing with all laser systems is the presence of no further visible tissue shrinkage with the final laser application. This holds true with the technique of festoon treatment described in this chapter. The effect of the initial 1 or 2 passes by most ablative systems has been showed histological to be largely confined to vaporizing epithelium and superficial papillary dermis [23, 24]. When additional laser passes are made, progressive thermal injury to the underlying tissue has been demonstrated histologically [15, 24, 25, 28–30]. By extrapolating from studies of burn pathology, this represents thermal damage to the reticular dermis [31]. Our clinical endpoint at which no further tissue shrinkage results suggests that the resolution of festoons occurs as a result of changes induced by thermal damage within the skin.

Modified laser skin resurfacing offers a predictable, rapid (10 min per lid), and safe treatment for lower eyelid festoons. Standard intraoperative laser safety guidelines, prudent post-operative care, and detailed management of the healing process are necessary to achieve the optimal clinical result. Laser skin resurfacing in general, and laser assisted festoon reduction, when needed, can add greatly to the overall aesthetic outcome in rejuvenation of the lower eyelid–cheek complex.

References

1. Furnas DW. Festoons of orbicularis muscle as a cause of baggy eyelids. Plast Reconstr Surg. 1978;61:540–6.
2. Kikkawa DO, Lemke BN, Dortzbach RK. Relations of the superficial musculoaponeurotic system to the orbit and characterization of the orbitomalar ligament. Ophthal Plast Reconstr Surg. 1996;12(2): 77–88.
3. Mendelson BC, Muzaffar AR, Adams Jr WP. Surgical anatomy of the midcheek and malar mounds. Plast Reconstr Surg. 2002;110: 885–96.
4. Goldberg RA, McCann JD, Fiaschetti D, Ben Simon GJ. What causes eyelid bags? Plast Reconstr Surg. 2005;115(5):1395–402.
5. Esmaeli B, Prieto VG, Butler CE, et al. Severe periorbital edema secondary to STI571 (Gleevec). Cancer. 2002;95:881–7.
6. Furnas DW. Festoons, mounds, and bags of the eyelids and cheek. Clin Plast Surg. 1993;20:367–85.
7. Baker SS, Woodward JA. Carbon dioxide laser blepharoplasty, ptosis correction, and treatment of festoons. In: Alster TS, Apfelberg DB, editors. Cosmetic laser surgery. 2nd ed. New York: Wiley-Liss; 1999. p. 121–39.
8. Patel CKN. Continuous-wave laser action on vibrational rotational transitions of carbon dioxide. Phys Rev. 1964;136:A1187–93.
9. Anderson RR, Parrish JA. Selective photothermolysis: precise microsurgery selective absorption of pulsed radiation. Science. 1983;220:524–7.
10. Walsh Jr JT, Flotte TJ, Deutsch TF. Er:YAG laser ablation of tissue: measurement of tissue ablation rates. Lasers Surg Med. 1989;9: 327–37.
11. Baker SS, Muenzler WS, Small RG, Leonard JE. Carbon dioxide laser blepharoplasty. Ophthalmology. 1984;91:238–43.
12. David LM. The laser approach to blepharoplasty. J Dermatol Surg Oncol. 1988;14:741–6.
13. David LM. Laser vermillion ablation for actinic cheilitis. J Dermatol Surg Oncol. 1985;11:605–8.
14. Weinstein C. Ultrapulse carbon dioxide laser removal of periocular wrinkles in association with laser blepharoplasty. J Clin Laser Med Surg. 1994;12:205–9.
15. Schomacker KT, Walsh JT, Flotte TJ, Deutsch TF. Thermal damage produced by high-irradiance continuous wave CO_2 laser cutting of tissue. Lasers Surg Med. 1990;10:74–84.
16. Zweig AD, Meierhofer B, Muller OM, et al. Lateral thermal damage along pulsed laser incisions. Lasers Surg Med. 1990;10: 262–74.
17. Lask GP, Keller G, Lowe N, Gormley D. Laser skin resurfacing with the Silktouch flash scanner for facial rhytides. Dermatol Surg. 1995;21:1021–4.
18. Chernoff G, Schoenrock L, Cramer H, et al. Cutaneous laser resurfacing. Int J Aesth Rest Surg. 1995;3:57–68.
19. Weinstein C, Alster TS. Skin resurfacing with high energy, pulsed carbon dioxide lasers. In: Alster TS, Apfelberg DB. Cosmetic Laser Surgery. New York: Wiley-Liss, 1996.
20. Alster TS. Comparison of two high energy, pulsed carbon dioxide lasers in the treatment of periorbital rhytides. Dermatol Surg. 1996;33:541–5.
21. Alster TS, Garg S. Treatment of facial rhytides with a high-energy, pulsed carbon dioxide laser. Plast Reconstr Surg. 1996;98:791–4.
22. Kirsch KM, Zelickson BD, Zachary CB, Tope WD. Ultrastructure of collagen thermally denatured by microsecond domain pulsed carbon dioxide laser. Arch Dermatol. 1998;134:1255–9.
23. Fitzpatrick RE, Ruiz-Esparza J, Goldman MP. The depth of thermal necrosis using the CO_2 laser: a comparison of the super pulsed mode and conventional mode. J Dermatol Surg Oncol. 1991;17: 340–4.
24. Waldorf HA, Kauvar AN, Geronemus RG. Skin resurfacing of fine to deep rhytides using a char-free carbon dioxide laser in 47 patients. Dermatol Surg. 1995;21:940–6.
25. Walsh JT, Flotte TJ, Anderson RR, Deutsch TF. Pulsed CO_2 laser tissue ablation: effect of tissue type and pulse duration on thermal damage. Lasers Surg Med. 1988;8:108–18.
26. Hobbs ER, Balin PC, Wheeland RG, Ratz JL. Super pulsed lasers: minimizing thermal damage with short duration, high irradiance pulses. J Dermatol Surg Oncol. 1987;13:955–64.
27. David LM, Lask GP, Glassberg E, et al. CO_2 laser abrasion for cosmetic and therapeutic treatment of facial actinic damage. Cutis. 1989;43:583–7.
28. Hruza GJ. Skin resurfacing with lasers. Fitzpatrick's J Clin Dermatol. 1995;3:38–41.
29. Cotton J, Hood AF, Gonin R, Beeson WH, Hanke CW. Histologic evaluation of preauricular and post auricular skin after high energy, short-pulse carbon dioxide laser. Arch Dermatol. 1996;132:425–8.
30. Fitzpatrick RE, Tope WD, Goldman MP, Satur NM. Pulsed carbon dioxide laser, trichloroacetic acid, Baker-Gordon phenol, and dermabrasion: a comparative clinical and histologic study of cutaneous resurfacing in a porcine model. Arch Dermatol. 1996;132:469–71.
31. Monafo WW. Initial management of burns. N Engl J Med. 1996;335: 1581–6.

Part V

Midface Rejuvenation

20 Midface and Lower Eyelid Rejuvenation

Oscar M. Ramirez

Key Points

- Endoscopic midface rejuvenation is a scarless procedure accessed through small hidden incisions.
- It can be performed on the young, middle aged, and elderly. In middle aged and elderly individuals, it is often part of a larger procedure (brow lift, facelift, blepharoplasty, etc).
- Appropriate knowledge of relevant clinical anatomy, surgical planes, and endoscopic instrumentation and technique, is critical to the success of surgery.
- Surgery is performed in the subperiosteal plane which provides excellent safety, visualization, and access for tissue remodeling.
- In my technique, multiple tissues (SOOF, Bichat's fat pad, etc.) are sequentially engaged, elevated, and secured to a common fixation point (temporal fascia proper).
- This imbrication of tissue cumulatively creates the youthful convexity of the midface and reestablishes the natural cheek contour (ogee line).
- Adjunctive procedures such as placement of facial implants, autologous fat grafting, and laser skin resurfacing can be safely and effectively added to surgery.
- Midface rejuvenation is often combined with lower lid blepharoplasty. I have found that the combined procedures act synergistically to improve the overall surgical outcome, and to enhance the individual results of each procedure.

20.1 Introduction

The periorbital region is the area of the face that people focus on when they engage socially and intimately. It is also the most expressive area of the face. All the natural human feelings of anger, sorrow, happiness, despair, etc. are manifested in this small area of facial anatomy. The aging process tends to produce an appearance of sadness and anger. This occurs despite that fact that the individual may have different feelings internally. Occasionally, some younger individuals may have this expression of sadness as a natural or acquired trait. However, when patients come for consultation to correct these features, very rarely will they make allusion to the changes of facial expression. Instead, they talk about lines, creases, sagging, etc. It is up to the surgeon to approach surgical rejuvenation in a dimension beyond the static morphology to which we are accustomed. It is also imperative that the surgeon does not worsen existing positive facial expressions and does aim to restore the happy face that is inherent to the young person.

From the surgical point of view, the aging manifestations on the face should be corrected by functional and anatomical units. From my personal perspective, the forehead and upper eyelids are one unit. The lower eyelids and midface another unit. The lower face and neck is the last unit. Surgery on one unit usually facilitates and enhances the correction of an adjacent unit. With this in mind, my approach to midface rejuvenation usually involves some procedure on the lower eyelid. Conversely, surgery of the lower eyelid may require a procedure on the adjacent midface. These combined procedures act synergistically to attain superior correction and rejuvenation of any one unit. Therefore, to be complete, I will describe my combined technique of endoscopic midface lift with lower blepharoplasty.

20.2 The Midface

Despite the numerous techniques described over the decades, the best approach to midface rejuvenation has, and continues to be, an area of constant surgical debate. The endoscopic technique that I described in the early 1990 approaches the deep layers of the midface in the safest plane of dissection using only small incisions. This approach allows more-soft tissue remodeling than any other technique. While I have used multiple access points for surgery, I have consistently performed this procedure in the subperiosteal plane. My current

O.M. Ramirez (✉)
Director, Sanctuary Plastic Surgery, Boca Raton, FL, USA
e-mail: drramirez@spsboca.com

G.G. Massry et al. (eds.), *Master Techniques in Blepharoplasty and Periorbital Rejuvenation*,
DOI 10.1007/978-1-4614-0067-7_20, © Springer Science+Business Media, LLC 2011

preference to access the midface involves a temporal slit incision (2 cm) and an intraoral mucosal incision (2 cm). These approaches prevent all the potential complications of prior techniques using eyelid incisions [1].

20.3 Why I Prefer the Subperiosteal Face Lift

I have been performing subperiosteal facelifts since my years as a Senior Resident at the University of Pittsburgh (1983–1984). I have not changed my preference for this approach since that time. Moreover, continued evolution, refinement, and improvement in the technique have occurred over the years [2–5] which has further substantiated my belief in this approach. I will enumerate what I have learned over time.

The subperiosteal dissection allows en-block mobilization of the soft tissues. Once dissection is done, in the forehead, the midface or the entire jaw line, the tissues are lifted in a vertical or superolateral direction. Key suspension sutures are applied to maintain the desired elevation. Some surgeons prefer the use of fixation devices such as endotine (Coapt), or barbed sutures such as the Quill brand etc., to anchor mobilized tissue. I have tried these and other methods of suspension. However, I have not seen that they offer any significant advantages over the simplest and less expensive methods of tissue fixation that I described originally: percutaneous screw fixation for the forehead, and polydioxanone (PDS) suture suspension for the midface. Of critical importance is to allow this en-block mobilization lift and fixation in the subperiosteal plane, it is essential to release the periosteal attachments in key anatomical areas usually in the lowermost boundaries of the area of dissection.

The subperiosteal dissection facilitates soft tissue remodeling. This can be accomplished by imbricating the entire mass of the dissected tissues, by transposition of vascularized fat flaps, or by injection of free fat to the entire thickness of the elevated soft tissues (Fig. 20.1).

The subperiosteal dissection leaves exposed the underlying bony skeleton. This allows skeletal contouring by bone reduction with osteotomies or by augmentation with implants (Fig. 20.1). There is no need for dissection in different planes, which is the case if one proceeds with a subcutaneous, sub-SMAS (sub-superficial-musculo-aponeurotic system), or intermuscular dissection.

The subperiosteal plane has better visibility and orientation than the more superficial planes, particularly when one

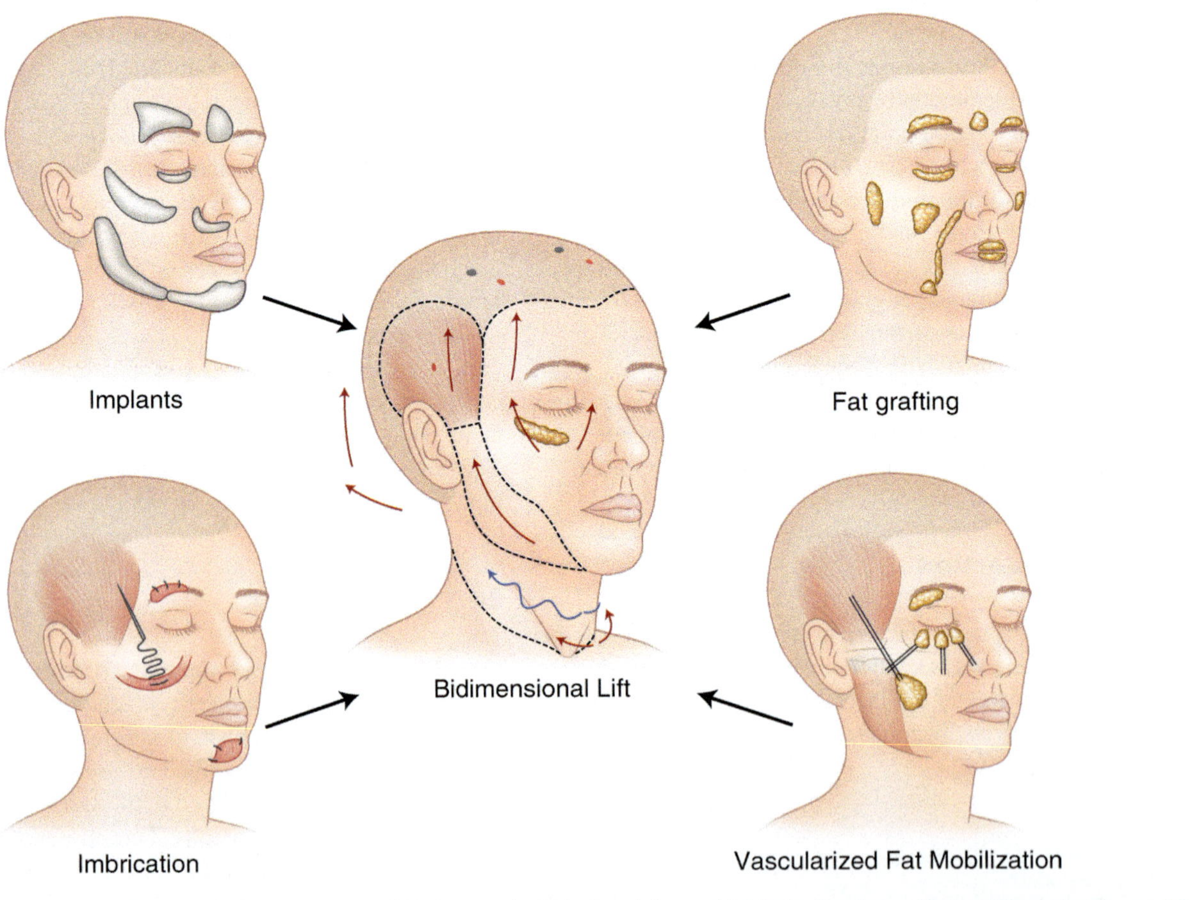

Fig. 20.1 The subperiosteal dissection of the central oval of the face, particularly the midface, which is the foundation for the tridimensional remodeling of the face. To the basic bidimensional manipulation you can add any of the different maneuvers of volumetric or tridimensional augmentation

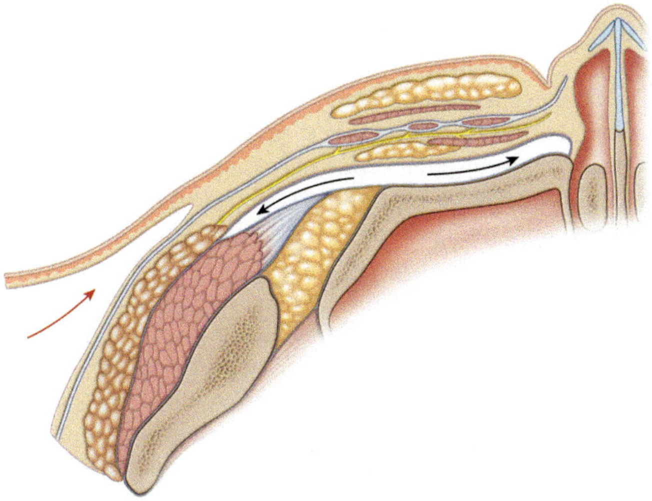

Fig. 20.2 My biplanar technique combines the safest planes of dissection: the subperiosteal dissection in the central oval of the face (*black arrows*) and the subcutaneous dissection in the periphery (*red arrow*)

uses endoscopic techniques. The bony surface reflects the light better and the bone surface provides good landmarks for orientation.

The subperiosteal plane is a safer plane for the facial nerves. Despite the unfounded claims that the subperiosteal plane of dissection has a high incidence of nerve injury, I strongly believe that this plane is as safe as the subcutaneous plane of dissection and definitively safer than the intermediate plane of dissection. This assumption is based on my vast experience of many years of surgery with this technique. My personal rate of nerve injury is about 2%, and all injuries have been temporary. For this reason, in my biplanar techniques, I combine the safest planes of dissection: subperiosteal and subcutaneous (Fig. 20.2).

The subperiosteal approach is probably more durable than other more superficial techniques. Once you have repositioned the block of soft tissues, and allow healing in the elevated position, the result will remain over time. In over 25 years of performing subperiosteal facelifts (open and endoscopic), I have seen that the operation on the central oval of the face, the forehead, and the midface, lasts for over 10 years at a minimum. The area that tends to relapse earlier is the lower face and the neck, in which a more superficial dissection has been performed. This usually last about 5 years.

Finally, the more superficial planes of dissection in this surgery usually pull the soft tissues in a horizontal or oblique direction. Using these techniques the central midface soft tissues are pulled indirectly by the tension applied to the peripherally dissected flaps. These two characteristics create tension bands and more pull on the periphery than in the centrally located tissues giving the typical "windswept" or "motorcyclist" appearance to the face.

20.4 Patient Selection

Most patients are candidates for minimal incision midface rejuvenation including young, middle aged, and elderly individuals. It is equally applicable to male and female patients, and can be performed on those with good as well as poor skeletal support.

In young individuals, I apply the principles of three dimensional facial rejuvenation of the midface for purposes of enhancement. For strategic and conceptual reasons, I do not call this facial rejuvenation. Instead I use the term of "facial beautification." I have performed these procedures of lifting and reshaping the face for beautification purposes on individuals as young as 18 years of age.

When a man or woman starts developing the first signs of aging in their middle thirties, it usually manifests with the development of an early tear trough deformity (naso-jugal groove), sagging of the cheeks, and the presence of a nasolabial fold. These are the group of patients that benefit the most from the endoscopic midface rejuvenation. This is because the results to surgery are superior, yet not dramatic or obvious to the casual observer. Even in those with more dramatic changes, the natural results and the lack of telltale signs of "face lifting" are advantageous when patients want to integrate to their working activities as quickly as possible.

Individuals of middle age, late middle age, and the elderly, are also excellent candidates for the procedure, because the endoscopic midface lift can be easily incorporated into more extensive and complete facial rejuvenation procedures. For those requiring additional volume augmentation, or correction of soft tissue asymmetries, fat grafting techniques are added. For those requiring skeletal augmentation in the pyriformis, malar or orbital areas, facial implants fabricated for these areas are used during surgery. Males are equally good candidates for the procedure. The only difference with the female counterpart is that the final aesthetic shape of the cheek is a bit different. This will be elaborated on later.

20.5 Indications

Patients with either early or considerable aging or ptosis of the structures of the central oval of the face can benefit from the endoscopic minimal incision midface lift. Eyelid commissures, nasolabial folds, cheeks, the angle of the mouth etc. are effectively addressed with this approach. Moderate tear trough deformities and infraorbital hollows are also correctable with endoscopic techniques. Endoscopic midface procedure allows recreation of the "ogee" of the midface [5]. This reciprocal multicurvilinear line is associated with a youthful and beautiful appearance. The endoscopic minimal incision midface lift is quite effective in conjunction with patients requiring secondary or tertiary face lift procedures, for those patients requiring deep chemical peel or CO_2 laser resurfacing, and for patients requiring soft tissue augmentation via fat grafting. In the first case, dissection of the midface is performed in areas usually not touched by prior procedures; therefore dissection is done in a virgin (subperiosteal) plane. In the second case, the thick composite flaps fashioned in surgery have excellent vascularity, and ablative procedures on the skin do not affect the skins survival. In the last case, the intermediate and superficial lamellae of the face are intact, and fat can be injected in as many tunnels as needed.

Patients with skeletal/soft tissue disproportion can also benefit from endoscopic techniques of the midface. The exposed bony structures can be augmented via implants or reduced by osteotomies or bone burring without the need to open a different plane of dissection, as is the case when one performs surgery in the superficial or the intermediate planes of the face.

20.6 Preoperative Preparation

A full medical workup and cardiac clearance are requested as needed. In this age of significant influence by fashion and the media, patients will do anything to maintain their slim figures, including restrictive diets. In this respect, many young patients present to their plastic surgeons with an undiagnosed or untreated condition of anorexia and/or bulimia. These patients, despite a deceptively normal appearance, might be in severe metabolic and electrolyte imbalance, including hypokalemia and hypomagnesaemia. These disorders can lead to an unexpected cardiac arrest during or after surgery, among other complications. Surgeons, particularly plastic surgeons, should be aware of this potential situation. They should also be aware of the ever-increasing incidence of patients with body dysmorphia syndrome.

Photographs are taken several days before surgery without, or with minimal makeup. The hair is moved from the face with hair bands, clips and elastic "ponytail" bands. No superior tension of the brows or temples should be exerted to prevent "photo-surgery." The ears, temples, forehead, and neck should be fully exposed in the photographs. For the neck, a low-cut V, a circular T-shirt or no shirt at all should be used.

Markings are made with the patient in a standing or sitting position. The orbital rim outline is marked in blue. The area of maximal midface projection, which is at the zygomaxillary point, is marked in green. The nasolabial fold, tear trough deformities, and other areas of contour deficit are marked in red. Areas of contour excess are marked in black. The jaw line and the cervicomental break are marked in blue.

20.7 Aesthetic Considerations

The goals of the surgical procedure are to: efface the tear trough deformity, lift the cheek, efface the nasolabial fold, enhance the projection of the cheek, and lift the corner of the mouth. Most importantly is to recreate the aesthetic and youthful appearance of the cheek mound. The cheek seen in a three quarter view has a specific outline that has the shape of Sigma or Greek S also called the "ogee line". In reality the entire facial outline is a "double Ogee-line" (Fig. 20.3). This starts with a slight concavity on the forehead, continues with a convexity on the lateral brow, a concavity on the lateral orbital area, and gradually changing to a significant convexity on the cheek. This convexity gradually goes down at the level of the upper lip to converge into a slight concavity lateral to the paracomissural area. The highest point of the cheek convexity seen in a three quarter view is located at the so-called "zygomaxillary point." This is a new anthropometric soft tissue point that can be located by the intersection of two lines: one traced vertically on the lateral external orbital rim and another line horizontally oriented extending from the upper lateral cartilage of the nose to the tragus. The intersection of these two lines determines the maximum point of projection of the convexity, the zygomaxillary point [5–7].

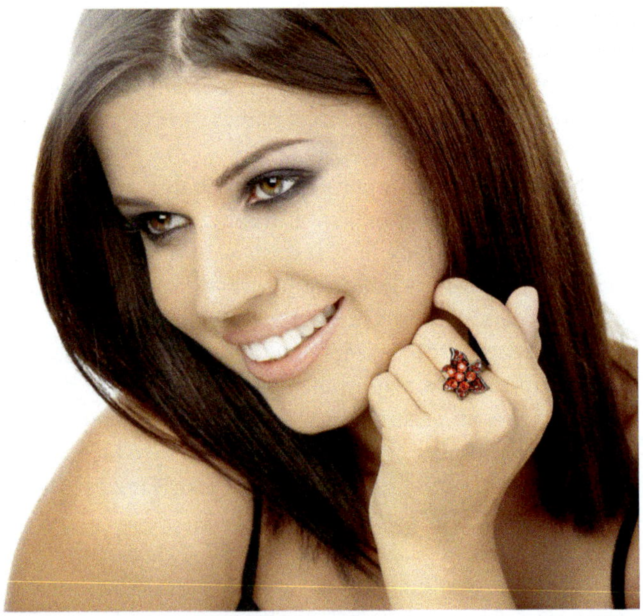

Fig. 20.3 Observe the reciprocal multicurvilinear outline of the face that I have been calling the *double ogee-line of the face*. This is seen better in a 3/4 view (*left side* of photo, *right side* of face). For many decades, artists, photographers, and glamor models have been using this view to emphasize beauty and youth. Photo © Shutterstock Images LLC; used with permission

The convexity in the male and female differs significantly in extent and projection. In a female, the convexity, as mentioned, extends to the upper lip. However, in the male, the convexity is short and ends at the level of the projection of the nasal ala. In general, this outline gives to the male midface a more angular and bony look. Conversely, in the female, the large convexity gives an impression of softer and delicate features without significant angularity, or a rounder look. It also shows a less bony facial appearance. As I mentioned, one of the important goals of midface rejuvenation is to create this reciprocal multicurvilinear line of beauty, or ogee line. The first step in this goal is to identify that you are creating a female or on a male – midface appearance.

20.8 Technique

Midface remodeling and lifting via an intraoral incision alone can be used in younger patients. This procedure called an endomidface lift can be done via a single intraoral 2.5 cm incision. However, the inclusion of the temporal component of the forehead provides superior results. This procedure is called an endotemporo-midface lift. This is used in most of the older patients because you will need the added lift and remodeling of the lateral periorbita and the temple, otherwise crowding and folding of tissue in those areas can be an unsightly appearance after the surgery. For logistic reasons, the most common endoscopic facial procedure that I perform is the combination endoforehead/endomidface lift. For the purposes of this chapter, I will only describe the endotemporo-midface lift which is the optimal technique for midface rejuvenation and beautification. Before going into the technique, it will be important to become familiar with the author's relevant anatomical nomenclature (Table 20.1), instruments (Ramirez Endoscopic Instrument Set, Snowden Pencer and Black & Black, Tucker, GA), and relevant anatomy (see Chap. 2).

Table 20.1 Ramirez anatomical nomenclature of the temporal and midface areas

Initials	Author's preferred name	Other name
TLF	Temporal line of fusion	None
TFP	Temporal fascia proper	Temporalis fascia Deep temporal fascia
ITF	Intermediate temporal fascia	Superficial layer of the deep temporal fascia
DTF	Deep temporal fascia	Deep layer of the deep temporal fascia
STF	Superficial temporal fascia	Temporo-parietalis fascia
BFP	Bichat's fat pad	Buccal fat pad
SOOF	Suborbicularis oculi fat	None

Surgery starts with a 2 cm temporal incision done within the hair-bearing portion of the temporal scalp (Fig. 20.4). This incision is normally located perpendicular to a line joining the nasal ala and lateral orbital rim extending into the temple. The incisions should be 2 cm posterior to the temporal hairline, and directed parallel to the hair follicles to prevent alopecia. Caution is advised not to make the incision too anterior in patients with significant and excess temporal hair. In these cases, the incision can be at or close to where the branches of the frontal nerve travel, and inadvertent injury is possible. In patients with sparse hair or with high temporal hairlines, do not make the incision too posterior or superior, to prevent overshooting the location of the temporal fascia proper (TFP) which will effect tissue suspension. After the skin incision, continue dissection to the white glistening surface of the TFP and proceed with dissection under direct visualization (directly on top of the TPF and below the superficial temporal fascia (STF)) for several centimeters in radius. The Guyuron's Endoscopic Access Device (Applied Medical Technologies, Brecksville, OH) is introduced at the incision for protection

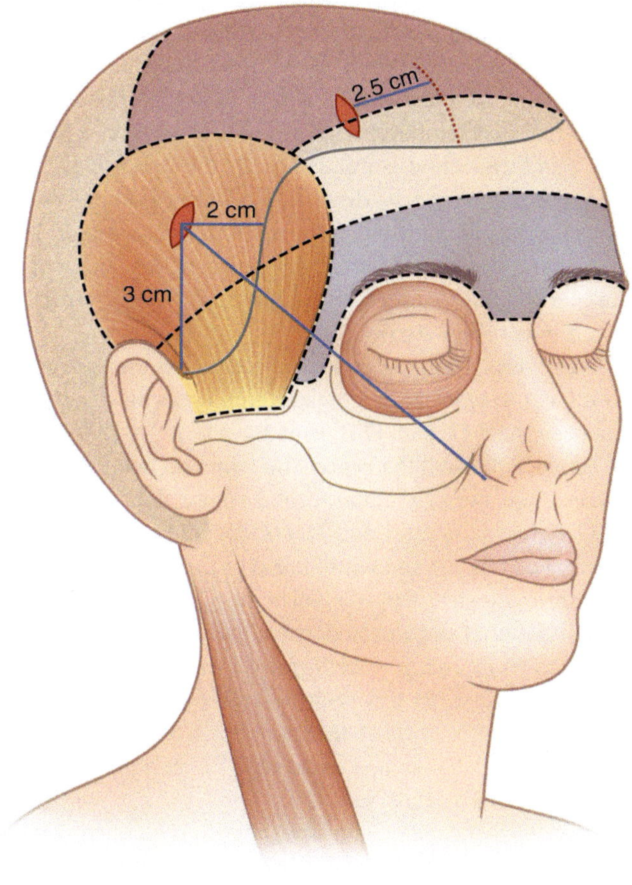

Fig. 20.4 The midface portion of the surgery starts with the temporal component for which a 2 cm incision is made. This is located in the temporal scalp on a line tangent to a line that joins the nasal ala and the lateral canthal area

of the hair follicles and to avoid penetration of hair into the surgical wound. Further dissection is done under endoscopic visualization. I use a 5 mm diameter, 30° down-angled endoscope over which the "Ramirez cobra sleeve" is applied (Snowden Pencer, Tucker, GA; Black and Black, Tucker, GA).

With a No. 4 Ramirez periosteal elevator, in the same surgical plane, the soft tissue is elevated until the temporal line of fusion (TLF) and the area of the sentinel vein, or temporal vein No. 2 (TV2), are identified. The TLF is a curvilinear linear structure extending from the level of the lateral margin of the superior orbital rim superiorly toward the parietal bone. It is present approximately 3 cm above the zygomatic arch and consists of a horizontal line of fascial blending where the TFP splits into a superficial and deep layer, with the intermediate temporal fat pad in-between (see Table 20.1). Posterior to the axis where the temporal branch (frontal nerve) of the facial nerve is located, dissection can continue to the root of the helix and posterior zygomatic soft tissue area.

Although the central forehead is not usually entered in standard midface surgery, most of the time elevation of the tail of the brow and crow's feet area are preferred. Therefore, dissection should continue for 1–2 cm medial to the TLF, and to the lateral one third of the brow. To do this, a curved Ramirez periosteal elevator No. 8 is used. This splits the periosteal and temporal fascia attachments (conjoined tendon), and dissection continues under the periosteum of the frontal bone. Inferiorly, dissection continues subperiosteally to incise the lateral extent of the arcus marginalis at the superior orbital rim, and to elevate the galea off the lateral orbital rim periosteum, but the periosteum of the lateral orbital rim is left intact (Fig. 20.5).

The "zero" Ramirez periosteal elevator is then introduced to dissect toward the zygomatic arch again in a safe plane between the STF and TFP. Tunnels anterior to the TV2 and in between this and the zygomatic temporal nerve (ZTN) are made. Near the zygomatic frontal suture line, a small vein (TV1) is usually split and electrocoagulated. Through the mentioned tunnels and with the aid of the endoscope and the Ramirez periosteal elevator No. 9, the zygomatic arch periosteum is entered and elevated just at the superior border of the arch and on its anterior one third. When this plane of dissection (subperiosteal) has been indentified, lateral dissection over the middle third of the zygomatic arch is performed. This subperiosteal plane is needed to protect the frontal branch of the facial nerve.

Rarely, the lateral one third of the arch is elevated. This lateral zygomatic arch dissection is needed when a more lateral vertical lift of the cheek is required. If the masseter tendon/muscle fascia is easily elevated from the temporal approach this can be continued 1–2 cm inferiorly. If not, this part of the dissection should proceed from the intraoral approach.

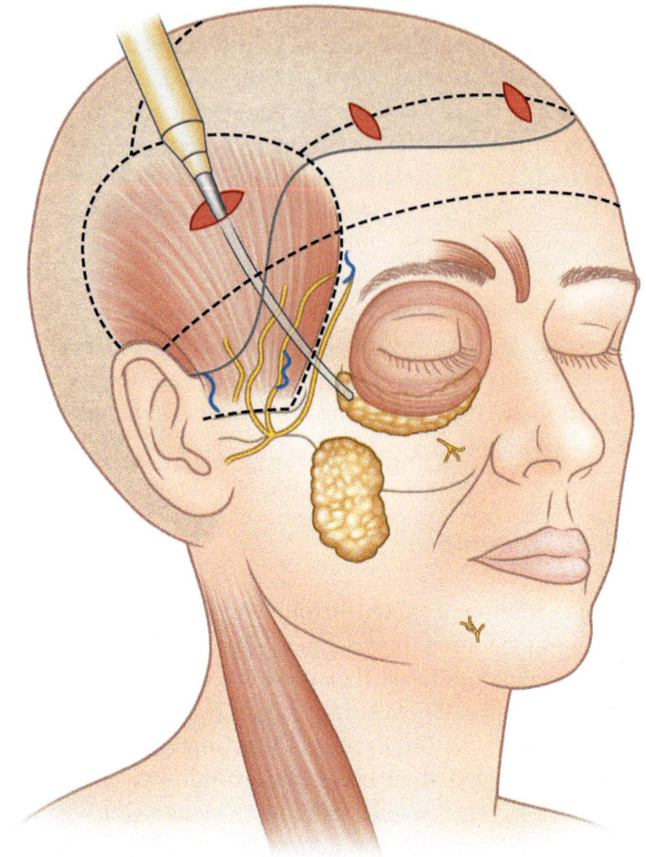

Fig. 20.5 On the lateral orbital rim, the subperiosteal dissection continues with a supraperiosteal dissection. This ensures periosteal integrity if canthopexy procedures are added to the operation. Laterally, a superiosteal dissection is done to connect the temporal and midface pockets across the zygomatic arch

The sequential endoscopic views in Fig. 20.6 show the midface dissection. The intraoral incision is obliquely/vertically oriented at the level of the first and second premolar, away from the opening of the Stenson's duct. The ends of the incision can be extended in a Z-shape if additional access is needed. Initially, the mucosa is incised with a No. 15 blade. The underlying buccinator muscle is bluntly separated during deepening of the incision toward the maxillary bone. With a No. 9 Ramirez periosteal elevator and with the aid of an Autfricht lighted retractor, a subperiosteal dissection ensues until the infraorbital nerve is identified. The dissection continues medially to the piriformis aperture and laterally to the masseter tendon insertion to the malar bone. If the visualization becomes cumbersome or difficult, the endoscope and the Ramirez periosteal elevator No. 8 are introduced and the dissection is continued laterally, elevating the fascia of the masseter muscle in continuity with the subperiosteal plane of dissection above the malar bone. Superolaterally, the periosteum of the zygoma body is elevated until the pre-dissected section (coming from the temporal approach) of the zygomatic

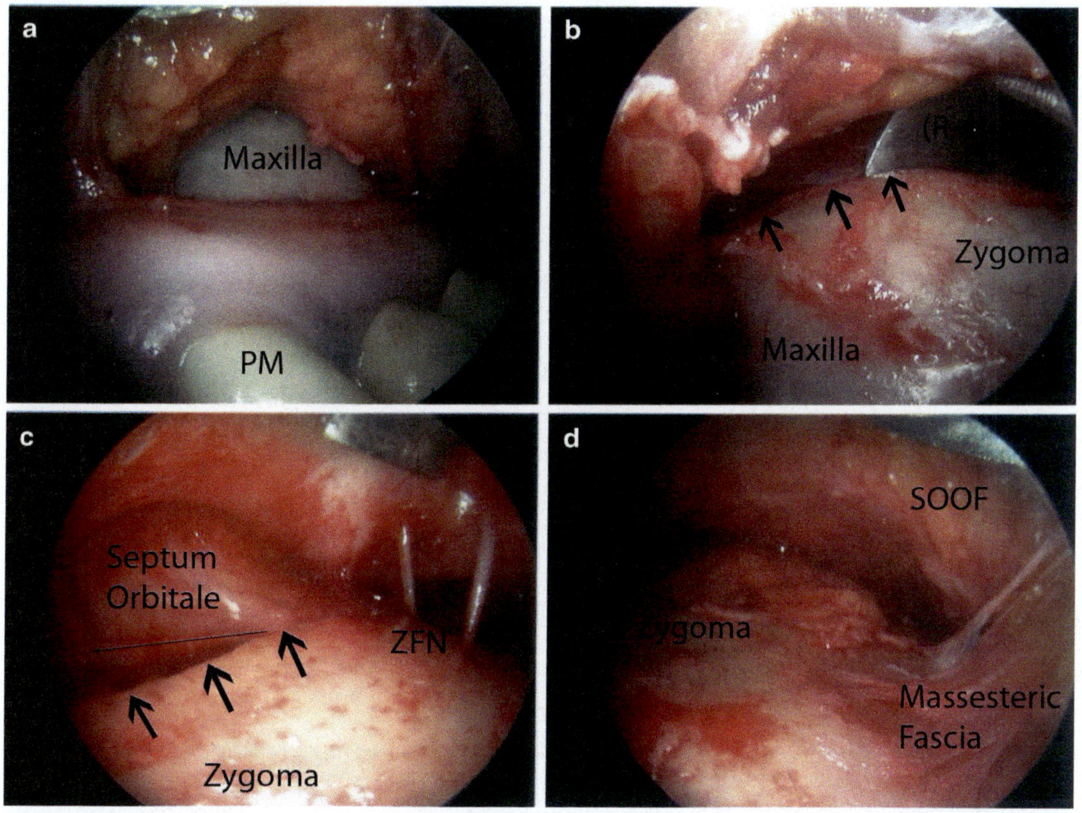

Fig. 20.6 This sequential endoscopic view on the left side of the patient shows: (**a**) Intraoral incision at the level of first premolar (pm). (**b**) Dissection over the maxilla and zygoma towards the infraorbital rim (*arrows*) with the Ramirez minus 4 (R–4) elevator. (**c**) The infraorbital rim (*arrows*) is exposed after the arcus marginalis (*interrupted points*) has been elevated. More laterally observe two branches of the zygomatico facial nerve (ZFN). (**d**) More laterally and inferiorly the masseter fascia is being elevated off the masseter tendon/muscle. Observe the location of the SOOF (Suborbicularis oculi fat)

arch (also in a subperiosteal plane) is made continuous with the malar dissection. Extension of the surgery around the inferior and lateral orbital rim should preserve the zygomatico facial nerve (ZFN).

In most cases, a 2–3 cm dissection over the masseter tendon is required. A wide connection between the midface and temporal pockets facilitates vertical lift and repositioning of the tissue elements that produce volumetric changes (Bichat's fat pad, imbrication of SOOF, etc.) at the zygomaxillary point. Superiorly, the periosteum and soft tissue attachments to the inferior orbital rim are manipulated using a combination of No. 9 and a –4 (minus 4) Ramirez periosteal elevators. The inferior arcus marginalis is elevated as is the periorbita 2 or 3 mm inside of the inferior orbital rim (Fig. 20.7). Dissection superior and medial to the infraorbital nerve is not yet performed. This portion of the procedure is completed after all the midface suspension sutures are applied and just before anchoring the midface to the temporal fascia is carried out. The attached surrounding muscles and soft tissues will protect the infraorbital nerve from inadvertent excessive traction during the midface manipulation. Traction is usually the cause for neuropraxia and numbness of the cheek, and upper lip postoperatively. The levator labii superioris and the orbicularis oculi muscle attachments to the medial and infraorbital rim are detached using the –4 (minus four) or the "zero" elevator.

The next critical step is the fixation of the midface. The number of fixation sutures placed and tension applied to these sutures is individualized. Only experience will dictate this part of the procedure. The inferior arcus marginalis is grasped with a 4–0 PDS suture on an RB1 needle. This is done in a vertical plane of the lateral limbus of the eye. The suborbicularis oculi fat (SOOF) is grasped approximately 1.5 cm inferior to the orbital rim and at the level of the medial limbus (Fig. 20.8). Both ends of the suture are either tied or driven to the temple pocket through a tunnel in between the orbital rim and ZFN and anterior to the temporal vein No. 2 (TV2). This suture is then anchored to the most anterior portion of the TFP using the sliding endoscopic "Peruvian" fisherman's knot [8]. This will vertically elevate the infraorbital SOOF (as opposed to the next suture – the lateral SOOF) in a superior and superolateral position over the infraorbital rim.

Fig. 20.7 This drawing illustrates the intraoral dissection of the periorbita to the inferior orbital rim. The insert shows the alternative access for extrusion of the intraorbital fat pads that can also be sutured to the SOOF for effacement of the tear trough

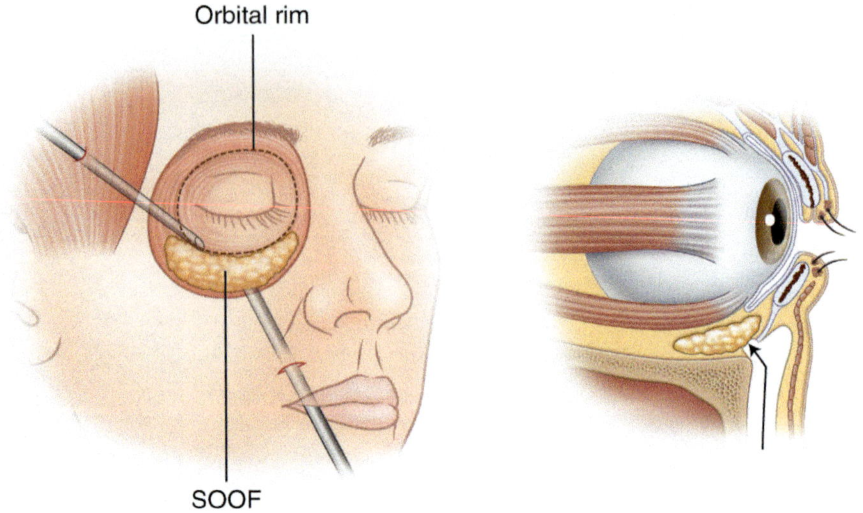

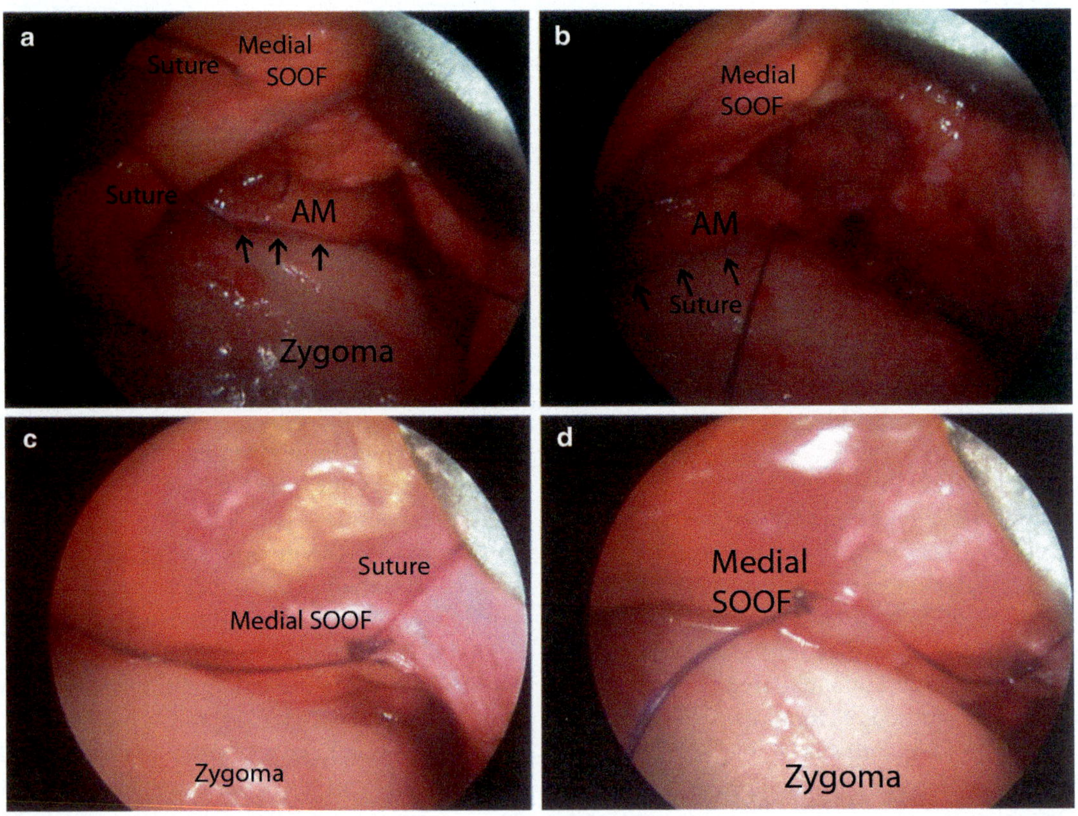

Fig. 20.8 These sequential endoscopic views (**a–d**) show the elevation of the Medial (infraorbital) SOOF towards the arcus marginalis (AM) using 4–0 PDS suture. Arrows show the orbital rim. The suture engages the fixed AM at the level of the lateral limbus, and the mobile Medial SOOF at the level of the medial limbus. As the suture is tied, the Medial SOOF is elevated superolaterally to efface the tear trough

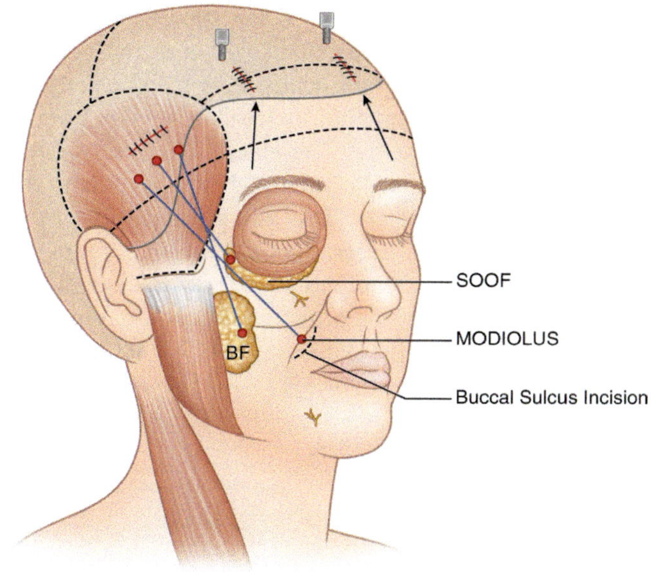

Fig. 20.9 Diagram showing the additional three suspension points for midface remodeling: the lateral SOOF, the Modiolus, and Bichat's fat pad (BF). Observe the decussation and orientation of the sutures. All are suspended in the temporal fascia proper (TFP) below the endoscopic entrance point. Also observe the frontal fixation (when endoscopic browlift is added) with the Ramirez self stabilizing percutaneous screws (Synthes, Paoli, PA)

In addition to the infraorbital SOOF suture above, three additional suspension sutures are applied (Fig. 20.9). These are anchored after final dissection medial to the infraorbital nerve is completed (as described previously). The first of these suspension sutures is to the lateral SOOF. This tissue is located 3–4 cm inferior to the lateral canthal tendon and is the bulkiest portion of the cheek mound. It is engaged with a 3–0 PDS suture on an RB1 needle.

The next suspension suture (modiolus suspension) is applied to the fascio-adipose tissue just superior to the modiolus, using a 4–0 PDS suture with an RB1 needle. The tissue is engaged near the mucosa, just anterior at the intraoral incision. The suture is woven 2 or 3 times tangentially to the plane of exposure to prevent catching a branch of the buccal nerve. (I have not had a neuropraxia related to this suture.)

The last suture is applied to Bichat's fat pad (BFP also called the buccal fat pad); BFP is exposed and extruded from the buccal space after the modiolus stitch is applied. If either of the cheeks, inferior orbital rim and/or piriformis implants, are used, these implants are fixated before BFP is mobilized. Inadvertent exposure of Bichat's fat pad prior to carrying out all these maneuvers will interfere with visualization as the fat pad will constantly protrude from the buccal space. BFP is extruded from its containment box with a blunt scissors, dividing the buccal space fascia between the anterior border of the masseter tendon and the lateral aspect of the maxilla. The constitution of the fat pad is very similar to that of eyelid fat, and its associated fascia is finely vascularized. The fat pad is mobilized using two blunt and smooth forceps or by similar neurosurgical forceps. With one forceps, BFP is pulled gently and with the other forceps, the fascia of the buccal space is teased away. This maneuver is similar to the mobilization of an inguinal hernia's sac from the peritoneal wall. It is critical to maintain BFPs fine protective fascia to allow its mobilization as a pedicle flap.

BFP tends to herniate down in front and anterior to the masseter tendon and muscle and lateral to the zygomatic major muscle in a trajectory from deep to superficial. This triangle is bounded inferiorly by the mandibular bone. This is a weak area of the midface covered only by thin SMAS layer. The buccal space fascia is similar to the peritoneal sac and tends to follow the migration of the "hernial content" in this case the BFP. This entity has been described by Matarasso in the past [9]. Gently pushing with the index finger from the outside of face at the level of the jowl toward the maxillary bone helps to further mobilize the low lying fat pad. The fat pad is mobilized for about 3 cm outside the buccal space into the intraoral incision. Here, it is grabbed with two or three woven 4–0 PDS sutures on an RB1 needles. A trial of mobilization toward the upper dental arcade outside the intraoral incision is made pulling the anchoring suture very gently. This is done to check if the fat pad is free without obstruction. The buccal fat pad is pushed back into the buccal space and both ends of the suture are driven to the temporal area and are brought out through the temporal incision. If the goal is to fill the submalar space with the uppermost projection at the level of the SOOF, then the suture is tied "piggy back" to the loop of the SOOF suspension suture. This will limit the upper ascent of the fat pad. If the goal is to give a more generalized volumetric augmentation of the cheekbone then the suture is anchored to the TFP.

As you have noticed, the sequence of suture placement in the midface started with a vertical (infraorbital) SOOF suspension which is secured to the TFP. Then the lateral SOOF, the modiolus, and BFP are secured as described. The sequence of anchoring and tying the last three sutures to the TFP is reversed. BFP is anchored first, then the modiolus, and the lastly the lateral SOOF. The placement of the sutures in the temporal plane also follows a sequence: the BFP suture is located anteriorly, the modiolus suture in the center, and the SOOF suture more laterally. This way, all the sutures are crisscrossed at the level of the zygomaxillary point with a maximum volumetric augmentation at this desired maximal point of projection. The effect of each one of the sutures is different, and when they are combined, the effect is synergistic.

As I mentioned, the vertical suborbital SOOF lift effaces the tear trough and periorbital V deformity. The BFP elevation gives a significant volumetric augmentation of the cheek, increases the convexity of the upper midface, and concomitantly increases the concavity of the lower midface. This will accentuate the reciprocal multicurvilinear line of beauty of the midface – the ogee line.

The cases in which BFP is excised, it will accentuate the concavity of the lower midface. Excision of BFP is done with a similar technique as its mobilization. The fat is extruded intact towards the intraoral incision. A moistened 2×2 gauze is applied in between the maxillary bone and the neck of the mobilized pedicle flap (BFP). Using a mono-polar needle point cautery, the pedicle is cauterized at the base of the extruded portion. This way there is no bleeding, associated facial ecchymosis or edema that is common with the piecemeal approach to remove this fat pad.

The modiolus stitch will lift the corner of the mouth and imbricates the lower cheek toward the upper cheek. The endpoint of lateral upper lip mobilization with the modiolus stitch is exposure of the entire canine tooth with the patient in a supine position. If this is done on both sides, it will secure symmetry of the corner of the lip elevation. Obviously, in cases of asymmetry, the lower lying lip and corner of the mouth are overcorrected. The lateral SOOF suspension also imbricates the cheek towards the zygomaxillary point, and suspends the entire cheek reducing the load of weight on the other suspension sutures.

Each one of the sutures except in the BFP suture is tied using the sliding locking endoscopic "Peruvian" fisherman's knot [8]. This will provide graded tension on the elevated tissue until the desired level is attained. If the tension of the suture is excessive the initial loop of knot can be loosened and tissue will descend. After appropriate midface position is achieved, a single square knot will lock the entire system. The BFP suture is then anchored with its own square knot while the assistant locks the first knot to prevent excessive traction on this delicate structure. BFP is transposed freely without undue tension.

Using this technique in several hundred cases I have had only two cases of disruption of the fat pad. If this happens, remobilize the fat pad from the buccal space, apply two woven sutures from the center of the flap, and anchor it as a piggyback to the lateral SOOF suture.

Any residual asymmetry is usually due to a preexisting asymmetry that becomes more obvious after the cheek feature are elevated and imbricated. This can be addressed with microfat injection in the intermediate layer of the face. A 2 mm butterfly drain is guided to each cheek and the intraoral incisions are closed which will be described.

The temporal flap is suspended from the STF to the TFP using three interrupted 3–0 PDS suture. The suture placement has a trapezoidal shape with a larger base located at the TFP and the shorter base at the superficial temporal fascia. If the shape is made quadrangular or the trapezoid inverted, the lifted temporal scalp will bunch up at or near the incision. The orientation of the flap tension is either vertical or vertico-medially oriented. This will give an effective vertical lift of the lateral cheek, zygomatic arch of soft tissues and temple. This will also open the crow's feet area with forces directly opposite to the forces of contraction and ptosis. This particular orientation will also prevent lateral pull of the brows and excessive separation between the lateral periorbital soft tissues and the temporal hairline.

20.9 Lower Eyelid Blepharoplasty

This is an added technique to midface rejuvenation that significantly enhances the final results. Treating the midface and the lower eyelid as one aesthetic and anatomical unit improves the aesthetic result and diminishes the complications of an isolated lower blepharoplasty. Younger patients may not require a lower blepharoplasty when undergoing a midface lift. In these cases, minimal excess skin can be treated with one pass of CO_2 laser or a chemical peel. In older patients, the vertical lift of the cheek will recruit skin to the lower eyelid. In these cases, I perform skin-only lower eyelid blepharoplasty. The orbicularis oculi muscle is also suspended to maximize the periorbital aesthetic improvement. I take advantage of the fact that the attachments of the orbicularis oculi muscle to the orbital rim have been elevated during the endomidface lift, and the composite soft tissues can be redraped further with oblique traction on the preseptal portion of this muscle. Furthermore, the tensions exerted on the muscle will retro-place the herniated lower lid fat into the orbit, while simultaneously reducing inherent laxity of the muscle.

I make a horizontal incision 2 mm inferior to the subciliary margin and extend it in a horizontal direction into a temporal rhytid (crow's feet). The skin is dissected off the pretarsal and preseptal orbicularis oculi muscle for approximately 1–1.2 cm inferiorly. The lateral orbicularis oculi muscle is spread open to create a tunnel into the most anterior portion of the TFP. The lateral extension of the preseptal orbicularis oculi muscle is grabbed with 5–0 Prolene suture. The suture is anchored to the TFP in a mattress fashion through the tunnel previously described. This allows superior and superolateral suspension of the muscle. This also creates a roll of muscle in the pretarsal area, which is a favorable feature typical of the youthful eye. If there is hypertrophy of the preseptal orbicularis muscle, then the muscle is trimmed in a tangential fashion preserving the vertically oriented motor nerves that travel deep to the orbicularis oculi muscle. If the treatment of the crow's feet is needed, the lateral orbital orbicularis oculi muscle can be excised as described by Viterbo [10].

The lower eyelid skin is now redraped in a vertical direction and its excess is removed conservatively. If significant laxity of the lower eyelid was present preoperatively, either a canthoplasty or canthopexy can be added through the same incision. I have found that the combination of a vertical orbicularis oculi muscle suspension and a canthopexy is usually adequate in the majority of patients. Very rarely I need to perform a canthoplasty or horizontal lid shortening type of procedure. The skin is closed with 6–0 Prolene suture with a vascular needle.

20.10 Fat Grafting

This is a technique that can be easily incorporated into the operation as fat can be injected at any level from the subdermis to the periosteum. Fat is usually obtained from the periumbilical area, spun in a centrifuge, and the fluid elements separated. Using a 1 cc Luer Lock syringe, with the Ramirez Super-Luer-Lock micro-cannulas (Tulip Medical, San Diego, CA), the fat is injected to correct any residual asymmetries, to erase the dermal creases resulting from the chronic folding of the nasolabial folds, and to inflate the brow area as needed. I use an average of 30 cc of fat for the entire face as an adjunctive technique. However, I do not typically rely on fat grafting for the volumetric augmentation of the cheek. I only do this when the patient's face is too thin and does not have enough soft tissues (including BFP) to create volume with the imbrication techniques described.

20.11 Drains, Closure, Taping, and Dressing

In my technique there are no significant areas of closure because the incisions are small. However, taping of the face is a very important maneuver. The skin of the scalp in the temporal areas is closed in a single layer with skin staples. In this area, there is usually no tension due to the vertical advancement of the lower flap. It is important to evert the edges of the wound to prevent overlapping of the skin edges with subsequent in growth of hair into the wound. Generally, three to five staples are used to close the temporal wounds on each side. All staples but the central one are removed at the fourth or fifth postoperative day. The remaining staples are removed at the seventh to tenth postoperative day. The intraoral incision is closed in a looped mattress fashion using a 4–0 chromic suture. This will prevent inversion of the mucosal edges or potential cheese wiring of the mucosa. Furthermore, this mattress closure provides a one-way valve (from internal to external), that in cases of excessive bleeding, or fluid collection, will allow fluid to seep out, but will prevent saliva from entering the wound. Prior to closure of the temporal incision, a 2 mm butterfly drain is introduced through a mini-puncture in the temporal scalp, with its tip left in the midface. The drain is fixated with an interlooped 4–0 PDS suture and connected to a Vacutainer tube. At 24–36 h postoperatively, the drain is advanced by pulling about 1 in. from the scalp exit. The drain is removed at 48–72 h postoperatively.

The forehead and midface are taped with half inch brown micropore tape. The initial taping is applied from the glabrous portion of the temple to the forehead in a superomedial direction. The lower eyelid and cheeks are taped horizontally and then in an oblique direction towards the temple. Both sites of taping are interconnected without creating creases or ripples in the skin of the lateral periorbital area. The facial taping is another stabilizing and splinting element that prevents motion, facial edema, and ecchymosis. The tape is left for about 10 days. The initial tape is removed at the fifth postoperative day, and a less aggressive taping is reapplied. Taping of the lower eyelid helps prevent edema and mechanical eyelid malposition by a swollen conjunctive (chemosis) if this exists. A circumferential helmet type dressing is applied to the forehead, face, and neck for about 24 h. This is mostly for comfort and to catch any fluid from the ice compresses to the cheeks and eyelids. These compresses are applied for 24–48 h.

20.12 Summary

The minimal incision midface lift is a safe and effective procedure for midface rejuvenation. It can be performed via only an intraoral incision. However, the endotemporo-midface lift (described herein), or the endoforehead-endomidface procedure, are more effective in remodeling the midface and periorbital areas. A wide subperiosteal dissection allows excellent surgical visualization, better remodeling of tissues, a safe plane of dissection, and improved outcomes. In addition, the imbrication of tissue and suture lift via this approach allows superior volume augmentation of the cheek. Bichat's fat pad is an essential element needed to create the convexity in the cheek, and the concavity in the paracomissural area. This simultaneously creates the ogee of the midface (Figs. 20.10–20.25) The surgery can be incorporated with any additional techniques of facial rejuvenation and can be performed in conjunction with the use of facial implants and or fat grafting. The midface procedure also allows optimization of lower blepharoplasty surgery to obtain better aesthetic and functional results.

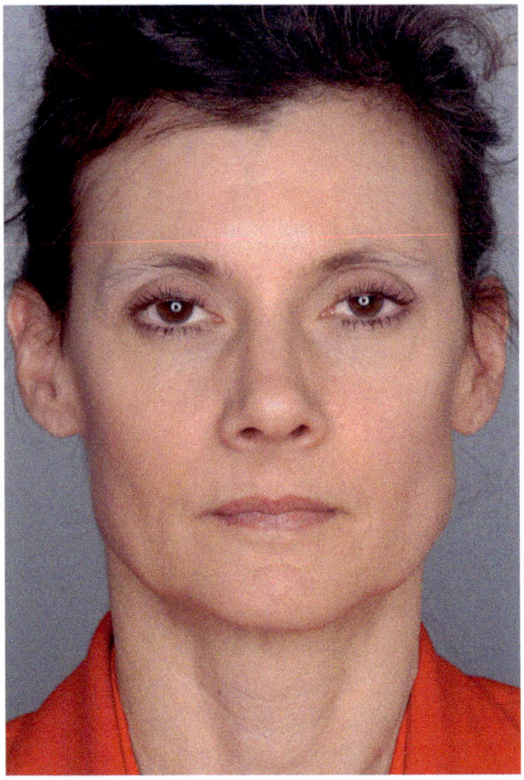

Fig. 20.18 Preoperative view of a woman who looks tired with midface sagging. Notice the bilateral eyelid ptosis

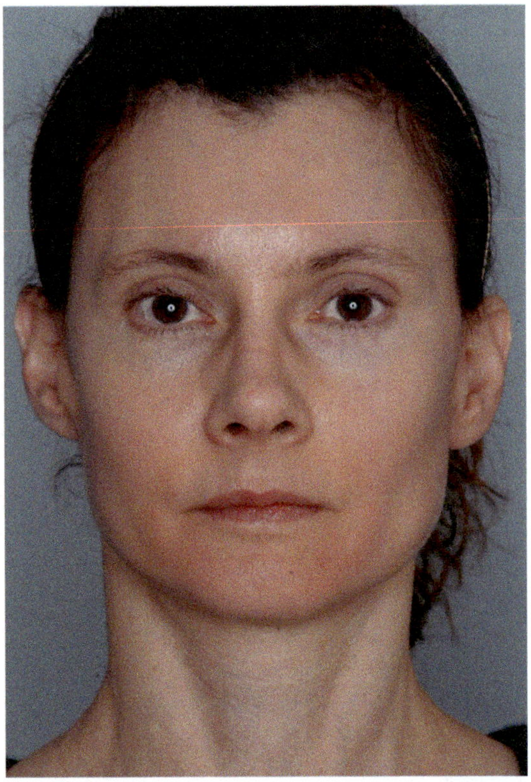

Fig. 20.19 Following ptosis repair, endoforehead and endomidface lift, lower blepharoplasty, fat grafting as well as cervicofacial lift

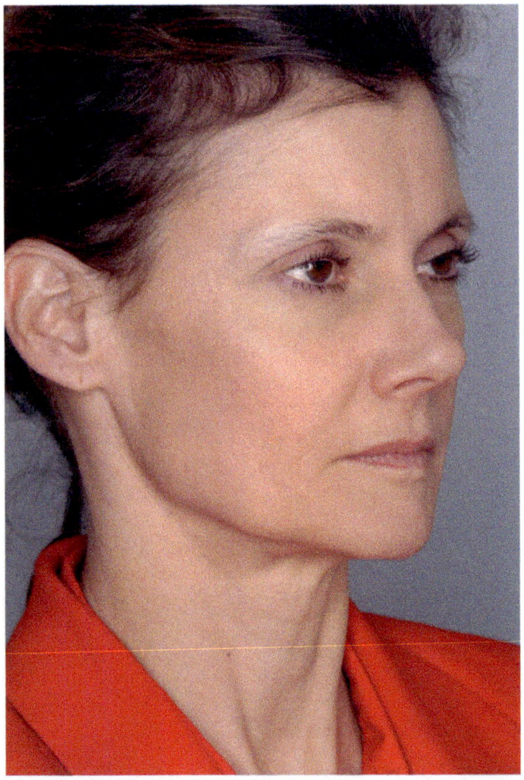

Fig. 20.20 Preoperative 3/4 view. Observe the subtle but generalized sagging of the face and the flattening of the cheeks

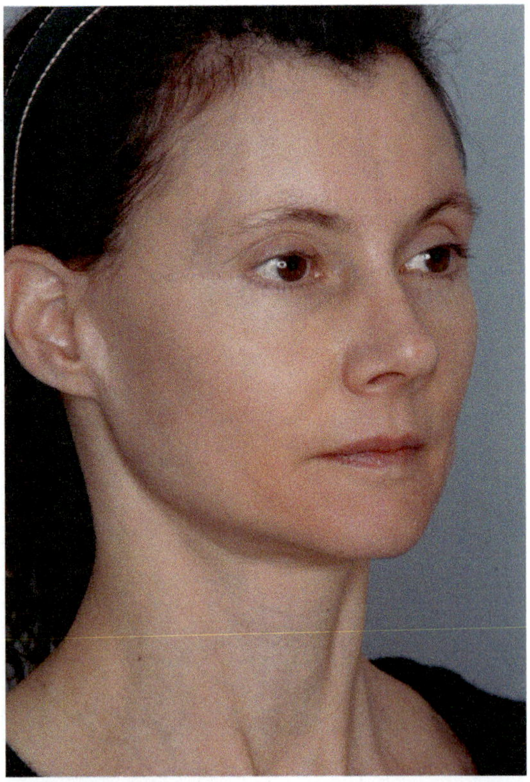

Fig. 20.21 Postoperative 3/4 view. Notice the subtle but definitive rejuvenation with the shape and beauty of a younger counterpart. There are no telltale signs of surgery

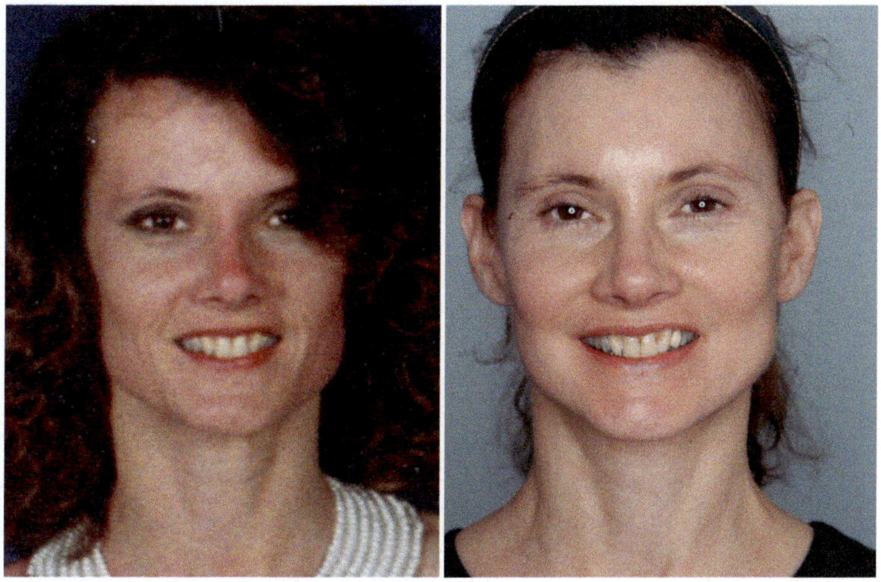

Fig. 20.22 These comparative photos show the patient (from Figs. 18–21) 20 years earlier on the left and 1 year after her surgery on the right. The shape of youth is the same if not better after surgery

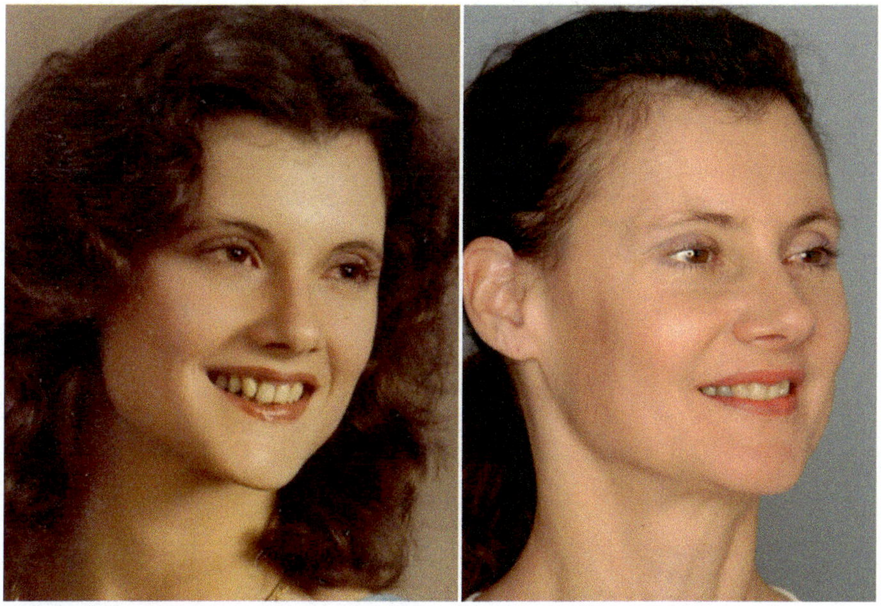

Fig. 20.23 Theg lamorp hoto (again of patient from Figs. 18–21) on the left is 30 years before. The nonglamor photo on the right is 1 year after her surgery. The facial shape and expressions are the same

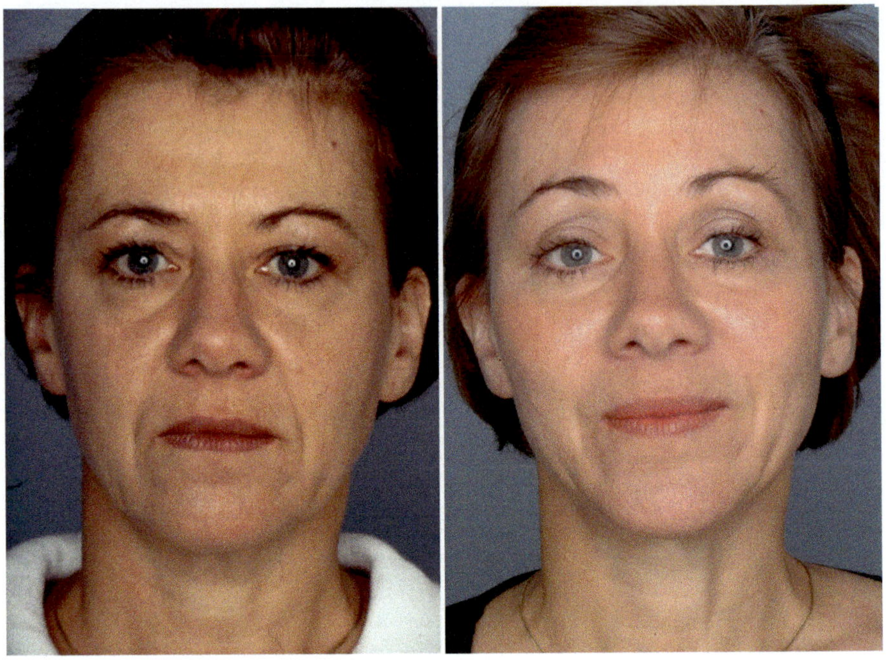

Fig. 20.24 Pre- and postoperative views of a woman who underwent endoforehead-endomidface lift, lower blepharoplasty, and fat grafting. Observe the improvement of the periocular depressions (*circles*) and the volumetric improvement of the cheeks

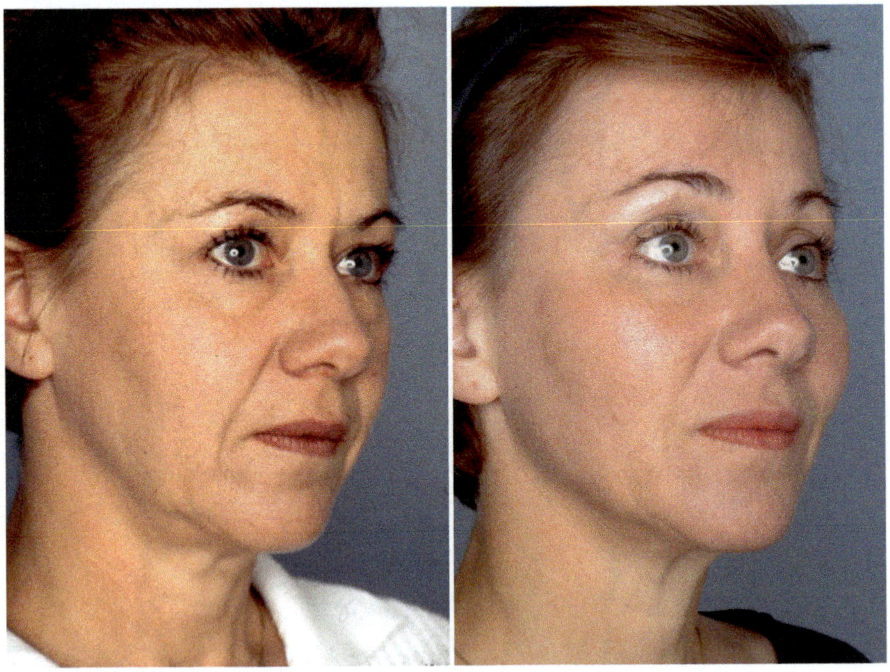

Fig. 20.25 Pre- and postoperative 3/4 views (of patient from Fig. 24) show the changes previously mentioned. Particularly observe the "ogee" of the midface and the correction of the lower eyelid deformities

References

1. Hurwitz DJ, Raskin EM. Reducing eyelid retraction following subperiosteal face lift. Aesthet Surg J. 1997;17:149.
2. Ramirez OM. The central oval of the face: tridimensional endoscopic rejuvenation. Facial Plast Surg. 2000;16:283–98.
3. Ramirez OM. Full face rejuvenation in three dimensions: a "face lifting" for the new millennium. Aesthet Plast Surg. 2001;25: 152–64.
4. Ramirez OM. Three-dimensional endoscopic midface enhancement. A personal quest for the ideal cheek rejuvenation. Plast Reconstr Surg. 2002;109:329–40.
5. Ramirez OM, Volpe CR. Double ogee facial rejuvenation, Chap. 43. In: Panfilov DE, Panfilov DE, editors. Aesthetic surgery of the facial mosaic. Berlin: Springer; 2007. p. 288–99.
6. Ramirez OM, Heller L. Facial rejuvenation. In: Peled IJ, Manders EK, editors. Esthetic surgery of the face. London: Taylor & Francis; 2004. p. 73–90.
7. Ramirez OM, Volpe CR. Tridimensional endoscopic facelift, Chap. 11. In: Azizzadeh B, Murphy MR, Johnson CM, Azizzadeh B, Murphy MR, Johnson CM, editors. Master techniques in facial rejuvenation. Philadelphia, PA: Elsevier Saunders; 2007. p. 173–96.
8. Ramirez OM, Tezel E, Ersoy B. The Peruvian fisherman's knot: a new, simple, and versatile self-locking sliding knot. Ann Plast Surg. 2009;62:114–7.
9. Matarasso A. Pseudoherniation of the buccal fat pad: a new clinical syndrome. Plast Reconstr Surg. 2003;112(6):1716–8.
10. Viterbo F. New treatment for crow's feet wrinkles by vertical myectomy of the lateral orbicularis oculi. Plast Reconstr Surg. 2003; 112:275.

Face Implants in Aesthetic Surgery

21

Joe Niamtu III

Key Points

- Midface volume loss is a consistent feature of facial aging.
- Cheek implants provide numerous advantages over other procedures which address midface volume loss.
- Cheek implants are available in numerous sizes and anatomic configurations.
- The intraoral route provides the best method for insertion of midface implants.
- The micro-screw system can be used to secure midface implants to the facial skeleton.
- Midface implants are easily and quickly inserted and can be removed or adjusted rapidly with minimal morbidity.

21.1 Introduction

Midface augmentation with alloplastic implants is a powerful tool in modern facial rejuvenation [1–12]. It can significantly improve the outcome of facial cosmetic surgery, and if ignored can equally detract from the final result. Often times surgeons omit the midface evaluation and subsequent intervention, while routinely performing brow lifts, blepharoplasty, and rhytidectomy for facial and periorbital aesthetic surgery. After surgery, this omission leads to potentially glaring discrepancies in facial proportions to the trained eye. These patients look "different" or "done" and can demonstrate classic stigmata of plastic surgery. This concept is further magnified when a volume depleted midface is elevated over a face devoid of appropriate skeletal support. The results are less than ideal.

J. Niamtu III (✉)
Cosmetic Facial Surgeon, Private Practice,
Midlothian, VA, USA
e-mail: niamtu@niamtu.com

To achieve a more natural outcome, there must be an understanding of the importance of restoring facial volume, especially in the midface. No other region of the face contributes as much to youthfulness, as a rounded and volumized midface which is a hallmark of both youth and beauty [1]. Virtually all patients in their late 40s and 50s will become volume deficient in the midface. With this progression, what once was the midface now become the jowls (Fig. 21.1). As a result, midface augmentation must be discussed with all cosmetic facial surgery patients over 40 years of age [3, 4, 10]. Since, most patients are not aware of this aspect of facial aging, a hand-held mirror is used to allow careful inspection of the cheek region with the patient in repose, as well as smiling. The act of smiling simulates the addition of midface volume that usually imparts a youthful appearance. Supporting the elevated cheek with the thumb and forefinger, and asking the patient to relax their smile, then demonstrates how the midface volume retreats to the jowl region (Fig. 21.2).

Another means of showing a patient the importance of midface volume restoration is to recline the examination chair, placing the patient in a supine position. The patient then holds a mirror above them. The gravitational influence will fill the gaunt midface in a similar fashion to the results achieved with midface implants (Fig. 21.3). Finally, midface deficiency can be illustrated by simply holding a submalar implant over the patient's cheeks. The implant usually is an exact match for the volume deficit and the patient can see firsthand how the implant can fill the midface hollow (Fig. 21.4).

By using one, or all, of these techniques for patient demonstration, the surgeon can increase patient awareness and acceptance for the placement of midface implants. Even the most conservative of patients will consider this option in their treatment plan, if they understand and visualize the mechanism of midface aging and volume restoration.

G.G. Massry et al. (eds.), *Master Techniques in Blepharoplasty and Periorbital Rejuvenation*,
DOI 10.1007/978-1-4614-0067-7_21, © Springer Science+Business Media, LLC 2011

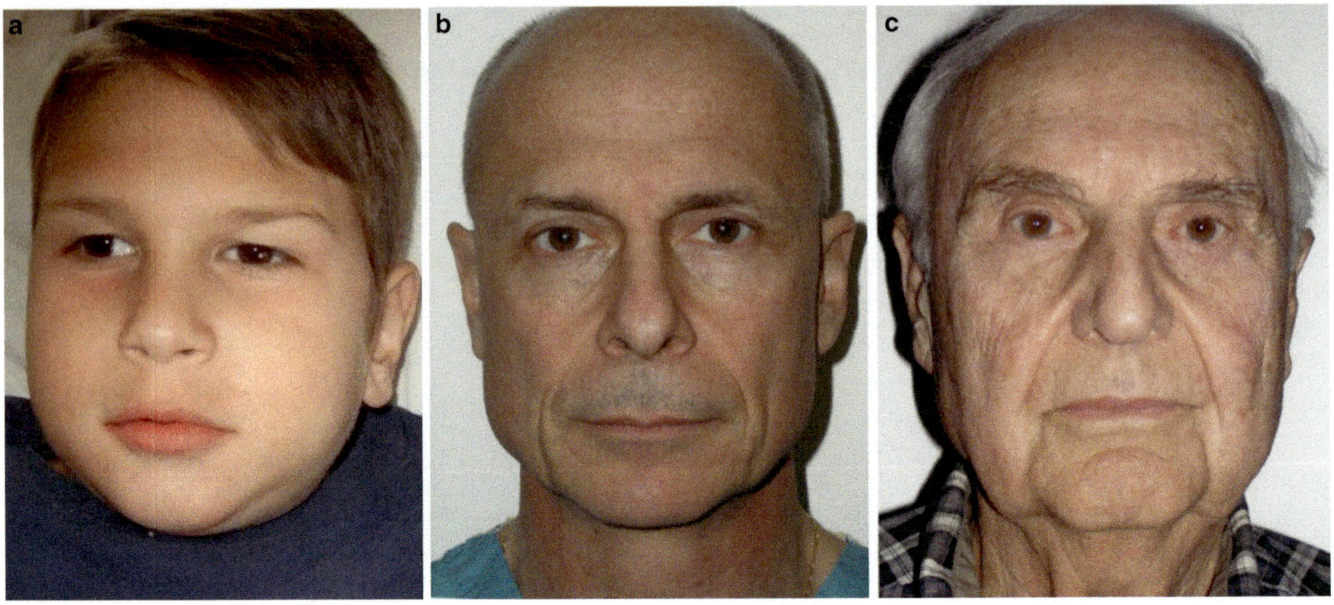

Fig. 21.1 This image shows the author's son (*left*-age 7), the author (*center*-age 56) and the author's father (*right*-age 79). These pictures illustrate the continual progression of midfacial volume loss with aging. (Photos courtesy Joe Niamtu III. (**b**) Reprinted from Niamtu [13], with permission from Elsevier)

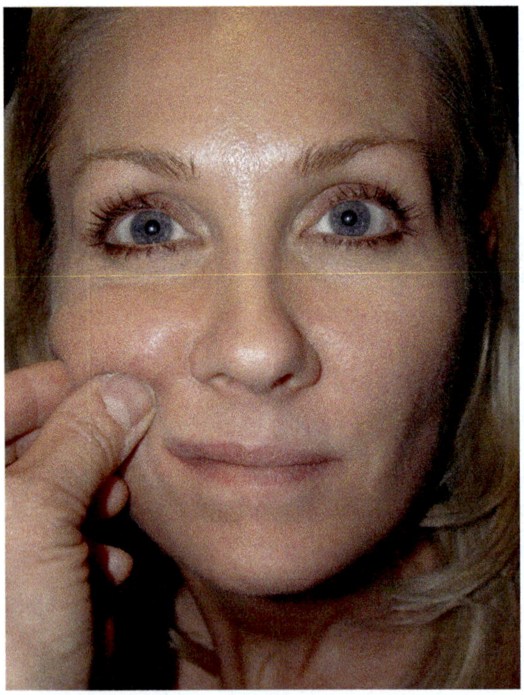

Fig. 21.2 To educate patients about midface volume loss, the cheek is elevated to show where the volume once existed, then released to show the gaunt midface as it exists. (Photo courtesy Joe Niamtu III)

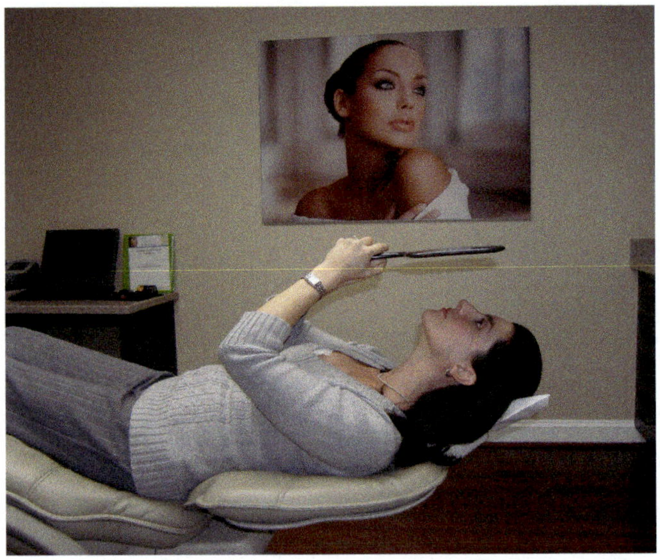

Fig. 21.3 Placing the patient in the recumbent position will enable gravity to fill the midface and give the patient an idea of how cheek implants may contribute to facial rejuvenation. (Photo courtesy Joe Niamtu III. Reprinted from Niamtu [13], with permission from Elsevier)

21.2 Midface Treatment Options

These are various options available for midface volume restoration including fillers, autologous fat grafting, endoscopic midface lifting, and alloplastic implants [1]. Fillers and fat grafting do enhance midface volume; but the techniques are rarely permanent and typically require repeat treatments and maintenance. Fat grafting and fillers can also contribute to tissue ptosis. An endoscopic midface lift can be a powerful procedure in the hands of an appropriate surgeon. However, the surgery is intricate, requires experience with technical equipment, and the results are frequently short-lived, and often do not adequately restore volume to the region.

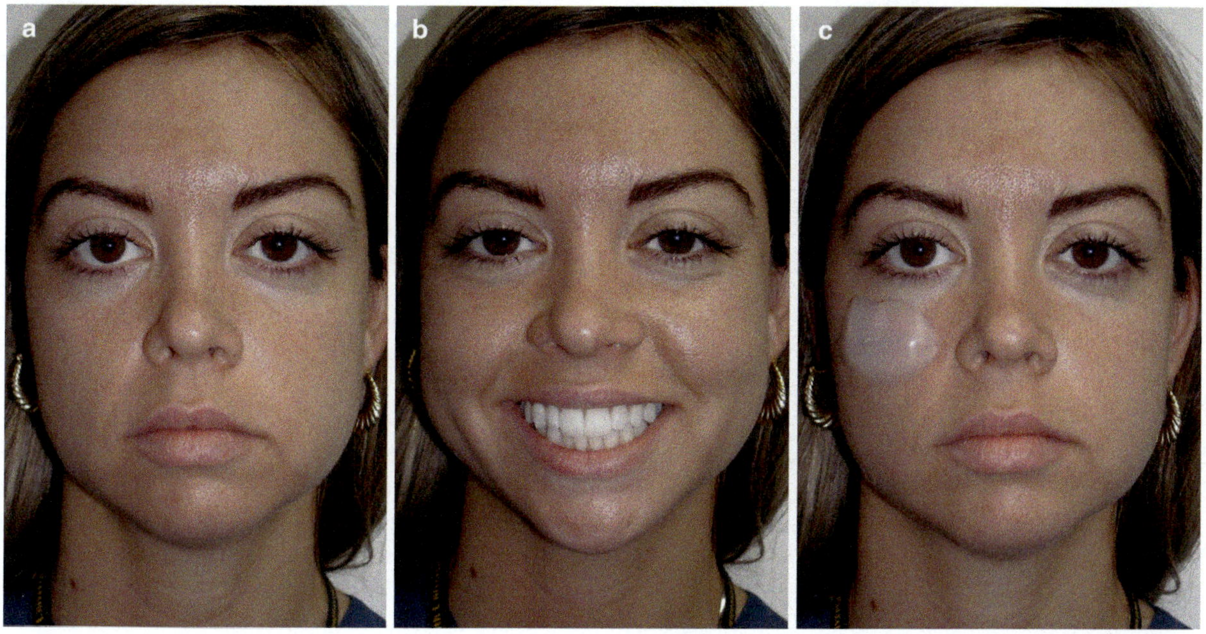

Fig. 21.4 This patient is shown in repose which shows moderate malar deficiency (**a**). She is also shown smiling which repositions the facial volume to a more natural state (**b**). A combined submalar shell implant is placed on the patient's cheek to illustrate the anticipated area of augmentation (**c**). (Photos courtesy Joe Niamtu III)

Table 21.1 Silicone midface advantages

Hidden incision
Simple to place
Permanent (when fixated)
Anatomic configurations
Numerous sizes and shapes
3D volume restoration
Reversible

Silicone cheek implants differ from filling or lifting in that they are permanent, three dimensional, reversible, and simple to place (Table 21.1). When they are placed and retained with a bone screw, migration is extremely rare. With time, they become encapsulated yet do not integrate into surrounding soft tissues, and are thus simple to remove.

21.3 Diagnosis and Implant Selection

For the novice implant surgeon, appropriate facial analysis as well as implant selection can be intimidating and confusing. From a diagnostic standpoint, one must understand midfacial anatomy and aging to properly select the correct implant. Changes in the skin, muscle, fat, and bone contribute to the aging midface and can vary from patient to patient. The midface can be subdivided into an infraorbital, submalar, and malar region (Fig. 21.5).

Most individuals begin to lose submalar volume in their early 40s. There is usually a concomitant component of infraorbital volume loss manifesting as a nasojugal groove or "tear trough" (Fig. 21.6a). These patients will benefit from a submalar implant which is the most commonly utilized midface implant in the author's practice (approximately 95% of cases) (Fig. 21.7a). Other patients have volume loss in the zygomatic superolateral "malar" region but have adequate submalar volume (Fig. 21.6b). This population benefits from the placement of a malar shell type implant as this configuration adds more volume to the superiolateral zygomatic region and little to the submalar region (Fig. 21.7b). This is also the style of implant for patients who request a "high cheekbone" appearance. Finally, some patients manifest volume loss in the submalar and malar regions and require dual site augmentation (Fig. 21.6c). These patients respond well to the combined submalar shell implant that is an amalgamation of the two previously described implants (Fig. 21.7c).

The infraorbital region is a more challenging region to treat with implants only. Although "tear trough" silicone implants exist, they demonstrate variable degrees of success and are thus less commonly used. In the author's experience, many patients will achieve some degree of infraorbital volume improvement from submalar implants, especially when performed with lower blepharoplasty and skin resurfacing.

It is also important to note that implants can also address issues other than midface aging. Some implants are placed to enhance midface features in youthful patients in the same manner that breast implants are used for augmentation. This is also true of youthful patients with genetic or developmental maxillary or malar hypoplasia.

As each patient has a different anatomic need, custom-made three-dimensional implants would lead to a more optimal outcome. These implants, commonly used for reconstructive and asymmetric cases, are typically developed from computerized tomographic scans (Fig. 21.8). The numerous sizes and shapes available of silicone implants enable "off the shelf" treatment for the vast majority of patients presenting for aging or augmentative treatment. The experienced surgeon can customize these implants by carving or trimming the edges to produce a more customized result.

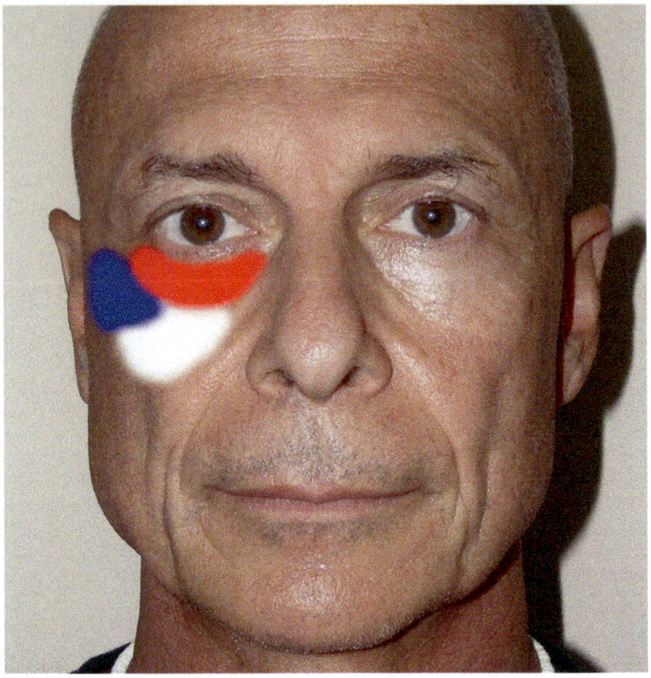

Fig. 21.5 This image shows three regions of the midface that can be augmented. The *red region* is the tear trough (infraorbital region), the *white region* is the submalar area and the *blue region* is the malar area

After trying almost every implant material over the years, including silicone, ePTFE and porous polyethylene, silicone has become my primary implant preference. In theory, any bio-compatible implant will suffice if it maintains stability over time. Porous polyethylene implants have gained popularity, but in the author's experience, are rigid, and do not conform to the underlying osseous anatomy. Their biggest drawback is that they are extremely difficult to remove as their porous structure leads to tissue integration. Removal of this type of implant is traumatic and results in adjacent tissue loss and severe implant fragmentation. Rigid plastic implants are hard, do not contour to bone well, and can be difficult to modify. Their utility is limited compared to silicone implants. Silicone rubber is soft and malleable. The implant curves around the cheek, from the surrounding weight of the soft tissues, without creating contour irregularities or obvious external signs of placement. Another advantage of silicone, over a rigid plastic implant, is that it does not fragment and is extremely easy to trim or carve. They also resist cracking or shattering if a screw is placed too tightly. Finally, these implants become well encapsulated, making removal or replacement easy if desired.

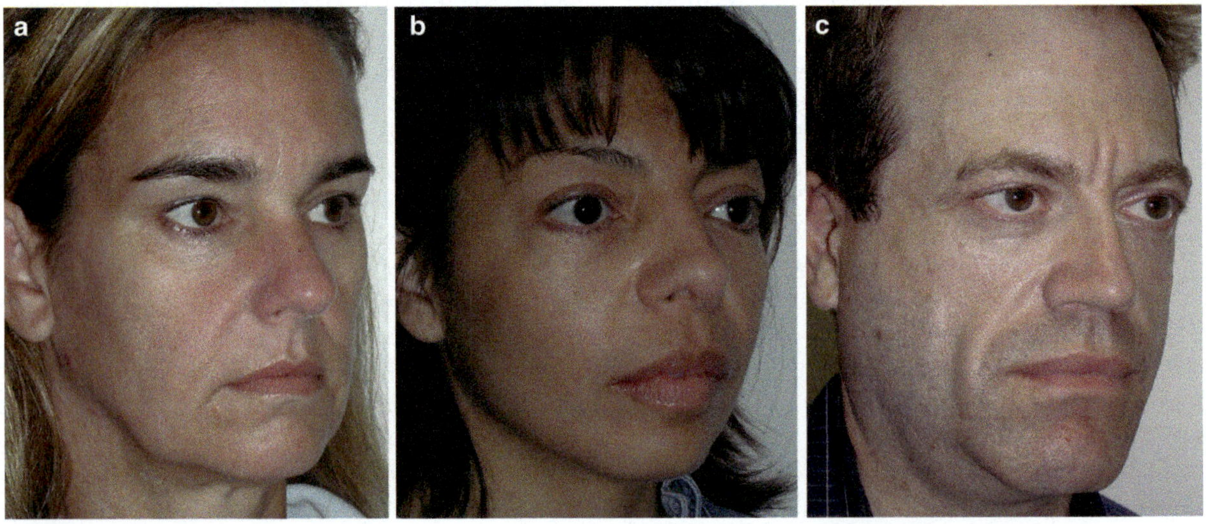

Fig. 21.6 (**a**) A patient with submalar volume loss and a candidate for simple submalar implants. (**b**) A patient with adequate submalar fill but with hypoplasia of the malar region who would be a good candidate for a malar shell implant. (**c**) A patient who lacks volume in both the submalar and malar regions and is a good candidate for a combined submalar shell implant. (Photos courtesy Joe Niamtu III. Reprinted from Niamtu [13], with permission from Elsevier)

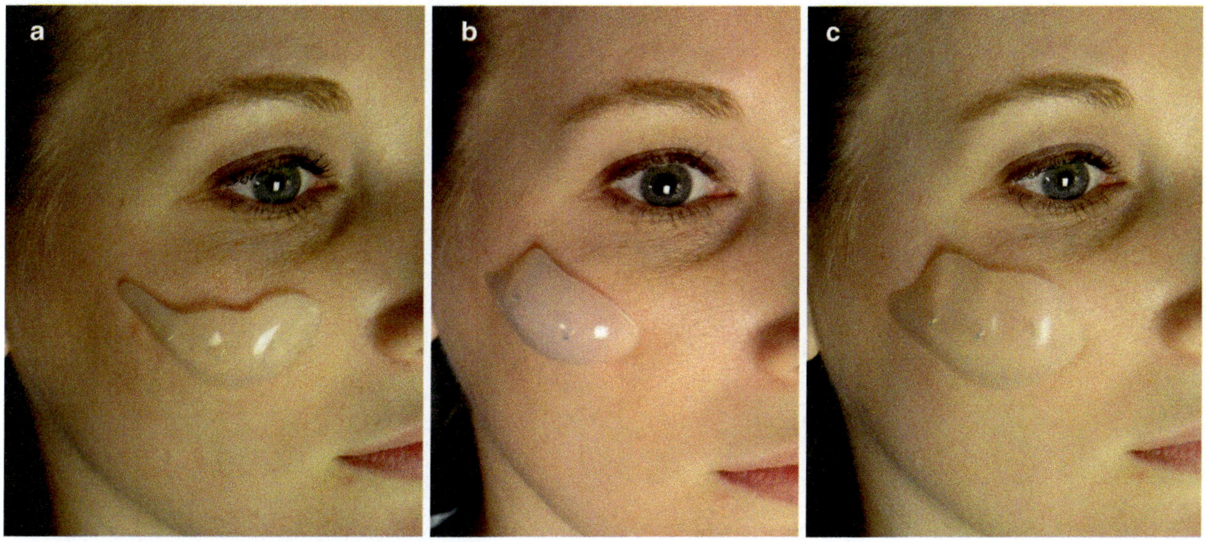

Fig. 21.7 (**a**) Submalar implant; (**b**) malar shell implant; (**c**) combined submalar shell implant. (Photos courtesy Joe Niamtu III. Reprinted from Niamtu [13], with permission from Elsevier)

Fig. 21.8 This image shows a 3D CT office scanner (**a**) with a CT scan (**b**) and a computer generated model with custom chin implant formulated specifically for this patient (**c**). (Fig. 21.8a courtesy i-CATA, used with permission, Fig. 21.8b, c, courtesy Joe Niamtu III. Reprinted from Niamtu [13], with permission from Elsevier)

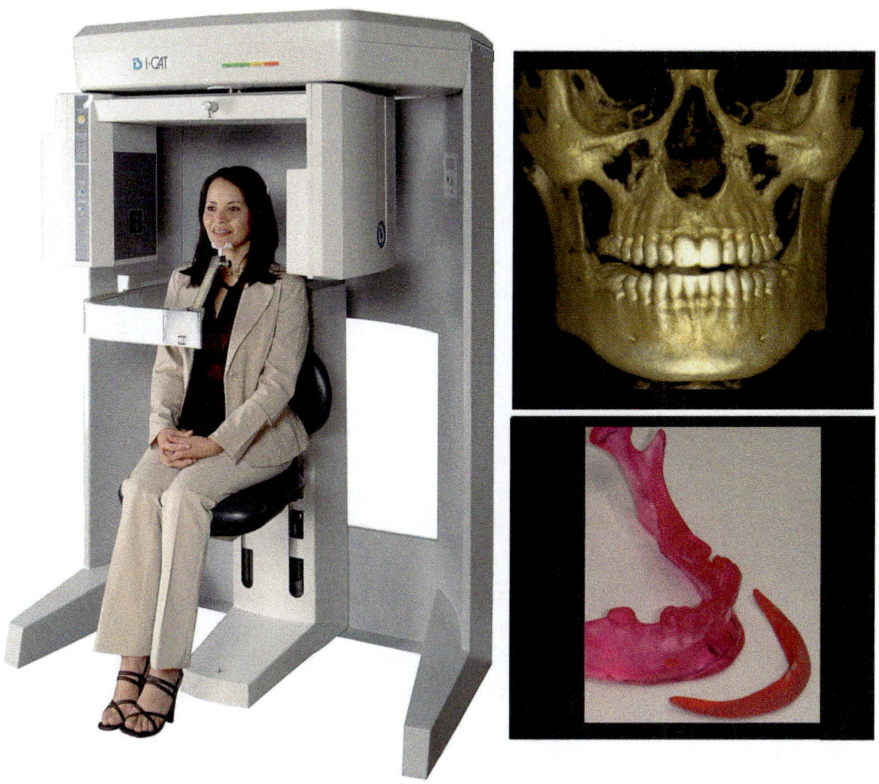

21.4 Surgical Procedure

Implant placement, in experienced hands, is relatively simple and should take about 10 min per side. As with all aesthetic and reconstructive procedures, there are technical nuances that can significantly impact the final surgical outcome. While cheek implants can be placed with local anesthesia alone, the author's preference is the addition of intravenous sedation, as cheek implants are commonly inserted as a part of more involved cosmetic facial procedures. Local anesthesia is infiltrated intraorally in the subperiosteal plane with 2% lidocaine with 1:100,000 epinephrine. Infiltration proceeds

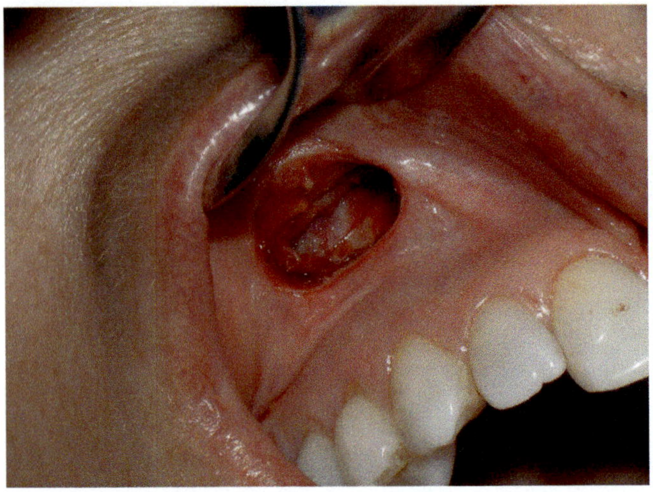

Fig. 21.9 A 10 mm incision is made about 10–12 mm above the gingival margin of the canine tooth just beneath the maxillary sulcus to the level of the periosteum. (Photo courtesy Joe Niamtu III)

over the maxilla from the infraorbital rim to the root of the teeth, and from the pyriform aperture to the zygomatic region. Percutaneous infiltration follows over the lateral malar region and tapers over the zygomatic arch.

The incision for cheek implant placement is made into the sulcus above the canine tooth about 10–12 mm above the gingival margin. The mucosa in this region is extensile and easily stretches so there is no need to make a large incision. A 10 mm incision is made with a scalpel, cautery, or radiowave electrode (Fig. 21.9). The subperiosteal plane is immediately identified. It is imperative that the incision and dissection remain subperiosteal as this is the plane in which the implants are placed. A periosteal elevator is used to elevate the periosteum and identify the infraorbital nerve, the only anatomic landmark of concern in the field of dissection. As tissue is elevated, the attachments of some of the lip elevator muscles are stripped from their osseous origins. They reattach as a consequence of normal healing.

The confines of the dissection are dictated by the size and shape of the implant placed. The dissection pocket should be slightly larger than the size of the implant and requires dissection that tapers over the zygomatic arch (Fig. 21.10). A larger pocket serves no purpose and may increase edema, potential hematoma formation, and excessive implant mobility. Larger implants, with larger dissections, will portend longer recoveries with more postoperative swelling and bruising. There is no need to dissect superior to the infraorbital rim or medially to the pyriform aperture as most implants are placed inferior and lateral to these landmarks. Most implants do not encroach on the infraorbital nerve, but occasionally, if this is an issue, the implant is trimmed to accommodate the nerve. This is more common in patients who use dentures as they can have significant bone resorption

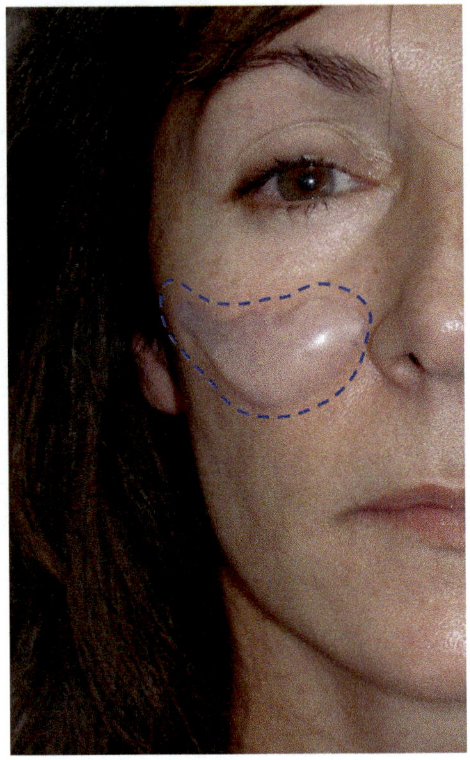

Fig. 21.10 The implant dissection pocket should be just slightly larger than the actual implant. More generous dissection serves no purpose and can encourage displacement and seroma. This image shows an outline in blue of the size of the dissection pocket in relation to the implant. (Photo courtesy Joe Niamtu III)

and the nerve is more easily encountered due to a vertically shortened maxilla.

With larger implants, that require more lateral and inferior dissection, the surgeon will encounter the masseter tendon where the muscle originates on the zygoma. There is no reason to violate this structure. The soft tissue is dissected off the tendon and muscle to accommodate the implant. There is no consequence of the implant lying partially on the masseter tendon or muscle in this area (Fig. 21.11).

When the implant pocket dissection is complete, an implant sizer may be utilized to evaluate the potential aesthetic outcome. These devices are silicone analogues of the actual implants and can be "tried in" to evaluate the appearance of a given implant size or shape. For novice surgeons, this can be a valuable tool. Even with sizers, it can be difficult to estimate the final surgical result on the operating room table, due to gravity and tissue swelling. Accurate judging of implant size and shape is an acquired ability that comes with experience.

It is always better to err on the side of placement of a smaller implant. The most common implant I place in women (90% of my cases) is a medium Binder Type II submalar implant (Implantech, Inc., Ventura, CA). The smaller submalar

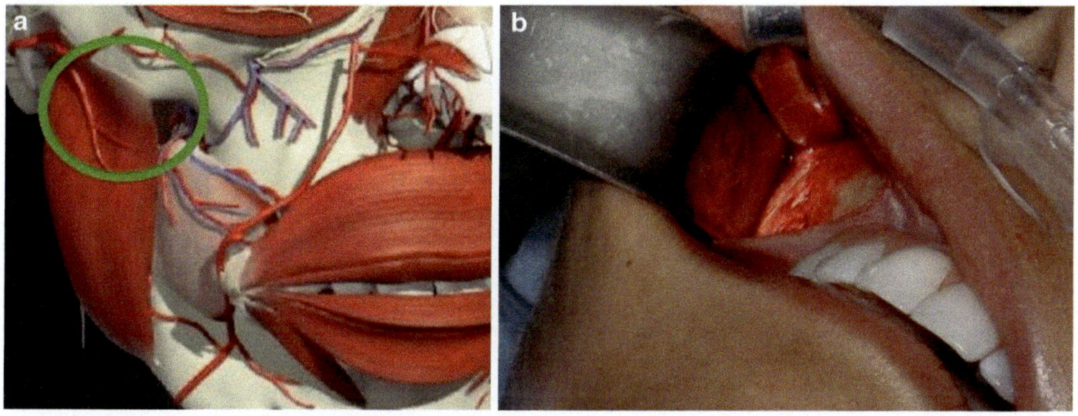

Fig. 21.11 The masseter tendon is frequently visible during midface implant dissection and no release of this structure is necessary. The implant periphery can lie over the tendon and related muscle without consequence. (**a**) An anatomic representation of the masseter tendon; (**b**) intraoperative view of the masseter tendon. (Photos courtesy Joe Niamtu III. Reprinted from Niamtu [13], with permission from Elsevier)

implant is typically inadequate for most patients. The large submalar implant is appropriate for bigger (taller) patients and those with significant volume deficit. The combined submalar shell implant is a very large implant, and even a medium size frequently requires trimming. In general, dissection for malar shell or combined submalar shell implants is more extensive to accommodate for the larger size or more superiolateral augmentation.

Midface implants are available in two configurations. The standard configuration has a smooth and more rigid posterior surface. A variation, known as the Conform Implant, provides increased implant flexibility and surface area by employing numerous flexible feet that protrude on the underside of the implant. The author's preference is to use the standard implant as its rigidity makes it easier to place through the tunnel. Implantech also makes implants that are coated with an ePTFE material, but I do not see an advantage in this addition over solid silicone.

The surgeon must strike a balance between the size of the implant and the size of the dissection pocket as the implant needs to sit passively in the pocket. Most contemporary facial implants are anatomic in form which means they have been made to conform to underlying normal anatomic contours. As a result, they will frequently fall into place and stabilize over the underlying bony contours.

After the implant is placed in the final pocket, the cheeks and upper lip are manipulated externally to simulate facial animation. If these maneuvers extrude the implant, then the pocket is poorly sized and a correction of one or both is necessary. A well-placed implant is one that passively sits on top of the maxilla and is not easily displaced from the incision pocket.

Once the correct implant placement is confirmed, the pocket is irrigated with antibiotic solution and the implant is secured with a single fixation screw. Many surgeons omit this step, but the author feels this is an extremely important step. After placing hundreds of implants, the author has never seen migration or significant underlying bone resorption with a stabilized implant. A single 6-mm self-drilling screw (eliminates the need for drills) is placed through the thinner periphery of the implant over the dense zygomatic buttress potion of bone (Fig. 21.12).

As stated, some surgeons believe fixation is not necessary. When patients begin early postoperative facial animation, an unsecured implant can become displaced. Empirically, a secured implant is less likely to migrate, cause bone resorption, or become infected. Many surgeons fabricate a complex bolster system to stabilize the implant where fixation sutures are placed intraorally, through the implant and exit the cheek where they are secured around a cotton roll or bolster. While this may stabilize the implant in some vectors, it may pull the implant away from bone, creating a potential space, and allowing the formation of a seroma, hematoma, and predisposing to infection. Once the implant becomes encapsulated, the chance of migration is less likely, but stabilizing the implant until that point is prudent.

The fixation screw should not be placed over the thinner antral bone at the canine fossa. When placing screws in the anterior sinus wall, the operator must not exert excessive pressure or the entire screw can be pushed into the maxillary sinus. If a sinus perforation occurs, the implant can still be placed. In the author's experience, numerous implants have been placed over antral perforations from previous sinus or maxillofacial surgery without consequence. Before the implant is screwed into final position, the operator must assure that the implants on both sides are in a similar and suitable position. This is more art than science, as it is difficult to accurately index the implants to fixed structures.

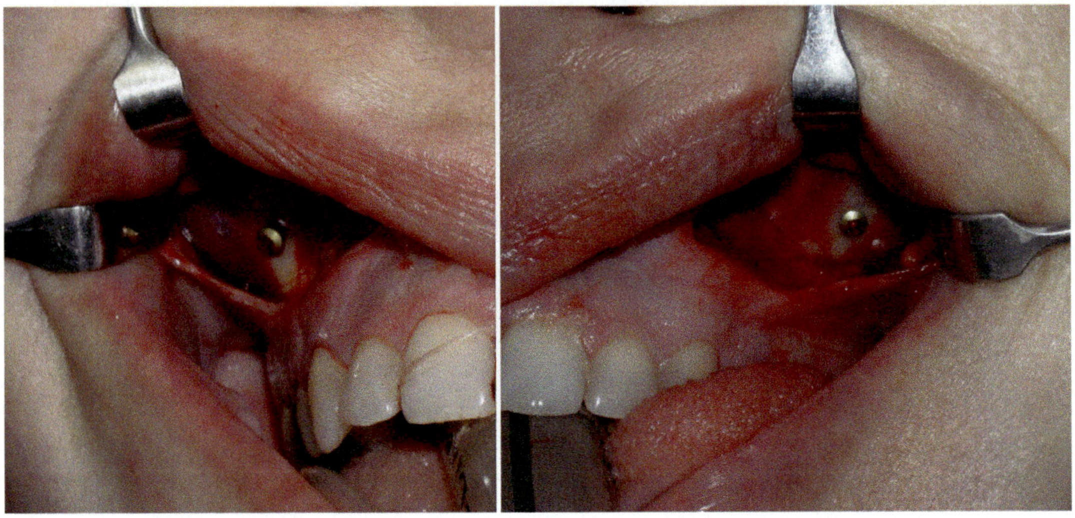

Fig. 21.12 This image shows implants in place with screw fixation. A single self drilling 6 mm bone screws is placed through the thinner periphery of the implant over the more dense zygomatic buttress bone. (Photos courtesy Joe Niamtu III. Reprinted from Niamtu [13], with permission from Elsevier)

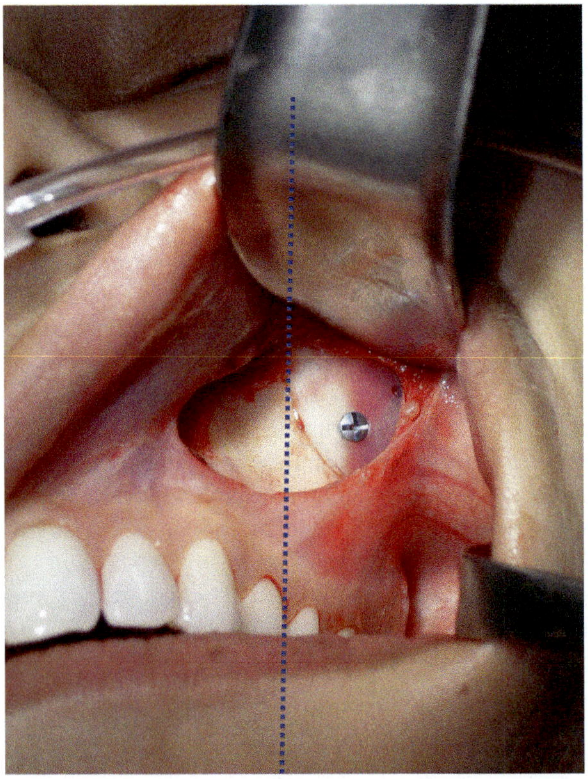

Fig. 21.13 Indexing the medial border of the implants to the first or second premolar region can assist in positional harmony and symmetry. (Photo courtesy Joe Niamtu III. Reprinted from Niamtu [13], with permission from Elsevier)

One means of identifying symmetry is to observe the medial edge of the submalar implant, as it typically is in vertical alignment with the first or second premolar teeth (Fig. 21.13). Another means of approximate alignment is to trace the implant in its approximated position on the face preoperatively and use those marks to index the intraoperative position (Fig. 21.14). Prior to the fixation, the surgeon should make sure that the implant edge or tail is not folded on itself. Since many of the implant configurations have a thinner leading edge or periphery, it is possible to roll the thin edge under the implant body during placement (Fig. 21.15). If this happens, a palpable and visible prominence will appear. Direct observation or running a periosteal elevator under the implant is the best means of confirming proper placement.

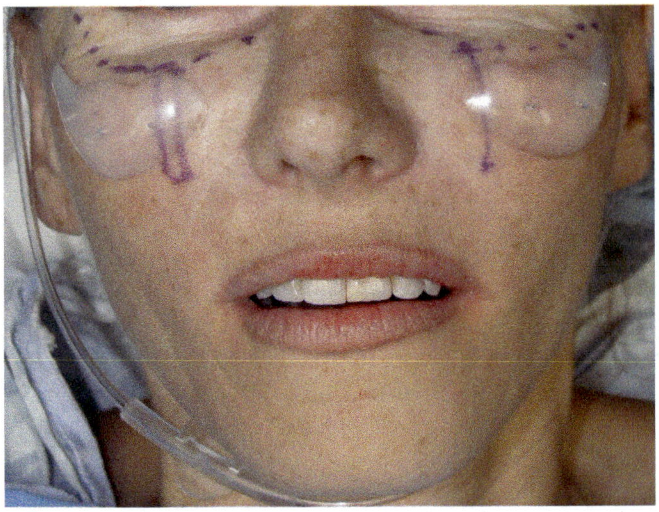

Fig. 21.14 Preoperative tracings can be referenced intraoperatively to assist the surgeon in symmetric implant placement. (Photo courtesy Joe Niamtu III. Reprinted from Niamtu [13], with permission from Elsevier)

After the implants have been properly placed, indexed, and secured, the wound can be closed. Antibiotic solution should be irrigated again prior to closure. The wound is closed in a single layer by taking big "bites" with a 4–0 chromic gut suture (Fig. 21.16). Facial dressing is not required.

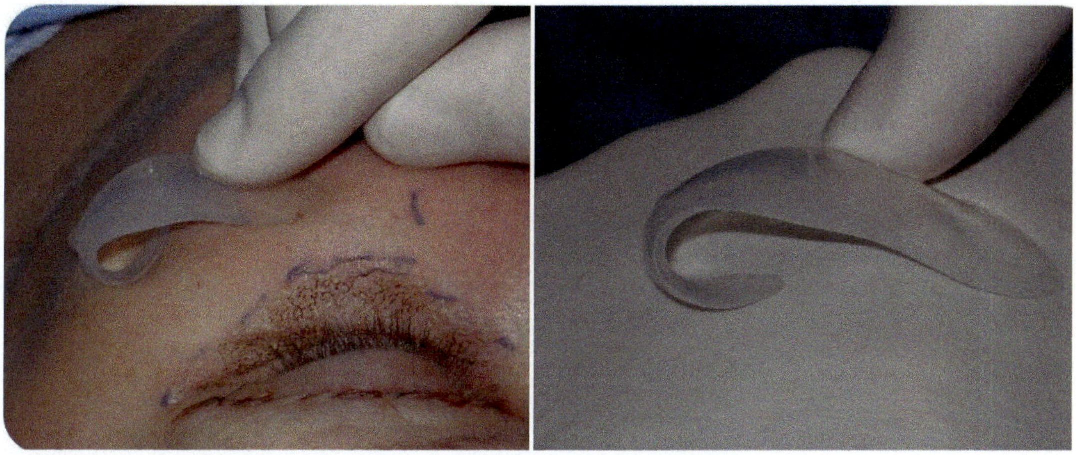

Fig. 21.15 This image shows the potential problem of an implant tail folded under itself during insertion. (Photo courtesy Joe Niamtu III. Reprinted from Niamtu [13], with permission from Elsevier)

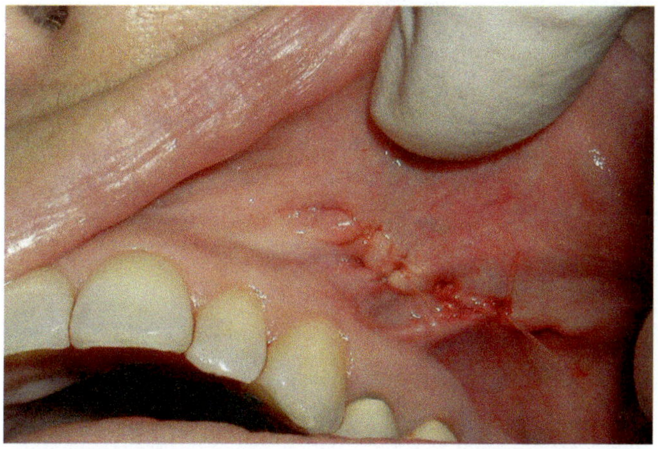

Fig. 21.16 A simple 4–0 gut suture is used to close the mucosal incision after implant placement. (Photo courtesy Joe Niamtu III. Reprinted from Niamtu [13], with permission from Elsevier)

21.5 Postoperative Care and Healing

As stated above, a dressing is not placed after cheek implant surgery. All patients receive antibiotic coverage beginning the day before surgery and continuing for 6 days after. An analgesic suitable for moderate discomfort is prescribed, as well as a steroid regimen if excessive swelling is anticipated. Patients are asked to refrain from excessive facial animation for 72 hours and are placed on a liquid or soft diet for the first 48 hours. Ice is applied to the midface intermittently for 48 hours, followed by warm compresses for the next several days.

Patients are told that the recovery period is typically 1–2 weeks with a qualification that most people will typically miss only one work week. Swelling is the primary complaint after surgery. Although this can take several weeks to resolve, most patients are presentable in a week or sooner. Ecchymosis is rare. Most patients will experience transient numbness of the infraorbital region which will spontaneously resolve over 1–2 weeks. Patients are also informed that their smile and/or pucker will appear unnatural for the first 7–10 days after surgery. This results facial edema, and disruption of the lip elevator musculature from the subperiosteal dissection.

Patients must be aware that the implants may look unnatural and large in the initial phase of recovery. They are encouraged to wait at least 6 weeks before deciding to remove the implant, as it takes time for subtle swelling to settle and for the patient to accommodate to the augmented midface.

21.6 Implant Complications

Significant complications have been rare in my practice but can include the following:

- Bleeding
- Hematoma/seroma
- Acute infection
- Late or chronic infection
- Implant migration
- Implant extrusion
- Permanent dysesthesia
- Overcorrection
- Undercorrection
- Asymmetry
- Facial pain

Many complications can be prevented by judicious preoperative screening [12]. Patients should be questioned for possible sources of infection such as dental or sinus disease. Oral hygiene should also be evaluated to assure there is no active dental or periodontal disease. Smokers may have problems with wound dehiscence, implant migration associated with puckering, and infection.

Subjective postoperative dissatisfaction can be avoided by appropriate patient selection. Various "red flags" can

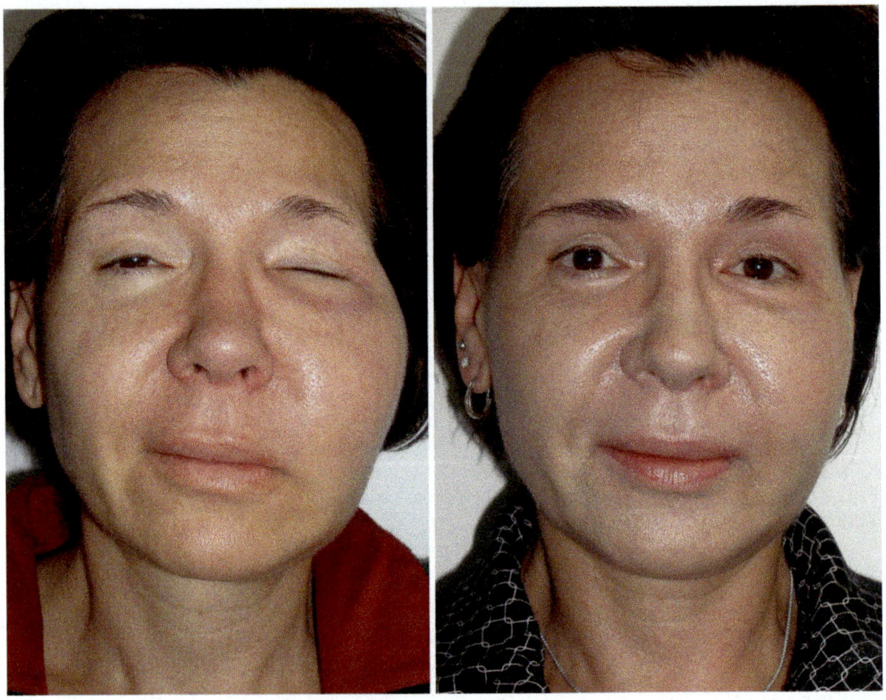

Fig. 21.17 This image shows a patient 48 h after implant placement with early rapidly progressing infection. She is shown 24 h after implant removal with almost total resolution of infection. (Photos courtesy Joe Niamtu III. Reprinted from Niamtu [13], with permission from Elsevier)

signal potential problematic patients. Caution should be employed when considering surgery on patients under 30 years of age who have had multiple cosmetic procedures. These patients often have components of body dysmorphic disorder and can be impossible to please. In addition, patients (especially males) who at consult requesting a "chiseled" face, or those who bring in numerous pictures of celebrities or models (who they want to look like) are very concerning. The best candidates for cheek implants, in my opinion, are those patients with midface aging or hypoplasia who will be happy with moderate improvement after surgery.

Over- or under-correction should be treated by exchanging the prostheses with a more appropriate implant. Again, waiting 6 weeks after placement may reduce the revision rate. Asymmetries are not unusual, given that many patients have preexisting facial asymmetries. Gross asymmetry should be recognized preoperatively and pointed out to the patient. In these cases, the surgeon may elect to place different size implants on either side of the face. For more subtle asymmetry, trimming or shaving the implants may be sufficient.

In the author's experience, infections after surgery are rare. This is most likely related to the stabilization technique described which reduces the risk of seroma formation and foreign body reaction. Fixation also allows the retained implants to better respond to "salvage" procedure if infection occurs. Implant infections, when present, typically occur in the first several days after placement. An infection must be considered if a patient develops unilateral pain, discharge, and/or periorbital swelling (Fig. 21.17). If an infection is present in an implant not secured with a screw, my preference is removal and replacement 4–6 weeks later. For screw retained implants, incision and drainage, antibiotic lavage, and oral antibiotics may salvage the implant.

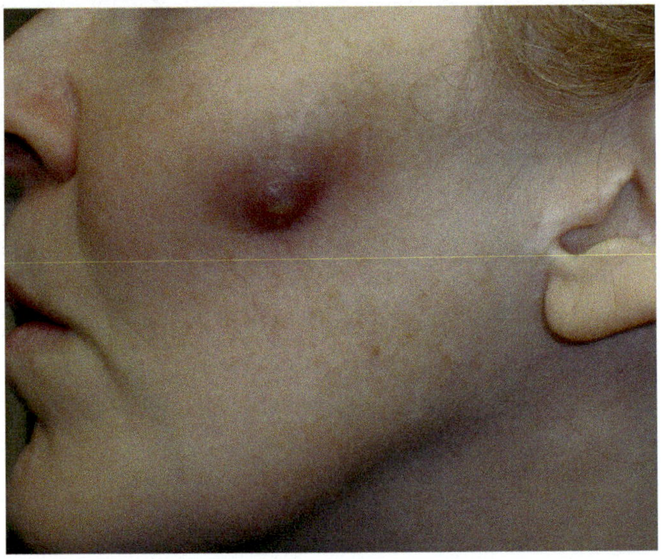

Fig. 21.18 This patient had a chronic recurrent subclinical infection that was treated with antibiotics numerous times. An oro-facial fistula finally formed requiring implant removal. Chronic infections of this nature are quite rare. (Photo courtesy Joe Niamtu III)

Some patients may present with recurrent swelling that is consistent with infection but clears with oral antibiotics. If this cycle recurs, the surgeon should remain suspicious that a chronic infection or implant inflammatory reaction is present. Figure 21.18 shows a patient with an external perforating fistula from a chronically infected left cheek implant that continued with a subclinical course. In these instances the implant should be removed.

Persistent facial pain, especially shooting pain into the lip or teeth, can signify implant compression on the infraorbital nerve. If these symptoms continue after several weeks, exploration with implant modification for relief of impingement should be considered.

21.7 Conclusion

Midface aging leads to significant facial changes that must be considered in the evaluation of the aesthetic patient. These changes include tissue deflation, descent, flattening, and resultant contour irregularities and depressions (tear trough, nasolabial fold). It is important for the cosmetic surgeon to identify these deficits and plan accordingly to address them in surgery. Silicone midface implants are an effective tool in attaining this goal. They are easy to place, reversible, and have few postoperative complications. As with any procedure, expertise comes with time and experience. The results to surgery are excellent and patient satisfaction high.

21.8 Case Presentations

Figures 21.19–21.25 show before and after images of various facial rejuvenation cases employing facial implants.

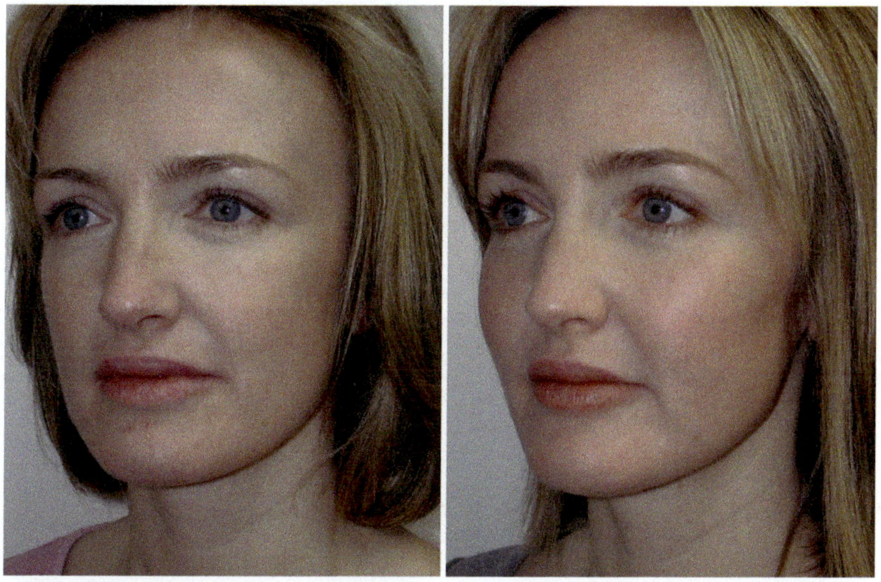

Fig. 21.19 This 45-year-old female desired a very subtle cosmetic change and underwent placement of medium submalar implants as a stand-alone procedure. (Photos courtesy Joe Niamtu III)

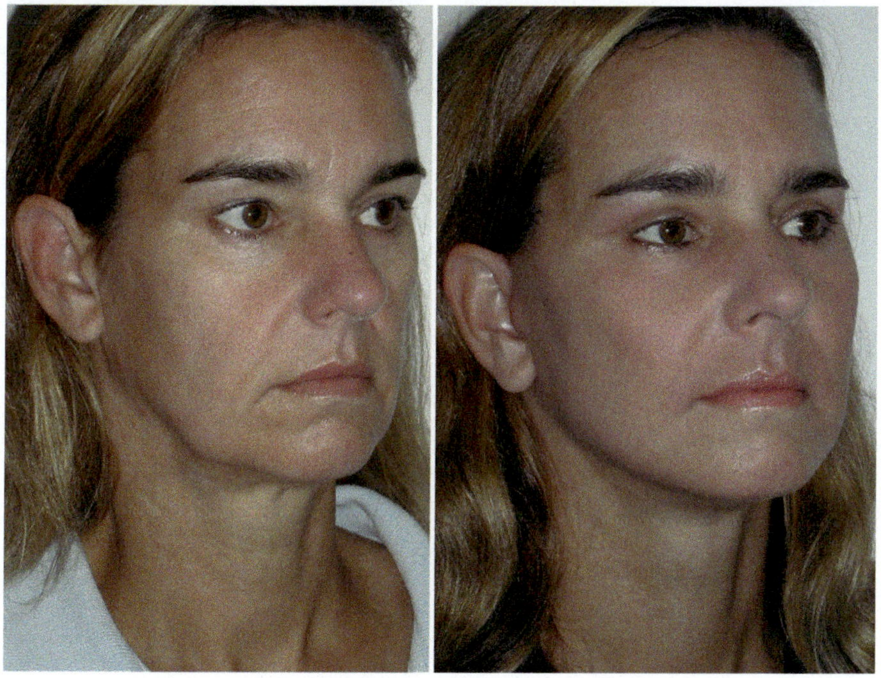

Fig. 21.20 This patient underwent upper blepharoplasty, facelift, and medium submalar cheek implants. The addition of midface volume is dramatically apparent in this case. (Photos courtesy Joe Niamtu III. Reprinted from Niamtu [13], with permission from Elsevier)

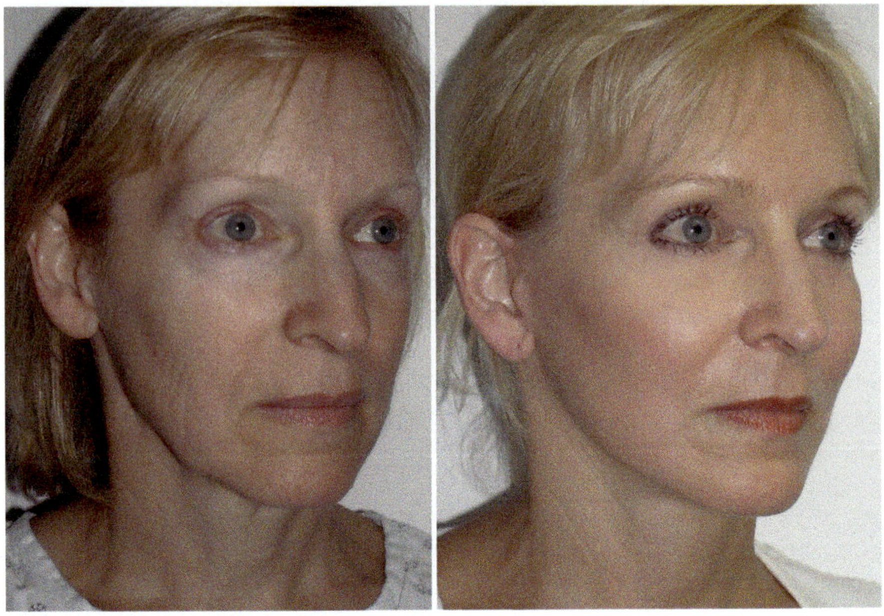

Fig. 21.21 This patient underwent medium submalar cheek implants with simultaneous facelift and CO_2 laser resurfacing. (Photos courtesy Joe Niamtu III. Reprinted from Niamtu [13], with permission from Elsevier)

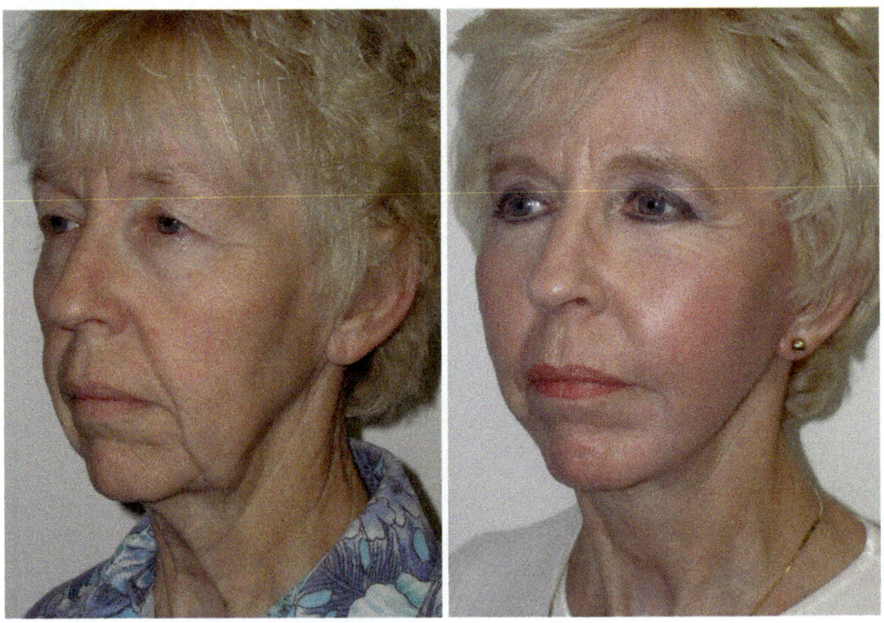

Fig. 21.22 This 65-year-old patient is shown before and after large submalar cheek implants, facelift, blepharoplasty, and full face CO_2 laser resurfacing. (Photos courtesy Joe Niamtu III. Reprinted from Niamtu [13], with permission from Elsevier)

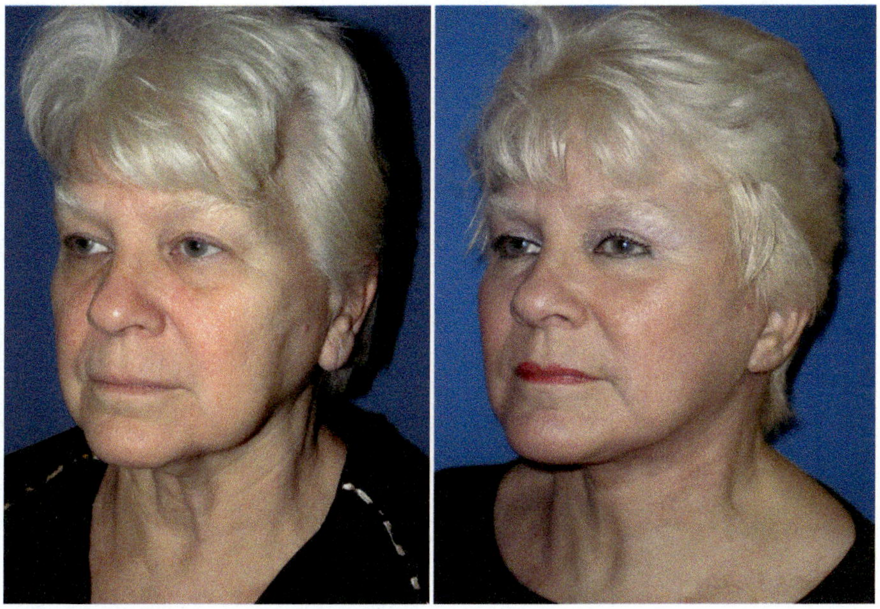

Fig. 21.23 This 67-year-old female is shown before and after medium submalar cheek implants and facelift. (Photos courtesy Joe Niamtu III)

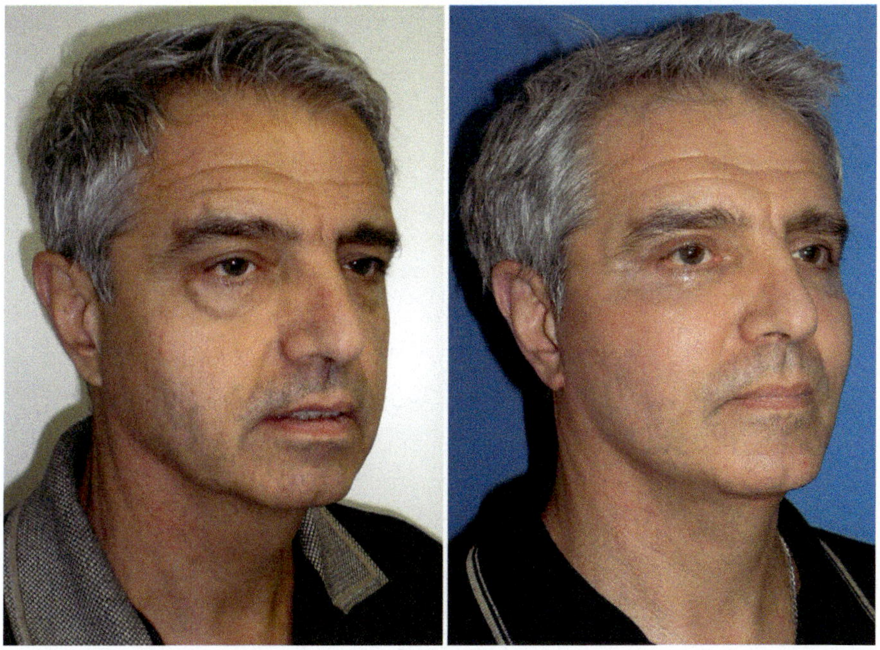

Fig. 21.24 This 58-year-old male is shown before and after medium combined submalar shell implants, facelift, blepharoplasty, and full face CO_2 laser resurfacing. (Photos courtesy Joe Niamtu III. Reprinted from Niamtu [13], with permission from Elsevier)

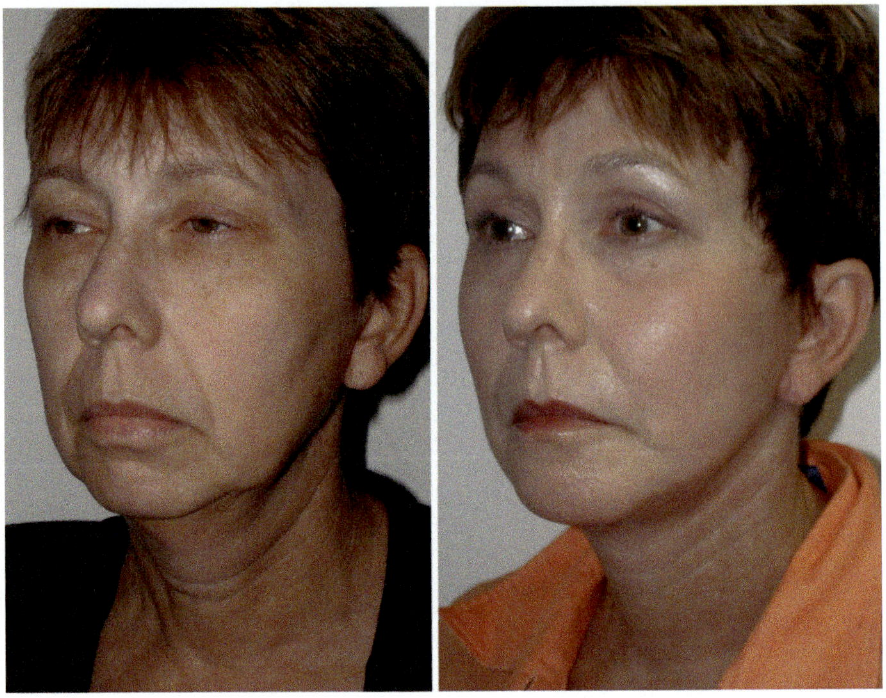

Fig. 21.25 This 53-year-old female patient is shown before and after medium submalar cheek implants, facelift, blepharoplasty, and full face CO_2 laser resurfacing. (Photos courtesy Joe Niamtu III)

References

1. Niamtu J. Essentials of cheek and midface implants. J Oral Maxillofac Surg. 2010;68:1420–9.
2. Niamtu J. New lip and wrinkle fillers. Oral Maxillofac Surg Clin North Am. 2005;17(1):17–28.
3. Binder WJ, Azizzadeh B. Malar and submalar augmentation. Facial Plast Surg Clin North Am. 2008;16(1):11–32, v.
4. Terino EO, Edward M. The magic of mid-face three-dimensional contour alterations combining alloplastic and soft tissue suspension technologies. Clin Plast Surg. 2008;35(3):419–50; discussion 417.
5. Louis PJ, Cuzalina LA. Alloplastic augmentation of the face. Atlas Oral Maxillofac Surg Clin North Am. 2000;8(2):127–91.
6. Yaremchuk MJ, Kahn DM. Periorbital skeletal augmentation to improve blepharoplasty and midfacial results. Plast Reconstr Surg. 2009;124(6):2151–60.
7. Matros E, Momoh A, Yaremchuk MJ. The aging midfacial skeleton: implications for rejuvenation and reconstruction using implants. Facial Plast Surg. 2009;25(4):252–9.
8. Downs BW, Wang TD. Current concepts in midfacial rejuvenation. Curr Opin Otolaryngol Head Neck Surg. 2008; 16(4):335–8.
9. Yaremchuk MJ. Secondary malar implant surgery. Plast Reconstr Surg. 2008;121(2):620–8.
10. Terino EO, Edwards MC. Alloplastic contouring for suborbital, maxillary, zygomatic deficiencies. Facial Plast Surg Clin North Am. 2008;16(1):33–67.
11. Roy D, Mangat DS. Facial implants. Dermatol Clin. 2005;23(3):541–7, vii–viii.
12. Cuzalina LA, Hlavacek MR. Complications of facial implants. Oral Maxillofac Surg Clin North Am. 2009;21(1):91–104, vi–vii.
13. Niamtu III J, editor. Cosmetic facial surgery. Philadelphia, PA: Elsevier Mosby; 2011.

Part VI

Special Considerations

Periorbital Fat Grafting

22

Robert A. Glasgold, Samuel M. Lam, and Mark J. Glasgold

Key Points

- Traditional blepharoplasty techniques have focused on excision of skin/muscle and fat.
- While tissue excision has an important role in blepharoplasty surgery, it alone can lead to a hollowed, aged, and unnatural appearance.
- A detailed understanding of periorbital esthetics and how aging affects this esthetic is an essential component of blepharoplasty surgery.
- We now understand that volume loss is an important part of the periorbital aging process.
- Volume preservation/augmentation is equally important in esthetic rejuvenation of the periorbital region.
- Fat grafting allows periorbital volume augmentation with autologous tissue.
- Autologous fat grafting is an excellent stand-alone or adjunctive procedure to cosmetic blepahroplasty to recreate youthful appearing eyelids and adjacent structures (eyebrows/midface).
- In experienced hands, fat grafting yields excellent results with few complications.

22.1 Introduction

Implementation of fat transfer for periorbital rejuvenation relies foremost on understanding patterns of soft and hard tissue (i.e., fat and bone) volume loss. Focusing volume rejuvenation on these areas of tissue deflation is a crucial step in achieving a natural and esthetically pleasing result.

Most patients seeking facial rejuvenation emphasize a desire for a natural and younger appearance; a goal which should be shared by the esthetic surgeon. Many traditional approaches to periorbital rejuvenation have fallen short of attaining this objective. The downfall has been in the lack of understanding of what defines the naturally youthful periorbita. Traditionally, there has been a reflex action of excising skin, muscle, and fat in response to upper lid hooding or lower lid bags. These procedures were not driven by the esthetic goal of recreating a youthful eye, but rather, by a procedure-oriented mentality founded on tissue subtraction. The results of these procedures did not lead to a natural or youthful appearance. To the contrary, patients often appeared altered, skeletonized (deflated), and "done" (Fig. 22.1). Both patients and surgeons are to blame for this cycle by staying focused on hooding and bags, and not on the natural and youthful result that everyone aims for.

Over the last decade, our understanding that volume loss is a major component of facial and periorbital aging has become increasingly accepted, particularly in the region of the lower lid and midface [1–4]. This paradigm shift, and the implementation of volume augmentation in these areas, has led to more natural results and less stigmata of plastic surgery. Critical evaluation of upper lid surgery in regard to volume replacement has been lagging behind despite increasing use of volume augmentation to the lower lid and midface region.

To appropriately rejuvenate the periorbital area, we must have patients look away from the mirror and focus on photos of themselves at a younger age, as well as photos of other youthful faces. This will help patients appreciate what defines a youthful periorbital region and what the goals of facial and eyelid rejuvenation surgery should be (Fig. 22.2).

In this chapter, we will discuss the concepts of age-related volume loss and review autologous fat grafting techniques to the periorbital region. Off-the-shelf fillers such as hyaluronic acids (HA) provide an alternative means of periorbital volume replacement and will also be addressed.

R.A. Glasgold (✉)
Clinical Assistant Professor of Surgery, Department of Surgery, UMDNJ-Robert Wood Johnson Medical School, Highland Park, NJ, USA
e-mail: drrobert@glasgoldgroup.com

G.G. Massry et al. (eds.), *Master Techniques in Blepharoplasty and Periorbital Rejuvenation*,
DOI 10.1007/978-1-4614-0067-7_22, © Springer Science+Business Media, LLC 2011

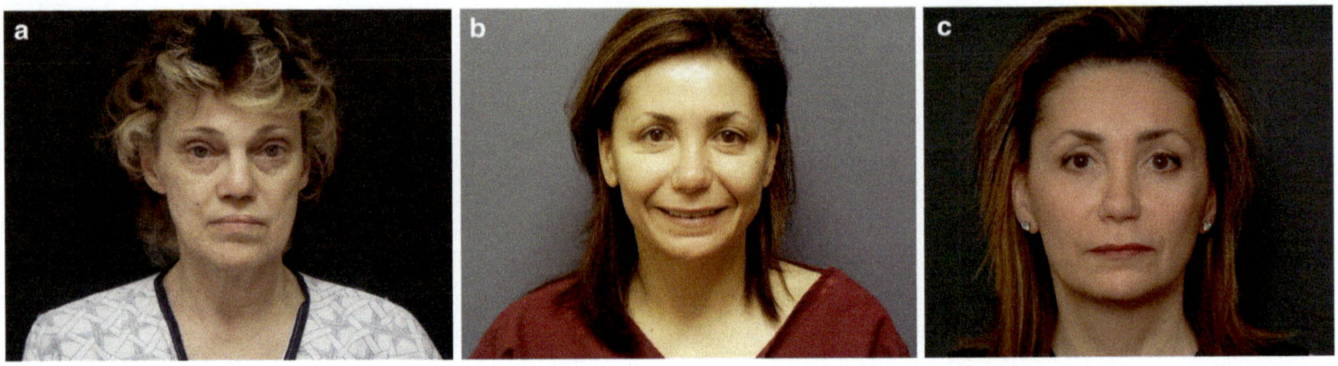

Fig. 22.1 (**a**) Patient demonstrating the outcome of prior traditional subciliary blepharoplasty without volume restoration resulting in skeletonization of the inferior orbital rim. (**b**) Preoperative photo of a patient who underwent browlift and upper blepharoplasty with removal of skin and fat. (**c**) Postoperatively, photo of the patient demonstrates skeletonization of the superior orbital rim and an exaggerated A-frame deformity

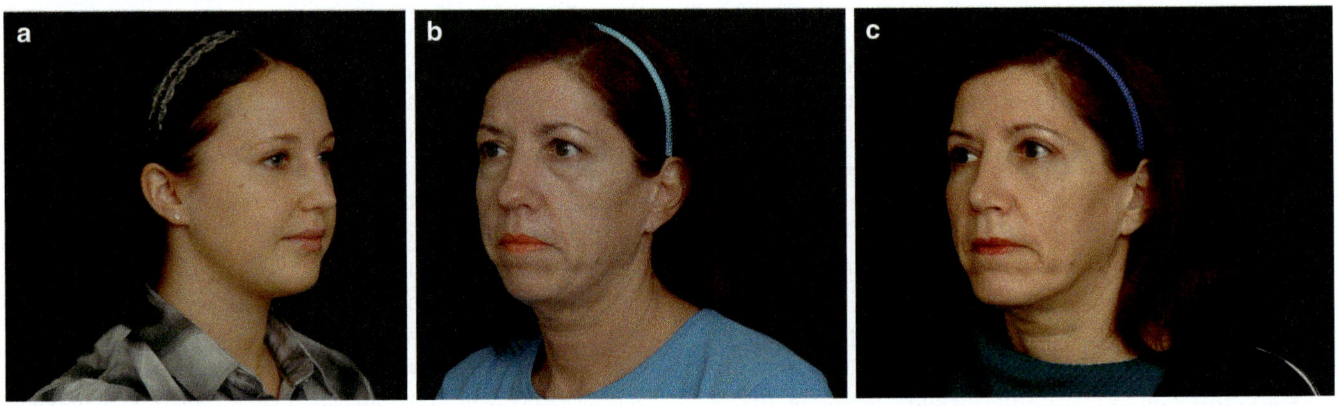

Fig. 22.2 (**a**) A woman in her early 20s demonstrates the characteristics of a youthful periorbita. (**b**) Preoperative photo of a woman seeking periorbital rejuvenation. (**c**) Following skin-only upper lid blepharoplasty, transconjunctival lower blepharoplasty with conservative fat excision, and fat transfer to the inferior orbital rim and midface. (**b**, **c**, Adapted from Carniol and Sadick [13])

22.2 Analysis

It is useful to think of the eye as the centerpiece of the periorbital region, with the bone and soft tissue surroundings providing the frame in which it sits. Aging results in a deterioration of the frame's integrity. The youthful periorbita, or frame, is soft and curvaceous, with an ample cushion of soft tissue hiding the underlying bony foundation. This voluminous base of tissue creates smooth transitions to the adjacent regions: the cheek, temple, and forehead (Fig. 22.3a). As age-related volume loss progresses, the facial contours and their resultant highlights and shadows change. This results in an older facial appearance dominated by shadows and harsh transitions between adjacent areas (Fig. 22.3b).

22.2.1 Lower Eyelid

Classically, the youthful lower eyelid (the lower frame of the eye) is indistinct from the cheek. The lid flows smoothly into the cheek forming a convexity ending inferomedially at the nasolabial fold (see Fig. 22.3a). The span from lower lid to nasolabial fold is devoid of shadows and graced with a highlight at the apex of the cheek prominence. Volume loss along the inferior orbital rim exposes the bony orbital rim, creating a shadow that isolates the lower lid from the cheek (see Fig. 22.3b) [5]. The role of pseudoherniated lower lid fat in aging of the eye should not be overlooked. As this fat bulge increases, the concavity below, and the degree of shadowing, becomes more pronounced. The traditional surgical approach of merely removing fat from the lower lid reduces the depth of the concavity (and its associated shadow), but often has the deleterious effect of further unmasking the bony orbital rim. The result is a skeletonized and unnatural appearing eye that looks neither younger nor refreshed (see Fig. 22.1a). Rejuvenation should focus on restoring the soft, voluminous midfacial appearance where the lower lid flows smoothly into the cheek. This requires adding volume to the concavity at the lid–cheek junction and, when necessary, reducing the protrusion of pseudoherniated lower lid fat (see Fig. 22.2).

Although we are emphasizing volume restoration, our goal is not to completely discard traditional procedures, but

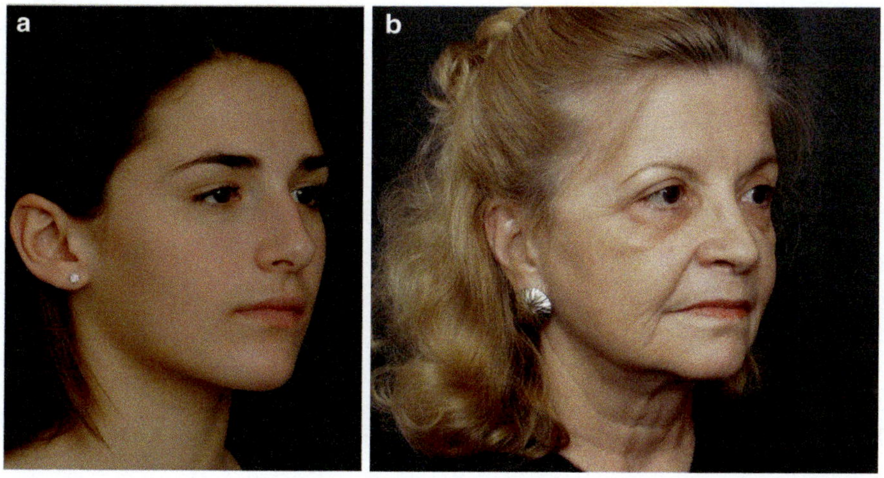

Fig. 22.3 (**a**) Young woman demonstrating the characteristic youthful lower lid: lack of pseudoherniated fat, minimal inferior orbital rim or midfacial volume loss, no separation of the lower lid from the cheek, and an uninterrupted convexity from lower lid to the nasolabial fold. (**b**) With advancing age, the combination of pseudoherniated lower lid fat and volume loss in the inferior orbital rim creates a shadow demarcating the lid from the cheek. The single youthful midface convexity is broken by volume loss at the inferior orbital rim and malar septum. (**b**, Adapted from Lam et al. [1], used with permission)

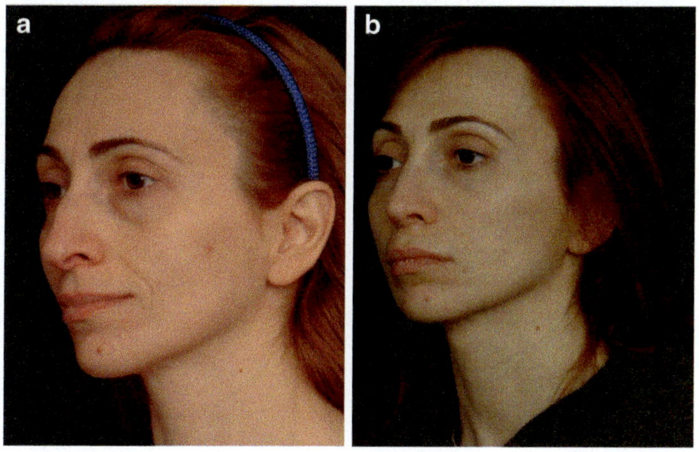

Fig. 22.4 (**a**) Preoperative photo demonstrating significant inferior orbital rim and midfacial volume loss. Despite appearing to have lower lid "bags", the patient does not actually have prominence of the lower lid fat pads. (**b**) Following fat transfer to the inferior orbital rim, malar, and submalar regions, the appearance of "bags" under her eyes is eliminated without removing any fat. Of note, she did have concurrent rhinoplasty and her nasolabial folds were addressed at a separate setting with a hyaluronic acid-based filler

rather to supplement them and to optimize results. In some cases, fat transfer alone will be adequate to accomplish this goal (Fig. 22.4). Other times, however, adding fat to eliminate the shadow effect is inadequate. When faced with the presence of prominent pseudoherniated fat, relying on volume augmentation alone can create an overinflated appearance to this area. These patients will best be served with supplemental conservative reduction of the relevant fat compartments (Fig. 22.5). Our procedure of choice for fat reduction is a transconjunctival lower lid blepharoplasty. This can be done at the same setting, just before or after the fat transfer.

Malar mounds present a uniquely difficult problem, and a full discussion of their management is beyond the scope of this chapter [1, 6]. Patients who have malar mounds or edema preoperatively should be made aware of the complexity of their issue. Otherwise, they may only become aware of their existence postoperatively. Patients should be counseled that no procedure will predictably get rid of malar mounds and that, when present, the goal is to both minimize their appearance and avoid exacerbating them. During volume restoration, the malar mounds should be worked around in order to minimize trauma and prolonged postoperative edema. Despite a careful approach, patients with prominent malar mounds should understand that they might have a prolonged postoperative course requiring oral or intralesional steroids.

22.2.2 Upper Eyelid

The youthful upper lid-brow complex should have soft rounded contours. As with the youthful lower lid, which is

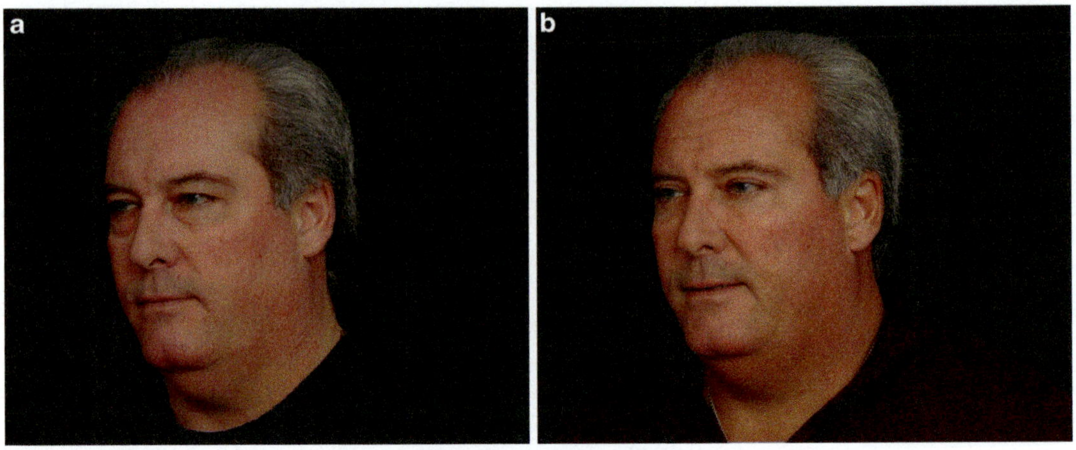

Fig. 22.5 (**a**) Preoperative photo demonstrating the presence of significant pseudoherniated fat in all lower lid compartments combined with volume loss across the inferior orbital rim. (**b**) Following transconjunctival blepharoplasty to reduce medial, central, and lateral lower lid fat pads combined with fat transfer to the inferior orbital rim. Of note, an upper lid blepharoplasty was performed simultaneously removing only skin, not fat

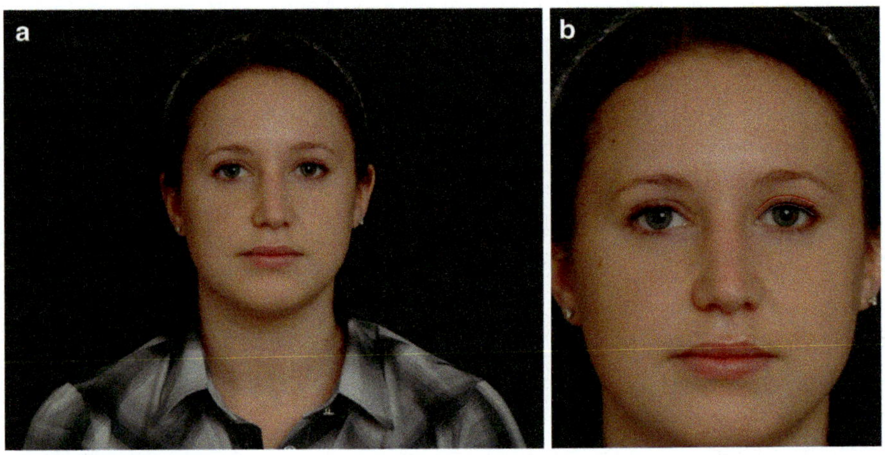

Fig. 22.6 Type 1 upper eyelid structure. (**a**) This woman in her early 20s demonstrates the youthful Type 1 upper lid. There is a convexity from brow to lid fold and a small separation between lid fold and lash line. (**b**) This illustration demarcates the narrow space between the two parallel lines: the inferior aspect of the lid fold (*red*) and the lash line (*blue*)

seamlessly joined with the adjacent midfacial units, the upper lid should have a similar relationship with its surroundings (the brow and temple). The soft tissue cushion overlying the superior orbital rim (SOR), which provides volume, also elevates the brow off of the orbital rim. As volume loss progresses, the gentle curves are lost and become dominated by harsh shadowing between the upper lid and brow (just as we see between the lower lid and cheek). Temporal volume loss will also contribute to an older and less healthy periorbital appearance. Before detailing the specific goals for obtaining a natural, youthful upper lid, we need to recognize that there are two primary variants of upper lid architecture that are very distinct. The analysis and rejuvenation plan will be different for each type of upper lid.

The first, and more common, type of upper lid (Type 1) is characterized by a full convexity running from the lid crease inferiorly to the brow above (Fig. 22.6a). The bony prominence of the SOR is completely masked by the soft tissue cushion underlying the brow. The distance between the upper lid crease and lash line is minimal (usually only several millimeters); with these two “lines” running parallel to one another (Fig. 22.6b). Age-related volume loss, although affecting the entire upper lid-brow complex, is more significant in the medial half of the upper lid in the area just below the brow. This can be partly attributed to the presence of the lacrimal gland, under the lateral portion of the SOR, which reduces skeletonization in that area. The predominance of medial upper lid volume loss creates what is referred to as an “A-frame” deformity. The overall effect of upper lid volume depletion is to unmask the bony SOR, creating a concavity and shadowing between the upper lid crease inferiorly and brow superiorly (Fig. 22.7). The progression from soft curves and highlights to harsh angles and shadowing is responsible for the aged appearance.

In the Type 1 eyelid, volume loss contributes to the development of upper lid hooding. Patients will often complain of a

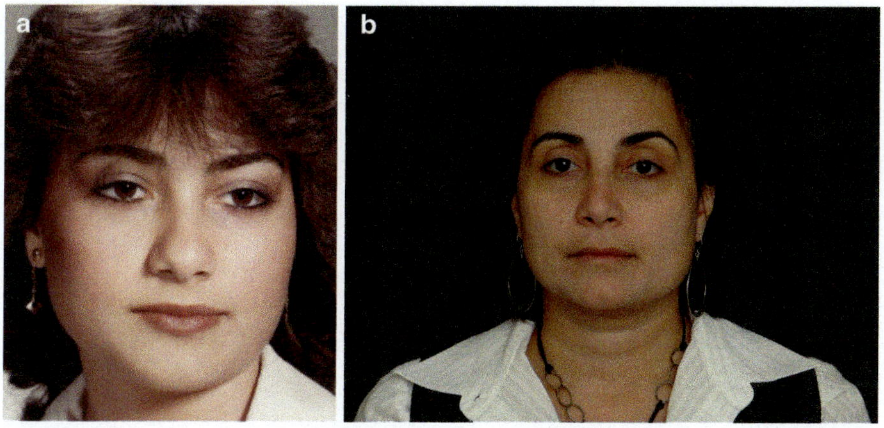

Fig. 22.7 Aging in the Type 1 upper eyelid structure. A high school yearbook photo (**a**) of an 18-year-old woman demonstrating the typical appearance of a youthful Type 1 upper lid. (**b**) The same woman, now in her early 40s, demonstrates the effects of aging, dominated by volume loss, on the upper lid. Loss of upper lid volume causes skeletonization of the superior orbital rim and a visible concavity between the brow and upper lid fold. Additionally, she demonstrates the A-frame deformity due to greater loss of medial volume.

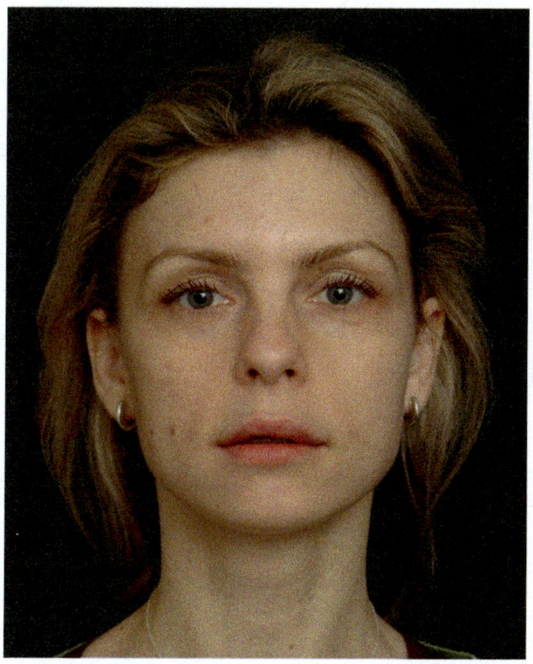

Fig. 22.8 The lateral fold of upper lid skin, particularly when draped out during examination, is nearly abutting the lash line. Despite the obvious volume deficit in the central half of the upper lid (A-frame deformity), failure to address the skin redundancy will likely lead to a dissatisfied patient

"flap of skin" sitting on the lid. The question that must be answered in evaluation is whether this "extra skin" is secondary to loss of skin elasticity and/or loss of volume. The answer is found in comparing the patient's old photos to their current status. During the examination, it is helpful to drape out the upper lid skin to see what actual separation remains between lid fold and lash line. When compared to pictures of themselves when younger, this distance will be either the same, greater, or less. If the distance has narrowed, meaning the skin is draping onto the lash line, then skin removal will be a necessary component of upper lid rejuvenation. The patient in Fig. 22.2b,c demonstrates this type of upper lid aging without volume loss. Preoperatively, the upper lid skin is draping onto the lash line. Following upper blepharoplasty with isolated skin removal, the gap between lid and lash line is restored as is the parallel relationship between these two lines. In comparison, some Type 1 upper eyelids will have a partial decreased distance between lid and lash line in combination with volume loss (Fig. 22.8). If the distance between lid and lash line has increased due to volume loss retracting the upper lid superiorly, then volume addition is essential. When this volume is restored, thereby reinflating the upper lid, the appearance of a flap is addressed without having to remove skin (Fig. 22.9). If there is minimal change, the patient will probably benefit from a combined approach of skin removal and volume augmentation. Caution should be taken in this last group of patients to not aggressively remove skin (Fig. 22.10). This can result in an increased distance between the lid fold and lash line, which does not represent a more youthful appearance.

In the upper lid, even more so than the lower, obtaining natural volumized results depend as much on preserving volume (upper lid fat), as it does on restoring volume. It is the rare patient that has significant upper lid pseudoherniation of fat. When present, it is most commonly seen in the medial. However, we believe that this generally represents a "pseudo-pseudo herniated fat." Most likely, there is deflation above the fat at the superior medial orbital rim, thereby creating a relative fat protrusion. This fat pocket should be surgically reduced in the rare circumstance that volume addition alone along the SOR will not sufficiently mask its presence.

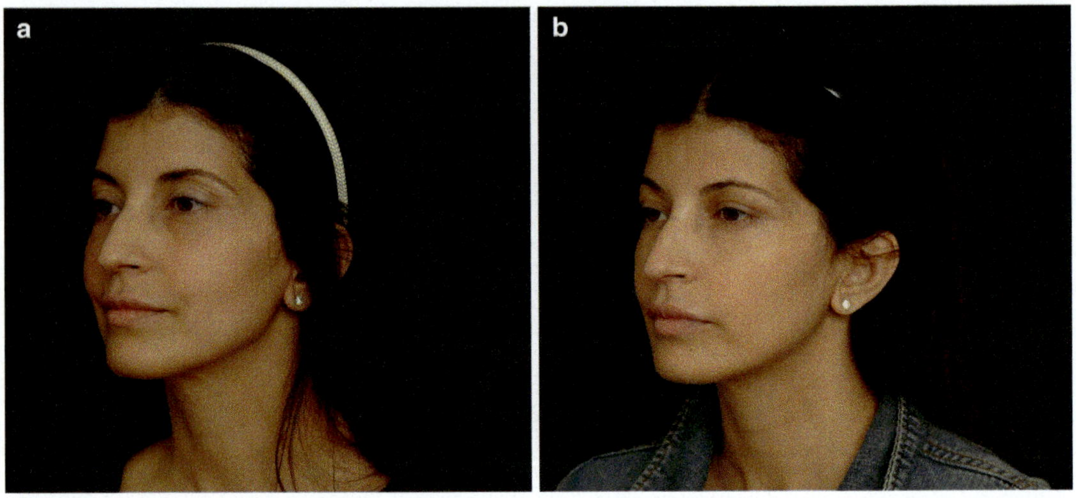

Fig. 22.9 (**a**) This patient demonstrates the loss of volume, which not only creates the upper lid concavity, but also gives the appearance of a "flap of skin" despite a more than adequate distance from the lid fold to lash line. (**b**) Following volume augmentation to the upper lid, staying inferior to the brow, the youthful convexity from brow to lid fold is restored. Additionally, by inflating the upper lid, the appearance of a redundant skin flap has been reduced

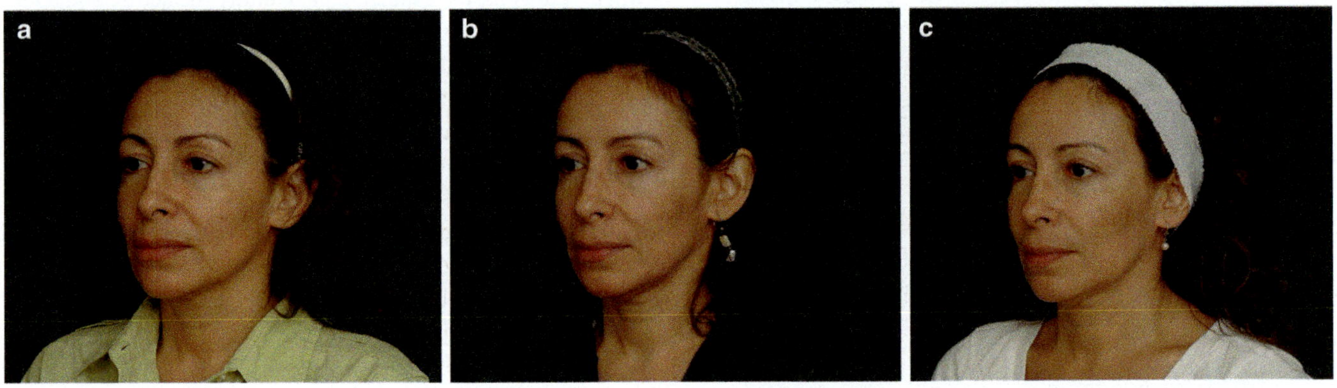

Fig. 22.10 (**a**) This patient with a Type 1 upper eyelid initially complained of the appearance of upper lid hooding, emphasizing the appearance of the visible flap of skin. (**b**) Following upper lid blepharoplasty, with removal of skin (no fat removal). Although there was slightly less skin draping, the end result was an increase show of pretarsal skin and a persistent appearance of a flap of upper lid skin. (**c**) After volume augmentation, filling the concavity between the medial half of the brow and the upper lid fold, the natural youthful appearance of the upper lid was restored. Filling the concavity inflated the skin flap and removed the shadow between lid fold and superior orbital rim

The central fat compartment should almost never be reduced. Further deflation, by surgical removal of fat, will magnify (or create) the upper lid concavity that is seen in the aged eye. Again, the goal of upper lid rejuvenation in these patients should focus on restoring a parallel line between the lid fold and lash line, creating a small pretarsal platform (pretarsal skin show) and forming a convex contour from lid crease to brow without skeletonization of the SOR (see Fig. 22.9). Traditional brow lifts and upper blepharoplasty that remove excess skin and fat do little to achieve these goals. These interventions are more likely to result in creating the impression of someone who had plastic surgery.

The second, and less common, upper eyelid (Type 2) is characterized by a natural concavity in the gap between brow and lid. The outline of the SOR is visible but, in youth, is softened due to soft tissue padding (Fig. 22.11a). In contrast to the Type 1 lid, the lid fold to lash line relationship is less central in defining the appearance. There is often a greater distance separating these two landmarks. The more important relationship in the Type 2 upper eyelid is that of the lash line and the shadow under the SOR. In contrast to the Type 1 eyelid where the lid and lash line run parallel to each other, the Type 2 eyelid demonstrates a parallel relationship between the lash line and the SOR shadow (Fig. 22.11b). These two "lines" appear as stacked semicircles. As these individuals age, volume loss occurs across the entire SOR, again more medial than lateral.

As with Type 1 upper lids, the Type 2 patients will often demonstrate an "A-frame" deformity as a result of the disparate eyelid volume loss. The natural evolution of the Type 2

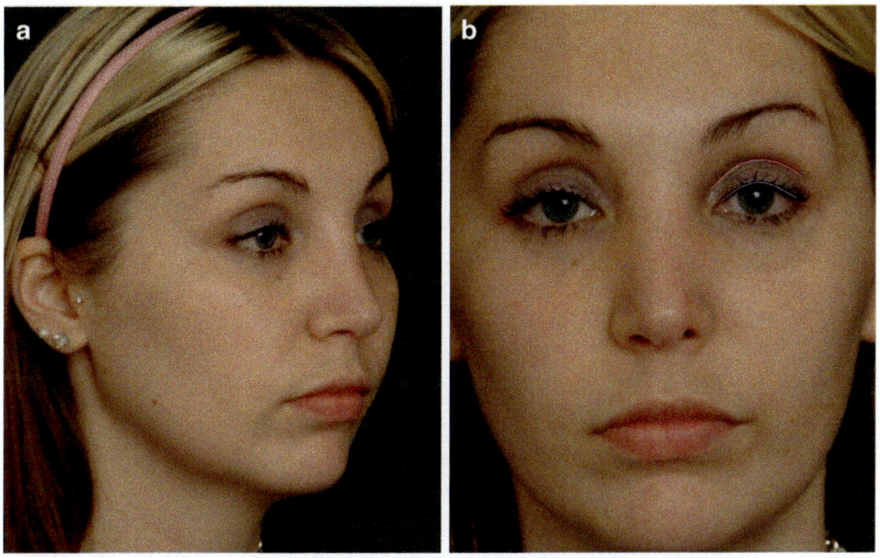

Fig. 22.11 (**a**) The youthful Type 2 upper lid has visible definition of the superior orbital rim, but it is not skeletal due to adequate soft tissue cushioning. (**b**) In these patients, the important linear relationship is between the superior orbital rim (*red line*) and the lash line (*blue line*); these two lines are parallel to each other and there is no A-frame deformity. This is in contrast to the Type 1 upper lid in which the height of the lid fold is more variable and not integral in defining the age of the person

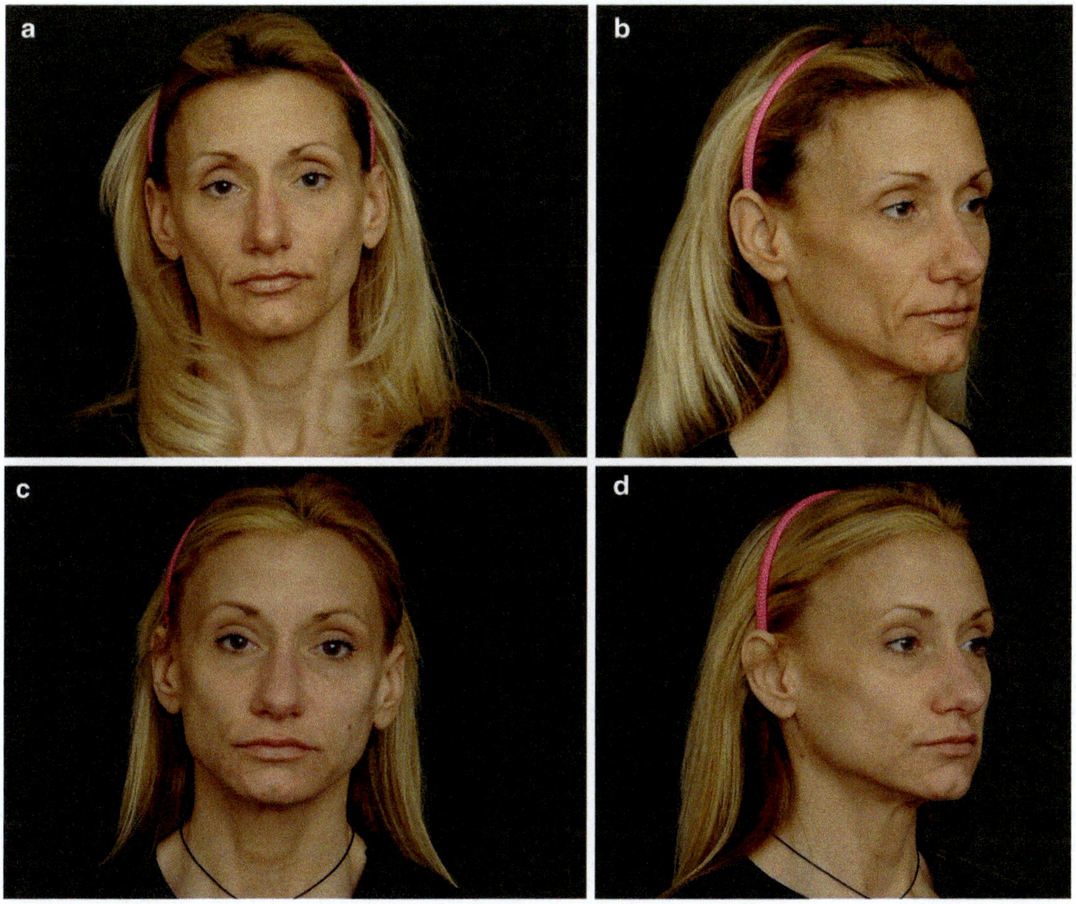

Fig. 22.12 (**a, b**) Baseline photo of a woman with a Type 2 upper lid showing the skeletonization of the superior orbital rim. The relatively greater volume loss medially clearly demonstrates the A-frame deformity. (**c, d**) Following augmentation along the entire superior orbital rim, the appropriate relationship of superior orbital rim and lash line is reestablished and a healthier and youthful Type 2 lid is achieved

eyelid, particularly in a thin individual, is that of a skeletonized and unhealthy appearance. Although the youthful Type 2 upper lid is normally concave, the progressive age-related volume loss creates a deep upper lid sulcus, significant shadowing, and a more pronounced concavity. Loss of soft tissue surrounding the SOR leads to a harsher appearance as bony definition is revealed (Fig. 22.12). In these individuals, there is no reason fat should be removed from the upper lid.

Upper lid hooding also tends to be much less significant in these patients. Rarely will it drape to the point of hitting the lash line. Volume rejuvenation generally takes on an even greater importance in the Type 2 patient.

22.3 Volume Source: Fat Versus Filler

This chapter emphasizes the use of autologous fat transfer for volume restoration, but for many patients HA fillers provide an excellent alternative. In the periorbital region, HA fillers routinely give a result lasting from 1.5 to 2.5 years. Patients are informed that by 1.5 years they will often see some resorption [7]. For patients, the advantages of HA fillers over fat transfer include previewing the results of volume restoration before opting for a more permanent solution, avoiding prolonged recovery associated with fat transfer and providing a nonsurgical alternative. From the physician perspective, the HA fillers may also be preferable for patients with smaller volume requirements, where a very precise result is needed. The analogy used for educating patients on the difference between the two is that an HA filler provides the precision of a fine drawing pencil, whereas fat is more akin to the broad strokes of a paintbrush.

When counseling patients on the option of HA filler or autologous fat transfer, there are several factors to consider. In patients requiring larger volume rejuvenation, extending throughout the face (pan facial volume augmentation), we recommend using fat transfer. When surgical procedures such as blepharoplasty (with its associated need for anesthesia and recuperative period) are added to obtain the optimal result, we also recommend using fat for volume augmentation. In patients with small volume deficiencies in the inferior orbital rim, and little to no pseudoherniated fat, we feel HA fillers will provide a greater degree of satisfaction based on the precision of the result.

In Type 1 upper eyelids, we suggest HA fillers for two reasons. First, many patients are attuned to removing eyelid skin and are not focused on the importance of volume loss in the aging upper lids. Despite viewing photos of themselves and others to demonstrate the role of volume, they may only reluctantly buy into these concepts and feel more comfortable using a reversible material. Secondly, Type 1 upper lids generally require smaller volumes that require precise placement. The reversibility and precise filling provided of HA fillers make this a great option in these patients.

Restylane® (Medicis Pharmaceutical Corporation, Scottsdale, AZ) and Juvederm® (Allergan Inc., Irvine, CA) are the primary HA filler options for periorbtial rejuvenation. We strongly recommend the use of Restylane® for this area. We have experience using both products, and while both have an excellent track records for facial filling, we have seen a significant number of issues with Juvederm® in the periorbital region. Often times, patients will note worsening of "bags" under the eyes or too much puffiness in the upper lids. In our experience, Juvederm® does not have the precise filling effect of Restylane®. We believe the source of the problem is that Juvederm® is more hydrophilic than Restylane® resulting in more edema and therefore less precise volumetric effect.

22.4 Surgical Technique

22.4.1 General Considerations

Once the preoperative analysis has been completed and the surgical plan reviewed, patients are marked in an upright position to delineate the fat recipient sites. In most cases, we perform these procedures using intravenous conscious sedation combined with infiltration of the surgical sites with local anesthetic. If upper or lower lid blepharoplasty is being performed concurrently, we will generally begin with fat harvest, followed by upper and/or lower lid blepharoplasty and ending with fat injection.

22.4.2 Fat Harvest

The most commonly used donor sites are the lower abdomen, inner thigh, outer thigh, and hip. Determination of the donor site is generally based on where the patient has the most abundant fat stores. A secondary factor is the depth of anesthesia. Certain donor sites (outer thigh and hip) require repositioning the patient, which is more cumbersome with deeper levels of anesthesia. As such, these sites are preferred in the awake patients. Finally, patients are evaluated for the presence of prior surgical incisions and/or hernias (umbilical or incisional). If present, these are avoided.

The surgical field is sterilely prepped and draped prior to beginning the procedure. The area of fat harvest is infiltrated with a 20 mL solution of local anesthetic on a 22-gauge spinal needle. If intravenous sedation is used, the 20 mL mix injected into each donor site consists of 5 mL of 1% lidocaine with 1:100,000 epinephrine and 15 mL of normal saline. If only local anesthetic is used, then the 20 mL mix contains 10 mL of 1% lidocaine with 1:100,000 10 mL of normal saline. Local anesthetic is injected by concentrating 10 mL superficially in the immediate subdermal plane and 10 mL at the deeper aspect of the fat, just superficial to the muscle. The rationale for this is to minimize the potentially destructive effect of the local anesthetic solution on the target adipocytes.

Fat is harvested via a stab incision placed in a relatively concealed location. For example, the lower abdomen access incision is placed in the umbilicus and the inner thigh entry incision is in the crease in the inguinal fold. These entry sites are anesthetized with a bleb of 1% lidocaine with 1:100,000 epinephrine. The incision is then made with a 16-gauge Nokor needle or a No. 11 blade. One of two fat harvesting cannulas are generally used: a 3.0 mm bullet-tip harvesting cannula or a 2.1 mm multiport harvesting cannula (Tulip Medical, Inc., San Diego, CA) (Fig. 22.13). The 2.1 mm multiport is a less-aggressive cannula and is useful for areas where there is greater concern of contour irregularity. In addition, when performed under local anesthetic, harvesting with the 2.1 mm multiport cannula is less painful and better tolerated.

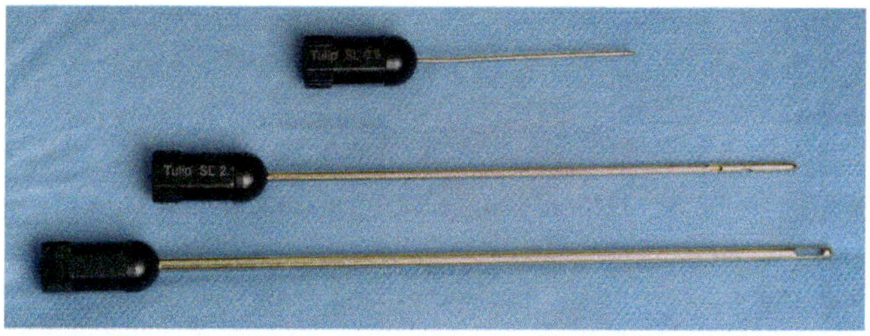

Fig. 22.13 Fat transfer instruments (Tulip Medical, Inc., San Diego, CA), from *top* to *down*. The 0.9 mm (4 cm length) injecting cannula is used to infiltrate local anesthetic and is the primary cannula for all periorbital fat injections. The 2.1 mm multiport harvesting cannula. The 3.0 mm bullet-tip harvesting cannula. (Adapted from Lam et al. [1], used with permission)

A 10-mL syringe is used with the harvesting cannula, and fat is suctioned while placing only 1–2 mL of manually applied negative pressure on the plunger. The cannula is gently passed back and forth through the midlayer of fat, avoiding superficial (which will appear as tethering on the skin) or deeper (which will elicit significant pain from muscle irritation) manipulation. Fat harvest should be performed uniformly over the region so as to avoid contour irregularities.

As each 10-mL syringe is filled, it is passed off to an assistant for preparation under continued sterile conditions. In determining the amount of fat to harvest, each 10-mL syringe will, on average, yield 5–7 mL of usable fat.

22.4.3 Fat Processing

A plug is fastened onto the Luer-Lok end of each syringe and the plunger is removed. A cap is then placed on the plunger end of the syringe. A balanced number of syringes are placed in sterile sleeves that fit into a centrifuge. This maintains the sterility of the syringes for subsequent steps in preparation. The centrifuge is turned on for 1–2 min at 2,000–3,000 rpm (Fig. 22.14). Upon completion of centrifugation, the syringes are removed and placed back on the surgical field. The syringes now demonstrate three layers: a supranatant, made up of free fatty acids; an infranatant, consisting of blood and lidocaine; and a central core of viable fat. With the cap still on, the Luer-Lok

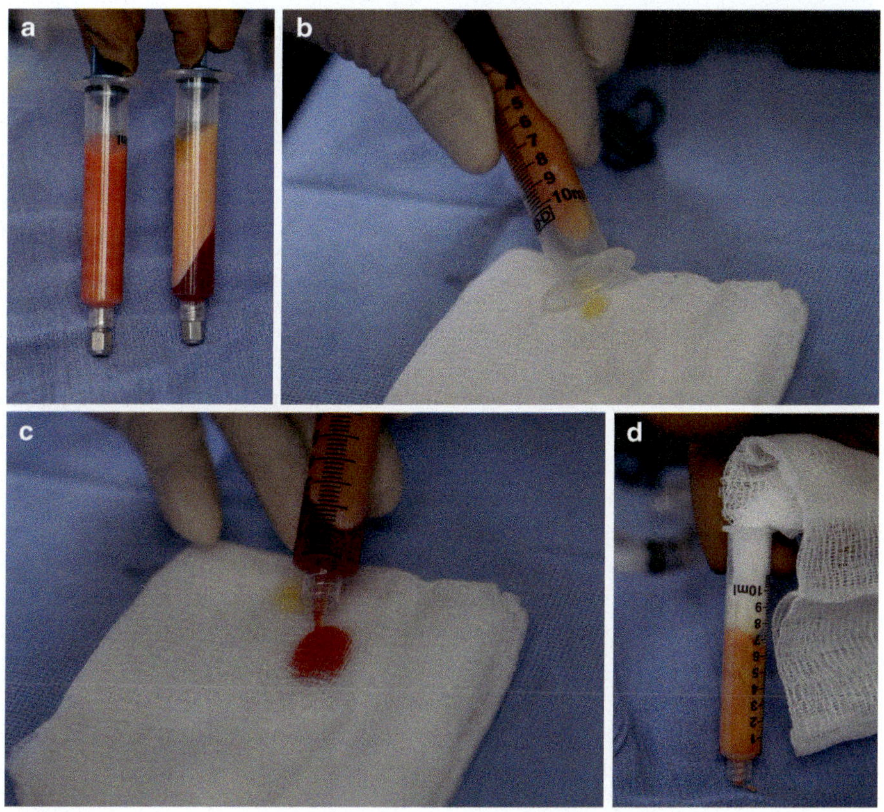

Fig. 22.14 (**a**) Immediately following fat harvest (*left*) and upon completion of centrifugation (*right*). The supranatant is poured off into a gauze (**b**), the infranatant drained (**c**), leaving an isolated layer of fat. The fat is then wicked with a sterile guaze to remove residual supranatant. (**d**, Adapted from Lam et al. [1], used with permission)

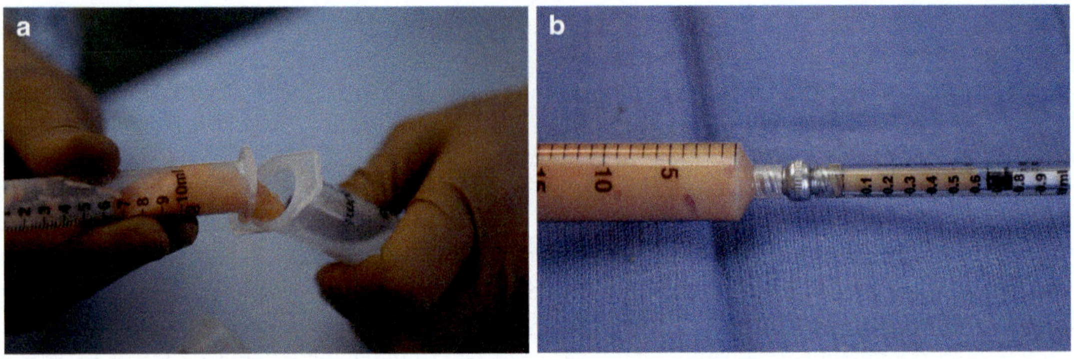

Fig. 22.15 (**a**) The fat is poured from the 10-mL syringes into a 20-mL syringe. (**b**) Fat is transferred from the 20 mL syringe into individual 1 mL Luer-Lok syringes in preparation for injection. (Adapted from Lam et al. [1], used with permission)

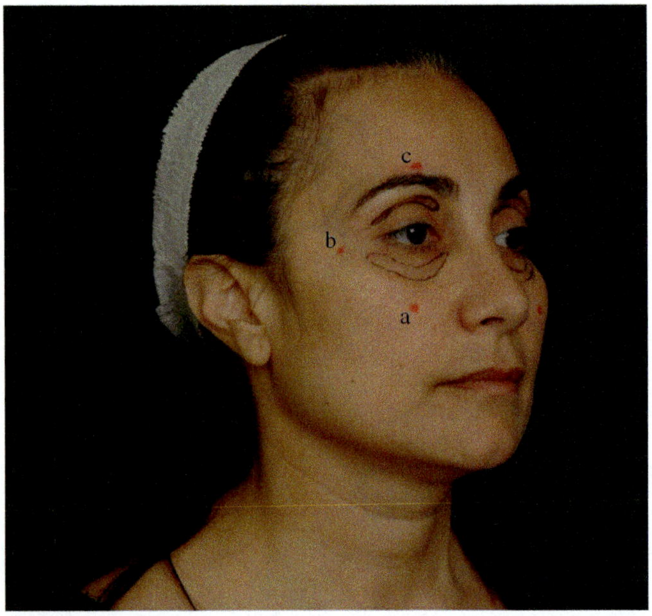

Fig. 22.16 Preoperative markings demonstrate the entry points (in *red*) for periorbital fat transfer. Moving from inferior to superior they include: (**a**) the midcheek entry site for inferior orbital rim augmentation; (**b**) the lateral canthal entry site for filling the lateral superior orbital rim and the depression in the region of the lateral canthus; and (**c**) the brow entry site for filling the superior orbital rim/upper eyelid

end is opened to allow the infranatant to drain out. The cap is then removed from the plunger end and the supranatant is poured off. The syringes are stood upright in a cup or test tube holder and the supranatant end is wicked using a cotton guaze. After several minutes, the individual 10-mL syringes are consolidated to facilitate the injection process. The plunger is removed from a 20-mL syringe and fat is poured from the plunger end of the 10-mL syringes into the 20-mL syringe (Fig. 22.15). The 20-mL syringes should not be filled with more than 15 mL of fat. A transfer hub is placed on the Luer-Lok end of the 20-mL syringe and the plunger is carefully placed back into the syringe. Fat is then transferred into individual 1-mL Luer-Lok syringes for injection.

22.4.4 Fat Injection

Local anesthetic consisting of 1% lidocaine with 1:100,000 epinephrine is administered at the planned entry site. An infraorbital and/or supraorbital nerve block (depending on the area addressed) is also given. Entry sites for the cannulas are created with a 20-gauge needle. Using a 0.9 mm injecting cannulas (Tulip Medical, Inc., San Diego, CA), local anesthetic is infiltrated into the recipient bed via the needle stick entry ports. Fat is then injected using blunt cannulas on 1-mL Luer-Lok syringes (see Fig. 22.12). The preferred cannula for fat infiltration in the periorbital region is a 0.9-mm injecting cannula, 4 cm in length (Tulip Medical, Inc., San Diego, CA). Small parcels, 0.03–0.05 mL, of fat are placed with each pass of the cannula.

The inferior orbital rim is approached through a midcheek entry point so that all fat is placed with the cannula passing perpendicular to the orbital rim (Fig. 22.16). The degree of volume loss will dictate the amount of fat to be placed. As a general rule, we recommend the total amount of fat injected in this area does not exceed 4 mL. We typically distribute the fat as follows. The initial injections of fat are placed in the immediate supraperiosteal plane. These are placed not with the intent of filling the visible defect, but following the bony landmarks by feel to build a foundation volume. The first milliliter is placed with the cannula passing back and forth across the medial half of the bony inferior orbital rim (Fig. 22.17). The fat is deposited in tiny parcels over the bone. The second milliliter placed at this depth is along the lateral half of the bony inferior orbital rim. The next set of injections is placed more superficially, just deep to the orbicularis oculi muscle. With the more superficial injections, the fat is injected focusing on filling the visible, marked out, volume deficit. We strongly recommend not placing fat superficial to the orbicularis oculi muscle, as this will significantly increase the risk of contour irregularities. The first of the superficial injections is directed at the medial half of the inferior orbital, or the "tear trough." The second superficial

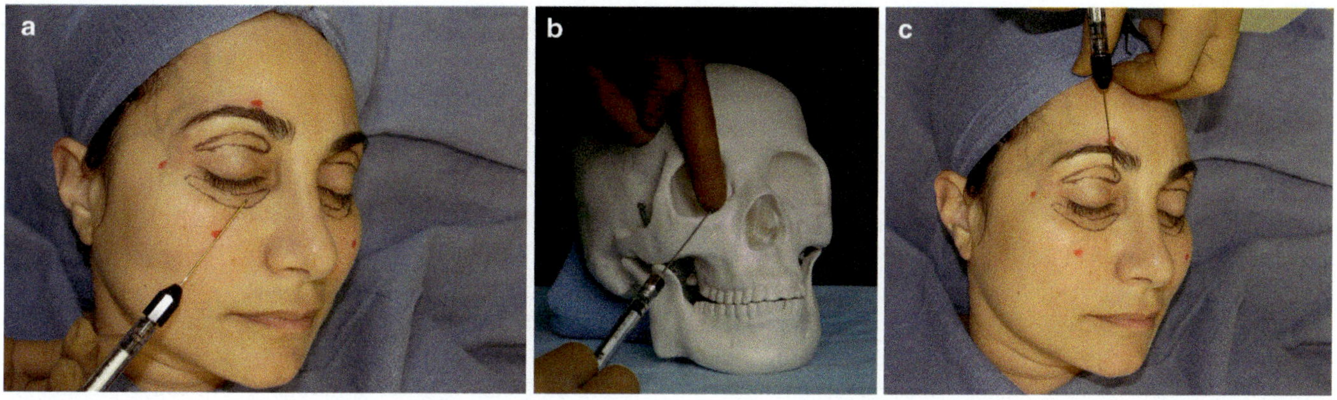

Fig. 22.17 (**a**) The cannula is positioned to demonstrate the orientation of the cannula passing perpendicular to the inferior orbital rim from the midcheek entry point. (**b**) The initial deep injections placed just superficial to the periosteum of the inferior orbital rim. The index finger of the surgeon's nondominant hand gives tactile feedback on the location of the bone and also serves to protect the globe. (**c**) The superior orbital rim is approached from an entry point just superior to the midportion of the brow. (**b**, Adapted from Lam et al. [1], used with permission)

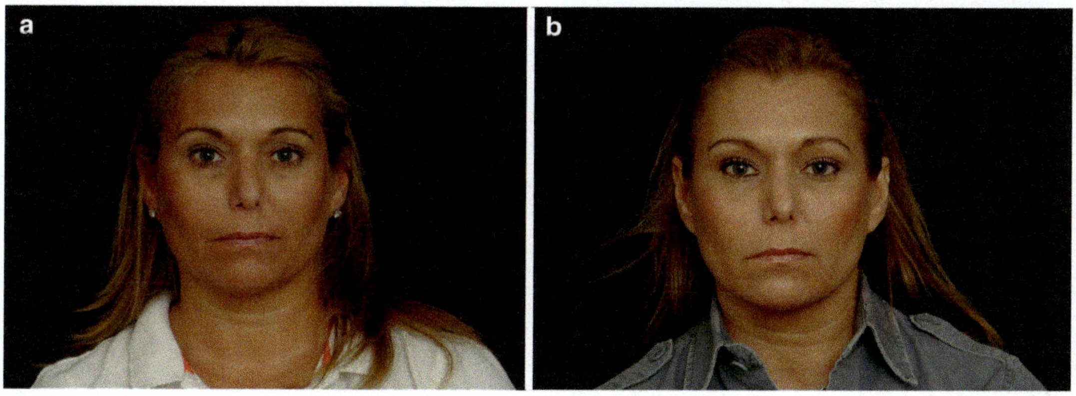

Fig. 22.18 By adding volume below the left superior orbital rim in this patient with a Type 1 upper lid, the A-frame deformity is corrected; the lid fold is pushed inferiorly, reestablishing the parallel relationship of lid fold and lash line. Pre- (**a**) and post- (**b**) volume augmentation of the left medial superior orbital rim. (Adapted from Glasgold et al. [14])

injection is placed to fill the lateral half of the visible inferior orbital rim depression.

The technique for approaching the SOR is the same as its lower lid counterpart. The goals of adding volume will depend on the individual's upper lid structure, Type 1 or 2, as delineated earlier. The medial half of the SOR is preferentially approached through an entry point superior to the brow. This allows very direct and precise placement of the fat. The fat is injected perpendicular to the orbital rim, as was done at the inferior rim. Filling of the lateral SOR is also performed from an entry point above the brow with the cannula passing perpendicular to the bony rim. Alternatively, the lateral SOR can be approached from a lateral canthal entry point (see Fig. 22.16). From this direction, the fat is placed with the cannula running parallel to the orbital rim. In the upper lid, this is an acceptable approach not associated with the contour problems inherent to inferior orbital rim grafting from a lateral entry point. As with the lower lid, fat is infiltrated in staged levels, supraperiosteal, and just deep to the orbicularis oculi muscle. As is prudent anywhere in the periorbital region, a conservative approach is suggested. Patients are happier with a slight undercorrection of volume, versus the potential prominence and contour irregularities and prolonged recovery of an overcorrection.

Type 1 upper lids generally require less volume augmentation, as these individuals have a fuller upper lid at baseline. The tendency in Type 1 lids is to concentrate the most volume in the medial half of the SOR. The ultimate goal is to eliminate the concavity from the brow to lid fold and to correct the A-frame deformity. Across the entire SOR, fat can be placed at and below the orbital rim. This allows the deflated brow to be minimally elevated off the bone while also putting volume at the level of the concavity inferior to the brow. Filling below the rim is very important medially where correction of the A-frame deformity requires pushing the lid fold inferiorly to reestablish the parallel relationship of the lid fold and lash line (Fig. 22.18).

Type 2 upper lids, characterized by skeletonization of the entire SOR, need larger volume augmentation. Fat is placed across the entire SOR, with greater attention placed on filling inferior to the bony orbital rim and not deep to the brow (Fig. 22.19). In these eyes, the brow is already isolated by the surrounding volume loss and brow position is usually felt to be relatively good. In order to lessen the apparent depth and hollowing of these upper lids, the lid is essentially unfolded from the depth of the sulcus. This leads to a greater span of visible upper lid skin below the brow and a reduction of the upper lid concavity (Fig. 22.20). The goal is not to create a Type 1 lid, which is neither realistic nor representative of the Type 2 patients' youthful upper lid. Rather the aim is to appropriately reinflate the lid back to its prior appearance.

After completing upper and lower lid fat augmentation, there is usually an apparent volume deficit at the lateral canthal region of the orbital rim. Through the entry point at the lateral canthus, a very small amount of fat (0.5 mL) is placed subcutaneously to soften the transition.

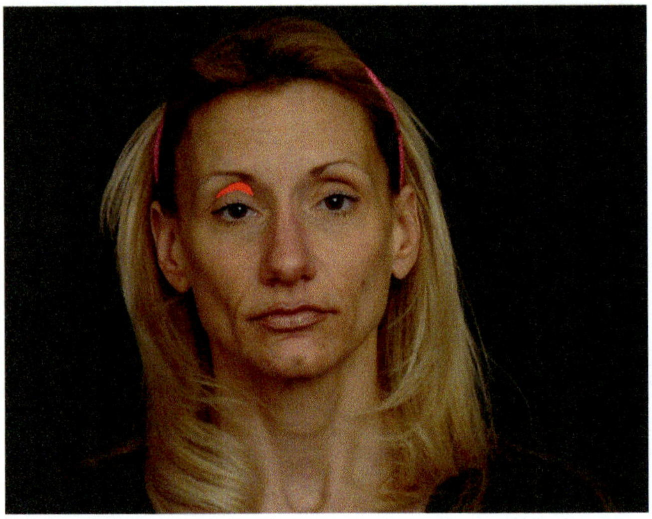

Fig. 22.19 The highlighted area (in *red*) demonstrates the focal point of volume augmentation in the Type 2 upper lid. Volume is added inferior to the superior orbital rim to unfold the upper lid skin and reduce the degree of visible shadowing. A greater amount is usually required medially to correct the A-frame deformity

22.5 Postoperative Considerations

No dressings are applied at the harvest or injection site. All entry sites made with a needle are small enough that they need not be closed with sutures. We recommend applying ice to the transfer sites intermittently for the first 48–72 hours. Patients are also instructed to keep their head elevated to reduce swelling during this time. If just fat transfer is performed, strenuous physical activity is discouraged until 1 week after surgery, at which time patients may gradually begin to return to normal activities. If other surgical procedures are performed at the same time, the patients are encouraged to wait 3 weeks to resume strenuous activity.

It is very important that the postoperative recovery phase is reviewed carefully prior to the operation in order to better manage patient expectations. Patients are instructed that they will have significant swelling and bruising in the immediate postoperative period, more than if they had a traditional upper or lower lid blepharoplasty alone. After 2 weeks, most patients feel as if they can return to work or daily activities. But at this point, they should expect to feel their face is fuller than what they hoped for. Over the subsequent 2 weeks, patients will begin to attain what they wanted. The end result is really not known for up to 12 months. Patients are cautioned that, on average, 30% of the fat injected is retained [8].

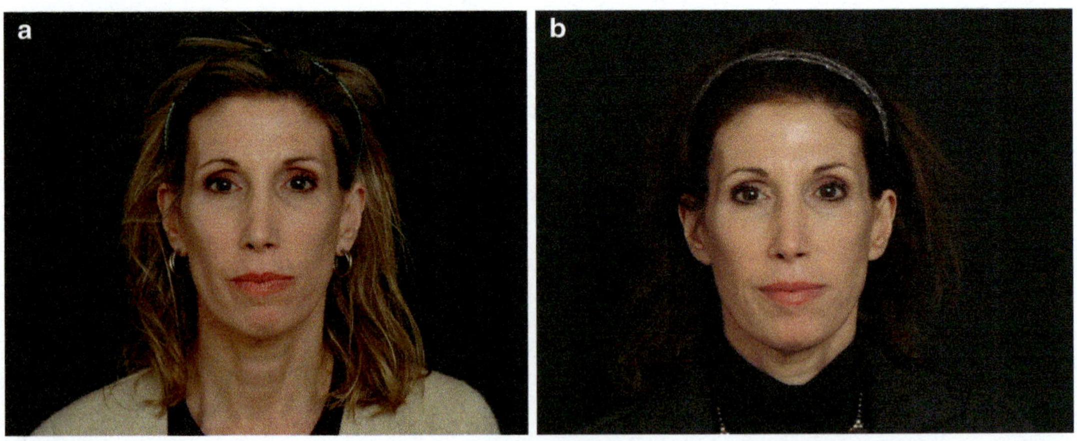

Fig. 22.20 Pre- (**a**) and postoperative (**b**) results of fat transfer to the superior orbital rim for a Type 2 upper lid. This result demonstrates how the upper lid skin is unfolded and brought inferiorly so that there is a greater degree of visibility of the upper lid, particularly medially. The harsh shadows are lessened, creating a younger and rejuvenated appearance, and the parallel relationship of the superior orbital rim shadow and the lash line is reestablished

It is essential that patients understand that a secondary touch-up procedure may be needed to obtain the ideal result. A touch-up procedure is generally not performed until at least 6 months, and frequently closer to 1 year, after the initial fat transfer.

22.6 Complications

The primary complications of fat transfer are related to contour irregularities and unpredictable volume retention. Less common complications include entry site irregularity and surgical site infections. Neurovascular complications are exceedingly rare [9]. Most of these potential complications can be minimized with appropriate planning and technique.

Contour irregularities typically appear as an isolated lump, from fat deposited in an area where it is visible, or as an elevated roll of tissue [10]. Isolated lumps are generally the result of poor technique in the periorbital region. They can be prevented by carefully depositing small parcels of fat (no more than 0.03 mL per pass), placing fat only deep to the orbicularis oculi muscle, and an overall conservative approach to fat injection. Some surgeons recommend fat infiltration superficial to the orbicularis oculi muscle. This maneuver will significantly increase the risk of contour problems while providing little potential benefit. When a periorbital lump occurs, intralesional kenalog injection can be attempted but is typically not as effective or precise as a direct excision.

A thickened roll of tissue along the inferior orbital rim, and less likely along the SOR, is a complication we have only seen when injecting strands of fat parallel to the orbital rim from a lateral entry point. Fat should always be placed with the cannula passing perpendicular to the inferior orbital rim. Adoption of this technique has all but eliminated this complication. These rolls often respond to intralesional kenalog injection, starting with very dilute (0.05 mg/mL) amounts, with gradual increases in concentration and spacing injections at 4-week intervals. If kenalog fails, direct transcutaneous excision can be performed. The incision heals very well when placed in a natural lower lid skin crease, or in the tear trough, at the junction of the thin lower lid skin and the thick cheek skin.

Overcorrection is a complication avoided by grafting conservative amounts of fat. Surgical intervention can include microliposuction. However, in the periorbital region, direct excision is more like to be successful. When overcorrection is present, we recommend waiting at least 6 months, and preferably a year, to assess if intervention should proceed. This delay allows swelling to fully dissipate and a truer assessment of volume status. Undercorrection is not a complication, but an inherent aspect of fat transfer that must be explained to patients in advance. It is much better to be faced with having to augment fat than having to excise it.

Although uncommon, there have been reports of intravascular injection and associated complications with any type of facial injections [11]. This complication should not occur if blunt infiltration cannulas are used, small volumes are injected, and minimal force is applied when injecting. Furthermore, by not forcing the cannula through significant tissue resistance; one is less likely to cause damage to neurovascular structures. We have not seen sensory or motor nerve injury with the technique described.

The fat infiltration entry sites are made with a 20-gauge needle and typically heal well without closure. On two occasions have we seen an entry site divot formation. In each case the divot was successfully treated by subcision with a 20-gauge needle. Persistent erythema, or discoloration, at facial entry points are generally not an issue. In contrast, the entry points on the body, where a larger cannula is used for harvesting, more commonly demonstrate persistent erythema that resolves over months. Placement of the entry site into a well-concealed location will help prevent patient concern regarding prolonged erythema. Should discoloration present a significant issue, resolution can be accelerated with the use of a pulse dye laser or intense pulse light (IPL) treatment.

Infection following fat transfer is exceedingly rare, and appropriate sterile technique aids in preventing its occurrence [12]. We use one dose of ancef, or clindamycin if penicillin allergic, preoperatively. We have only seen postfat transfer infection in two cases. In both patients, the infection was delayed (weeks after surgery) and manifested erythema and mild discomfort. Both were diagnosed as atypical mycobacterial infection and successfully treated with clarithromycin.

22.7 Conclusion

Over the last decade, our understanding that volume loss is a major component of facial/periorbital aging has become increasingly accepted. This paradigm shift, and the implementation of volume augmentation in periorbital region, has led to more natural results and less stigmata of plastic surgery. Fat grafting and fillers such as hyaluronic acids should be a key component to the treatment algorithm for any patient seeking periorbital rejuvenation. Overall, they provide a safe and effective approach to volume augmentation of the upper lid/brow and lower lid/midface regions.

References

1. Lam S, Glasgold M, Glasgold R. Complementary fat grafting. Philadelphia, PA: Lippincott Williams & Wilkins; 2007.
2. Coleman S. Structural fat grafting. St. Louis, MO: Quality Medical; 2004.

3. Lambros VS. The dynamics of facial aging. Paper presented at the Annual Meeting of the American Society for Aesthetic Plastic Surgery, Las Vegas, NV, April 27–May 3, 2002.
4. Donath AS, Glasgold R, Glasgold M. Volume loss versus gravity: new concepts in facial aging. Curr Opin Otolaryngol Head Neck Surg. 2007;15(4):238–43.
5. Pessa JE. An algorithm of facial aging: verification of Lambros's theory by three-dimensional stereolithography, with reference to the pathogenesis of midfacial aging, sclera show, and the lateral suborbital trough deformity. Plast Reconstr Surg. 2000;106:479–88; discussion 489–90.
6. Mendelson BC, Muzaffar AR, Adams WP. Surgical anatomy of the midcheek and malar mounds. Plast Reconstr Surg. 2002;110(3): 885–96.
7. Donath A, Glasgold R, Meier J, Glasgold M. Quantitative evaluation of volume augmentation in the tear trough with a hyaluronic acid-based filler: a 3-dimensional analysis. Plast Reconstr Surg. 2010;125:1515–22.
8. Meier JD, Glasgold RA, Glasgold MJ. Autologous fat grafting: long term evidence of its efficacy in midfacial rejuvenation. Arch Facial Plast Surg. 2009;11(1):24–8.
9. Kranendonk S, Obagi S. Autologous fat transfer for periorbital rejuvenation: indications, technique, and complications. Dermatol Surg. 2007;33:572–8.
10. Glasgold RA, Glasgold MJ, Lam SM. Complications following fat transfer. Oral Maxillofac Surg Clin North Am. 2009;21:53–8.
11. Murillo J, Torres J, Bofill L, et al. Skin and wound infection by rapidly growing mycobacteria. Arch Dermatol. 2000;136: 1347–52.
12. Feinendegen D, Baumgartner R, Vuadens P, et al. Autologous fat injection for soft tissue augmentation in the face: a safe procedure? Aesthet Plast Surg. 1998;22:163–7.
13. Carniol PJ, Sadick NS, editors. Clinical procedures in laser skin rejuvenation. London: Informa Healthcare; 2007.
14. Glasgold M et al. Volumetric rejuvenation of the periorbital region. Facial Plastic Surg. 2010;26:3.

Periorbital Laser Resurfacing

23

Douglas G. Hamilton

Key Points

- Lasers are an excellent nonsurgical treatment option for periorbital rhytids and lower lid laxity.
- Four categories of resurfacing lasers exist: traditional ablative lasers (CO_2 and erbium laser), traditional nonablative lasers (Cool Touch, N-lite), fractionated nonablative lasers, and fractionated ablative lasers.
- Fractionated lasers are less effective for periorbital treatment of lower lid laxity and deep rhytids as compared with the traditional ablative Ultrapulsated CO_2 and erbium lasers.
- Proper pretreatment of skin with hydroquinone and Retin-A is essential for avoidance of adverse effects with all laser technologies.
- The results of ablative resurfacing are immediate, improve with time, and are long lasting.
- The incidence of ablative laser complications such as dyschromia is greater with extreme skin types: Fitzpatrick I and V–VI.
- Laser resurfacing can be an extremely useful adjunct to blepharoplasty and other lower lid rejuvenation techniques in the periorbital region.

23.1 Introduction

Lower lid rejuvenation remains one of the more challenging problems in cosmetic surgery. Other chapters in this book have elegantly discussed multiple surgical approaches to addressing lower lid laxity and pseudoherniation of orbital fat. The *surgical* management of deeper lower lid rhytids and fine lines remains elusive. Although, aggressive skin care regimen and chemical peels can improve the appearance of fine lines, periorbital laser skin resurfacing is still the gold standard for attaining excellent long-term improvement of this very difficult problem.

23.2 History

Laser technologies for resurfacing procedures fall into four basic categories in chronological order of their development:

1. Traditional ablative lasers (Ultrapulsated CO_2; Erbium)
2. Traditional nonablative lasers (Cool Touch; N-Lite)
3. Fractionated nonablative lasers (Relient's Fraxel SR750, 1500 (Re:store): Cynosure's Affirm 1440/1320; Palomar Lux)
4. Fractionated ablative lasers (Fraxel Re:pair CO_2; Affirm CO_2; Palomar Lux 2940 erbium: Lumenis CO_2: Cutera Pearl)

The traditional ablative lasers were introduced in the mid-1990, with great enthusiasm, for full and segmental facial resurfacing. CO_2 was the first ablative laser introduced to the market. Erbium ablative laser technology was later introduced as a "less invasive" option. They were both shown to be efficacious for the treatment of wrinkles and scars, with Ultrapulsated CO_2 being more efficacious in improving lower lid laxity. Clinical improvements with these traditional ablative lasers were shown to continue for 5 years. Despite the significant aesthetic improvements with traditional ablative lasers, the prolonged recuperation time with significant erythema reduced overall patient acceptance. As a result, multiple technologies subsequently came to market in an attempt to achieve similar results with reduced downtime.

The search for a no-downtime procedure to resurface the face resulted in the development of the second category of lasers (traditional nonablative lasers) such as Cool Touch and

D.G. Hamilton (✉)
Private Practice, Dermatologist and Assistant Clinical Professor,
David Geffen School of Medicine at UCLA,
Beverly Hills, CA, USA
e-mail: dgh@ucla.edu

G.G. Massry et al. (eds.), *Master Techniques in Blepharoplasty and Periorbital Rejuvenation*,
DOI 10.1007/978-1-4614-0067-7_23, © Springer Science+Business Media, LLC 2011

N-lite. Unfortunately, the pendulum swung significantly with this category of lasers. Although, downtime and side-effects were generally inconsequential, these lasers were significantly less effective in effacing lower lid rhytids.

Fractionated nonablative lasers were a major advance in laser skin resurfacing appearing in 2004 with the production of Reliant's Fraxel 750 developed under contract by Wellman Laboratories at Harvard Medical School. Other fractionated nonablative lasers soon followed. Treatment with these types of lasers resulted in minimal downtime and an extremely low incidence of dyschromia, allowing use on all skin types. Efficacy with acne scars, fine rhytids, and overall skin texture has been significant with this category; however, improving deeper (nondynamic) rhytids as well as lower lid laxity has been limited. To improve the treatment of static rhytids, a second generation of ablative, fractionated lasers using the CO_2 and Erbium technologies has since been developed. These fractionated lasers offered some of the advantages of the traditional CO_2 and Erbium lasers with slightly less downtime as well as lower risk of dyschromia.

23.3 Use of Resurfacing Lasers for Periorbital Resurfacing

Periorbital cosmetic concerns generally involve anatomic changes, cutaneous laxity, and rhytids. *Anatomical changes* typically include true or pseudoherniation of orbital fat, tissue deflation, sagging, and loss of eyelid tone. Correction of these concerns is addressed elsewhere in this book.

Periorbital *rhtyids* are primarily a result of photodamage, loss of elasticity, and dynamic expression (facial animation). These issues need to be addressed with appropriate treatments such as chemodenervation, skin care, sun protection as well chemical and laser resurfacing. Skin resurfacing results are more predictable with the use of lasers than chemical peels. All laser categories will produce improvement but the most substantial improvement comes from the use of traditional ablative CO_2 and erbium lasers.

Surgery is the optimal treatment for *cutaneous laxity* of the upper eyelids. For the lower lids, however, lid tightening can also be addressed with lasers. While traditional surgical approaches can remove excess skin, they do not alter the quality of remaining skin. Ultrapulsated CO_2 laser skin resurfacing not only enhances the quality of rhytids, it can additionally improve skin laxity and may be the treatment of choice for the appropriate skin type. The clinical skin tightening produced by the traditional CO_2 is immediate and long lasting. Erbium laser with appropriate treatment protocol can achieve similar improvements in deep rhytids as Ultrapulsated CO_2 laser but falls short in causing skin tightening. The ablative fractionated CO_2 and Erbium lasers will produce some skin contraction but not enough to justify their use for this purpose.

23.4 Traditional Ablative Laser Resurfacing

Although erbium lasers were first introduced as a less invasive option to CO_2 lasers, both technologies are effective for periorbital rhytids. The downtime and complication rates are also similar for both lasers at settings that garner the same aesthetic outcome. Typically, erbium laser will require additional passes to achieve the rhytid results of CO_2. The main difference between the two technologies is that the CO_2 application is more efficacious in tightening the lower eyelid skin.

The potential complications with ablative laser resurfacing include dyschromia (hyperpigmentation, hypopigmentation), prolonged edema/erythema, hypertrophic and atrophic scarring. Tables 23.1–23.3 summarize the preoperative evaluation for appropriate patient selection. Each patient must first be clearly classified into the Fitzpatrick skin classification, which has an excellent correlation with laser candidacy and potential complications. Absolute contraindications include active infectious disease, oral retinoids, connective tissue disorder, propensity for keloid formations, suspicion for cutaneous malignancy, and pregnancy. Relative contraindications

Table 23.1 Fitzpatrick skin classification system

Skin type	Skin color	Characteristics
I	White; very fair; red or blond hair; blue eyes; freckles	Always burns, never tans
II	White; fair; red or blond hair; blue, hazel, or green eyes	Usually burns, tans with difficulty
III	Cream white; fair with any eye or hair color; very common	Sometimes mild burn, gradually tans
IV	Brown; typical Mediterranean Caucasian skin	Rarely burns, tans with ease
V	Dark brown; mid-eastern skin types	Very rarely burns, tans very easily
VI	Black	Never burns, tans very easily

Table 23.2 Pretreatment analysis for ablative CO_2 and erbium laser procedures

Absolute contraindications	Relative contraindications
• Active infectious disease	• Fitzpatrick skin type I-hypopigmentation
• Connective tissue disorders	• Fitzpatrick skin type V–VI-hyperpigmentation
• Patients with propensity for keloid formations	• Immune compromised patients
• Pregnancy	• Poor lid distraction test
• Oral retinoids	
• Suspicion for cutaneous malignancy	

Table 23.3 Pretreatment medications for ablative CO_2 and erbium laser procedures

Skin preparation: Hydroquinone (in the morning) and Retin-A (at night) are initiated one month prior to the procedure
Antibiotics: Cefuroxime 250 mg BID starting 12 h before procedure through evening after
Antiherpetic: Valacyclovir 500 g BID starting 3 days before procedure through postoperative day 4
Pain medications: Extra Strength Tylenol for mild to moderate pain; Tylenol with codeine for severe pain
Sleeping pills: Dalmane 15 mg
Specifications and technology information were taken from the following websites
Lumenis aesthetic: http://www.aesthetic.lumenis.com/ultrapulse
UltraPulse specifications data sheet: http://www.aesthetic.lumenis.com/pdf/UltraPulse_Encore_datasheet.pdf
Cynosure affirm specs: http://www.cynosure.com/products/affirm/specs.php
Fraxel.com: http://www.fraxel.com/physicians.cfm
Fraxel laser skin treatments and resurfacing procedures: http://www.fraxel.com/Fraxel-Lasers-Compare-Technology/

include immune compromise status, poor lid distraction test, Fitzpatrick skin type I (hypopigmentation), and V–VI skin (hyperpigmentation). Patients with darker skin complexion are at a higher risk of hyperpigmentation. As a result, individuals with Fitzpatrick skin type V and VI require significant diligence in pretreatment protocol including one month of daily application of 0.025% trentinoin cream and 4% hydroquinone. Patients should be made aware that hyperpigmentation is treatable in most individuals. On the contrary, skin types I and II are at a higher risk of developing hypopigmentation with ablative lasers. Hypopigmentation, unlike hyperpigmentation, has no great solution and can be a serious complication. As a result, patients with very light complexion must be approached with extreme caution.

23.5 Technical Considerations: Ablative Ultrapulsated CO_2 Laser Resurfacing

Patients are instructed to avoid sun 2 weeks prior to the procedure and are pretreated for one month with daily application of 0.025% trentinoin cream and 4% hydroquinone. Oral prophylaxis with antibiotics and antiviral medication is also recommended. Infraorbital and supraorbital nerve blocks are administered using 2% xylocaine with epinephrine 10 min prior to beginning the procedure. Tetracaine ophthalmic drops are administered prior to beginning the procedure.

The CO_2 laser is performed on Hibiclens or alcohol prepped skin. With the Lumenis Ultrapulse CO_2 laser (Lumenis Inc., Santa Clara, CA), a setting of 300 mJ at a fluence of 5 J/cm^2 is used with a rectangular pattern. All personnel should wear laser-specific protective goggles. The upper lid and brows are typically treated at the same time as the lower lids. A laser safe Jaeger lid plate (or similar type protective shield) is inserted under the lids as a protective measure after application of lacrilube ophthalmic ointment. This specific Jaeger lid plate has a dull surface, removing its capacity to dangerously reflect the laser beam. The contralateral eye is covered closed with water-soaked gauze.

The white char created by the first pass is removed using wet gauze and the face is dried again. The first pass generally removes about 80–100 μm of tissue reaching the superficial dermis. Pinpoint bleeding may begin depending upon the area of the face. The first pass is merely a facilitator for the second and/or third pass when collagen remodeling and substantial long-term benefits can be achieved. On the second pass, the aesthetic benefit of the laser is observed with the ablation of the shoulders of the wrinkles and collagen contraction. Even though further beneficial effects may be achieved by a third pass, many experienced laser surgeons avoid further treatment with the eyelids. Third passes, if performed, should be done in a "spot" fashion. One wants to avoid the development of a grayish hue, which indicates imminent penetration of subcutaneous fat. Airborne debris is evacuated throughout the procedure with a vacuum device handled by an assistant. After a final removal of char, refrigerated plain Aquaphor is applied. Vigilon Primary Wound Dressing (Bard Medical, Covington, GA) may be used as an alternative for 24–48 h. Unlike other parts of the face, Wound dressing is fairly difficult to keep around the eyes. Figure 23.1 illustrates a typical outcome for crow's feet with ablative laser resurfacing.

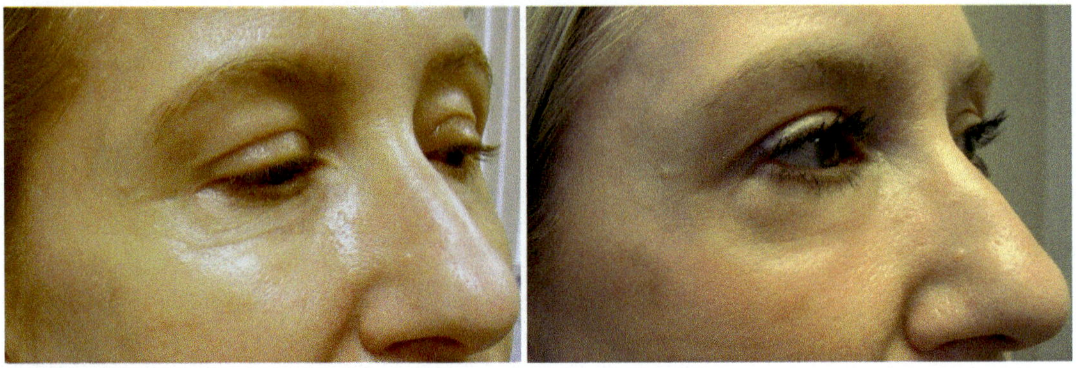

Fig. 23.1 Before and after (2 weeks) ablative laser resurfacing with CO_2

23.6 Posttreatment Care for Ablative CO_2 and Erbium Laser

Pain following the skin treatment is usually mild to moderate and can often be controlled by Extra Strength Tylenol. The patients are encouraged to apply cold compress continuously on the day of procedure until bedtime and 20 min per hour the day following the procedure. The head should be elevated between 30 and 45° for 4–5 days after the procedure. The patients can take a bath or shampoo their hair.

The treated area should be soaked for 10–15 min (4–6 times a day) with a mixture of 1 teaspoon of white vinegar in one 8 oz cup of cool water using a fine sponge or wash cloth. The skin should be kept lubricated with aquaphor in between soaks to prevent crusts and scabs. Dead skin or scabs should not be picked, rubbed, or removed by the patient as this may increase the risk of scarring. There should be no vigorous or strenuous activity which would raise the blood pressure or pulse for 2 weeks.

There may be considerable swelling, some bruising, and mild discomfort for up to a week following the procedure. There may be oozing of a pinkish/yellow serous fluid for the first several days following the procedure. The skin will be very smooth and quite reddish/pink in color in the first few weeks. The redness may last as long as 8–12 weeks before gradually fading.

Reepithelization starts immediately after laser resurfacing. The epidermis continues to thicken for several weeks; however, the region can be treated like normal skin about a week after the treatment. Although the area remains sensitive to wind and potential irritants for weeks, make-up and concealers can be applied at the 1-week time period. Sunscreen should be applied after 3 weeks and excessive sun exposure should be avoided.

23.7 Fractionated Laser Resurfacing

Although fractionated laser resurfacing can be an excellent option for dyschromia and photodamage in the periorbital region; this technology has yet to produce the superior results of the Ultrapulsated CO_2 technology for lower lid laxity. Although the postoperative erythema does not have as long duration as traditional ablative lasers, the perioperative management and complication profile for *ablative* fractionated lasers is very similar to erbium and Ultrapulsated CO_2 technology. The techniques for *ablative* fractionated laser will depend on the device type and therefore should be optimized with the help of the manufacturer and their representatives.

Nonablative fractional lasers have a lower risk profile and significantly decreased recovery time as compared with their ablative counterparts. Specifically, they have minimal downtime and an extremely low incidence of dyschromia, allowing use on all skin types. These class of lasers, however, require multiple treatments to achieve the desired outcome. In the following section, we will focus on the treatment protocol and postoperative management of Fraxel SR750, one of the most commonly used *nonablative* fractional lasers. Most light-based devices in this category will require a similar treatment algorithm.

23.8 Technical Considerations: Nonablative Fractionated Laser

Contraindications for fractionated lasers are similar to other lasers which include active use of oral retinoid, predisposition to keloid formation, or excessive scarring as well as lesions suspicious for malignancy. Prior to the procedure, the patients are pretreated with hydroquinone and Retin-A for one month and encouraged to stop 5 days prior to treatment. The area is prepped 30 min to 1 h in advance with a high potency topical betacaine anesthetic. After the topical anesthetic is removed, Opti-Guide Blue is applied followed by a low potency topical anesthetic that allows the treatment tip to navigate easily. The dye (not used with the SR1500) serves to enhance contrast for the optical mouse. Eight nonoverlapping passes are performed with a density of 250 Mtz/cm^2

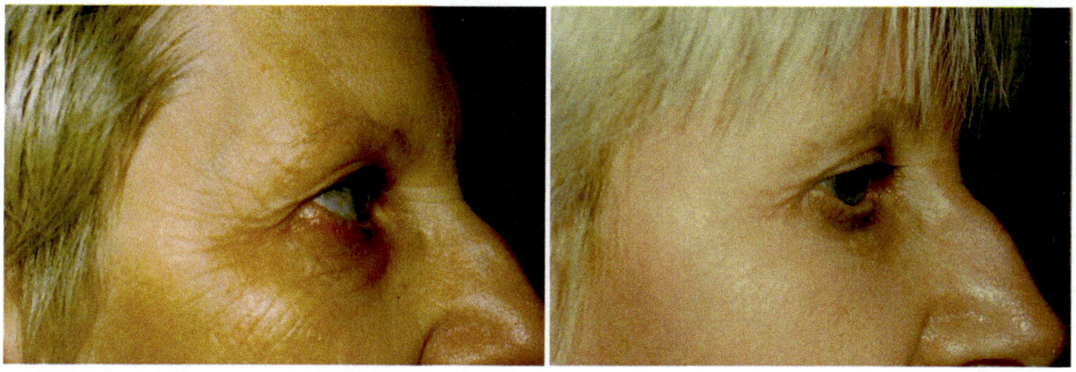

Fig. 23.2 Before and after 2 Fraxel treatments

(any energy level of 10 mJ). Sensation is similar to a feeling of needles on the skin.

No bandage is required after the procedure. Figure 23.2 illustrates an outcome with fractionated laser resurfacing.

Nonablative fractionated lasers maintain the structural integrity of the epidermis. Repeat treatments are required at one month intervals (three to five since each treatment affects about 20% of the treated surface). The energy level is increased by 2 mJ per treatment session though development of petechia may occur in this area, requiring a lowering of energy levels.

23.9 Posttreatment Care for Nonablative Fractionated Laser

Patients typically have swelling and erythema for 24–48 h. The facial area should not be manipulated with the exception of cold compresses. They are also encouraged to keep their head elevated in the first night and avoid vigorous activity. Normal skin care regimen may be resumed if skin irritation is not present. Strict adherence to sun protection with use of total sunscreen and avoidance of direct sun exposure is encouraged for at least 3 months.

23.10 Conclusion

Periorbital laser resurfacing is an excellent option for lower lid rhytids, fine lines, and laxity. Ultrapulsated CO_2 laser remains the gold standard in "tightening" of the lower lid as well as improving static rhytids and fine lines albeit with lower patient acceptance and higher morbidity. Fractionated ablative and nonablative lasers represent a newer generation of light-based devices with limited down-time and decreased risk of dyschromia. These lasers, however, also have not been able to achieve the same degree of lower lid improvement as traditional ablative lasers.

24 Laser Incisional Eyelid Surgery

Julie A. Woodward and Amina Husain

Key Points

- Incisional surgery with the CO_2 laser reduces intraoperative surgical time, potential patient expenses, and provides a clear view of relevant anatomy.
- Incisional CO_2 laser surgery of the eyelids minimizes the risks of intraoperative bleeding and possibly orbital hemorrhage.
- The technique also has the advantage of not conducting electric current throughout the patient's body which is safer for the orbit and in patients with implantable cardiac devices.
- Laser surgeons should understand how lasers work and attain basic knowledge regarding the laser physics of their machine.
- Both the surgeon and staff must become familiar with laser use and safety.
- There is a learning curve for the various eyelid and periorbital procedures that can be performed with the laser. Spend time with an experienced laser surgeon to master these techniques.
- Proper laser safety protocols must be followed including laser safe drapes, a smoke evacuator, and protective eyewear.
- Supplemental oxygen must be turned off during surgery.
- Laser incisional surgery can be useful not only with blepharoplasty but also ptosis repair, midface-lifting, canthoplasty, and a variety of other ancillary procedures.

24.1 Introduction

Carbon dioxide (CO_2) laser incisional surgery for upper lid blepharoplasty was first described by Baker in 1984 [1]. The advantages of this technique include reduced surgical time (Most standard four-lid blepharoplasties can be performed in less than an hour under local anesthesia.) with resultant decreased facility and anesthesia fees. There is improved hemostasis with decreased risk of intraoperative and postoperative hemorrhage, potentially reduced healing time, a clearer view of the relevant anatomy, and more precise surgical incisions, making surgery simpler and more efficient. In addition, there is an appreciation by patients of a more advanced surgical technique. Saving on procedural costs, potentially faster healing, and adding "modern" technology are strong motivation tools for patients to consider in selecting the surgeon with whom to proceed.

The disadvantages of the technique are the expense of the laser and the initial investment of time and effort needed to educate and train the surgeon and staff on laser use and safety. It is not necessary to purchase a laser as many surgery centers have a CO_2 laser that is maintained for other services (such as otolaryngology or gynecology). Familiarization with these lasers is an appropriate way to get started with laser surgery before making an investment in the machinery.

24.2 History

The first human laser procedures performed was with ruby and neodymium lasers in 1962 to create thermal necrosis of a malignant melanoma prior to excision [2]. Nonpigmented tissue ablation followed in 1964 when Patel described the use of the 10,600-nm continuous wave CO_2 laser [3]. The first reported case of incisional CO_2 laser in the periorbital region was published by Beckman et al. in 1980, who described laser-assisted removal of small skin lesions [4]. Histologic studies revealed that the CO_2 laser was able to seal lymphatic vessels and coagulate blood vessels that are 1 mm in diameter and smaller [5, 6]. This is especially relevant in eyelid surgery because most blood vessels in the periorbital region are less than 0.5 mm in diameter.

J.A. Woodward (✉)
Associate Professor, Chief Division of Oculofacial Surgery, Department of Ophthalmology, Duke University, Durham, NC, USA
e-mail: juliewoodward1@mac.com

G.G. Massry et al. (eds.), *Master Techniques in Blepharoplasty and Periorbital Rejuvenation*,
DOI 10.1007/978-1-4614-0067-7_24, © Springer Science+Business Media, LLC 2011

By the late 1970, CO_2 lasers were being used by gynecologists, otorhinolaryngologists, neurosurgeons, plastic surgeons, and dermatologists. However, one of the major problems with these continuous wave CO_2 lasers was that the diameter of the laser beams was too large (1 mm). This resulted in laser energy dispersed into a relatively large surface area, creating a shallow cut, too much thermocoagulation, and a broad zone of thermal injury at the wound edges (200–500 μm), making skin excisions problematic [7]. Plastic surgeons and dermatologists, in particular, became dissatisfied with the high incidence of wound dehiscence and poor aesthetic outcome with the use of these lasers. Today, modern CO_2 lasers employ high frequency pulsed beams (suprapulsed or ultrapulsed) which are just 0.2 mm in diameter, with the same amount of energy focused into a smaller surface area. This allows a more precise incision with deeper vaporization of tissue, reducing thermocoagulative damage at the wound edges and the problems associated with cutaneous thermal tissue damage [8, 9].

Incisional devices used in periorbital surgery have included traditional cold steel, radiofrequency and monopolar cutting devices, the Erbium:Yag (Er:Yag) laser, and the CO_2 laser. The steel scalpel is often considered the gold standard for cutaneous surgery as it is inexpensive and readily available. However, scalpel or scissor incisions inevitably cut through blood vessels in the surgical field, requiring thermal cautery to assure hemostasis. This prolongs surgical time and may increase the risk of bruising, swelling, and tissue distortion associated with intraoperative hemorrhage [5]. The CO_2 laser reduces the incidence of all these potential problems.

The radiofreqency (RF) and monopolar cautery devices can both be used with a fine tip needle for cutting and coagulation (i.e., Colorado tip). This reduces bleeding when compared with a steel blade but provides less thermocoagulation than a laser. Therefore RF and monopolar cautery devices may be associated with more bleeding and increased surgical times than the CO_2 laser. More importantly, the devices that use a Colorado needle do not have a sturdy dissection tool at the tip of the instrument as a CO_2 laser does. Without this tool, the surgeon will spend more time switching back and forth between different instruments. This dissection tool on the laser is called a *laser finger*. The laser finger is useful not only for dissection but also to titrate the dispersion of laser energy and allow switching from precision cutting to coagulation modes. When the tip is close to tissue and the beam is focused (2-mm spot size), precise cuts can be made. Alternatively, when the tip is pulled back the beam becomes defocused; the spot size is larger with wider dispersion of energy. This defocused spot size is more appropriate for coagulation of bleeding vessels. Finally, with monopolar units, propagated energy may cause damage to orbital structures and potentially to patients with implanted cardiac devices (ICDs). To their credit, RF devices are more economical than lasers.

Attempts have been made to create Er:Yag lasers that can incise tissue. These lasers successfully cut tissue; however, they do not provide useful hemostasis. This is because the laser wavelength is too precisely absorbed by water. The surrounding proteins do not absorb sufficient laser energy to create thermocoagulation [10]. This limits the utility of the Er:Yag laser as an incision tool.

The ideal incisional instrument should provide patient safety, minimal tissue trauma, hemostasis, and rapid surgical time while allowing appropriate wound healing. The wound should have excellent tensile strength, superior final appearance, and lead to high patient satisfaction. This is especially true in the delicate area of eyelid surgery. The CO_2 laser meets these criteria. Total intraoperative time is reduced as the laser handpiece acts as both a cutting and a cautery tool, obviating the need for excessive movements and tissue manipulation. The laser finger can be used for blunt dissection. This again reduces the time needed for switching to additional instruments. As eyelids tend to bleed, the superior hemostasis that is achieved with the CO_2 laser is especially useful in reducing intraoperative surgical time in these particular cases. Hemorrhage can rapidly obscure the anatomic detail of eyelid structures. The hemostasis achieved with laser surgery greatly enhances the visualization of important anatomy and increases the efficiency and precision of surgery. The great precision of the CO_2 laser and excellent dissection of tissue planes produces superior exposure of the relevant anatomy. This allows laser surgery to be performed on delicate vascular structures in the periorbital region, such as the levator palpebrae superioris and Mueller's muscle, and reduces the risk of tissue distortion, hematoma formation, and potential functional impairment [11]. CO_2 lasers are also invaluable for rapid fat sculpting and shrinkage. A potential drawback of the CO_2 laser surgery is the lack of tactile feedback inherent to traditional surgery with the scalpel blade. This difference is quickly adapted to as the surgeon becomes accustomed to visual recognition of tissue planes. High cost of equipment is another potential drawback.

24.3 Laser Incisions

Surgeons who operate with lasers should understand the basic physics of the machines that they work with. Joule = J = energy, watts = W = power, and fluence is the number of joules delivered per area. The fluence required for the CO_2 laser to vaporize tissue is only about 5–7 J/cm^2 [12]. This would be just enough to remove a few microns of the epithelium as is needed for laser skin resurfacing. In order to make a full thickness skin incision, the fluence of a 0.2 mm diameter beam at 6 W drawn at 1 cm/s is about 300 J/cm^2. This is demonstrated by the calculation below.

$$\text{Beam iadmeter} = 0.2\text{mm} = 0.02\text{cm}$$

$$\text{Area} = 0.02\text{cm} \times 1\text{cm} = 0.02\text{cm}^2$$

$$\text{Joules} = \text{watts} / \text{second} = 6\text{W} / 1\text{s} = 6\text{J}$$

$$\text{Fluence} = \text{Joules} / \text{cm}^2 = 6\text{J} / 0.02\text{cm}^2 = 300\text{J} / \text{cm}^2$$

The chromophore for the CO_2 laser is water, which is demonstrated on the laser absorption curve [11] (Fig. 24.1). The burn is the zone of thermo-coagulation that allows hemostasis on either side of the wound. This area measures about 115–250 μm. The laser incision is time dependent: a fast cut makes a shallow incision while slow cut makes a deep incision. As previously described, the operator must rely on visual feedback when performing surgery.

Most laser systems deliver the laser energy through an articulated arm that bounces the laser beam along reflecting mirrors, through a condensing lens, and then along a 125 mm handpiece before targeting tissue. Some lasers have a fiberoptic arm, but these systems may lose coherence of the beam. It is important for the condensing lens to create a small spot size. A spot size of 0.2 mm or less is recommended. Most condensing lenses have a focal length of 125 mm. For this lens, incisions are divided into three modes:

- Focused: 1–2 mm from the skin; to make precise incisions.
- Slightly defocused: 1–2 cm from tissue; to remove skin/muscle flap or incise fat.
- Defocused: 5–8 cm from tissue; to coagulate a bleeding vessel or to shrink fat via laser lipolysis.

If the laser's condensing lens has a focal length of less than 125 mm, the laser will be more sensitive to defocusing the beam, and above recommended distances will all be smaller. This is the case with the Nidek laser that has a condensing lens with a focal length of 50 mm to produce a 0.05 mm spot.

24.4 Laser Safety

The CO_2 laser is a class 4 laser. This means it is hazardous to view and requires protective goggles for use. The wavelength of the laser is 10,600 nm. It is highly specific for absorption by water but is also absorbed by some proteins. In contrast, the 2,940 nm Er:Yag laser is almost 20 times more specific for its absorption by water and is less absorbed by proteins. This makes the Er:Yag less useful for incisions because it so precisely vaporizes the water in tissue that it doesn't create enough heat to seal the finer vessels. Consequently there is more bleeding when using the Er:Yag laser.

It is important to have anodized instruments that create specular instead of focused (mirror-like) reflections. The sterile field should have nonflammable drapes of wet towels and gauze and/or sterile aluminum foil. Metal eye shields are required for patients and protective lenses are required for all staff members. A smoke evacuator must be present in the room and a laser sign on the door. Trip-and-fall precautions must be placed for the pedals and wires. Communication is critical with the laser. The nurse should be advised each time the laser is switched between "standby" and "ready" modes. All supplemental oxygen should be turned off during laser use. For general anesthesia, a laser-safe metal intubation tube should be used.

24.5 Upper Blepharoplasty

Patients are marked sitting in an upright position. The lid crease is first marked. If a lid crease is higher than 10 mm in a woman or 8 mm in a man, consider lowering it to a more aesthetically pleasing position (Fig. 24.2). If the patient has a very low crease, it is important to elevate it 1–2 mm to avoid suturing the thick skin near the brow to the thin skin

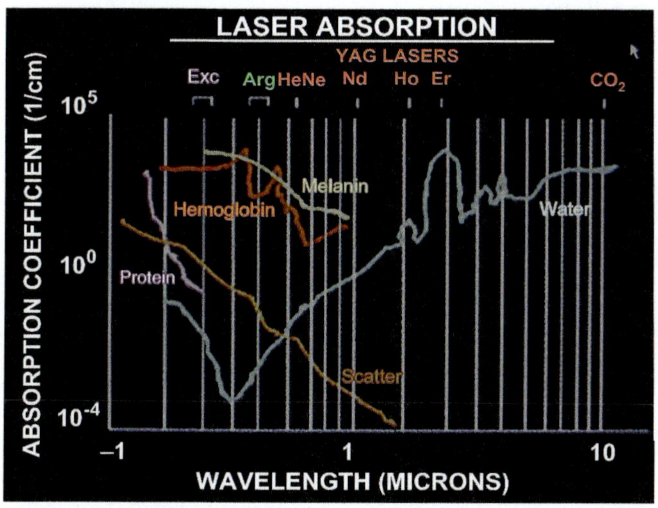

Fig. 24.1 Laser absorption curve

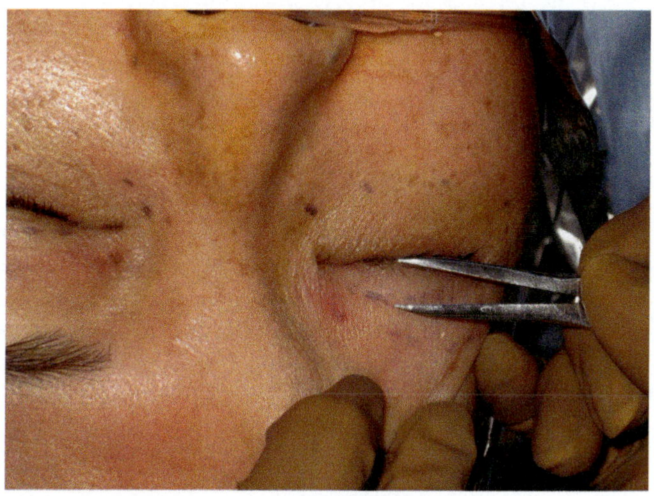

Fig. 24.2 Lid crease being measured with calipers

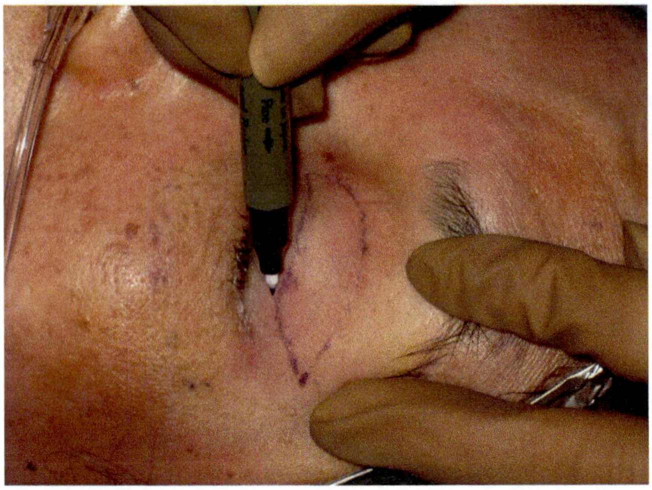

Fig. 24.3 Marking is incorporated into rhytid laterally and curved upward

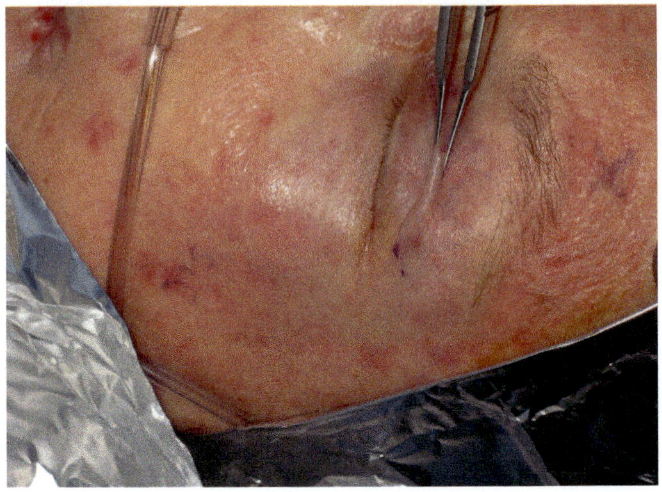

Fig. 24.4 The pinch technique to ensure no lagophthalmos postoperation

over the tarsal plate. In order to reestablish a higher crease, the laser can be used to undermine the skin inferiorly to release levator attachments passing through the orbicularis muscle. This will encourage the lid to favor the newly established crease. If the crease is too high, it should be lowered to the level of the tarsal plate. If in doubt, flip the upper lid and measure the central height of the tarsal plate from the gray line. This distance can be used as the new crease height.

Mark the crease along the top of the tarsal plate. In Asians, this must be modified as their creases are typically 6 mm or lower. Carry the markings along the curvature of the tarsal plate medially, but do not extend beyond an imaginary vertical line drawn through the punctum. Operating medial to the punctum increases the risk of webs, scarring, and bleeding from damage of trochlear vessels. Carry the incision laterally and sweep upward into a preexisting rhytid (Fig. 24.3). The amount of skin and orbicularis to be excised is measured via the pinch overlap or "pinch technique" in which the forceps are used to grasp the tissue above the marked crease incision and the location of the proposed upper incision until the lashes are gently everted without producing eyelid opening or pulling the brow down (Fig. 24.4). This is marked nasally, centrally, and temporally to assure an appropriate and safe excision of skin. The tissue excision demarcation is then made continuous in an ellipse. If ptosis repair is also planned, a mark is placed in the lash line just above the pupil for reference for levator suture placement.

A local anesthetic mixture consisting of 5 cc of lidocaine 2% with epinephrine in a 1:1 ratio with marcaine 0.75% with 0.5 cc hyaluronidase is infiltrated into each upper lid subcutaneously with a 30 gauge needle (Fig. 24.5). The hyaluronidase aids in anesthetic spread through the tissue so only one or two needle sticks are necessary.

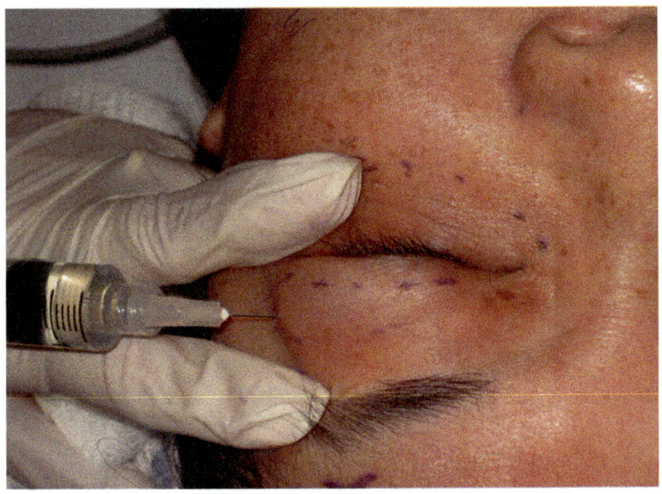

Fig. 24.5 Injection of local anesthetic subcutaneously

The patient is then prepped and draped with full face exposure to reduce potential claustrophobia and allow surgical comparison of each eye. In order to avoid eye burning from the prep solutions, one drop of topical anesthetic (Tetracaine or Proparicaine) is placed into each eye. The O_2 cannula, if used, is also prepped. Notify the anesthesiologist to discontinue O_2 during the case. The presence of flowing O_2 can lead to fire when the laser is in use. Drape the patient's head with laser-safe materials such as a turban made of wet towels or sterile aluminum foil. Use the same to drape the patient's chest. Sterile aluminum foil may be fashioned into a very useful tray that will hold surgical instruments on the patient's chest. After the patient is anesthetized, prepped, and draped, the surgical incision markings can be fine-tuned as needed.

Before using the laser, place the David-Baker lid clamp (Oculoplastik, Canada) in the operative eye. Cover the

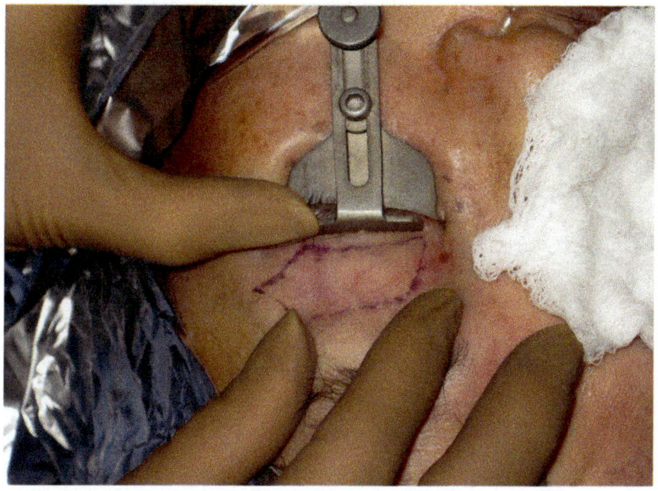

Fig. 24.6 Damp gauze covers nonoperating eye, while the David-Baker lid clamp protects the operative eye

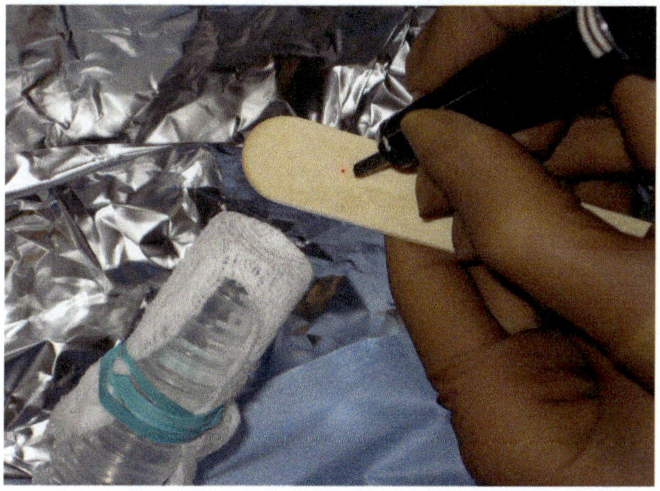

Fig. 24.7 Laser beam test on tongue blade

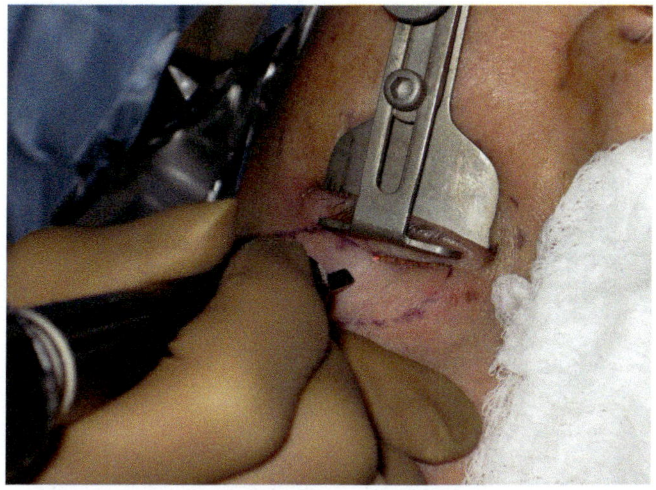

Fig. 24.8 With the David-Baker lid clamp in place and eyelid put in stretch, incision is carefully made

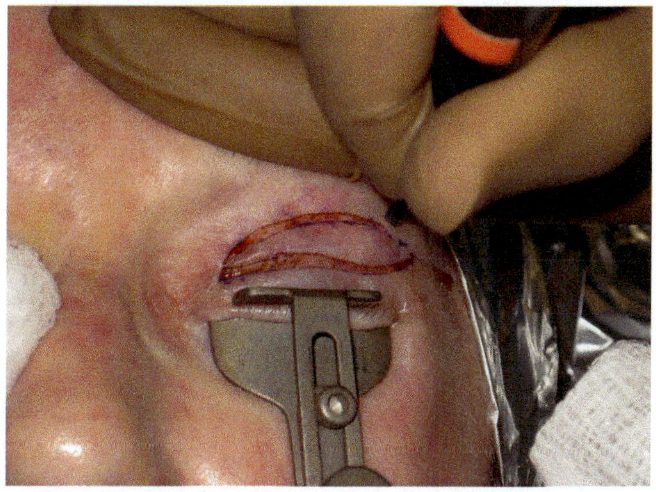

Fig. 24.9 Skin incision complete

opposite eye with damp gauze (Fig. 24.6). Make sure that all personnel in the OR are wearing protective eyewear and assure that supplemental oxygen is off. Set the laser at 6 W in continuous wave. Check the condensing lens and laser handpiece to make sure the spot size is 0.2 mm or less. Turn the smoke evacuator on. Test the laser on a wet tongue blade to assure the aiming beam is coaxial with the incision beam. Practice your first few incisions on the tongue blade (Fig. 24.7). Remember to release the foot pedal prior to pulling the laser away from the target site, or inadvertent stray laser rays will result.

Put the brow on gentle stretch and make the inferior crease incision first (Fig. 24.8). The upper incision is then connected to the inferior one (Fig. 24.9). Make sure your positioning is always comfortable and that the laser beam is focused on the skin. It should be held no more than 1–2 mm from the target skin. The incision should be made at a constant and appropriate speed. Too rapid a pace will make the incision too shallow, and too slow will make the incision too deep. Remember that the surgeon relies on visual cues as there is no tactile feedback. The skin is then excised by elevating its lateral edge with a toothed forceps and dissecting it from the orbicularis muscle with the laser moving in a side to side fashion (Fig. 24.10). Deeper dissection below the orbicularis muscle will expose the orbital septum (Fig. 24.11). The laser may be held slightly defocused at 1 cm from the tissue to maintain a bloodless field (Fig. 24.12). If there is any bleeding, have the assistant roll a dry cotton swab over tissue to pressure clamp the vessel. The laser is held 5–6 mm from tissue in a defocused mode for coagulation. If the bleeding vessel is too large to coagulate with the laser, use bipolar cautery, which should be on the field for all cases. If fat

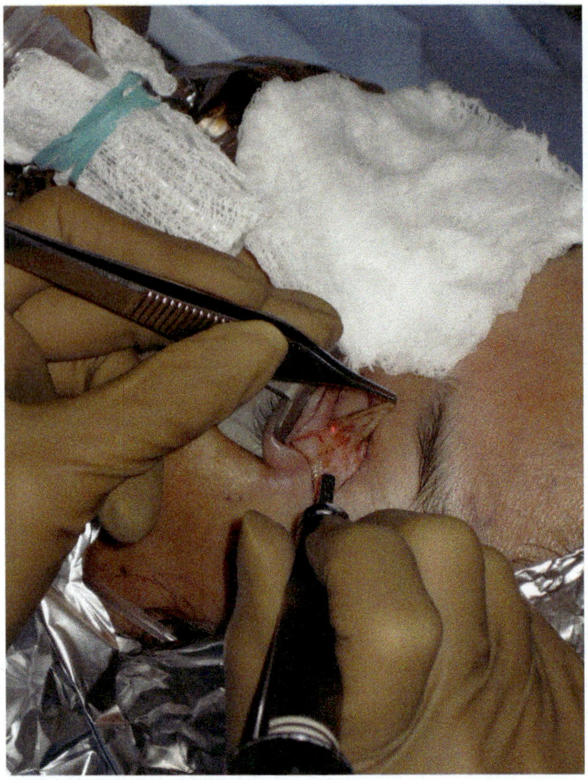

Fig. 24.10 Skin flap elevated and dissection started

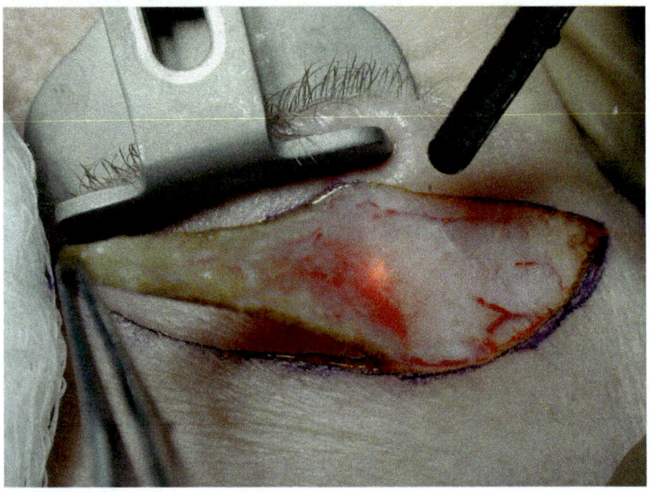

Fig. 24.11 Excision of flap in a to-and–fro manner

excision or combined ptosis repair is planned, open the orbital septum over a wet cotton swab (Fig. 24.13).

Fat can be resected with the laser in a slightly defocused mode over a wet cotton swab, or shrunken via laser-lipolysis technique also with the laser in the defocused mode. Finally, suture the wound with 6-0 monofilament suture in either an interrupted or running fashion. The suture is typically removed after 6–7 days. Instruct the patient to apply ice

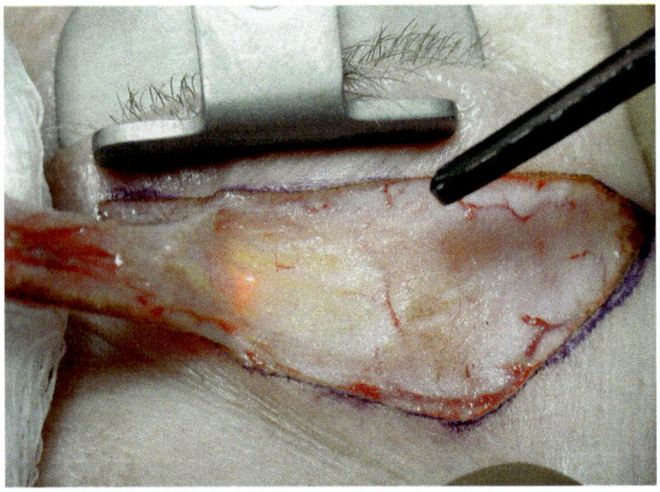

Fig. 24.12 Laser beam slightly defocused while flap is excised

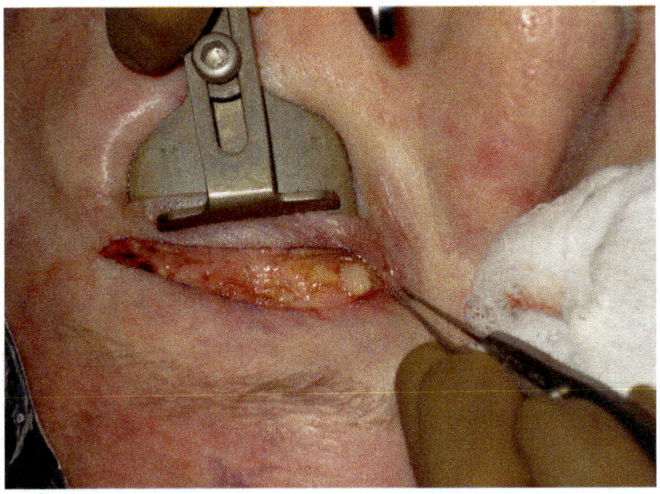

Fig. 24.13 The septum is incised and fat is prolapsed

packs and keep the head elevated for the first 48 h. Antibiotic ointment is applied to the sutures 4 times a day.

24.6 Lower Lid Transconjunctival Blepharoplasty

Inject each of the three fat pads transconjunctivally with the anesthetic mixture (Fig. 24.14) previously described. The surgeon's thumb is placed on the upper lid so that the patient cannot see the needle coming. The thumb is also used to push gently down on the globe while the third finger pulls the lower lid inferiorly. These maneuvers help evert the lower lid and expose the conjunctiva. Upon withdrawing the needle, a small amount of anesthetic is injected to minimally balloon the conjunctiva. The surgeon inserts a Jaeger lid plate to

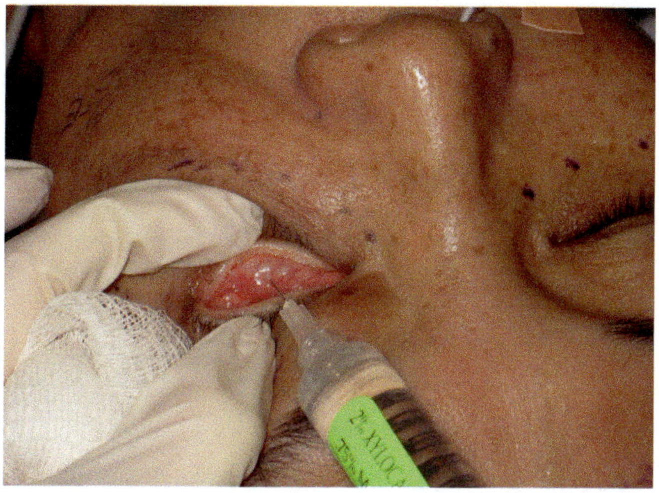

Fig. 24.14 Transconjunctival injection of fat pads with local anesthetic

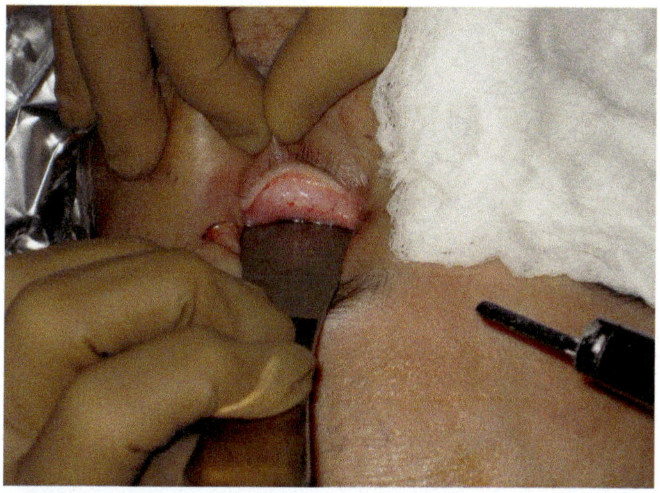

Fig. 24.15 The lower lid is everted by the assistant, exposing the conjunctiva, while the globe is protected with Jaeger lid plate in place

protect the globe as the assistant everts the lower lid with his or her fingers (Fig. 24.15). An incision is made with the laser at 6 W in continuous wave through the conjunctiva and the lower lid retractors, 3–4 mm from the inferior edge of the tarsal plate. The inferior vascular arcade, if visible, can be used as a guide (Fig. 24.16). Begin the incision 2 mm from the caruncle and carry it laterally, gently curving the Jaeger plate as the incision is made (Fig. 24.17).

The Jaeger plate is now passed to the assistant, who also retracts the lower lid with a Desmarres retractor with the opposite hand. This way, the surgeon can hold the laser in one hand and a forceps in the other hand. The laser is used to identify each of the three fat pads (Fig. 24.18).

The fat pads are elevated over the Desmarres retractor (used as a backstop) and excised in the defocused mode of the laser. Care must be taken to avoid injury to the inferior oblique muscle which separates the nasal and central fat pads (Fig. 24.19).

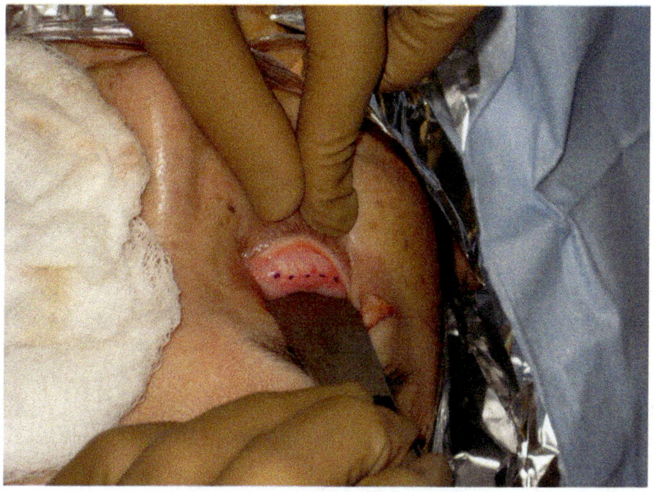

Fig. 24.16 Visualization of inferior arcade (demarcated)

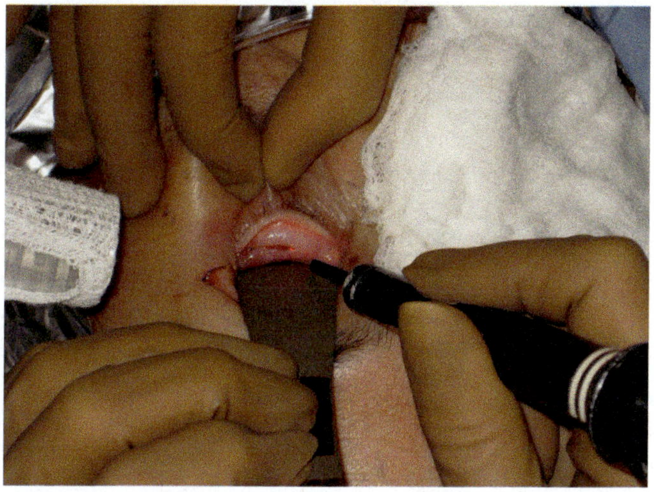

Fig. 24.17 Transconjunctival incision through the conjunctiva and retractors

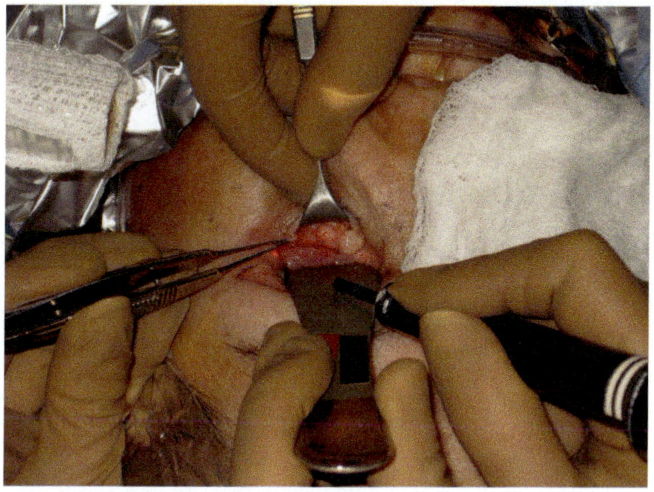

Fig. 24.18 Exposure of the fat pads

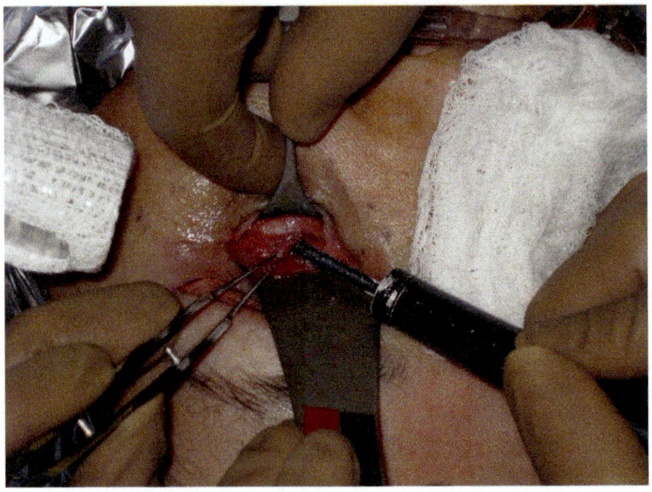

Fig. 24.19 Laser finger elevating inferior oblique muscle

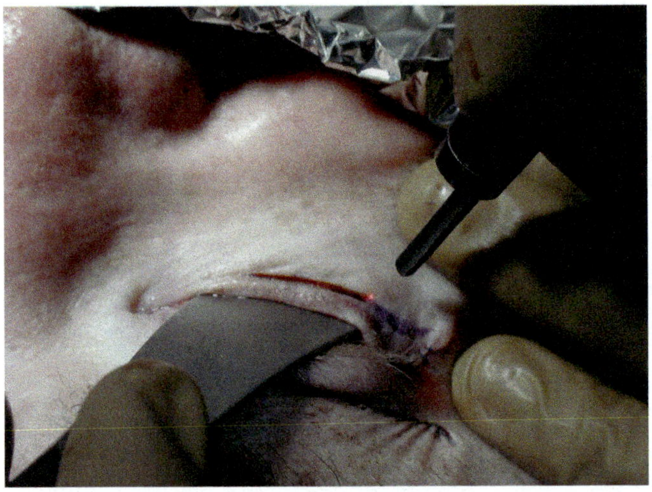

Fig. 24.20 Sub-ciliary incision for lower lid skin excision

The lid is repositioned, and retropulsion of the globe will identify the presence of residual fat. Further fat excision proceeds as need and the conjunctival wound is not sutured. If skin excision is planned it proceeds via a sub-ciliary incision (Fig. 24.20).

24.7 Ptosis Repair

Ptosis surgery can be performed on its own or added to patients undergoing upper eyelid blepharoplasty. In this setting, infiltrate anesthetic without hyaluronidase to avoid spread into the levator muscle and introducing potential error in judging lid height and contour. If planned, blepharoplasty is first performed. The orbital septum is then divided as previously described, inserting a wet cotton swab beneath it to protect surrounding tissue (Fig. 24.21). Fat is removed as needed. The orbicularis muscle is isolated from tarsal plate with the laser held at an oblique angle (Fig. 24.22). The undersurface of the

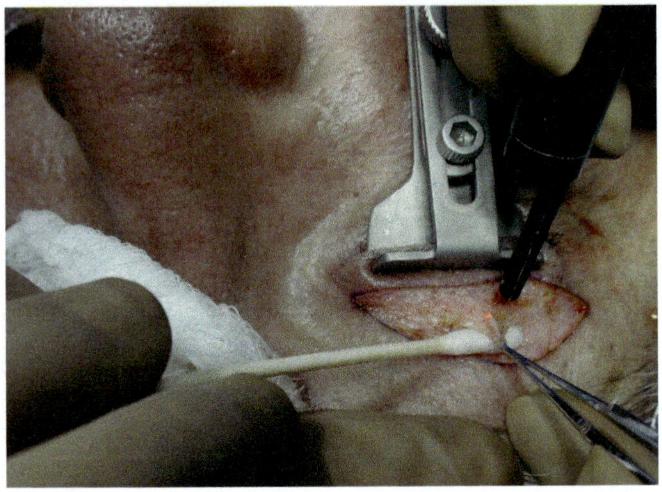

Fig. 24.21 Cotton tip applicator placed beneath septum as a backboard to laser beam

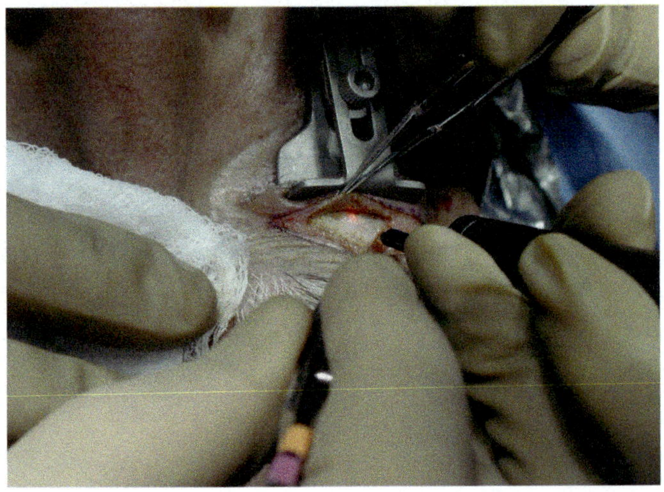

Fig. 24.22 Tarsus exposed with inferior dissection of orbicularis off tarsal surface

levator aponeurosis is dissected free from Mueller's muscle with the laser or bluntly with a cotton swab (Fig. 24.23). The levator aponeurosis is advanced and secured to the tarsal plate with a double armed 6-0 vicryl suture passed partial thickness (Fig. 24.24). Eyelid height and symmetry are noted and adjusted if necessary. The wound is closed with 6-0 Prolene suture.

24.8 Direct Brow Lift

A direct brow lift is useful in male patients with brow ptosis and a receding hairline, who are not good candidates for an endoscopic or pre-trichial lift. The supraciliary skin of the brows is marked in an appropriate elliptical fashion. Incise the skin with the laser in the focused mode. In this procedure the laser is moved more slowly across the skin to create a deeper incision, as the brow skin is much thicker than eyelid

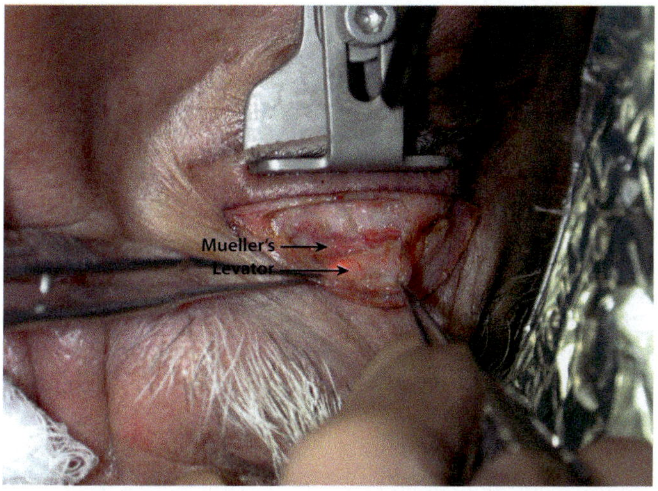

Fig. 24.23 Visualization of Mueller's and levator aponeurosis (labeled with *arrows*)

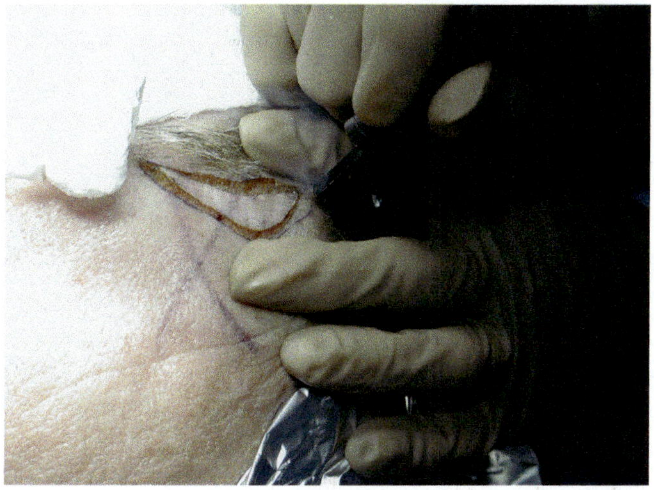

Fig. 24.25 Laser skin incision above the brow

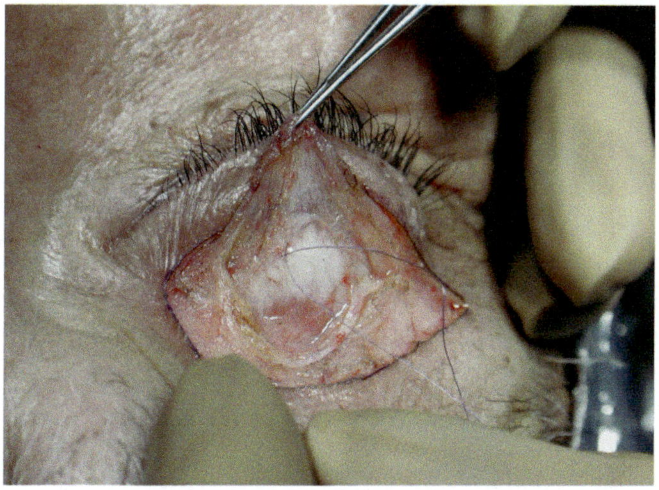

Fig. 24.24 Vicryl suture securing levator aponeurosis (white tissue) to tarsus

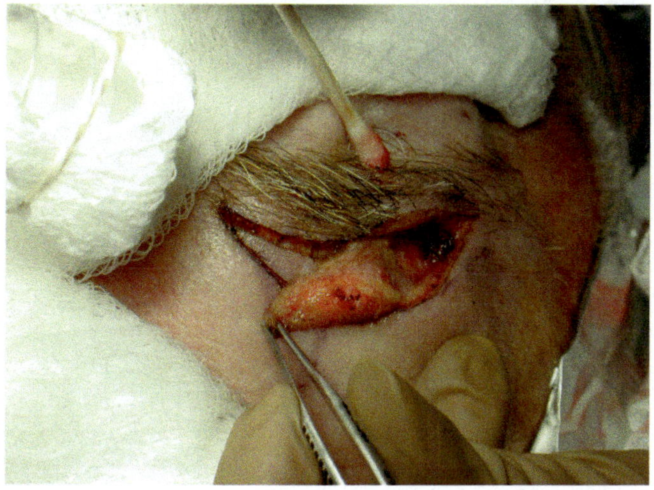

Fig. 24.26 Skin/subcutaneous tissue flap excision in side-to-side fashion

skin (Fig. 24.25). Incise with caution over the supraorbital neurovascular bundle. Remove the skin/subcutaneous flap in a side to side fashion with the laser in the slightly defocused mode (Fig. 24.26). Since the vessels are larger in this area, the bipolar cautery is necessary to attain hemostasis. Pinch the incision together to assess closure. Sculpt the subcutaneous fat with the laser in a slightly defocused mode. Close the wound with buried, interrupted 5-0 vicryl and a running/locking 5-0 prolene.

24.9 Laser-Assisted Tarsal Strip and SOOF Lift

A lateral tarsal strip and SOOF (midface) lift can be performed in conjunction with laser skin resurfacing (Chap. 23) or transcutaneous lower blepharoplasty (Chap. 15) to improve the appearance of festoons. The skin, inferior tarsal plate, and orbital rim are anesthetized. A tarsal strip is isolated as described in Chap. 17. Conversely an inverted triangular wedge of full thickness lid can be excised for lid shortening. The terminal lid (skin, muscle, tarsus) is clamped prior to incision to aid in hemostasis (Fig. 24.27). A Jaeger plate is tucked inside the lateral orbital rim and the lid is shortened (a wedge excised) with the laser at 6 W in continuous wave (Fig. 24.28). Dissection is carried to the periosteum so that access is easier when the deep suspensory sutures are placed. The inferior crus of the lateral canthal tendon is released if necessary.

If a midface lift is planned, the lateral canthal incision is continued in a transconjunctival fashion across the length of the lid. Dissection is then carried in the post-orbicularis plane to the level of the periosteum on the anterior surface of the inferior orbital rim, to avoid fat prolapse into the field. The Jaeger plate is placed over the globe while a Desmarres retractor is used to engage the lower lid tissue

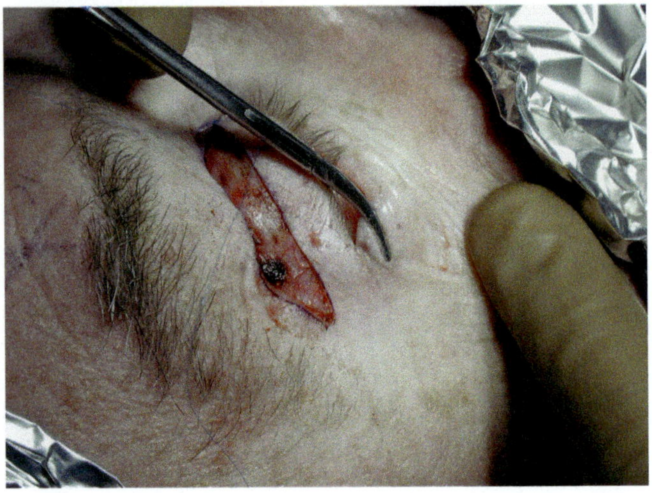

Fig. 24.27 The lateral eyelid (including tarsus) is clamped

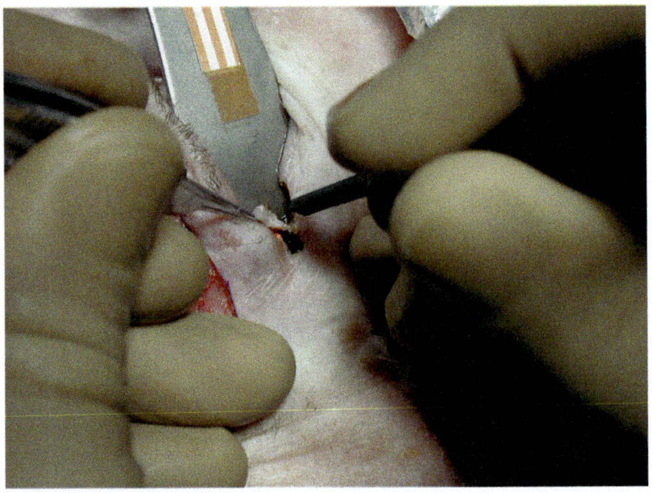

Fig. 24.28 Wedge (*inverted triangle*) resection of eyelid

and pull the lid inferiorly. The laser incision is continued in the sub- or pre-periosteal plane. Dissection continues inferiorly to mobilize the SOOF. The SOOF is then engaged and elevated with two 4-0 vicryl sutures anchored to the external aspect of the lateral orbital rim.

The previously fabricated tarsal strip is engaged with either 4-0 Merseline or Vicryl suture on a 1/2-circle needle (a P-2 needle). The suture is secured to the internal aspect of the lateral orbital rim periosteum in close proximity to Witinall's tubercle. The lid margin and skin are sutured with interrupted and running 6-0 plain gut suture.

24.10 Conclusion

Incisional laser surgery can be used for a variety of eyelid and periorbital procedures [13]. Once experience with the laser is gained, eyelid surgery can be accomplished more rapidly, patient's costs are reduced, hemostasis is better controlled, fewer instruments are needed, anatomy is more clearly visualized, and tissue distortion is reduced. The main drawbacks are the cost of a laser and the associated learning curve. With appropriate training and observation, all surgeons can become familiar with, and gain benefit from, laser technology and surgical techniques.

References

1. Baker SS, Muenzler WS, Small RG, Leonard JE. Carbon dioxide laser blepharoplasty. Ophthalmology. 1984;91:238–44.
2. Goldman I. Laser treatment of malignant melanoma. In: Goldman I, editor. Laser cancer research. New York: Springer; 1966.
3. Patel CKN. Continuous-wave laser action in vibrational-rotational transitions of carbon dioxide. Phys Rev. 1964;136:A1187–93.
4. Beckman H, Fuller TA, Beman R, Mandell G, Nathan LE. Carbon dioxide laser surgery of the eye and adnexa. Ophthalmology. 1980;87(10):990–1000.
5. David LM, Sanders G. CO_2 laser blepharoplasty: a comparison to cold steel and electrocautery. J Dermatol Oncol. 1987;13:110–4.
6. Baker SS, Hunnewell JM, Muenzler WS, Hunter GJ. Laser blepharoplasty: diamond laser scalpel compared to the free beam CO_2 laser. Dermatol Surg. 2002;28:127.
7. Ben-Bassat M, Ben-Bassat J, Kaplan I. An ultrastructural study of the cut edges of skin and mucous membrane specimens excised by carbon dioxide laser. In: Kaplan I, editor. Laser surgery II. Jerusalem: Academic; 1976.
8. Biesman BS. Lasers play a useful role in periorbital incisional surgery. Dermatol Surg. 2000;26:883–6.
9. Goldman MP, Fitzpatrick RE. Cutaneous laser surgery. St. Louis: Mosby; 1994.
10. Lieb WE, Klink T, Munnich S. CO_2 and erbium YAG laser in eyelid surgery. A comparison [German]. Ophthalmologe. 2000;97: 835–41.
11. Lessner AM, Fagien S. Laser blepharoplasty. Semin Ophthalmol. 1998;13:90–102.
12. Hruza GJ, Dover JS. Laser skin resurfacing. Arch Dermatol. 1996;132:451–5.
13. Wesley RE, Bond JB. Carbon dioxide laser in ophthalmic plastic and orbital surgery. Ophthalmic Surg. 1985;16:631–3.

25 Neuromodulators and Fillers for Periorbital Rejuvenation

Kenneth C.Y. Yu, Kartik D. Nettar, and Corey S. Maas

Key Points

- Hyperfunctional muscular activity, volume loss, and contour irregularities are the anatomic targets for neuromodulation and soft-tissue fillers in periorbital rejuvenation.
- Botulinum toxin A prevents presynaptic release of acetylcholine at the neuromuscular junction conveying temporary muscular paresis and reduction in dynamic rhytids.
- Neuromodulators are very effective in the treatment of lateral orbital rhytids (Crow's feet), horizontal forehead lines, and glabellar lines (eleven lines).
- Botox® Cosmetic and Dysport™ are the two commercially available neuromodulators in USA. While they function similarly, their reconstitution, dosage, and results differ.
- Dysport™ has been observed to have a slightly greater regional effect, which can be used to its advantage in treating lateral orbital rhytids.
- Complications of neuromodulators include brow or eyelid ptosis, diplopia, and dry eyes, while those of injectable fillers include skin necrosis, Tyndall effect, and heaved rows.
- Hyaluronic acid (HA) is a naturally occurring biopolymer molecule with a uniform structure throughout nature.
- Restylane-L™, Juvederm XC™, and Prevelle Silk™ are the most popular of the hyaluronic HA gel products and are quite effective in the rejuvenation of the periorbital region.
- The linear threading and serial puncture injection techniques are both effective in effacing the nasojugal groove.
- Unwanted side effects of HA fillers can be reversed with the use of injectable hyaluronidase.

C.S. Maas (✉)
The Maas Clinic, Associate Clinical Professor, University of California-San Francisco, San Francisco, CA, USA
e-mail: drmaas@maasclinic.com

25.1 Introduction

The periorbital region is one of the early and more dramatic regions demonstrating signs of facial aging. The appearance of the periorbital area projects impressions regarding one's health, energy, and emotion. Surgical and nonsurgical options such as blepharoplasty, browplasty, and skin resurfacing remain mainstays for primary management of age-related changes in the eyelids and adjacent areas. However, the authors strongly feel that such interventions can be significantly enhanced by the use of injectable cosmetic agents.

The goal of periorbital rejuvenation employing injectable cosmetic agents can be classified into three basic categories. These include the following:

1. Reduction in hyperfunctional or dynamic muscular activity (and the effects of chronic hypertonicity)
2. Correction of involutional or congenital volume-related contour irregularities
3. Improvement of surface irregularities (fine lines)

While age, gender, and ethnicity impart variation on treatment parameters, the techniques used are generally the same.

The nonsurgical adjuncts to treatment of the periorbital region include neuromodulators as well as injectable fillers. This chapter discusses their use, excluding fat, for the glabella, forehead, lateral orbital, and tear trough areas.

25.2 Review of Neuromodulators and Fillers: The Products

Botulinum toxin type A is the primary neuromodulator used today for treatment of lines due to hyperfunctional or dynamic muscular activity. Botulinum toxin, a naturally occurring protein, was originally described as the etiologic agent causing the illness botulism, which is associated with ingestion of large amounts of *Clostridium botulinum* contaminated food. Botulinum toxin type A (BoNTA) affects the

G.G. Massry et al. (eds.), *Master Techniques in Blepharoplasty and Periorbital Rejuvenation*,
DOI 10.1007/978-1-4614-0067-7_25, © Springer Science+Business Media, LLC 2011

neuromuscular junction at the presynaptic level and inhibits the release of acetylcholine. Its distinct beneficial action is selective weakening or relaxation of treated muscles or muscle groups. Unwanted facial lines and facial expressions can be suppressed or even eliminated by selective weakening of specific hypertrophic muscles in the face and neck.

There are seven serotypes of botulinum neuromodulator (A–G), and only A and B have been developed for routine clinical use [1, 2]. The B serotype neuromodulator rimabotulinumtoxinB (Myobloc, Solstice Neurosciences, Inc., Malvern, PA) is indicated for the treatment of cervical dystonia. It is less suitable and practical for cosmetic use due to its shorter duration of effect [3] and injection discomfort associated with its acidity (pH of 5.6) [4, 5]. The A serotype has demonstrated the longest duration of effect (90–120 days) and least discomfort with injection. Only two formulations of BoNTA have been studied and used extensively for cosmetic and therapeutic indications [3]. The mechanism of action for onabotulinumtoxinA (BotoxCosmetic™, Allergan Inc., Irvine, CA) and abobotulinumtoxinA (Dysport™, Medicis, Scottsdale, AZ) is the same, but the products differ in the composition of the surrounding hemagglutinins and complex size (BotoxCosmetic™: 900 kDa, Dysport™: 500–900 kDa).

BotoxCosmetic™ set the standard for neuromodulators by demonstrating a proven safety and efficacy record for over 15 years. Dysport™ was licensed for medical use in Europe in 1990 and has been used for cosmetic treatments for many years. In 2009, it received US Federal Drug Administration (FDA) approval for treatment of glabellar lines. While these two formulations are not interchangeable, and reportedly cannot be substituted by one another by any fixed-dose conversion ratio, most experienced investigators believe that a 2.5–3 abobotulinumtoxinA units (AU) to 1 onabotulinumtoxinA unit (OU) [3] can be utilized when comparing the two products. Based on both preclinical and clinical studies, it appears that Dysport™ has a slightly greater regional effect, which can be used to the product's advantage. Using a slightly higher concentration of Dysport™ provides the same or better benefits with lower volumes of injection. While the injection doses and volumes differ between Botox™ and Dysport™, the injection technique need not be altered.

Bovine collagen (Zyderm™ and Zyplast™, McGhan Medical Corporation, Fremont, CA) was the first commercially manufactured, syringe-supplied injectable approved for use as a soft-tissue filler. The need for skin testing, delay from initial consultation to treatment, and risk of delayed hypersensitivity reactions led to the development of human-derived "tissue engineered" collagen. Cosmoderm™ and Cosmoplast™ (Allergan Inc., Irvine, CA) are the only currently available dermal fillers made from cultured human fibroblasts. The cell lines are obtained from newborn foreskin and are screened for viruses, tumorigenicity, and other potential pathogens. One advantage compared to Collagen™ is that no skin testing is required. Additionally, Cosmoderm™ is, in the senior author's opinion, the best commercially available injectable product for the treatment of fine lines. Other fillers including the plethora of hyaluronic fillers currently available are not easily used as intradermal fillers without visible signs such as Tyndall effect and heaved runways elevating the target line. Unfortunately, this product is now being withdrawn from the market for economic reasons.

Hyaluronic acid (HA) fillers have also gained traction in the treatment of volume loss and surface irregularities. HA is a naturally occurring glucosaminoglycan biopolymer molecule made up of linked alternating residues of the monosaccharides D-glucuronic acid and *N*-acetyl-D-glycosamine, which coil around themselves [6]. This results in an elastic and viscous matrix. HA exhibits no species or tissue specificity, and its chemical structure is uniform throughout nature. The most common sources for HA-based product development are bacterial cultures and heterologous sources (e.g., rooster combs). Although, in theory, there is no potential for eliciting hypersensitiviy or allergic reactions, several case series have reported delayed reactions [7, 8]. These were probably related to residual trace streptococcal proteins from manufacturing.

The most popular HA fillers today are Restylane™, Perlane™ (Medicis, Scottsdale, AZ), Juvederm™ (Allergan Inc., Irvine, CA), and Prevelle Silk™ (Mentor, Santa Barbara, CA). The addition of lidocaine to several of these products (Restylane-L™, Juvederm XC™, Prevelle Silk™) has facilitated their ease of administration.

In addition to HA fillers, two other classes of fillers merit mention, though these products are generally not recommended in periorbital applications. Calcium hydroxylapatite (Radiesse™ , BioForm Medical, San Mateo, CA) and poly-L-lactic acid (Sculptra™, Sanofi Aventis, Bridgewater, NJ) are larger molecule fillers, ranging from 25 to 63 μm in particle size. These products work primarily by causing a foreign body reaction and an increase in fibroblasts and collagen deposition. Radiesse™ is composed of microscopic calcium hydroxyapatite particles suspended in a carboxymethyl-cellulose gel. Its mechanism of action is both in volume restoration and to act as a framework for fibroblastic ingrowth in soft tissue. In facial treatments, its duration ranges from 6 to 12 months depending on the site of injection and the technique used [9]. Sculptra™ is an injectable form of poly-L-lactic acid, a compound that has been used in absorbable suture material for over 40 years. It is nontoxic, synthetic, immunologically inactive, and biodegradable. Sculptra™ is supplied as a powdered form that must be reconstituted with sterile water (with or without lidocaine) and must sit for 2 h before injection. While the company advertises results lasting up to 2 years, opinion in Europe and USAis mixed. Multiple repeat injections, spaced months apart, are required to achieve desired enhancement. Granulomas, nodule formation, and drainage have been reported, and these can be difficult to manage [9]. The use of Sculptra™ and Radiesse™ is limited in the periocular region. Wrinkles in the periorbital area are generally fine to moderate, and these products are more suitable for treating deeper depressions, such as the nasolabial fold. Using these products to treat the typical periorbital wrinkles risks undesirable consequences.

25.3 Treatments

25.3.1 Lateral Orbital Rhytids (Crow's Feet)

The orbicularis oculi muscle is a flat, wide muscle that encircles each orbit and extends into the eyelids (Fig. 25.1). The muscle has been arbitrarily divided into two parts: orbital and palpebral. The palpebral portion is further subdivided into a preseptal and pretarsal segment. The orbital portion consists of the outermost part of the muscle overlying the orbital margins. The preseptal portion overlies the orbital septum. It originates from the medial canthal tendon and lacrimal diaphragm and passes across the lid, meeting at the lateral canthal tendon. The pretarsal portion is the innermost portion of the muscle that overlies the superior and inferior tarsal plates. The pretarsal orbicularis has a lacrimal portion that inserts into and around the medial canthal tendon. The part of the orbicularis oculi that is located along the lateral orbit is responsible for creating the lateral radial lines, known as "crow's feet." In addition, the orbital segment of the orbicularis oculi is a depressor of the lateral brow.

The most common treatment for lateral orbital rhytids is BoNTA. The use of BoNTA should keep two goals in mind: (1) relaxing the radial crow's feet lines by targeting the lateral, vertically oriented portion of the orbicularis oculi and (2) providing brow elevation by neuromodulation of the brow depressor function by treating the entire length of the lateral orbicularis oculi. Studies have demonstrated the effect of BoNTA treatment of the lateral orbicularis oculi on brow position [10, 11]. Since this muscle acts as a sphincter, careful attention must be paid to the vectors of force during contraction. The contraction vectors at 12 and 6 o'clock are predominantly horizontal, while the vectors at 3 and 9 o'clock are primarily vertical. The crow's feet wrinkles are treated by injecting the lateral orbicularis oculi at several sites lateral to the orbital rim. This reduces the risk of orbital complications. A typical dose of 10 units of BotoxCosmetic™ or 30 units of Dysport™ per side is injected, divided into four or five aliquots (Fig. 25.2). The injections should be placed carefully to achieve maximum effect on the orbicularis oculi, and avoid injecting or injuring any superficial blood vessels.

Fillers have a limited role in the thin skin of the lateral orbital area. Most patients have fine to moderate lines due to orbicularis oculi overactivity and respond well with BoNTA. More severe rhytids are difficult to efface with BoNTA and may be better addressed with skin resurfacing, such as chemical peels or laser resurfacing. Collagen fillers such as Cosmoderm can be considered to fill in persistent fine lines. When using Cosmoderm, the injections are delivered in more superficial levels of the mid to upper dermis. The serial puncture technique, whereby small aliquots of filler are given to achieve even distribution over a two dimensional area, is particularly effective in accurate filler placement.

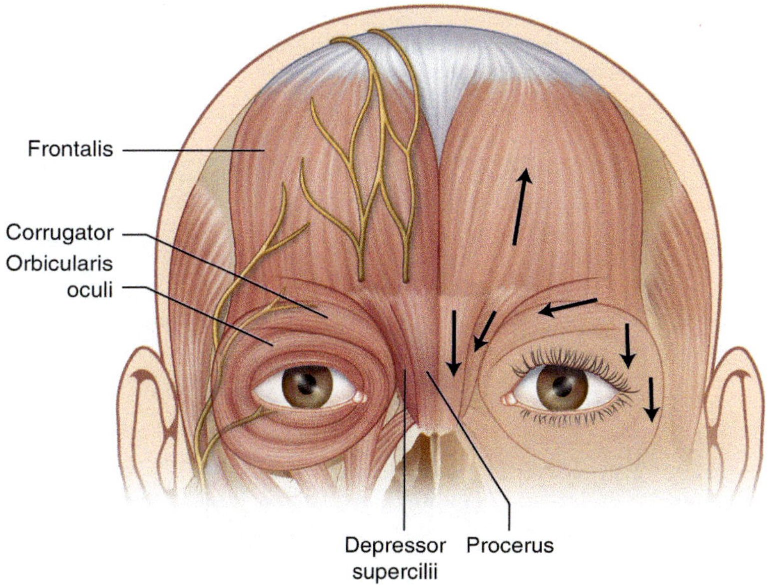

Fig. 25.1 Frontoorbital muscular anatomy demonstrating the origin, insertion and direction of action (*arrows*) of the orbicularis, frontalis, corrugator, depressor supercilii, and procerus muscles

25.3.2 Glabellar Complex

The vertical glabellar lines are primarily formed by the actions of the paired corrugator supercilii muscles. The inferior aspect of these vertical wrinkles may have an oblique or horizontal component caused by the procerus muscle. The corrugator supercilii originates from the procerus medially and insert, laterally, into the orbicularis oculi muscle and the soft tissue at and slightly above the medial eyebrow (Fig. 25.1). This muscle is nearly horizontal in most individuals; thus, contraction of the corrugator produces a vertical wrinkle. In some patients (<10%), the corrugator supercili muscle is oriented more diagonally; its contraction may result in an oblique wrinkle. It is crucial that BoNTA be injected properly in the corrugator supercili muscle to create a smoothing effect. More importantly, proper placement avoids any unnatural facial appearances. Many textbooks erroneously depict the corrugator supercilii muscle as a long vertically oriented muscle that inserts into the frontalis muscle in the mid forehead. Consequently, a common mistake is to inject the corrugator supercilii too far superiorly and actually treat the frontalis. The frontalis relaxation may cause a mephisto, or "Mr. Spock-like," unattractive appearance (Fig. 25.3). The correct placement of BoNTA into the corrugator supercilii muscle is more inferior, just at or slightly above the medial clubhead of the eyebrow. A second small dose is also given about 3–5 mm lateral to the first injection to treat the entire length of the corrugator muscle. Typically, 10 units of BotoxCosmetic™ or 30 units of Dysport™ to each side are employed (Fig. 25.2).

Furrows created at the base of the nose are created by the procerus muscle (Fig. 25.1). This muscle is anatomically larger in women than men [12]. It can be a powerful "wrinkler" of the nose. With chronic activity, the procerus can create deep furrows. Careful evaluation of the glabellar complex is important because many patients seeking treatment for the

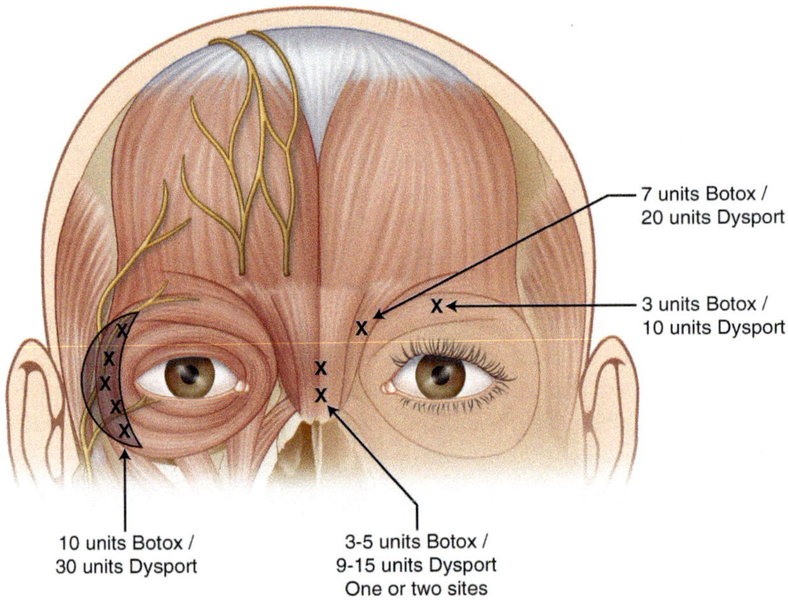

Fig. 25.2 Standard injection sites for treating lateral orbital rhytids and the glabellar complex. Crow's feet injections should be placed lateral to the orbital rim to reduce the risk of orbital complications. Avoid injecting or injuring any superficial blood vessels. The correct placement of BoNTA into the corrugator supercilii muscle is just at or slightly above the medial clubhead of the eyebrow. A second small dose is also given about 3–5 mm lateral to the first injection to treat the entire length of the corrugator muscle. The procerus is treated by injecting one or two aliquots at the belly of the muscle

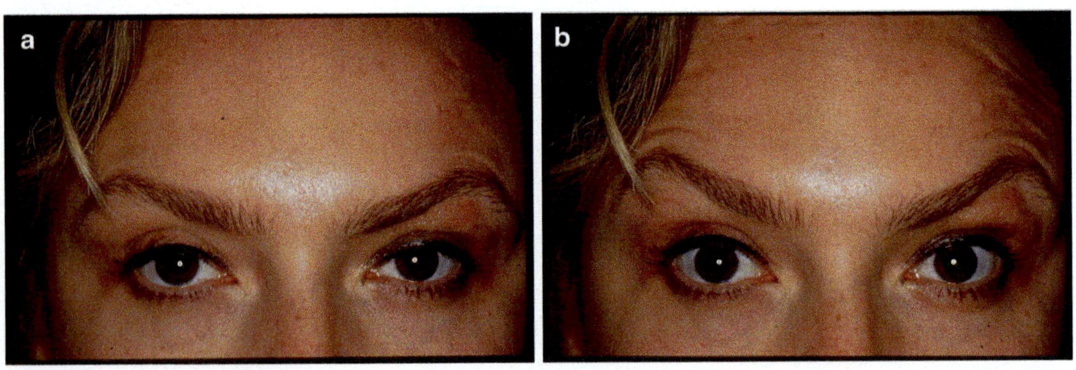

Fig. 25.3 Injecting the corrugator muscle too far superiorly and treating the frontalis may cause a mephisto or "Mr. Spock-like" appearance. (**a**) No brow elevation; (**b**) forced brow elevation

vertical glabellar furrows have very limited or nonexistent transverse lines. These patients, thus, do not need any treatment. Not all patients are the same; treatment formulas that are universal are wasteful and unnecessary. If a patient has transverse furrows, 3–5 units of BotoxCosmetic™ or 9–15 units of Dysport™ in one or two aliquots directed at the belly of this muscle are sufficient for most patients to achieve a satisfactory reduction in procerus activity (Fig. 25.2).

Occasionally, some superficial lines persist after BoNTA treatment to the glabellar area. It is wise to advise patients of the potential need for supplemental fillers if they present for neuromodulator treatment and have deeply ingrained dermal lines at rest. These lines are excellent candidates for correction with Cosmoderm [13]. Alternatively, Prevelle Silk™ can be used to treat superficial lines. In cases with deeper furrows, HA products can be used. When injecting HA product, one must stay superficial to the mid dermis. Ischemic necrosis of the glabellar skin, a rare and disastrous complication, can occur if any filler is injected intravascularly [14–17] (see Sect. 25.4). If combining BoNTA and filler, it is advisable to stage the treatment, particularly for new patients. Most experienced injectors will use BoNTA first; this allows for evaluation of residual lines or folds after BoNTA has taken effect [3]. Afterward, a better determination of filler application can be made.

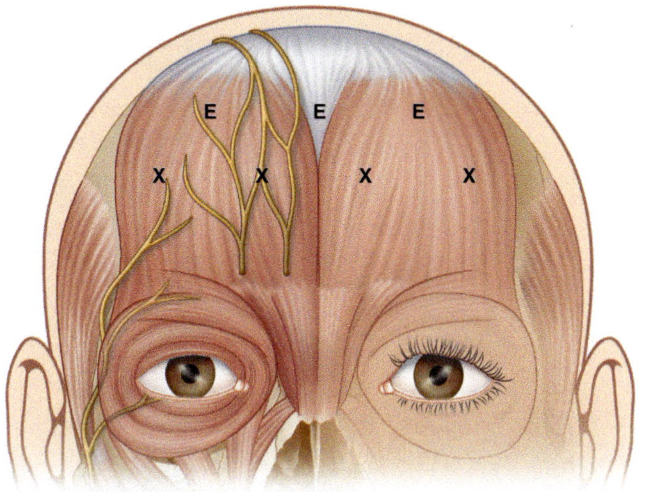

Fig. 25.4 Standard injection sites for treating the frontalis muscle. Injecting immediately above the most inferior horizontal line is recommended. Laterally, the point at which the forehead curves temporally is the lateral injection point. Medially, the medial canthus is the medial injection point. Three additional injection points can be added as extension therapy in patients with numerous forehead lines, or those with greater forehead height. One extension therapy injection is added in the midline, while the others are added between the medial and lateral injection points bilaterally. X, standard injection sites; E, extension therapy

25.3.3 Frontalis Muscle

The frontalis is a thin, quadrangular muscle originating from the galea aponeurotica below the coronal suture superiorly and inserting into the brow inferiorly (Fig. 25.1). While it has no bony attachments, it is contiguous with the procerus muscle centrally and interdigitates with the corrugator and orbicularis oculi muscles at the brow. Its fibers are vertical in orientation and contraction causes elevation of the brow. As such, hyperfunctional lines in this area cause classic horizontal forehead furrows.

BoNTA treatment of the frontalis muscle offers an excellent treatment for mild and moderate forehead lines. Ten units of BotoxCosmetic™ or 30 units of Dysport™, divided into four aliquots are used to treat the frontalis. The location of injections is critical to optimum results. To best identify appropriate injection placement, it is important to have the patient raise their brow to better define the forehead lines. Injecting immediately above the most inferior horizontal line is recommended. Laterally, the point at which the forehead curves temporally is the lateral injection point. Medially, the medial canthus is the medial injection point (Fig. 25.4). Three additional injection points (2 units BotoxCosmetic™/6 units Dysport™) can be added as extension therapy in patients with numerous forehead lines, or those with greater forehead height. One extension therapy injection is added in the midline, while the other is added between the medial and lateral injection points bilaterally (Fig. 25.4). When counseling a patient, it is important to explain that BoNTA treatment of the frontalis can result in brow ptosis. Therefore, treatment of the frontalis involves walking a fine line between undertreatment of the forehead and persistent lines versus ptosis of the brow.

With the advent of BoNTA, soft-tissue fillers have a more limited role in the treatment of horizontal forehead lines. It is important to distinguish between dynamic and nondynamic lines of the forehead. While the former is better treated with BoNTA, the latter, particularly in superficial lines caused by actinic damage, qualify for treatment with soft-tissue filling agents. Cosmoderm™, a human collagen agent, and Prevelle Silk™, an HA, offer the most superior results for these superficial lines without the risk of Tyndall effect.

25.3.4 Nasojugal Groove/Tear Trough

Contemporary periorbital rejuvenation techniques focus on improving the lower eyelid-mid-face contour [18]. As one ages, the mid-face structures become ptotic and expose the nasojugal groove and orbital rim. Often, pseudoherniation of orbital fat is also present, which accentuates the lower eyelid–cheek complex. Surgical options include blepharoplasty and mid-face lifts. However, volume replacement can be an effective option or supplement for patients with mild to moderate deformities [18]. Choices for volume replacement

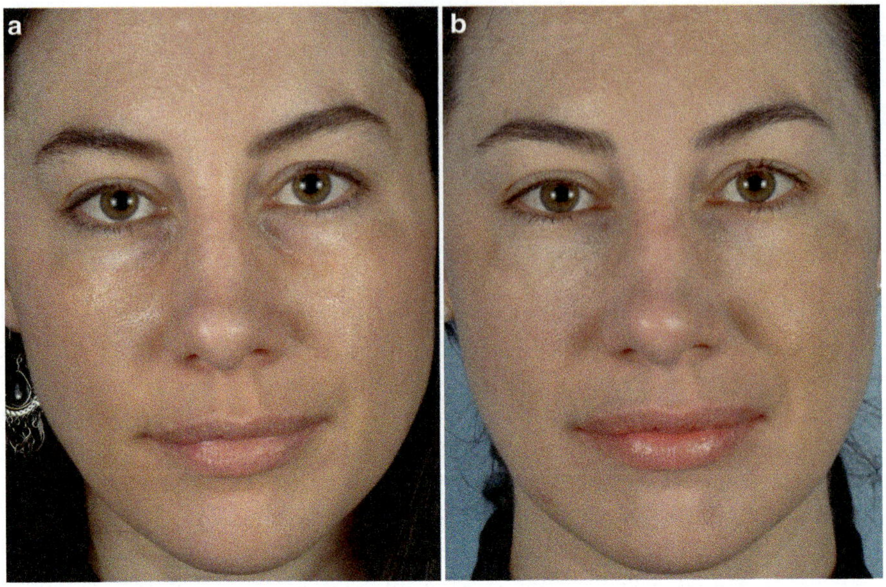

Fig. 25.5 (**a**) Before and (**b**) after photos of Restylane™ injection of the nasojugal groove area

include a variety of fillers, autologous fat, or solid implants. This section focuses on HA fillers.

HA products are commonly used to fill the tear trough (Fig. 25.5). The senior author prefers Restylane™ due to its firmer consistency. Juvederm Ultra™ and Ultra Plus™ have a smoother consistency but, in the senior author's experience, are more hydrophilic than Restylane™. Thus, these products will hold more water and result in more edema. This can confuse the correction and lead to eventual undercorrection and shorter duration than anticipated.

Filling the nasojugal groove is a delicate procedure requiring precision and artistry, and one must possess a clear understanding of the anatomy. Topical anesthetic creams and ice offer the best anesthesia. Anesthetic injections can distort the anatomy and interfere with proper filler injection. The patient is seated upright and a light is placed overhead to highlight the lower eyelid to mid-face contour.

Various injection techniques can be used. The senior author prefers to use the serial puncture and retrograde linear threading technique. Some feel the anterograde linear threading technique is easier to verify the proper depth of needle tip placement [3]. Other advantages include possible softer forward movement through tissues, blunting the impact of the sharp needle tip, pushing vessels out of the way, and reducing the chances for bruising. However, cannulization and intravascular injection are a greater risk with this technique. The retrograde technique is felt to avoid intravascular injection of filler as well as the creation of additional tracks or dissection planes [3]. This technique is often used for very soft, thin, or vascular areas present under the eyes. Regardless of the technique used, it is important to inject slowly (less than 0.3 mL/min) and avoid tissue tears. Most clinicians inject between 0.2 and 0.4 mL per side. Since injecting the nasojugal groove can be extremely volume sensitive, it is important to treat conservatively at first to avoid overcorrection. Reevaluation in 2–4 weeks and touch-up treatment can be performed if needed. In order to achieve an optimal aesthetic result, massage the filler at the time of injection to distribute it. Tyndall effect and water absorption are possible long- and short-term side effects.

25.4 Avoiding and Managing Complications

BoNTA injections have a long history of safety and efficacy. Since the dosages used in cosmetic treatments are small, serious adverse events are rare. Most adverse events are mild and temporary and include pain at injection sites, bruising, swelling, and flu-like symptoms [19]. Bruising and other adverse events can be decreased by advising patients to avoid taking medications that inhibit clotting. Vitamin E, aspirin, and nonsteroidal anti-inflammatory drugs should be stopped up to 2 weeks before treatments.

More significant complications can occur but are usually due to poor injection techniques, unfamiliarity with muscle anatomy, and injector inexperience. Most of these result from diffusion of toxin into adjacent musculature, which can lead to unexpected muscle weakening. Periorbital complications include an overtreated frontalis, brow ptosis, eyelid ptosis, asymmetry, cocked eyebrows, diplopia, ectropion, decreased strength of eye closure, and dry eyes. One should also carefully evaluate patients for any pre-existing low brow position or ptosis prior to treatment. Brow ptosis can generally be avoided by injecting no closer than 1 cm above the bony orbital rim in the mid-pupillary line and using lower doses in the frontalis [20].

One of the most common significant complications is eyelid ptosis. Publications have reported an average incidence of 6.5%, though in the senior author's experience, this is extremely high. Clinical trial data suggests an approximately 3% rate with BotoxCosmetic™ and 2% rate with Dysport™. Even these numbers are higher than those experienced by the senior author.

Upper eyelid ptosis can occur as early as 48 h after injection and as late as 14 days post treatment. The duration rarely lasts more than 3–4 weeks, but the problem can be particularly bothersome to patients. This complication most commonly occurs after BoNTA injections to the glabellar complex. Most authors believe the etiology of eyelid ptosis is diffusion of the toxin through the orbital septum into the levator palpebrae muscle. It is also felt that older patients, or those with loose skin or a weak orbital septum, are more susceptible to this complication. The senior author feels that ptosis is related to hydrostatic pressure from injection or localized edema, with subsequent diffusion of product via the supraorbital or supratrochlear foramina (or notch) or the superior orbital fissure. Eyelid ptosis may be avoided by using a higher concentration (lower volume) of BoNTA and by applying low plunger pressure during injection. In addition, one should avoid placing high levels of direct pressure at sites after injection.

While diplopia and dry eyes are well-described complications of BoNTA treatment for blepharospasm, facial spasm, and essential hyperlacrimation (crocodile tears), these are extremely rare complications from cosmetic applications and only reported in various case reports [21, 22]. Possible explanations for diplopia include incorrect placement of injections, larger volumes that lead to greater toxin diffusion, or a defective orbital septum that allows the toxin to reach extraocular muscles [22]. Dry eyes can result from diffusion of toxin into the lacrimal gland or paralytic lagophthalmos, leading to decreased blink strength. The case report attributed this complication to an injection site 0.5 cm from the superior orbital rim [21].

As mentioned previously, using fillers in the upper face is an advanced technique that should be undertaken by experienced injectors. Though rare, the most serious complication is necrosis, which can occur when any filler is inadvertently injected intravascularly [14–17]. Thus, injectors must have thorough knowledge of upper facial anatomy and blood supply. Additionally, one should inject slowly (<0.3 mL/min) and with low pressure. Blanching and sudden pain are symptoms and signs of possible blood-vessel occlusion. Injectors must be alert to these warning signs and immediately intervene to mitigate serious problems. If signs of occlusion occur, immediately stop and apply a topical vasodilator. Hyaluronidase should be given if an HA filler was used. One can also consider giving low-molecular-weight heparin daily for 1 week [14–17].

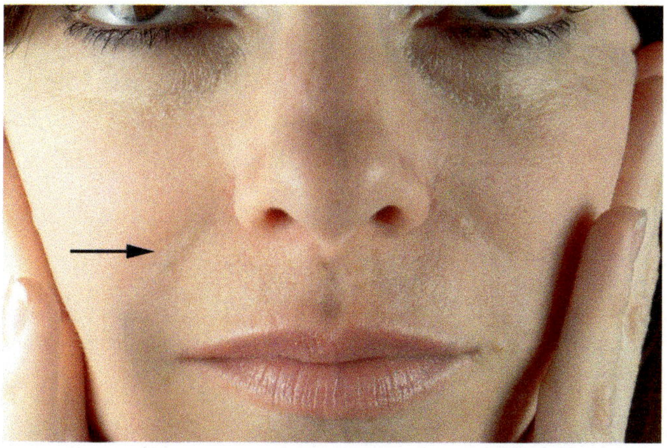

Fig. 25.6 Unpleasant bluish tint (Tyndall effect, *arrow*) seen in the nasolabial folds from injection of Restylane™ placed too superficially

Too superficial injection of hyaluronic acid filler can create visible ridges as well as an undesirable bluish tint known as the Tyndall effect [9] (Fig. 25.6). This complication can be avoided by injecting in the subdermis. Another helpful trick is to inject with the bevel down. Beading, clumping, and overcorrection are other potential complications with fillers. Massaging the area to distribute the filler can help in preventing this complication. Overcorrection can be minimized by using the multiple puncture serial technique. One can also consider using smaller gauge needles to control the amount of filler injected. Finally, hyaluronidase can be used to reverse unwanted effects of hyaluronic acid filler.

25.5 Conclusion

Neuromodulators and periorbital fillers offer an excellent means of periorbital rejuvenation and can also serve as an adjunctive treatment to surgery. While BoNTA remains the foundation of injectable treatment, soft-tissue fillers can enhance results, particularly the deep resting lines that persist after BoNTA treatment has been maximized. In addition, fillers alone improve depressions and contour irregularities, such as the nasojugal groove (tear trough).

Over the last decade, the burgeoning interest in minimally invasive aesthetic treatments has created a competitive and lucrative market for injectable cosmetic agents. The past several years has witnessed the introduction of numerous injectable fillers as well as an effective BoNTA competitor to Botox Cosmetic. This expansion of products offers both clinicians and patients more options for rejuvenation.

The goal of any aesthetic facial procedure should be the achievement of a refreshed, balanced, and harmonious aesthetic result. Attaining this requires a detailed knowledge of facial anatomy and facial aging. This is especially true in the very delicate periorbital region. A comprehensive understanding of the different clinical applications of BoNTA and the various filler agents available can help the clinician attain this goal by creating a customized approach for each patient.

References

1. Aoki KR, Guyer B. Botulinum toxin type A and other botulinum toxin serotypes: a comparative review of biochemical and pharmacological actions. Eur J Neurol. 2001;8 Suppl 5:21.
2. Aoki KR. A comparison of the safety margins of botulinum neurotoxin serotypes A, B, and F in mice. Toxicon. 2001;39:1815.
3. Carruthers J, Glogau RG, Blitzer A. Advances in facial rejuvenation: botulinum toxin type A, hyaluronic acid dermal fillers, and combination therapies – consensus recommendations. Plast Reconstr Surg. 2008;121(Suppl):5S–30.
4. Ramirez AL, Reeck J, Maas CS. Botulinum toxin type (MyoBloc) in the management of hyperkinetic facial lines. Otolaryngol Head Neck Surg. 2002;126(5):459–67.
5. Ramirez AL, Reeck J, Maas CS. Preliminary experience with botulinum toxin type B in hyperkinetic facial lines. Plast Reconstr Surg. 2002;109(6):2154–5.
6. Brandt FS, Cazzaniga A. Hyaluronic acid fillers: Restylane and Perlane. Facial Plast Surg Clin North Am. 2007;15:63–76.
7. Lowe NJ, Maxwell A, Lowe P, et al. Hyaluronic acid fillers: adverse reactions and skin testing. J Am Acad Dermatol. 2001;45: 930–3.
8. Micheels P. Human antihyaluronic acid antibodies: is it possible? Dermatol Surg. 2001;27:185–91.
9. Maas CS, Yu K, Egan KK. Neuromodulators and injectable soft tissue substitutes. In: Papel I, editor. Facial plastic and reconstructive surgery. New York: Thieme; 2009. p. 346.
10. Ahn M, Catten M, Maas CS. Temporal browlift using botulinum toxin. Plast Reconstr Surg. 2000;105:1129–35.
11. Maas CS, Kim EJ. Temporal browlift using botulinum toxin A: an update. Plast Reconstr Surg. 2003;112 Suppl 5:109S–12.
12. Macdonald MR, Spiegel JH, Raven RB, et al. An anatomical approach to glabellar rhytids. Arch Otolaryngol Head Neck Surg. 1998;124:1315–20.
13. Rostan E. Collagen fillers. Facial Plast Surg Clin North Am. 2007;15:55–61.
14. Born T. Hyaluronic acids. Clin Plast Surg. 2006;33:525.
15. de Boulle K. Management of complications after implantation of fillers. J Cosmet Dermatol. 2004;3:2.
16. Carruthers J, Carruthers A. Complications of botulinum toxin type A. Facial Plast Surg Clin North Am. 2007;15:51.
17. Schanz S, Shippert W, Ulmer A, et al. Arterial embolization caused by injection of hyaluronic acid (Restylane). Br J Dermatol. 2002;146:928.
18. Finn JC, Cox S. Fillers in the periorbital complex. Facial Plast Surg Clin North Am. 2007;15:123–32.
19. Alam M, Dover JS, Klein AW, et al. Botulinum A exotoxin for hyperfunctional facial lines: where not to inject. Arch Dermatol. 2002;138:1180.
20. Bailin PLBM. Collagen implantation: clinical applications and lesion selection. J Dermatol Surg Oncol. 1988;14:49.
21. Northington ME, Huang CC. Dry eyes and superficial punctate keratitis: a complication of treatment of glabelar dynamic rhytides with botulinum exotoxin A. Dermatol Surg. 2004;30:1515–7.
22. Aristodemou P, Watt L, Baldwin C, et al. Diplopia associated with the cosmetic use of botulinum toxin A for facial rejuvenation. Ophthal Plast Reconstr Surg. 2006;22:134–6.

Management of the Prominent Eye

26

John B. Holds

Key Points

- There are a variety of congenital and acquired causes of a prominent globe.
- Thyroid eye disease (TED-Graves exophthalmos) is the most common medical cause of a prominent eye.
- Identifying the etiology of globe prominence is critical before proceeding with eyelid surgery.
- Globe prominence poses unique risks with eyelid surgery and predisposes the patient to various potential postoperative ocular and eyelid complications.
- Understanding how to avoid the pitfalls of surgery on patients with prominent globes is essential to successful surgical outcomes.
- Familiarity with more complex orbital/eyelid procedures (i.e., orbital decompression, lid recession, mucosal grafting, and advanced lid suspension techniques) is necessary to appropriately perform surgery on patients with a prominent globe.
- If the surgeon lacks experience and comfort with these procedures, the assistance of a specialized eyelid/orbital surgeon is warranted.
- There are a number of variations to standard blepharoplasty surgery techniques in patients with prominent globes, which will prevent poor outcome and patient dissatisfaction. it is incumbent upon the surgeon treating these patients to understand these principles.

26.1 Introduction

The presence of a prominent globe poses a unique set of risks to the patient and eyelid surgeon, ranging from worsening aesthetic appearance to ocular exposure and visual disturbance [1]. For this reason, special attention must be given to this unique patient population in order to prevent poor outcomes. A prominent globe may be acquired with disease states, such as thyroid eye disease (TED-Graves exophthalmos), or be due to the congenital position of the globe and surrounding bony and soft tissue anatomy, as in craniofacial syndromes (Crouzon's disease) [2]. In addition, globe prominence may be seen with increased axial length of the globe (as in moderate to high myopia).

Eyelid retraction can independently create or enhance the appearance of globe prominence and may result from relative proptosis as described, or be due to trauma, or other congenital or acquired processes. For example, a patient with thyroid disease may develop eyelid retraction and the appearance of proptosis without any axial shift in the globe position. True proptosis adds to the eyelid retraction (upper and lower lids) in TED. The patient with proptosis of the eye and eyelid retraction is much more difficult to correct surgically.

A prominent globe should be diagnosed and managed prior to any aesthetic enhancement. For example, patients with TED commonly present with complaints relating to sagging of the pretarsal skin, fullness of the superior sulcus, or fat herniation in the lower eyelid. Proceeding immediately to a classic subtractive upper and lower blepharoplasty will at the very least give a suboptimal result, if not leave the patient with incurable exposure symptoms, tearing, or an unsightly cosmetic result. Cosmetic treatments in the periocular area, using modified techniques focused on achieving aesthetic improvement at minimal risk, must sometimes be preceded by surgery that directly addresses the globe and/or orbital rim position.

In this chapter, I will review the various treatment options which the eyelid surgeon should consider when evaluating the patient with globe prominence. I will focus on TED as this is the typical etiology of globe prominence that is most commonly encountered. However, the treatment modalities can be employed with other causes of globe prominence. Some treatments mandate referral to a specialist, while others are less complex but necessary procedures for any surgeon who commonly performs eyelid surgery.

J.B. Holds (✉)
Clinical Professor, Departments of Ophthalmology and Otolaryngology Head and Neck Surgery, St. Louis University School of Medicine, Director, Ophthalmic Plastic and Cosmetic Surgery, Inc., Des Peres, MO, USA
e-mail: jholds@sbcglobal.net

G.G. Massry et al. (eds.), *Master Techniques in Blepharoplasty and Periorbital Rejuvenation*,
DOI 10.1007/978-1-4614-0067-7_26, © Springer Science+Business Media, LLC 2011

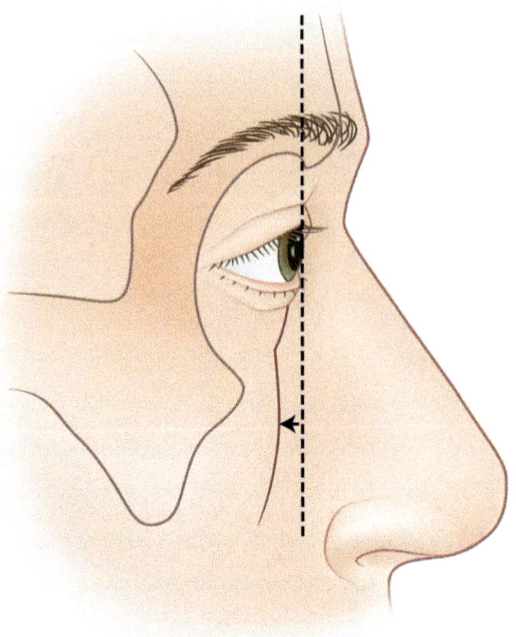

Fig. 26.1 Sagittal view of the orbit and midface demonstrating a negative vector eyelid as the tip of the globe protrudes more anteriorly than the midface

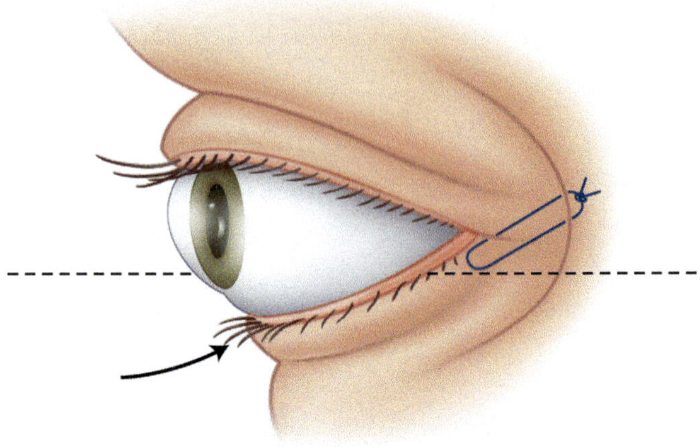

Fig. 26.2 The bowstringing effect encountered when tightening an eyelid in a patient with a prominent eye. The *arrow* demonstrates lid retraction (sclera show) created by the eyelid tightening

26.2 Anatomic Associations of the Prominent Eye

In addition to increased orbital soft tissue volume, as with TED, eye prominence may be associated with primary exorbitism (shallow orbit), a hypoplastic malar eminence, a congenitally enlarged globe, or other soft tissue and bony lesions. In all instances, a "negative vector eyelid" is present when the cornea protrudes further anteriorly than the malar area (Fig. 26.1). A negative vector eyelid is a set-up for postoperative complications in aesthetic eyelid surgery, as the lower lid must overcome an anatomic predisposition towards abnormal retraction [3]. The lower lid is anchored laterally and medially by canthal ligaments, and supported inferiorly by soft tissues and the bony facial skeleton, as well as the sphincteric action of the orbicularis oculi muscle. This creates a delicate balance that can easily swing toward lid retraction in normal surgical settings, but much more so when globe prominence is present. In this scenario (prominent globe with negate vector eyelid), canthal suspension (an integral part of lower lid blepharoplasty) may lead to "bowstringing" of the globe (Fig. 26.2).

Associated physical findings specific to the periocular area in the setting of globe prominence include eyelid retraction, a high eyelid crease, prominent fat prolapse in the eyelids, and an increased prominence of the tear trough or nasojugal fold. All of these features may be present in the patient without a prominent globe but tend to be more evident and thus cosmetically worse in the patient with the prominent eye. As such, each finding must be identified, evaluated, and addressed when necessary to appropriately and safely rejuvenate the periorbital area of the cosmetic patient with a prominent globe.

26.3 Surgical Treatment of the Prominent Eye

26.3.1 Orbital Decompression Surgery

TED often produces axial proptosis which is directly addressed only with techniques of orbital decompression surgery [4–9]. Orbital decompression surgery expands orbital volume or decreases the volume of orbital contents, which allows recession of orbital contents into the expanded space. Most patients with TED and proptosis want to look more normal. Sometimes, even with no ocular symptoms, the proptosis is severe enough that orbital decompression should be considered. In these instances, a referral to an experienced decompression surgeon is wise if you do not have the expertise needed to perform such a procedure on a cosmetic basis.

Orbital decompression surgery was traditionally performed only in the setting of severe visual loss caused by optic neuropathy or uncontrollable ocular exposure. As surgical techniques have improved, surgeons have been more willing to perform orbital decompression surgery for lesser symptoms or even on a purely cosmetic basis. Clearly, orbital decompression for only aesthetic reasons requires significant expertise with the surgical procedure, and should be reserved for more severe cases in which eyelid surgery will fail to camouflage the proptosis, or even worsen the cosmetic appearance. If there is no visual or exposure issues and eyelid surgery alone (lid recession and/or blepharoplasty) can mask the globe prominence, this is the patient's easiest, lowest risk, and often best cosmetic option.

Historically, every orbital wall has been addressed surgically. The transantral decompression technique, which removes the medial wall of the orbit and the orbital floor, is quite effective in reducing axial proptosis but is associated with potentially unattractive globe ptosis, diplopia, and sinus complaints [10, 11]. Many surgeons advocate a balanced approach to decompression by removing the medial and lateral orbital walls [6, 7]. The incidence of postoperative diplopia and globe ptosis is decreased with this approach. The medial orbital wall can be approached via a transnasal endoscopic approach or via a transconjunctival and transcaruncular incision. The lateral wall is often approached via a small canthotomy or temporal upper lid crease incision, although the deeper portions of the lateral wall of the orbit are better exposed via a coronal approach.

As fracturing the walls of the orbit for cosmetic purposes would be objectionable to the majority of patients, orbital fat decompression is a less invasive alternative. Orbital fat decompression techniques, which excise retrobulbar fat, captured the imagination of orbital surgeons when they were introduced by Olivari and Trokel in the early 1990 [4, 9]. Greater familiarity with the internal orbit, aided by high-resolution non-invasive imaging and better understanding of orbital soft tissue anatomy, encourages these approaches. These techniques have particular appeal in that they involve purely soft tissue surgery, avoiding special instrumentation and minimizing risks and morbidity. It is possible to combine surgical techniques, performing medial and/or lateral wall decompression in association with a graded amount of orbital fat decompression. The surgical approaches to the orbital fat readily facilitate simultaneous upper and lower blepharoplasty surgery, arcus marginalis release, various midface lifts, and lower eyelid fat repositioning on a cosmetic basis.

26.3.2 Cheek/Orbital Rim Implants

Orbital rim augmentation, either via osteotomy and bone advancement (Fig. 26.3) or more simply via the placement of an alloplastic implant, moves the orbital rim forward and lessens the prominence of the eye, thereby improving the patient's cosmetic appearance [12–15]. The association between orbital malar hypoplasia, a negative vector eyelid, and a prominent and cosmetically distracting tear trough deformity is striking.

An osteotomy may be performed with good results on a purely cosmetic patient but is a technique most applicable in patients with a true craniofacial syndrome or severe TED. The use of onlay silicone or porous polyethylene implants to the orbital rim and malar area is well described (Fig. 26.4) and often effective (Fig. 26.5). In some cases, fat repositioning blepharoplasty achieves much of the intended cosmetic improvement associated with these techniques, without the potential risks and complications of an implant.

26.3.3 Repair of Eyelid Retraction

The appearance of a prominent globe is enhanced by retraction of the upper and lower eyelids. Upper eyelid retraction generally relates to TED although it sometimes occurs primarily or in association with other medical conditions. Lower eyelid retraction is a product of globe position, orbital depth, malar projection, and factors innate to the eyelid and cheek soft tissues. Prior surgery may be a serious complicating factor in lower eyelid retraction requiring scar release, full thickness skin grafting, and other treatments. Additionally, surgery for lid retraction is generally undertaken only after

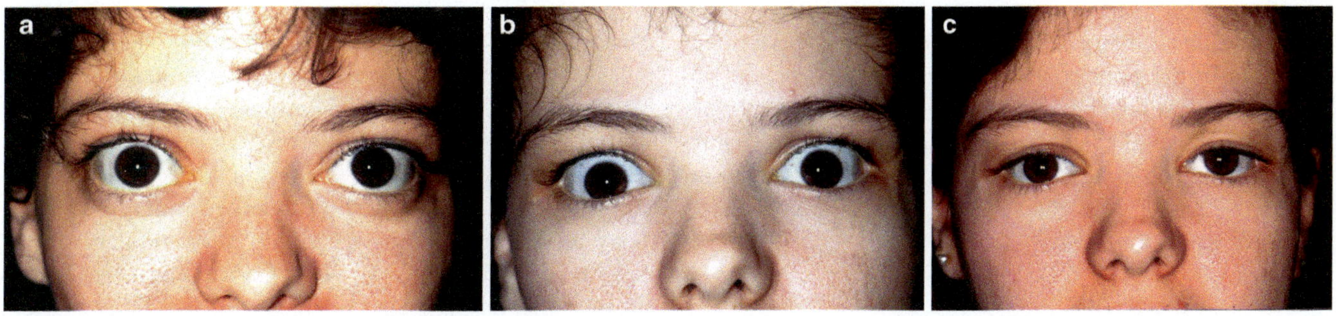

Fig. 26.3 Author's patient with congenitally shallow orbits, midface hypoplasia, and severe TED. (**a**) Preoperative; (**b**) after balanced medial/lateral orbital decompression with C-osteotomy and advancement of the lateral orbital rim; (**c**) after upper lid recession and lower lid hard palate mucosa spacer grafts

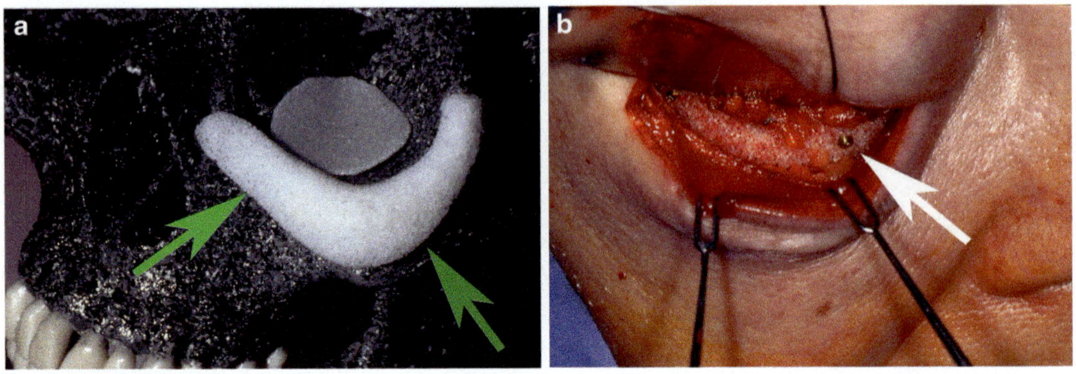

Fig. 26.4 Porex onlay orbital rim implant for orbital rim advancement. (**a**) Implant on model skull (*green arrows* demarcate implant); (**b**) Implant in place during surgery. *Arrow* to titanium screw fixing implant position

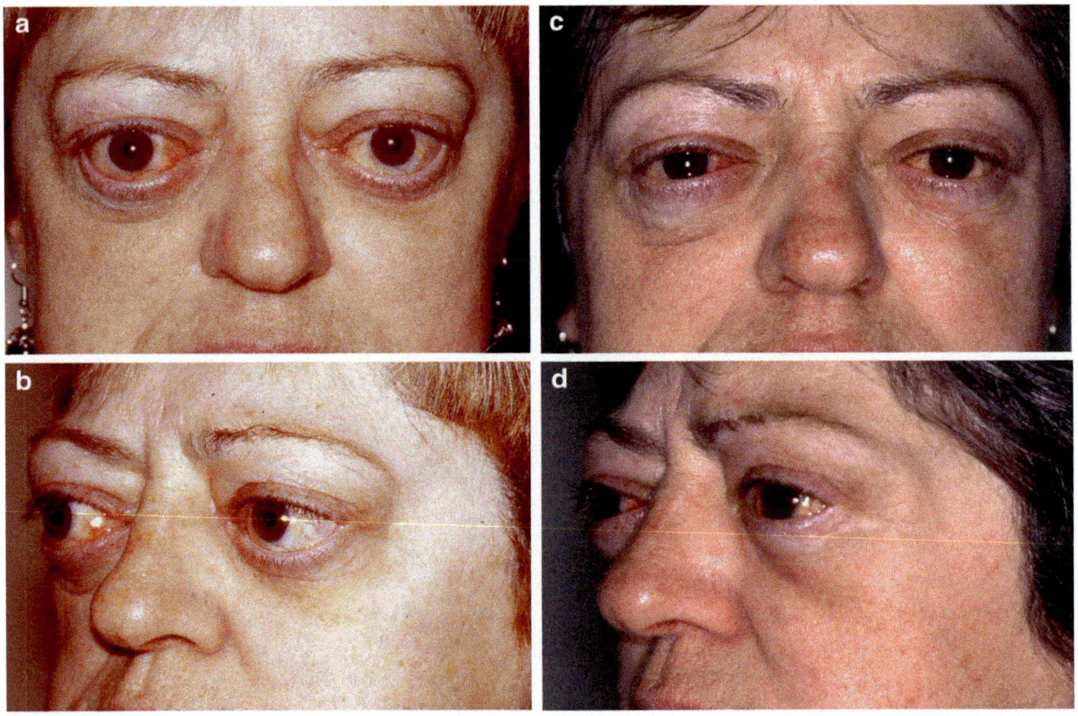

Fig. 26.5 Patient who underwent orbital decompression with onlay orbital rim implants and subsequent hard palate mucosa graft lower lid spacers; (**a**, **b**) preoperatively, (**c**, **d**) postoperatively

decompression surgery (if it is to be done) is performed. Alteration of the globe position with decompression surgery will alter eyelid position and may change the surgical plan for the treatment of eyelid retraction. Additionally, the shifting of orbital volume that occurs with orbital decompression surgery will often alter the surgical plan for any cosmetic treatment that is to follow.

26.3.4 Upper Lid Retraction

Upper eyelid recession surgery has traditionally relied on anterior approaches to the elevating structures of the eyelid generally recessing the levator aponeurosis and Mueller's muscle, and posterior approaches, which release or resect Mueller's muscle and/or levator aponeurosis [16, 17]. The treatment of upper lid retraction is best performed by surgeons with familiarity and expertise in the treatment of ptosis. The author has enjoyed predictable results for over 20 years using an anterior technique very similar to that described by Harvey et al. [16]. This approach is ideal in treating the cosmetically oriented patient, as concurrent upper blepharoplasty can be performed addressing redundant skin, prominent prolapsing fat, especially the medial fat pad, which is generally hypertrophic in the patient with TED (Fig. 26.6).

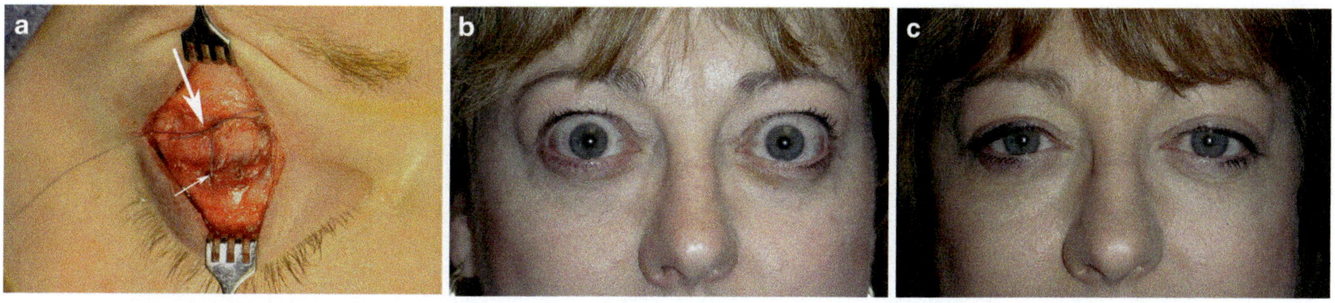

Fig. 26.6 (**a**) Surgical levator/Mueller's muscle recession showing inferior cut edge of levator aponeurosis (*small arrow*) and recessed edge of levator aponeurosis (*large arrow*). Suture stabilizing eyelid position in between arrows. (**b**) Preoperative lid recession; (**c**) 3 months postoperative lid recession

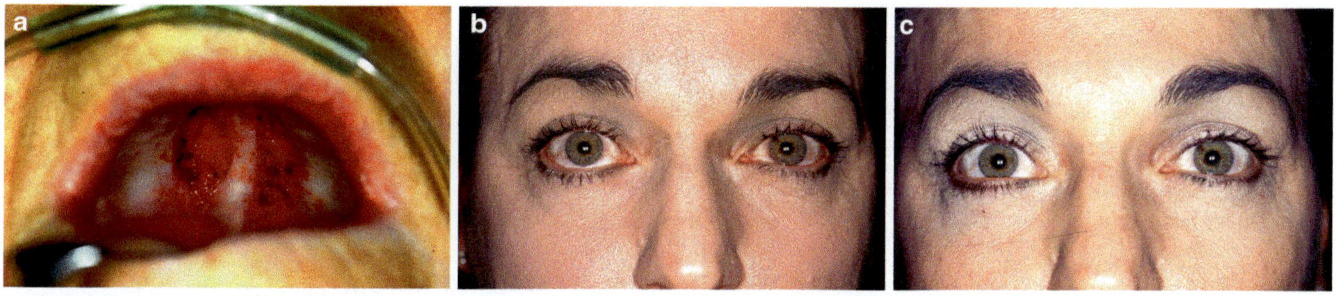

Fig. 26.7 (**a**) View of patient's hard palate showing defect immediately after harvest of hard palate mucosa graft (bilateral); (**b**) a different patient with right lower lid retraction preoperatively; (**c**) same patient postoperatively after placement of a hard palate mucosa graft as a right lower eyelid spacer graft

26.3.5 Lower Lid Retraction

Lower lid retraction is a more common and in many ways difficult condition to treat than upper eyelid retraction. The techniques used in the treatment of TED are generally applicable to the patient with primary or postoperative lower lid retraction.

Lateral canthoplasty of the tarsal strip variety by itself is generally long-term ineffective in the treatment of lower lid retraction. A posteriorly placed tarsal strip canthoplasty appropriate to the usual patient may even increase lower lid retraction (bowstringing effect) in the patient with a very prominent eye (Fig. 26.2). A canthotomy is performed when undertaking a transorbital lateral decompression surgery, and a simultaneous release of the conjunctiva and lower lid retractor layer allows the opportunity to improve the lower lid retraction, with recession of the eyelid retractors and an appropriate lateral canthotomy procedure. Long-term improvement is often obtained in this situation, aided by the placement for 3–5 days of reverse Frost traction sutures in the lower eyelids, which maintain an upward pull.

Attempts to treat lower lid retraction without the placement of a spacer graft are often difficult and unsatisfying. For this reason, spacer grafts to the lower eyelid are generally employed when attempting to permanently correct lower eyelid retraction. Various allografts of human and porcine collagen [18–20] have been utilized and are usually effective in treating small to moderate amounts of lower eyelid retraction. Hard palate mucosa has proven for over 20 years to be the premier posterior lamella spacer in the treatment of lower eyelid retraction [21–23]. Appropriately placed, hard palate mucosa accurately corrects lower eyelid retraction in a predictable and permanent fashion (Fig. 26.7).

Occasionally, patients present with eyelids lacking anterior lamella (skin) to a degree that full-thickness skin grafting is essential to reliably reposition the eyelid. Midface elevation is always a consideration in the treatment of lower eyelid retraction with various cosmetic and functional benefits. These lifts may be performed trans-eyelid, or via a transtemporal approach as an extension of the temporal dissection performed for endoscopic browlift surgery. Because of the cosmetically undesirable aspects of full-thickness skin grafting of the eyelid, it is appealing and oftentimes appropriate to perform midface lifts as part of a repair for eyelid retraction.

26.4 Cosmetic Treatment of the Tear Trough in the Prominent Eye

Fat repositioning techniques of blepharoplasty can be effective in safely treating the tear trough deformity in the patient with a prominent eye [24–26]. By necessity, these techniques generally incorporate a release of the arcus marginalis with undermining of the soft tissues of the orbital rim and cheek in an intra-suborbicularis oculi fat (SOOF) or subperiosteal plane. The fat repositioning tends to elevate and anteriorly

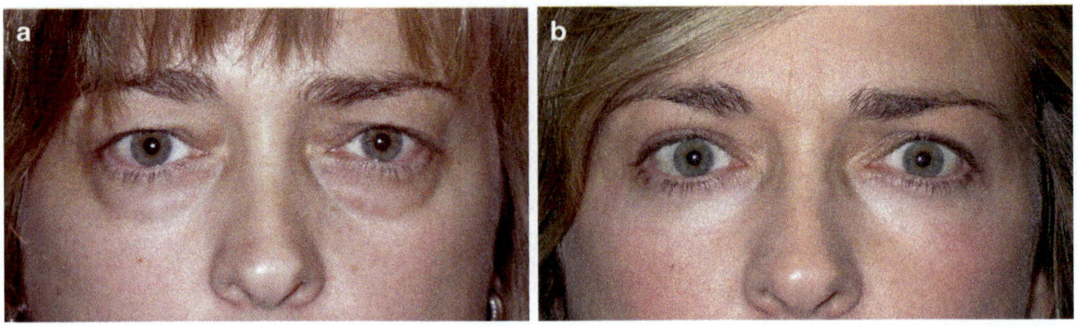

Fig. 26.8 Patient with TED and mild exophthalmos (**a**) before and (**b**) after lower blepharoplasty with intra-SOOF technique of fat repositioning. Lessening of fat pseudoherniation, preservation of eyelid margin position, smoothing of the tear trough, and an elevation in the apparent orbital rim position are all apparent in a cosmetically desirable way

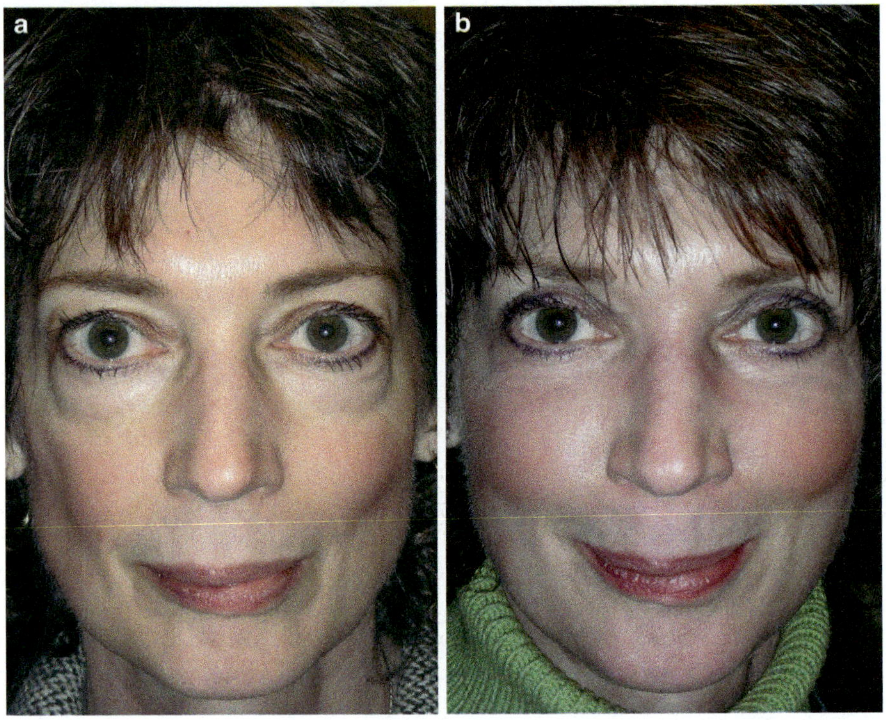

Fig. 26.9 Patient with prominent eyes, relative midface hypoplasia, and a prominent tear trough deformity (**a**) before and (**b**) 6 months after four-lid blepharoplasty with lower lid intra-SOOF fat repositioning, erbium-YAG laser skin resurfacing, and fat transfer to the midface

project the inferior orbital rim and eyelid–cheek junction, both desirable in the patient with eye prominence (Fig. 26.8). This is in contrast to purely subtractive techniques which do nothing to specifically address either of these facial defects.

Midface lifting is often beneficial from a cosmetic perspective in patients with prominent eyes that have no explanatory medical or surgical history. Elevation of the ptotic malar tissues to provide more coverage for the tear trough area may be performed in conjunction with implants or fat repositioning blepharoplasty techniques. Trans-lid techniques of SOOF or midface lifting are excellent adjuncts to blepharoplasty. The temporal approach to midface lifting as an extension of the temporal endoscopic browlift dissection is also an excellent method of elevating a ptotic midface in a patient with a prominent eye, while safely providing cosmetic correction.

Injectable fillers provide a straightforward and precise tool for augmentation along the orbital rim and tear trough, whether performed primarily in a patient "not ready for surgery" or as a postoperative adjunct [27, 28]. Hyaluronic acid fillers provide an excellent option for volume augmentation. Surgeons are cautioned to develop their skills gradually and use appropriate technique, introducing the filler from below and fanning into a deep plane along the orbital rim. It is tempting to simply parallel the tear trough with the needle pass; however, this technique markedly increases the risk for causing an undesirable thickening along the orbital rim that could necessitate reversal with an injection of the enzyme hyaluronidase, which rapidly eliminates contour issues related to excessive hyaluronate filler placement.

Autogenous fat grafting is also a helpful adjunct in treating prominent eye patient with cosmetic concerns. Fat may be used similarly to injectable fillers to increase the orbital rim projection and volumize the midface. It may be employed as a primary treatment or as an adjunct to other treatments such as fat repositioning blepharoplasty and/or midface lift procedures [3] (Fig. 26.9). Fat transfer carries the disadvantage of unpredictable resorption and may require multiple treatment sessions to obtain adequate results. Nonetheless, it is a useful tool in the surgeon's armentarium.

26.5 "Rescue" Techniques with the Prominent Eye

All too often inappropriate or misdirected surgery results in an undesirable functional or cosmetic outcome after eyelid surgery. This risk is especially high in the patient with a prominent eye. Ocular exposure symptoms and cosmetically unacceptable eyelid retraction are the most common postblepharoplasty complications in this patient population.

Recognition of the patient's anatomic features and the avoidance of "standard" subtractive techniques in at-risk patients will avoid most of these situations. When patients with these complications of surgery present, the treatment approaches are as described previously. The first surgery generally creates problems and impediments to correction. Surgical correction often focuses on replacing what has been removed. For example, excessive fat resection may leave no fat to drape the orbital rim and camouflage the tear trough. In such cases, the harvest of a dermis-fat graft from the abdomen as performed in anophthalmic socket surgery and placement of an appropriately-sized graft after surgical exposure may provide adequate volume to correct this element of the patient's condition.

Midface lifting via transeyelid or temporal approaches may be attempted to elevate ptotic midfacial tissues and recruit skin into the lower eyelid, correcting ectropion or lower lid retraction [29–31] (Fig. 26.10). Given the strong tendency for any vertical elevation to regress over the first year after surgery, the surgeon is advised to depend on this approach only as an adjunct or for the correction of mild degrees of anterior lamella deficiency.

Despite attempts to recruit anterior lamella tissue with midface lifting, the long-term treatment plan for patients with overdone "classic" blepharoplasty and a prominent eye often entails full-thickness skin grafting. In this regard, an ounce of prevention is worth a pound of cure, as the restorative surgery is much more difficult and complex than the initial misdirected procedure.

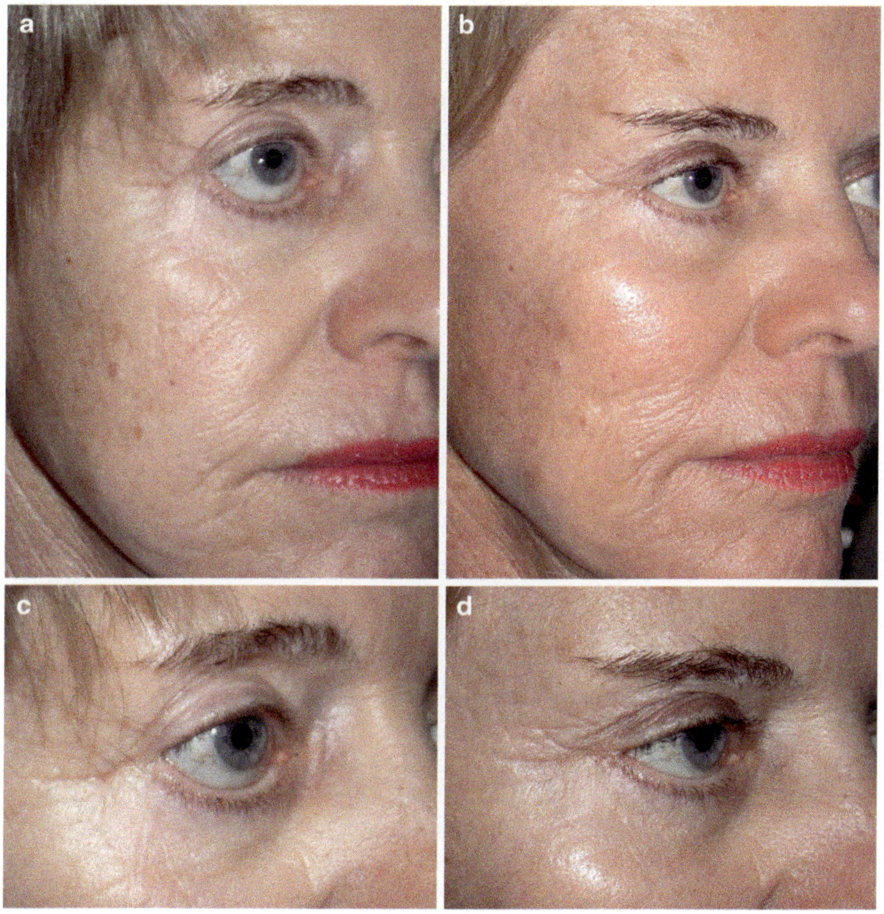

Fig. 26.10 This patient with prominent globes presented with cicatricial lower lid retraction after previous lower lid blepharoplasty. She underwent transconjunctival and temporal (endoscopic) approach to midface lifting (for multiple points of fixation) in addition to hard palate grafting and modified canthoplasty (hangback suture and supra-placement of tarsus). (**a**) Preoperative full face oblique view. (**b**) postoperative full face oblique view. (**c**) Preoperative periorbital oblique view. (**d**) postoperative periorbital oblique view. (Photos courtesy of Dr. Guy Massry)

26.6 Nuances In Blepharoplasty in Patients with Prominent Globes

Upper blepharoplasty should be conservative with an effort made to avoid excess skin removal, which is more likely to result in lagophthalmos and exposure keratitis. With prominent eyes, the vertical length of skin needed to drape the eye with the lid shut is increased. In this setting, there needs to be sufficient excess preseptal skin to allow for this closure. It is a good rule of thumb to mark the normal ellipse of skin to be excised, as with upper lid blepharoplasty in a normal globe projection, and then reduce the amount of skin excision by 20%. The common technique of pinching redundant skin until the lashes evert with mild lagophthalmos will result in an overly aggressive resection of skin in these patients. Backing off from these "normal" amounts of skin excision will allow a valuable window of safety during surgery. Similarly, do not aggressively excise (debulk) the orbicularis muscle in surgery. Orbicularis muscle weakness is a normal involutional change which can be iatrogenically enhanced or hastened with upper blepharoplasty. In the normal setting, corneal protective mechanisms such as the Bell's phenomenon (globe supraduction with lid closure), tear production, corneal sensation, and lid closure are adequate to overcome a slightly overzealous blepharoplasty. In patients such as those with TED, these compensatory mechanisms are reduced or absent. For example many of these patients sleep with their eyes open (nocturnal lagophthalmos), have exposure findings (dryness), and have reduced eye elevation on closure (Bell's phenomenon) from inferior rectus pathology inherent to the disease. These patients are often asymptomatic at presentation for aesthetic lid surgery. Any manipulation of these patients' eyelids can lead to exposure symptoms, even in the best of hands. Careful evaluation and conservative surgery should be the rule in these patients.

Special attention should be given to marking of the upper eyelid crease in the presence of prominent eyes. In these patients, there is tendency towards a higher eyelid crease than nonprominent globes. A conventional surgical approach with the eyelid crease marked at a high anatomic position may exaggerate the appearance of an elevated eyelid crease after surgery. As such, marking the crease at 8–12 mm above the lash line and often a few millimeters below the anatomic crease for the patient is recommended. In TED patients who undergo simultaneous upper lid recession, the crease can be higher and asymmetric after surgery as the recessed levator aponeurosis drags the preaponeurotic fat back and elevates the eyelid crease postoperatively. Generally, no preaponeurotic fat is removed centrally in these patients, and a very limited (if any) skin excision is performed to avoid the appearance of an overly elevated upper eyelid crease.

Fat removal during upper blepharoplasty must be conservative and appropriately directed. Topographically, when the globe protrudes, the surrounding fullness can mask or camouflage a degree of this prominence. When this soft tissue is reduced, the prominence may be unmasked to a further extent, leading to a sunken, surprised, and more proptotic appearance. TED patients often have abundant fat at surgery. It is important not to be misled by this exuberance of fat with aggressive excision. This can lead to very unhappy patients. Generally speaking, the medial fat pad is prominent and is judiciously debulked. The central fat should be preserved or minimally reduced. Laterally, the lacrimal gland may be prolapsed (sometimes excessively in TED patients) with associated temporal fullness. In these instances, it should be resuspended [32–34]. Simultaneous upper eyelid recession results in lengthening of the upper eyelid as previously noted, creating a hollower superior sulcus. Fat reduction should be less aggressive in this setting.

In the lower eyelid, great care in surgical technique is essential to avoid any cicatricial or other force that increases lower eyelid retraction. Fat preservation techniques with intra-SOOF or subperiosteal fat repositioning are excellent, especially when performed transconjunctivally [24–26]. The transconjunctival approach releases the lower eyelid retractors, providing much of the benefit of a postoperative traction suture, while avoiding trauma that can stimulate scarring to the anterior or middle lamella. Appropriate placement of malar implants can improve the relationship between the eyelid and globe and prevent eyelid malposition (vector correction) (Fig. 26.11).

Skin excision, if undertaken, must be very conservative in these patients, as is chemical or laser resurfacing of the skin. Canthal suspension can be quite challenging in patients with prominent eyes. "Bowstringing" of the globe can occur as a longer lower lid is needed to circumvent the added curvature imposed by the prominent globe. When sufficient vertical and horizontal length of the eyelid is not present, the lower lid will take the path of least resistance and ride down the globe (retract) with increased scleral show (Fig. 26.2). There are a few modifications of traditional canthoplasty which help prevent this eyelid malposition. First, the suture securing the lid to the lateral orbital rim can be left to hang back. This effectively horizontally lengthens the lid. The knot is tied after titrating its tightness and monitoring the lid position. Also the lid can be secured to a higher position on the lateral orbital rim (above Whitnalls tubercle) (Fig. 26.12). Finally, a graded translid midface suspension in addition to preseptal orbicularis muscle plication may be of added benefit in selected cases. As a general rule, staying out of harm's way is the best course of action. Canthoplasty in these cases (when primarily aesthetic in nature) can open a Pandora's box of problems, as patients will not concern themselves with case complexity and focus on immediate outcome only.

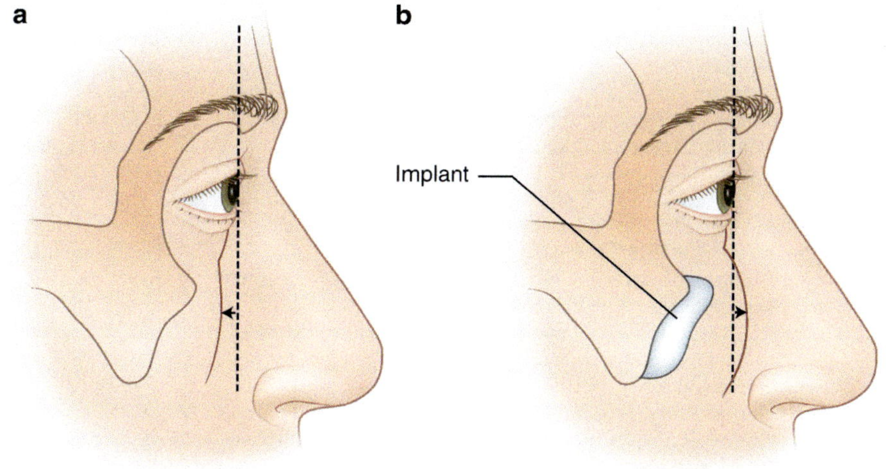

Fig. 26.11 (**a**) Negative vector eyelid as described in Fig. 26.1. (**b**) Surgical placement of malar implant to project cheek anteriorly and correct the negative vector

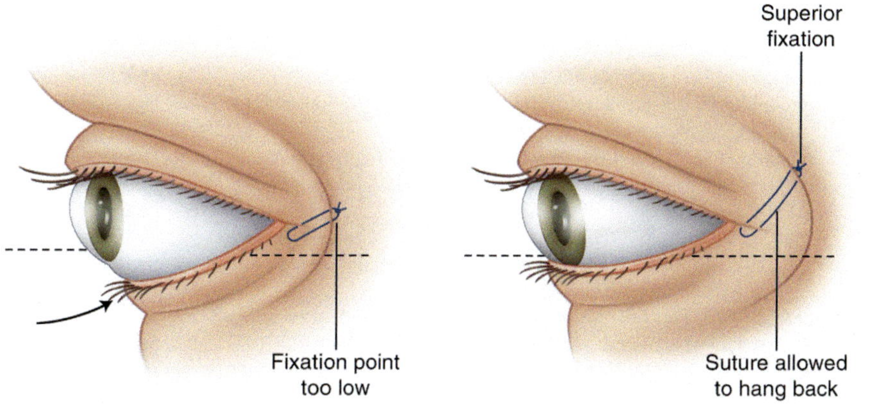

Fig. 26.12 (*Left*) Bowstringing of a prominent eye with lid tightening as is shown in Fig. 26.2. (*Right*) Modification of canthoplasty by hang-back and supra-placement of eyelid fixation suture. This prevents "the bowstinging" effect. Note elevation of lower lid and reduction of scleral show

The take-home message is to avoid skin excision and lid tightening if at all possible. In most cases, this can be accomplished.

26.7 Conclusion

The prominent eye may have important medical associations including congenital syndromes, myopia, and thyroid eye disease. A prominent globe is a common and significant complicating factor in performing cosmetic periocular surgery. Recognition of the cause of globe prominence and appropriately accounting for it are essential to avoid surgical complications when performing blepharoplasty and other eyelid surgery in such patients.

An armentarium of surgical corrective techniques combined with cosmetic approaches that prevent worsening of the underlying problem allow safe and cosmetically appropriate surgery in this challenging patient population. The treatment of complications of surgery is more challenging, and requires more complex reconstructive techniques than in similar patients without prominent eyes. It is hoped that the readers of this chapter embark on eyelid surgery on the patient with a prominent eye with a new respect for the problem and its potential to produce suboptimal results.

References

1. Goldberg RA, Weinberg DA, Shorr N. Management of the patient with a relatively prominent eye. Facial Plast Surg Clin North Am. 1998;6:11–9.
2. Hirmand H, Codner MA, McCord CD, Hester Jr TR, Nahai F. Prominent eye: operative management in lower lid and midfacial rejuvenation and the morphologic classification system. Plast Reconstr Surg. 2002;110(2):620–8; discussion 629–34.
3. Massry GG. Comprehensive lower eyelid rejuvenation. Facial Plast Surg. 2010;26:209–21.
4. Olivari N. Transpalpebral decompression of endocrine ophthalmopathy (Graves' disease) by removal of intraorbital fat: experience with 147 operations over 5 years. Plast Reconstr Surg. 1991;87:627–41; discussion 642–3.
5. Richter DF, Stoff A, Olivari N. Transpalpebral decompression of endocrine ophthalmopathy by intraorbital fat removal (Olivari technique): experience and progression after more than 3000 operations over 20 years. Plast Reconstr Surg. 2007;120:109–23.

6. Leone Jr CR, Piest KL, Newman RJ. Medial and lateral wall decompression for thyroid ophthalmopathy. Am J Ophthalmol. 1989;108(2):160–6.
7. Graham SM, Brown CL, Carter KD, Song A, Nerad JA. Medial and lateral orbital wall surgery for balanced decompression in thyroid eye disease. Laryngoscope. 2003;113(7):1206–9.
8. Schaefer SD, Soliemanzadeh P, Della Rocca DA, Yoo GP, Maher EA, Milite JP, et al. Endoscopic and transconjunctival orbital decompression for thyroid-related orbital apex compression. Laryngoscope. 2003;113:508–13.
9. Trokel S, Kazim M, Moore S. Orbital fat removal. Decompression for Graves orbitopathy. Ophthalmology. 1993;100:674–82.
10. Carter RD, Freuh BR, Hessberg TP, et al. Long term efficacy of orbital decompression for compressive optic neuropathy of Graves disease. Ophthalmology. 1991;98:1435–42.
11. Warren JD, Spector JG, Burde R. Long term follow-up and recent observation of 305 cases of orbital decompression for dysthyroid orbitopathy. Laryngoscope. 1989;99:35.
12. Gilliland GD, Clayton E. Beveled osteotomy with lateral wall advancement and interpositional bone grafting for severe thyroid orbitopathy. Ophthal Plast Reconstr Surg. 2007;23:192–6.
13. Weinberg DA, Goldberg RA, Hoenig J, Shorr N, Baylis HI. Management of relative proptosis with a porous polyethylene orbital rim onlay implant. Ophthal Plast Reconstr Surg. 1999;15:67–73.
14. Yaremchuk MJ. Infraorbital rim augmentation. Plast Reconstr Surg. 2001;107:1585–92; discussion 1593–5.
15. Yaremchuk MJ, Kahn DM. Periorbital skeletal augmentation to improve blepharoplasty and midfacial results. Plast Reconstr Surg. 2009;124:2151–60.
16. Harvey JT, Corin S, Nixon D, Veloudios A. Modified levator aponeurosis recession for upper eyelid retraction in Graves' disease. Ophthalmic Surg. 1991;22:313–7.
17. Putterman AM, Fett DR. Muller's muscle in the treatment of upper eyelid retraction: a 12 year study. Ophthalmic Surg. 1986;17:361–7.
18. Shorr N, Perry JD, Goldberg RA, et al. The safety and applications of acellular human dermal allograft in ophthalmic plastic and reconstructive surgery. Ophthal Plast Reconstr Surg. 2000;16:223.
19. Rubin PA, Fay AM, Remulla HD, Maus M. Ophthalmic plastic applications of acellular dermal allografts. Ophthalmology. 1999; 106:2091.
20. Fay AM, Pieroth L, Rubin PAD. An animal model of lower eyelid spacer grafting with acellular dermis. Ophthal Plast Reconstr Surg. 2001;17:270.
21. Siegel RJ. Palatal grafts for eyelid reconstruction. Plast Reconstr Surg. 1985;76:411.
22. Cohen MS, Shorr N. Eyelid reconstruction with hard palate mucosa graft. Ophthal Plast Reconstr Surg. 1992;8:183–95.
23. Kersten RC, Kulwin DR, Levartovsky S, et al. Management of lower-lid retraction with hard-palate mucosa grafting. Arch Ophthalmol. 1990;108:1339.
24. Espinoza GM, Holds JB. Evaluation and treatment of the tear trough deformity in lower blepharoplasty. Semin Plast Surg. 2007;21:57–64.
25. Nassif PS. Lower blepharoplasty: transconjunctival fat repositioning. Facial Plast Surg Clin North Am. 2005;13:553–9.
26. Mohadjer Y, Holds JB. Cosmetic lower eyelid blepharoplasty with fat repositioning via intra-SOOF dissection: surgical technique and initial outcomes. Ophthal Plast Reconstr Surg. 2006;22: 409–13.
27. Morely AM, Malhotra R. Use of hyaluronic acid filler for tear-trough rejuvenation as an alternative to lower eyelid surgery. Ophthal Plast Reconstr Surg. 2010;27(2):69–73.
28. Goldberg RA, Fiaschetti D. Filling the periorbital hollows with hyaluronic acid gel: initial experience with 224 injections. Ophthal Plast Reconstr Surg. 2006;5:335–41;discussion 341–343.
29. Shorr N. Madame Butterfly procedure with hard palate graft: management of post-blepharoplasty round eye and scleral show. Facial Plast Surg. 1994;10:90.
30. Edelstein C, Balch K, Shorr N, Goldberg RA. The transeyelid subperiosteal midface-lift in the unhappy postblepharoplasty patient. Semin Ophthalmol. 1998;13(3):107–14. Review.
31. Anderson RDA, Lo MW. Endoscopic malar/midface suspension procedure. Plast Reconstr Surg. 1998;102:2196.
32. Smith B, Petrelli R. Surgical repair of prolapsed lacrimal glands. Arch Ophthalmol. 1978;96:1132.
33. Beer GM, Kompatscher P. A new technique for the treatment of lacrimal gland prolapsed in blepharoplasty. Aesthet Plast Surg. 1994;18(1):65–9.
34. Smith B, Lisman RD. Dacryoadenopexy as a recognized factor in upper lid blepharoplasty. Plast Reconstr Surg. 1983;71(5):629–32.

Postoperative Wound Modulation in Aesthetic Eyelid and Periorbital Surgery

27

Mehryar Taban, Seongmu Lee, Jonathan A. Hoenig, Ronald Mancini, Robert A. Goldberg, and Raymond S. Douglas

Key Points

- Wound modulation in the postoperative setting of aesthetic eyelid and periorbital surgery is helpful in managing scar formation and wound contracture. This is a useful adjunct in determining the surgical outcome of the procedure.
- 5-FU is a versatile anti-metabolite that can be utilized for wound modulation after aesthetic eyelid and periorbital surgery. It can be used for scar therapy, eyelid retraction, and encapsulated injected autologous fat.
- Corticosteroids can be used along with 5-FU for optimal wound modulation and scar management.
- Injectable fillers, such as hyaluronic acid gels, are a reversible tool that can be used in the postoperative period to correct contour irregularities and to act as a tissue expander to minimize tissue contracture.

27.1 Introduction

Scar formation is a highly regulated tissue response following skin or tissue injury and is anticipated after surgical manipulation. However, exuberant scar formation on conspicuous areas of the face can be aesthetically disfiguring and functionally debilitating. The modulation of scar formation in the postoperative setting is a vital component of aesthetic eyelid and facial surgery. While numerous surgical approaches have been described to revise scars, nonsurgical adjunctive treatments which target the underlying biologic process are effective and safe. A variety of nonsurgical approaches including anti-metabolites, anti-inflammatory agents, and tissue volume expansion can provide substantial improvement.

A meticulous preoperative evaluation, including a complete physical examination, discussion of functional limitations, and a realistic appraisal of patient expectations, is paramount. We cannot stress enough that realistic expectations are especially important in the setting of scar revision. Factors to consider in formulating a treatment plan include the nature, anatomic location, and extent of the scar. In addition, it is critical to assess skin type and ethnicity of the patient, etiology of the scar, history of scarring tendencies, and all prior treatments and their relative efficacy. As scar formation is an evolution, the timing of all surgical and nonsurgical interventions is critical.

27.2 Anti-metabolites

In general, antimetabolites interfere with the proliferative mechanisms of scar formation, most notably by disrupting fibroblast biology. Anti-metabolites are not cell-type specific but rather target proliferating or synthetically active cells instead of quiescent cells. Interference with fibroblast proliferation and the production of collagen and other synthetic products has proven successful in scar prevention and reduction.

27.3 5-Fluorouracil

The anti-metabolite, 5-Fluorouracil (5-FU) (Fig. 27.1), has been used widely for decades in oncology and more recently in dermatologic management of skin lesions. The drug has a long track record of efficacy, safety, and mechanistic understanding. More recently, this anti-metabolite has gained popularity in the management of exuberant scar formation as it is efficacious and has an excellent safety profile.

R.S. Douglas (✉)
Associate Professor, Department of Ophthalmology and Visual Sciences, University of Michigan, Ann Arbor, MI, USA
e-mail: raydougl@med.umich.edu

G.G. Massry et al. (eds.), *Master Techniques in Blepharoplasty and Periorbital Rejuvenation*,
DOI 10.1007/978-1-4614-0067-7_27, © Springer Science+Business Media, LLC 2011

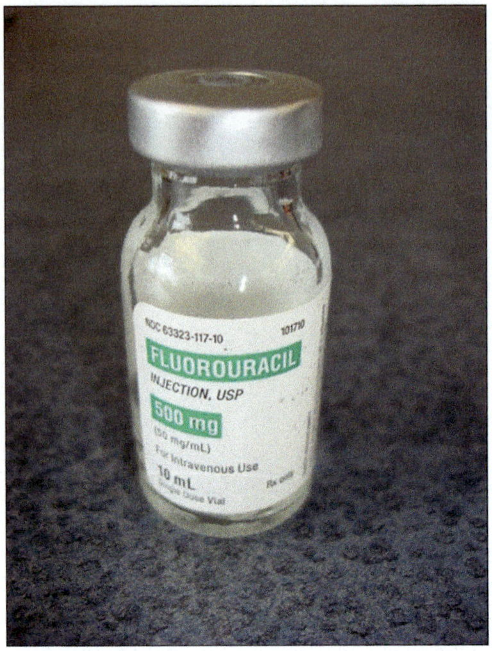

Fig. 27.1 5-Fluorouracil (5-FU) supplied in 50 mg/mL concentration

27.3.1 Mechanism of Action

5-FU minimizes scar formation by inhibiting cell proliferation through the disruption of DNA synthesis and inhibiting collagen production. As 5-FU is a fluorinated pyrimidine, it acts to inhibit DNA synthesis and cell proliferation by inhibition of thymidylate synthetase and direct misincorporation. Structurally, it is identical to uracil but with fluorine substituted for hydrogen at the C-5 position, which allows rapid cellular entry and utilization. 5-FU is converted into fluorodeoxyuridine monophosphate, which, through its interaction with thymidylate synthetase, inhibits the conversion of uracil into thymidylate. This results in a deficiency of thymidylate, a precursor of thymidine phosphate, one of the four deoxyribonucleotides needed for DNA synthesis and repair. Additionally, direct misincorporation into DNA leads to single strand breaks and aberrant incorporation into RNA, thereby interfering with normal RNA function [1–4]. 5-FU directly and specifically inhibits proliferating and synthetically active cells that cause fibrosis. The relative specificity directed to actively synthetic or proliferating cells minimizes clinical tissue toxicity.

The efficacy of 5-FU in the management of scars may also be related to its capacity to interfere with transforming growth factor-β (TGF-β) signaling and resultant type I collagen gene expression in dermal fibroblasts. Abnormally excessive accumulation of type I collagen has been found in keloids and hypertrophic scars, which is believed to play a pathological role in these exuberant scar responses [5, 6]. TGF-β is thought to be the main factor leading to tissue fibrosis secondary to its induction of collagen gene expression. 5-FU has been found to reduce intermediary cell signaling and prevent TGF-β induced gene transactivation and type I collagen production in human fibroblasts, thus providing a mechanism for the efficacy of 5-FU in the treatment of hypertrophic and keloid scars [7–10].

In glaucoma surgery, 5-FU is routinely used for its ability to inhibit and prevent scarring after trabeculectomy surgery [11]. Uppal et al. reported their results utilizing an external application of 5-FU soaked pledgets following extralesional excision of keloids. Biopsies 1 month following treatment showed a reduction in Ki-67 (a marker of cell proliferation), vascular cell adhesion molecule-1 (a marker of inflammation), and TGF-β compared to controls [12].

27.3.2 Management

Intralesional 5-FU has been described as an effective treatment modality in the management of dermal scars, particularly for the treatment of hypertrophic scars and keloids [10, 13–15]. However, as this is an off-label use for 5-FU , the indications, risks, benefits, and alternatives are explained in detail to the patient prior to treatment. For each treatment, an intradermal injection of approximately 0.2–0.3 mL (50 mg/mL, American Pharmaceutical Partners, Schaumburg, IL) is given at weekly or biweekly intervals for a course of one to three treatments based on response. Transient pain at the injection site is the main drawback. The pain of injection can be substantially reduced by mixing 5-FU and lidocaine 2% in the same syringe (2:1–5-FU:lidocaine) and using topical anesthetics. Placement of 5-FU is targeted to the areas of maximal scar density, usually the dermis and subcutaneous tissues. Placement of 0.2–0.5 cc in the skin and areas of maximal scar density using multiple passes is ideal. Given the short half-life of 5-FU, patients are discouraged from massaging the area for 8 h to allow maximal benefit. Softening and improvement in appearance can often be noted after as few as one or two treatment sessions, with continued improvement over the weeks to follow. The literature is mixed in terms of frequency of recurrence, but in the eyelid and face we have noted longstanding results with minimal regression (Fig. 27.2).

Postsurgical eyelid scarring and contracture can result after any eyelid surgery, particularly following lower eyelid reconstruction or blepharoplasty [16, 17]. It can manifest as lower eyelid retraction, ectropion, or entropion depending on the state of the anterior and posterior lamella and is usually apparent as the postoperative edema is regressing (1–2 weeks postsurgery). Resultant signs and symptoms include ocular irritation, photophobia, excessive tearing, and nocturnal

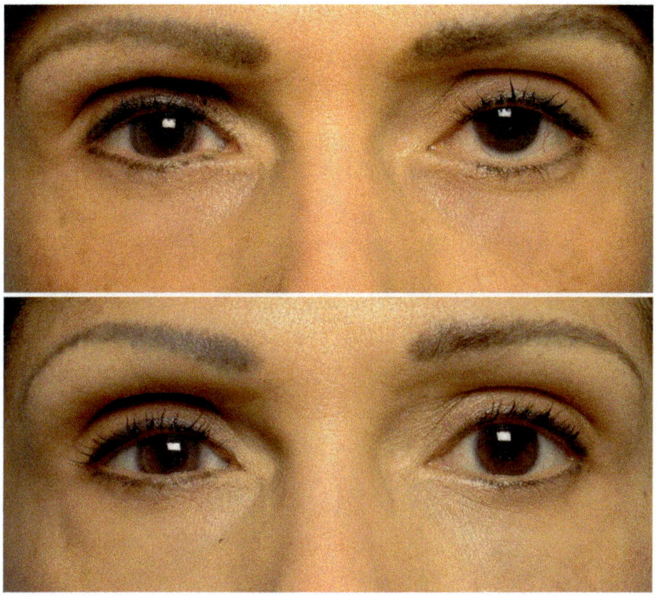

Fig. 27.2 Cicatricial left lower eyelid retraction improved after two 5-FU injections

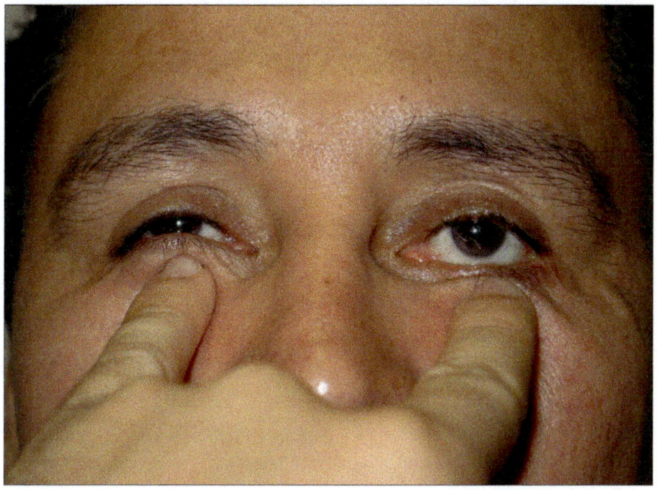

Fig. 27.3 Photograph illustrating cicatricial left lower eyelid retraction, as demonstrated by positive forced upward traction test

lagophthalmos. While aggressive lubrication of the ocular surface with artificial tears and ointments may alleviate some of these symptoms, surgical intervention is usually necessary for management.

Cicatricial wound healing of the lower eyelid can result in significant lower eyelid scarring with subsequent progressive retraction (Fig. 27.3). This can be especially problematic when combined with temporary or permanent localized facial nerve paresis (orbicularis weakness). The injection of anti-metabolites such as 5-FU at the earliest signs of contracture (typically 1–2 weeks after surgery) may minimize this process. Administration of 0.2–0.3 mL of 5-FU mixed with

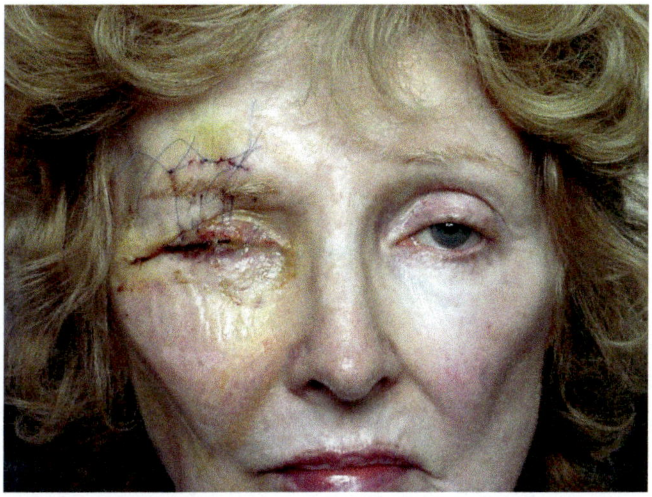

Fig. 27.4 A middle-aged woman with left eyelid Frost suture immediately after lower eyelid surgery

lidocaine in the middle eyelid lamellae surrounding maximal areas of contraction can be carried out via the transcutaneous or transconjunctival route depending upon the areas of contracture at weekly or biweekly intervals. The goal is to maximize 5-FU concentration in the scarred area so that modulation of the healing process can occur in a beneficial way, leading to less cicatrization with maintenance of normal anatomy. Patients can be carefully followed up during the postoperative period, and adjunctive treatments such as placing the eyelid on stretch (i.e., Frost suture) can be utilized (Fig. 27.4). In situations of persistent or significant scarring, we routinely treat the eyelid retraction with scar lysis and middle lamellar stenting with a tissue matrix graft (Alloderm, Lifecell, KCI, Branchburg, NJ) (Fig. 27.5) utilizing a small conjunctival incisional approach. We have found that when a tissue matrix graft is reconstituted in 5-FU, there is dramatic improvement of the cicatrix. The graft likely elutes antimetabolite over an extended time period, reducing the fibrotic process.

Autologous facial fat injections are commonly utilized for soft tissue augmentation to address contour irregularities and volume deflation associated with aging. Encapsulation of autologous injected fat with inflammatory tissue, however, is a relatively common and disfiguring complication, particularly under the thin skin of the periocular region. Attempts at surgical excision or disruption have limited success, unpredictable outcome, and can lead to irregular scars [18]. The authors routinely treat encapsulated fat with intralesional injection of 5-FU. Typically, 0.2–0.3 mL of 5-FU is injected into the fat granuloma, with repeat treatment at 2–3 week intervals. We have found improvement of these lesions with softening, and in a subset of patients, complete resolution of encapsulation of autologous injected fat.

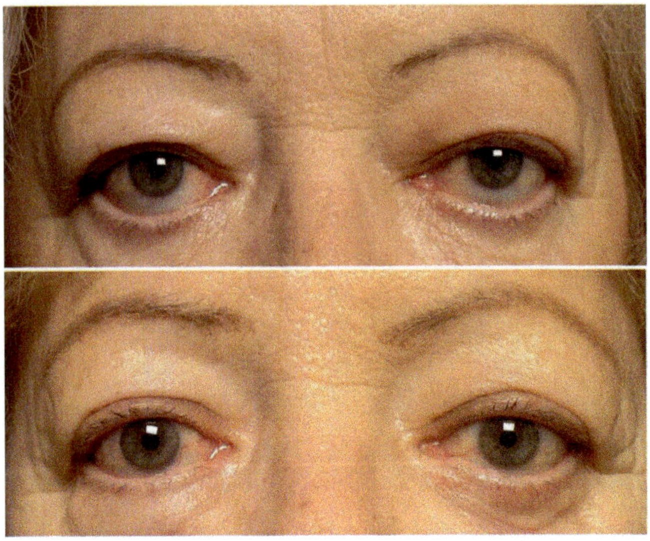

Fig. 27.5 A middle-age female patient, before (*top*) and 3 months after (*bottom*) bilateral cicatricial post-blepharoplasty lower eyelid surgery utilizing a small conjunctival incision approach with scar lysis and middle lamellar stenting with 5-FU soaked Alloderm graft

27.3.3 Safety

Intralesional injections of 5-FU are usually well tolerated, with rare adverse side effects that are typically mild to moderate and localized to the site of treatment. Adverse effects include transient pain, local erythema, edema, and erosions. Hyperpigmentation and occasional ulceration at the site of treatment have been reported, with occasional secondary infections [19, 20]. Rare cases of contact dermatitis have also been described. Serious side effects are rare and have not been experienced by the authors. They include myocardial ischemia, systemic toxicity, and bullous pemphigoid [2, 21–23]. The use of lower doses of injectable 5-FU in conjunction with combination therapy such as concurrent triamcinolone has reported higher success rates and may reduce the incidence of side effects [14, 23].

27.4 Corticosteroids

Corticosteroids have been regularly used for the treatment of pathological scars. Corticosteroid injections have resulted in reduction in scar dimensions, volume, and pliability. However, there has been significant variability in efficacy of treatment, and relatively high rates of recurrence have been reported [24].

27.4.1 Mechanism of Action

While there is a long history of intralesional corticosteroid use for the management of hypertrophic scars [25, 26] and

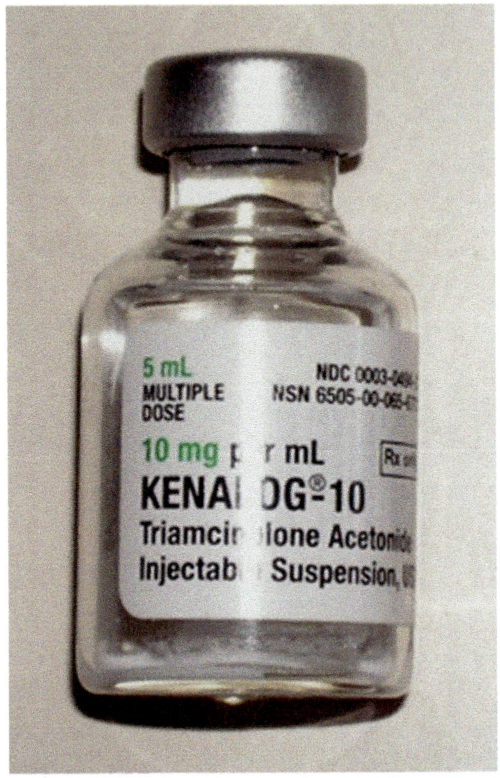

Fig. 27.6 Kenalog is supplied either in 10 mg/mL concentration as shown, or in 40 mg/mL concentration

keloids [27–30], the precise mechanism of action remains unclear. Possible mechanisms of action include inhibition of inflammatory cell migration, vasoconstriction with resultant disruption of nutrient and oxygen supply, antimitotic activity on proliferating fibroblasts and keratinocytes, and promotion of collagen degradation [25–27]. Another study showed that the mechanism of action of intralesional steroid injections may involve suppression of vascular endothelial growth factor expression and fibroblast proliferation [28].

27.4.2 Management

A variety of corticosteroid preparations have been described for the reduction of scar formation, including hydrocortisone acetate, methylprednisone, dexamethasone, and triamcinolone. A commonly utilized regimen is an intradermal injection of 0.1–0.3 mL of triamcinolone directly into the lesion every 3–4 weeks (Fig. 27.6). The lower dosage of 10 mg/mL is used for darker complexions. Prior to treatment, topical anesthetic creams are applied, and distraction techniques used.

Treatment with corticosteroids, while effective, may have relatively high recurrence rates. Some authors have described a combined approach with adjunctive agents, including 5-FU, laser, and cryotherapy, with potentially enhanced efficacy and improved long-term results [31, 32].

27.4.3 Safety

Intralesional corticosteroids are well tolerated, and adverse effects are typically localized to the site of injection. Local side effects include pain and atrophy of skin and subcutaneous tissues, which may be reversible. The potential for contour irregularities within surrounding skin and soft tissue exists, and hyper/hypopigmentation may occur. Rare, more serious complications include local skin necrosis, vascular occlusion, ulcer formation, and systemic effects, including a Cushingoid response [25, 29–31].

27.5 Fillers

Injectable tissue fillers have been increasingly utilized as a treatment modality for soft tissue augmentation to address fat deflation associated with aging. This approach is also a viable treatment option to address contour deformities associated with scar formation, while also allowing for improvement of age-related periorbital hollows.

The authors have found that cross-linked hyaluronic acid gel (Restylane, Medicis Corporation, Scottsdale, AZ) works well as a filler for the management of contour deformities in the periocular area (Fig. 27.7) related to scarring. Topical 5% lidocaine is initially applied over the eyelid skin prior to the procedure. Hyaluronic acid gel is injected in a fanning pattern, with multiple passes made to create a layered, thread-like configuration. The entire length of the needle should be directed into the scar, and gel deposited along the length of the scar. A cotton-tipped applicator is used to apply gentle pressure to the injection site to minimize bleeding/bruising.

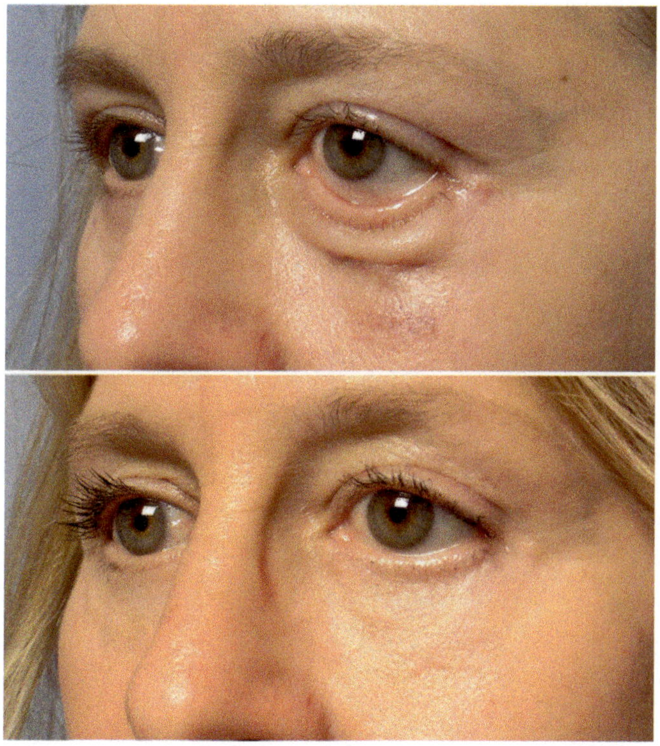

Fig. 27.7 A young female patient with left lower eye cicatricial retraction, treated with hyaluronic acid gel injection to stent the eyelid and correct the contour irregularity. Before (*top*); 3 months post-injection (*bottom*)

Post-injection contour irregularities can be treated with hyaluronidase, which may reduce the effect of the filler. The effect of the filler diminishes over time (typically 6 months), although persistence may be seen for longer periods. Also, progressive tissue molding and expansion may continue after loss of filler. Maintenance treatments may be performed as needed.

27.5.1 Safety

Hyaluronic acid gel filler is typically well tolerated, and adverse effects are usually limited to the injection site. Adverse effects include pain, bruising, swelling, and tenderness at the injection site. Rare but serious complications include vascular embolization with necrosis [33].

27.6 Conclusions

Wound modulation in the postoperative setting of aesthetic eyelid and periorbital surgery is critical in the final surgical outcome. While surgical advances in minimally invasive surgical techniques continue to evolve, there is a definite and necessary role for nonsurgical adjunctive methods, which address the underlying biologic process of wound healing and scar formation. These include the utilization of anti-metabolites and anti-inflammatory agents (5-FU, corticosteroids) and injectable tissue fillers with tissue volume expansion. In the future, we await the production of other modulators that can target the mechanisms for scar formation more specifically.

References

1. Danenberg PV, Shea LC, et al. Effect of 5-fluorouracil substitution on the self-splicing activity of tetrahymena ribosomal RNA. Cancer Res. 1990;50(6):1757–63.
2. Goette DK. Topical chemotherapy with 5-flurouracil. J Am Acad Dermatol. 1981;4(6):633–49.
3. Longley DB, Latif T, et al. The interaction of thymidylate synthase expression with p53-regulated signaling pathways in tumor cells. Semin Oncol. 2003;30(3 Suppl 6):3–9.
4. Longley DB, Harkin DP, Johnston PG. 5-fluorouracil: mechanisms of action and clinical strategies. Nat Rev Cancer. 2003;3(5):330–8.
5. Ehrlich HP, Desmoulière A, et al. Morphological and immunochemical differences between keloid and hypertrophic scar. Am J Pathol. 1994;145(1):105–13.

6. Uitto J, Kouba D. Cytokine modulation of extracellular matrix gene expression: relevance to fibrotic skin diseases. J Dermatol Sci. 2000;24 Suppl 1:S60–9.
7. Wendling J, Marchand A, et al. 5-Fluorouracil blocks transforming growth factor-beta-induced alpha 2 type I collagen gene (COL1A2) expression in human fibroblasts via c-Jun NH2-terminal kinase/activator protein-1 activation. Mol Pharmacol. 2003;64(3):707–13.
8. Bulstrode NW, Mudera V, et al. 5-Fluorouracil selectively inhibits collagen synthesis. Plast Reconstr Surg. 2005;116(1):209–21; discussion 222–3.
9. de Waard JW, de Man BM, et al. Inhibition of fibroblast collagen synthesis and proliferation by levamisole and 5-fluorouracial. Eur J Cancer. 1998;34(1):162–7.
10. Chin GS, Liu W, et al. Differential expression of transforming growth factor-beta receptors I and II and activation of Smad 3 in keloid fibroblasts. Plast Reconstr Surg. 2001;108(2):423–9.
11. The Fluorouracil Filtering Surgery Study Group. Five-year follow-up of the Fluorouracil Filtering Surgery Study. Am J Ophthalmol. 1996;121(4):349–66.
12. Uppal RS, Khan U, et al. The effects of a single dose of 5-fluorouracial on keloid scars: a clinical trial of timed wound irrigation after extralesional excision. Plast Reconstr Surg. 2001;108(5):1218–24.
13. Berman B, Viera MH, et al. Prevention and management of hypertrophic scars and keloids after burns in children. J Craniofac Surg. 2008;19(4):989–1006.
14. Fitzpatrick RE. Treatment of inflamed hypertrophic scars using intralesional 5-FU. Dermatol Surg. 1999;25(3):224–32.
15. Gupta S, Kalra A. Efficacy and safety of intralesional 5-fluorouracil in the treatment of keloids. Dermatology. 2002;204(2):130–2.
16. Seiff SR. Complications of upper and lower blepharoplasty. Int Ophthalmol Clin. 1992 Fall;32(4):67–77.
17. Baylis HI, Nelson ER, et al. Lower eyelid retraction following blepharoplasty. Ophthal Plast Reconstr Surg. 1992;8(3):170–5.
18. Eremia S, Newman N. Long-term follow-up after autologous fat grafting: analysis of results from 116 patients followed at least 12 months after receiving the last of a minimum of two treatments. Dermatol Surg. 2000;26(12):1150–8.
19. Miller BH, Shavin JS, et al. Nonsurgical treatment of basal cell carcinomas with intralesional 5-fluorouracil/epinephrine injectable gel. J Am Acad Dermatol. 1997;36(1):72–7.
20. Romagosa R, Saap L, et al. A pilot study to evaluate the treatment of basal cell carcinoma with 5-fluorouracil using phosphatidyl choline as a transepidermal carrier. Dermatol Surg. 2000;26(4):338–40.
21. Rozenman Y, Gurewich J, et al. Myocardial ischemia induced by topical use of 5-fluorouracil. Int J Cardiol. 1995;49(3):282–3.
22. Johnson MR, Hageboutros A, et al. Life-threatening toxicity in a dihydropyrimidine dehydrogenase-deficient patient after treatment with topical 5-fluorouracil. Clin Cancer Res. 1999;5(8):2006–11.
23. Apikian M, Goodman G. Intralesional 5-fluorouracil in the treatment of keloid scars. Australas J Dermatol. 2004;45(2):140–3.
24. Niessen FB, Spauwen PH, et al. On the nature of hypertrophic scars and keloids: a review. Plast Reconstr Surg. 1999;104(5):1435–58.
25. Wang XQ, Liu YK, et al. A review of the effectiveness of antimitotic drug injections for hypertrophic scars and keloids. Ann Plast Surg. 2009;63(6):688–92.
26. Reed BR, Clark RA. Cutaneous tissue repair: practical implications of current knowledge, II. J Am Acad Dermatol. 1985;13(6):919–41.
27. Kauh YC, Souda S, et al. Major suppression of pro-alpha1(I) type I collagen gene expression in the dermis after keloid excision and immediate intrawound injection of triamcinolone acetonide. J Am Acad Dermatol. 1997;37(4):586–9.
28. Wu WS, Wang FS, et al. Dexamethasone induction of keloid regression through effective suppression of VEGF expression and keloid fibroblast proliferation. J Invest Dermatol. 2006;126(6):1264–71.
29. Darzi MA, Chowdri NA, et al. Evaluation of various methods of treating keloids and hypertrophic scars: a 10 year follow-up study. Br J Plast Surg. 1992;45(5):374–9.
30. Manuskiatti W, Fitzpatrick RE. Treatment response of keloidal and hypertrophic sternotomy scars: comparison among intralesional corticosteroid, 5-fluorouracil, and 585 nm flashlamp pumped pulsed dye laser treatments. Arch Dermatol. 2002;138(9):1149–55.
31. Yosipovitch G, Widijanti SM, et al. A comparison of the combined effect of cryotherapy and corticosteroid injections versus corticosteroids and cryotherapy alone on keloids: a controlled study. J Dermatolog Treat. 2001;12(2):87–90.
32. Shaffer JJ, Taylor SC, et al. Keloidal scars: a review with a critical look at therapeutic options. J Am Acad Dermatol. 2002;46(2 Suppl Understanding):S63–97.
33. Burt B, Nakra T, et al. Alar necrosis after facial injection of hyaluronic acid. Plast Reconstr Surg. 2010;125(5):199–200.

28 Short-Flap Superficial Musculo-Aponeurotic System (SMAS) Rhytidectomy

Babak Azizzadeh and Kimberly J. Lee

Key Points

- Individuals who are seeking periorbital rejuvenation must also be analyzed for lower and midfacial aging changes; patients who are undergoing periorbital rejuvenation often require simultaneous rhytidectomy in order to create a balanced esthetic outcome.
- The superficial musculo-aponeurotic system (SMAS) is a fascial tissue layer between the subcutaneous fat and the parotidomasseteric fascia investing the muscles of facial expression and its incorporation in rhytidectomy has significantly improved surgical outcomes.
- The facial nerve is one of the most critical anatomic structures in facelift surgery.
- Short-flap SMAS rhytidectomy (SFR) is a facelift technique that can be mastered with appropriate training.
- The risk profile of SFR is generally lower than other rhytidectomy procedures that require significant SMAS, subcutaneous, deep plane, or subperiosteal dissections.
- Midface volume restoration with fat grafting or injectable fillers can be performed simultaneously with SFR.
- SFR has a high patient satisfaction and excellent esthetic outcome.
- Restoring a youthful appearance often requires more than just surgical intervention. It is the combination of surgery with nonsurgical modalities that is often required to yield optimal results.
- Individuals with poor chin projection and prominent prejowl sulcus may also require chin augmentation in order to obtain enhanced results.
- Rhytidectomy patients with a low and anteriorly positioned hyoid bone will not obtain satisfactory results in the neck.

B. Azizzadeh (✉)
Center for Advanced Facial Plastic Surgery, Assistant Clinical Professor of Surgery, Department of Facial Plastic and Reconstructive Surgery, David Geffen School of Medicine at UCLA, Beverly Hills, CA, USA
e-mail: md@facialplastics.info

28.1 History

Over the past century, facelift techniques have greatly evolved. Initially, in the early twentieth century, only skin excisions were performed with ephemeral results. In 1919, Bettman and Bourget simultaneously presented their experiences with subcutaneous rhytidectomy [1, 2]. Despite limited understanding of the facial anatomy, surgeons were attempting to improve facelift results by extending skin undermining, which increased the complication rates with only minimal esthetic improvement.

In due time, as surgical techniques evolved and the understanding of facial structures and layers advanced, surgeons obtained longer lasting results to satisfy the demands of their patients. Aufricht was the first to introduce the concept of deep tissue plication in 1960, while Webster used similar techniques of suturing the deeper layers for enhanced results [3–5]. During the same era, Skoog advanced facelift outcomes by using both the skin and platysma as a musculocutaneous advancement flap [6]. In 1976, Mitz and Peyronie described this deeper tissue layer in anatomic studies and named it the superficial musculo-aponeurotic system (SMAS) [7]. They proposed that this deeper fascial tissue layer between the subcutaneous fat and the parotid-masseteric fascia invested the muscles of facial expression, and its incorporation in rhytidectomy gained popularity [8–14]. In the 1980s and 1990s, the deep plane facelift [15–20] and subperiosteal facelift [21–30] were increasingly utilized. However, variations of the SMAS facelift continued to be commonly performed.

Richard Webster was the first to advocate rhytidectomy with conservative skin undermining to maintain the integrity of dermal-SMAS attachments. This concept was innovative for a few reasons. First, Webster demonstrated that this technique, combined with SMAS plication, resulted in a better outcome than more aggressive surgical techniques [5, 31–34]. Additionally, this method decreased the tension on the incision and increased the amount of facial suspension from the

G.G. Massry et al. (eds.), *Master Techniques in Blepharoplasty and Periorbital Rejuvenation*,
DOI 10.1007/978-1-4614-0067-7_28, © Springer Science+Business Media, LLC 2011

procedure. A recent cadaveric study compared different SMAS facelift techniques and found that wound tension increased significantly with increased skin undermining when compared to shorter skin flaps [35]. Webster's technique was further adapted by McCollough who advocated maintaining the skin adipose-SMAS integrity for even better results and coined the procedure "suspension rhytidectomy" [36].

28.2 Short-Flap SMAS Rhytidectomy

Having performed facelifts using a myriad of different techniques, including the standard, long-flap SMAS, deep plane, and "mini" facelifts, it appears that a modified version of the Webster SMAS facelift with limited skin undermining is a worthy option for obtaining excellent results. There are several key components of performing the SFR, which include undermining a conservative amount of skin in the facial region, imbricating the SMAS, performing platysmaplasty, and liposuctioning a limited amount of fat in the cervical region. The anterior dermal-SMAS attachments remain intact because of the conservative facial skin flap dissection, thereby allowing aggressive facial suspension while avoiding significant wound tension. The SMAS is an integral component of this procedure as the carrier of the rhytidectomy flap.

The SFR offers some distinct advantages over alternative rhytidectomy techniques. This technique minimizes the risk for facial nerve injury by limiting the area of dissection beyond the parotid gland as well as the possibility for postoperative hematoma formation. Because of the limited elevation of skin flap, the likelihood of vascular compromise is also diminished, especially in smokers, diabetics, and elderly patients [37, 38]. Furthermore, there is a significant decrease in the procedure duration and postoperative edema, which in turn minimizes recovery time. Another advantage of the SFR is high patient satisfaction and excellent esthetic outcome. Although prospective randomized long-term studies have not been performed, we have not found any difference between the longevity of results between the SFR and other more invasive rhytidectomy techniques. Our philosophy for elective esthetic surgery is to obtain outstanding results, reduce the risk of perioperative morbidity, and allow patients to resume their normal activity at the earliest possible time. Most patients undergoing this technique resume normal activity within 7–10 days postoperatively.

Over the past decade, we have gained a better understanding of the significant role of volume loss in midface and lower face aging process (Fig. 28.1) [39, 40]. Volume restoration has gained significant attention for treating this underlying cause of facial aging [41, 42]. Traditional rhytidectomy procedures often preclude the use of autologous fat grafting due to extensive undermining of midface and lower facial tissue layers. Since the midface and prejowl regions are not dissected during the SFR, these areas could safely undergo autologous fat grafting.

In contrast to the SFR, long-skin flaps (using SMAS or subcutaneous techniques) require extensive undermining of the skin to release the fascio-osteo-cutaneous ligaments [43–49]. However, during this process, the dermal-SMAS attachments are separated, thereby preventing the SMAS support required to accomplish the lift. Furthermore, careful attention needs to be directed to the anatomy of the facial nerve in order to prevent inadvertent damage to the distal branches. The facial nerve branches near the oral commissure

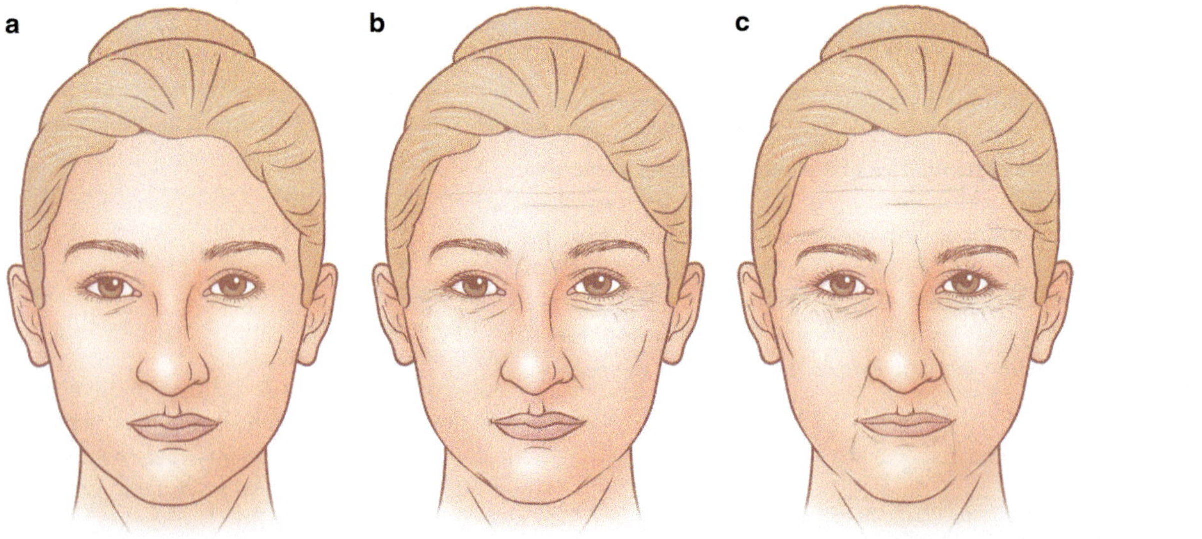

Fig. 28.1 The progression of the aging face. The aging process is illustrated in an individual in their 20s (**a**), 40s (**b**), and 60s (**c**). The face continuously and gradually changes resulting in prominent nasolabial folds, jowl formation, marionette furrows, neck laxity, volume loss, and rhytids in the perioral and periorbital region

and midportion of the zygomatic arch run in a more superficial fashion, endangering injury during long-skin flap dissection [50]. Muzzafar et al. and Mendelson et al. also demonstrated that releasing retaining ligaments in the prezygomatic space through extensive subcutaneous dissection can potentially cause nerve injury to the motor branch of the orbicularis oculi [48, 49].

Unlike the SFR, deep plane rhytidectomy does not involve aggressive undermining of the skin. Deep plane facelifts incorporate a sub-SMAS composite musculocutaneous advancement flap. The results of the deep plane facelift in the lower face (namely the jowls and neck) are very consistent because the SMAS serves as a carrier of the facelift. Midface enhancement, including the nasolabial folds, using the deep plane facelift is more controversial. Owsley and others have shown that the SMAS must be completely released beyond the melolabial fold over the zygomaticus muscle to truly obtain satisfactory nasolabial effacement [51–54]. Not only can a lengthy anteromedial dissection cause extensive postoperative edema, but it can also significantly endanger the branches of the facial nerve. Furthermore, the deep plane facelift does not address lipoatrophy associated with the aging process much like the SFR. Today, facial rejuvenation techniques are also less focused on effacing the nasolabial folds and more focused on volume restoration of the midface. While controversy exists as to the best technique to achieve the best outcome, the deep plane facelift may have better outcomes in older patients with extensive rhytidosis [55, 56].

Rhytidectomy procedures, including the SFR technique, are not without shortcomings. The SFR does not address several important issues, such as the double cheek convexity, infra-orbital rim hollowness, tear trough deformity, facial volume loss, and deep nasolabial folds. Injectable fillers (calcium hydroxylapatite, hyaluronic acids), subcutaneous volumizers (poly-L-lactic acid), fat grafting, and/or implants may need to be performed to address the aging process of the midface [57].

Over the past decade, patient demands for decreased postoperative recovery time has stimulated the resurgence of "limited," "mini," or "endoscopic" facelifts. In our experience, "mini" facelifts appear to be ideal only for a select group of patients with minimal signs of facial aging or those requiring minor revision touch-ups [56, 58–60].

28.3 Key Anatomic Features

Knowledge of the anatomy is critical for any surgical procedure to obtain outstanding results while avoiding inadvertent complications. The anatomical relationships of the tissues serve as the basis for rhytidectomy. The facial musculature in the face, midface, and neck is surrounded by the SMAS that extends to the preparotid region and continues with the neck platysma inferiorly and frontalis superiorly. In the anterior neck, the platysma may or may not interdigitate to form a sling. Laxity and/or dehiscence of this anteriorly in the neck can cause neck banding.

The SMAS is the key structural layer of tissue in rhytidectomies. Because of the inherent characteristic of creep phenomenon in the skin and rebound characteristics, skin-only rhytidectomy does not yield long-lasting results. Only when the SMAS layer is incorporated into the procedure are the effects of rhytidectomy longer lasting. The SMAS layer is connected to the skin in the middle and central portion of the face by strong dermal filaments such that lifting and pulling the SMAS layer, while still integrated to the platysma and facial muscles, lift and reposition the skin satisfactorily. The continuity of the skin and SMAS layer as a functional unit is also necessary to maximize the safety and longevity of rhytidectomies [31–34, 36]. This is a critical point because if the two are separated, the SMAS will lose the functional support of the skin layer. This principle guides the surgical outcome in short-flap and deep plane rhytidectomies [15–20]. Long-flap SMAS and extended SMAS facelifts, on the other hand, detach the skin from the SMAS layer and disrupt the skin-SMAS attachments.

In addition to the facial anatomy, a strong grasp of the fundamental knowledge of the neurosensory and neuromotor branches of the face is critical to avoid complications of mimetic dysfunction. Following rhytidectomy, temporary paresthesias and loss of sensation are expected in the auricular region. The trigeminal nerve (cranial nerve V) supplies cutaneous sensation to the face, head, and neck. Any type of rhytidectomy requires elevation of the preauricular and postauricular skin, which interrupts innervation in these regions of the face. Return of sensation is expected within the first 6–8 weeks if no damage is rendered to the major branch of the greater auricular nerve, but can occasionally take longer. If the sternocleidomastoid fascia is violated with damage to the greater auricular nerve, immediate nerve anastomosis is recommended and permanent loss of sensation is uncommon.

The facial nerve is one of the most critical anatomic structures in facelift surgery. Originating in the pons, the facial nerve exits extracranially through the stylomastoid foramen to enter the parotid gland, where it first divides into an upper and lower division before further subdividing into five main branches: frontal, zygomatic, buccal, marginal mandibular, and cervical branches (Fig. 28.2). Branches of the facial nerve course superficially once past the parotidomasseteric fascia. Due to the extensive arborization of the facial nerve, permanent iatrogenic facial paralysis is uncommon in the zygomatic and buccal region. However, the frontal and marginal mandibular are often terminal branches with limited arborization and injury to them has the highest risk of leading

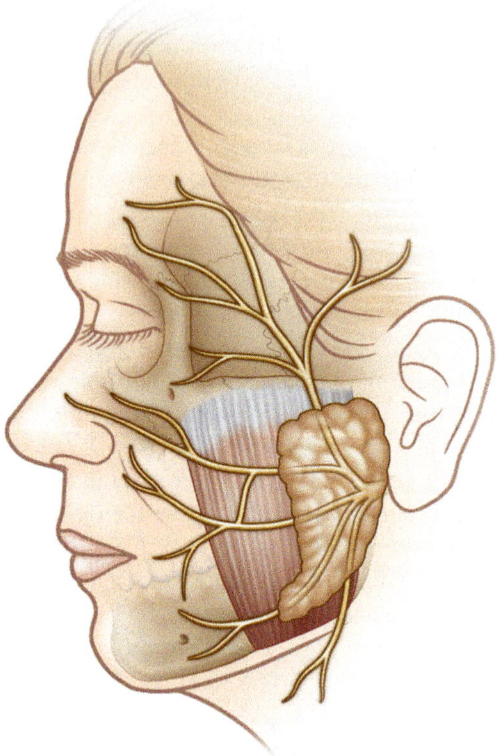

Fig. 28.2 The facial nerve. The facial nerve bifurcates in the parotid into an upper and lower division. It then divides into five main branches: frontal, zygomatic, buccal, marginal mandibular, and cervical

to permanent paralysis (0.53 and 2.6%) [38, 61, 62]. The marginal mandibular nerve is of risk as it courses over the mandibular margin. Deep plane elevation underneath the SMAS layer in the midface endangers facial nerve branches innervating the orbicularis, zygomatic, and buccinators muscles. Of the facial nerve branches, the frontal branch is the most commonly injured branch as it runs in the danger zone. The branch courses superficially at the level of the zygomatic arch, extending just beneath the subcutaneous tissues underneath the SMAS layer before reaching the frontalis muscle. To prevent injury to this region, it is critical that the surgeon comprehends the anatomical relationships of the layers of the face and temporal region. At the level of the zygomatic arch, the level of dissection needs to be either thin subcutaneous (traditional rhytidectomy) or subperiosteal (endoscopic midface lift) or else transection of the nerve will result. Innervation of the frontalis muscle is unpredictable following injury.

Lastly, attention towards the underlying bony framework of the face and neck is extremely important to maximize satisfactory results in cervicofacial rhytidectomy. Attention should be particularly focused on the key skeletal regions of the malar and submalar regions, dental occlusion, chin projection, and hyoid position. Patients with visible loss of elasticity in the jowl regions, as well as neck skin and platysma, are ideal for rhytidectomies. Patients with malar prominence, submalar fullness, and good chin projection will obtain enhanced results from SFR. If these areas are deficient, skeletal and/or volume enhancements should be considered prior to the rhytidectomy. Individuals with poor chin projection and prominent prejowl sulcus may require chin augmentation in order to obtain ideal results. Finally, patients with a low and anteriorly positioned hyoid bone will not obtain satisfactory results in the neck [63]. Unfortunately, the hyoid cannot be repositioned during rhytidectomy, thus limiting maximal results.

28.4 Preoperative Assessment

Individuals who are seeking periorbital rejuvenation must be also analyzed for lower and midfacial aging changes. Patients who are good candidates for periorbital rejuvenation often require simultaneous lower facial rejuvenation in order to create a balanced esthetic outcome. The typical facelift patient is one who is over 45 years old and is concerned with jowl formation, neck banding, and midface volume loss. During the preoperative consultation, an accurate assessment of the patient's concerns and expectations need to be understood and discussed. Often this discussion is facilitated with the use of mirrors and morphing equipment to allow the patient to clearly understand the aging process and potential surgical benefits. A comprehensive facial analysis with a clear understanding of the goals is mandatory for successful results.

Facial analysis needs to focus on four key components of the aging process: cutaneous photodamage, facial laxity, musculo-skeletal-lipoatrophy, and dynamic rhytids. Restoring a youthful appearance often requires more than just surgical intervention. It is the combination of surgery with other modalities that yield optimal results. A discussion of skin care, including an antiaging regimen, sun protection, and tobacco cessation, needs to be thoroughly addressed to enhance long-term results. Then, nonsurgical procedures, such as skin resurfacing, soft tissue fillers, and neuromodulators (botulinum toxin-A), are considered. The consultation then focuses on areas that will benefit from facial plastic surgery. To achieve a balanced and natural appearing esthetically pleasing outcome, all regions of the face need to be properly evaluated. Table 28.1 highlights the surgical and nonsurgical options discussed during the consultation process. Should the patient be a surgical candidate, a second consultation will be used to further discuss the risks, alternatives, and perioperative course of the surgical procedures. Photographs should be reviewed in detail with patients during the consultations.

Table 28.1 Comprehensive facial evaluation

Upper-third
Upper blepharoplasty
Endoscopic browlift
Neuromodulators
Dermal fillers and fat grafting
Middle-third
Dermal fillers, volumizers, fat grafting
Lower blepharoplasty
Endoscopic midface lift
Malar and submalar implant
Skin resurfacing
Lower-third
Short-flap SMAS rhytidectomy
Dermal fillers, volumizers, fat grafting
Chin and prejowl augmentation

Table 28.2 Medications to avoid preoperatively

A.P.C.	Darvon compound
Advil	Dristan
Alka-Seltzer	Doan's pills
Anacin	Duragesic
Anaprox	Ecotrin
Arthritis pain formula	Empirin
Ascodeen-30	Emprazil
Ascriptin	Equagesic
Aspirin suppositories (all brands)	Excedrin
Aspirin	Fiorinol
Bayer Aspirin	Four-way cold tablets
Buff-a-Comp	Indocin
Buffadyne	Measurin
Bufferin	Midol
Butalbital	Monacet with Codeine
Carna arthritis pain reliever	Motrin
Carna-Inlay tabs	Naprosyn
Cheracol capsules	Norgesic
Congespirin	Nuprin
Cope Coricidin	Os-Cal-Gone
Coricidin	Pamprin Pamprin (buffered)

28.5 Preoperative Care

Rhytidectomy may be performed under IV sedation or general anesthesia. To optimize results, patients are encouraged to avoid certain medications, especially blood thinners and herbal products, starting 2 weeks prior to surgery (Table 28.2). The patients are started on Arnica and Bromolin approximately 3 days prior to the surgery to reduce perioperative bleeding, edema, and ecchymoses as well as psychologically prepare patients for the upcoming surgery.

In the preoperative area, a marking pen is used to identify the incision areas as well as important landmarks for the SFR, blepharoplasty, and endoscopic browlift in the upright position as the landmarks can be distorted once supine.

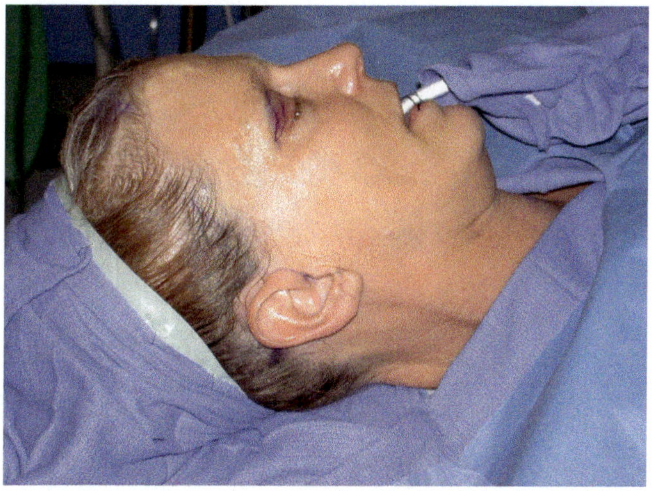

Fig. 28.3 The preparation. Autoclave tape is applied to the hair 2–4 cm posterior to hair line. Sterile towel is then stapled to the autoclave tape and the endotracheal tube is wrapped in a sterile manner

Table 28.3 Sequential order of procedures

Transconjunctival lower blepharoplasty
Endoscopic brow lift
Endoscopic midface lift
Upper blepharoplasty
Lower pinch blepharoplasty
Submental liposuction
Platysmaplasty
Chin implant
Rhytidectomy

Patients are given an opportunity to visualize the proposed incisions with a mirror.

28.6 Surgical Preparation and Technique

Patients can elect either general anesthesia or IV sedation. If general anesthesia is chosen, the endotracheal tube is sutured to the bottom teeth in the midline. Cefazolin and steroids are administered intravenously, and a foley catheter and lower extremity pulsatile compression stockings are placed. 1% lidocaine with 1:100,000 epinephrine is infiltrated using a 3-cc syringe and 27-g needle for the face or brow or a 1-cc syringe with 30-g needle for blepharoplasty prior to prepping and draping the patient. This will maximize time for vasoconstriction to occur. Next, autoclave tape is placed circumferentially around the head 2–4 cm behind the hairline to properly secure the hair away from the surgical field (Fig. 28.3). The entire face and anterior hairline are prepped using diluted betadine. A sterile blue towel is used as a head drape and secured to the autoclave tape via staples. The endotracheal tube is wrapped in a sterile manner using either blue towels or drapes.

Some patients elect to undergo multiple procedures simultaneously and Table 28.3 outlines the recommended order.

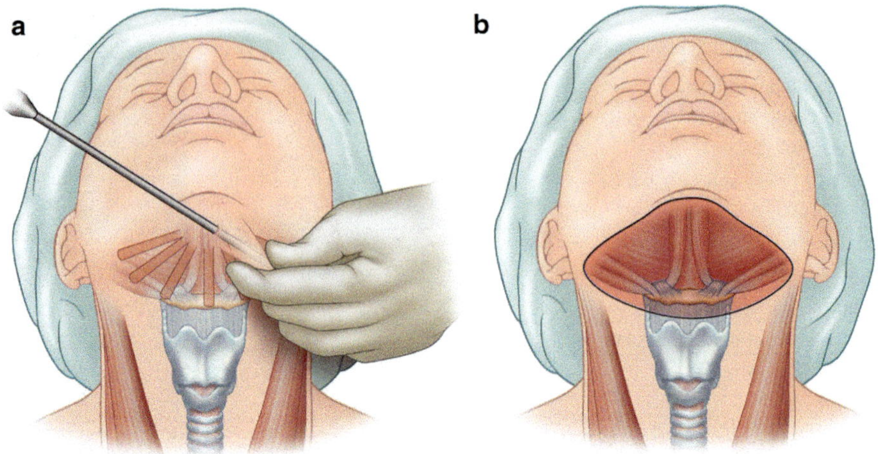

Fig. 28.4 Submental suction-assisted lipectomy. Suction-assisted lipectomy is usually performed through a submental incision (**a**). A fan-shaped region is aspirated (**b**). The body of the mandible is avoided in order to minimize the risk of marginal mandibular facial nerve injury

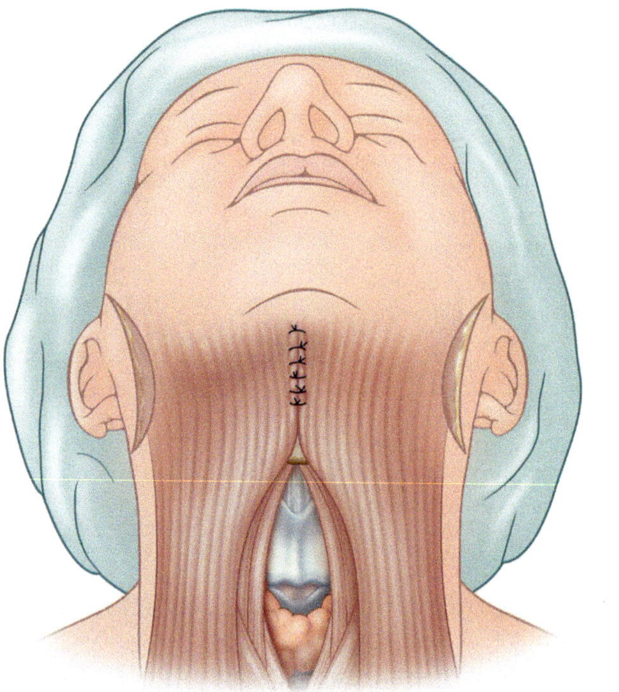

Fig. 28.5 Platysmaplasty. Platysmaplasty allows the lateral SMAS/platysma imbrication to lift the neck as a sling and create a more defined cervicomental angle. Three to six buried interrupted 3–0 Mersilene sutures are utilized to plicate the muscles together. The first suture is placed at the most anterior portion of the platysma

Prior to each portion of the procedure, a second round of local anesthetic using 1% lidocaine with 1:100,000 epinephrine can be considered depending on the time since the initial injection. The face procedures generally begin with suction-assisted lipectomy of the submental region if the patient has liposis. Either a stab incision or a 1–2-cm incision is made in the submental crease. Platysmaplasty or chin implants would require the longer incision to be made. A 1-mm liposuction cannula with multiple ports is used for suction-assisted lipectomy and is inserted deep to the dermis. Multiple passes of the cannula is performed rapidly in a folding fan-shaped fashion (Fig. 28.4). Caution is used to avoid overzealous fat removal to prevent the potential complication of cobra neck deformity. Attention should be directed towards avoiding the body of the mandible to prevent inadvertent marginal mandibular nerve injury.

Approximating the platysma creates a better-defined cervicomental angle by imbricating the lateral SMAS and platysma to lift the neck. If plastysmaplasty is to be performed, an Aufricht retractor is placed in the incision to visualize the platysma (Fig. 28.5), which is facilitated by vertical spreading with facelift scissors. Once the medial borders of the plastyma are identified, subcutaneous dissection is performed laterally. A small strip of the platysma muscle is excised medially to allow adhesion of the two sides after they are reapproximated. If necessary, backcut of the platysma in a horizontal fashion can be performed at the level of the cervicomental angle. Preplatysmal fat can be judiciously removed in a direct manner as needed at this point. The muscles are plicated using buried interrupted 3–0 PDS (Ethicon, New Brunswick, NJ) with the first of 3–6 sutures placed at the most anterior portion of the platysma extending down to the level of the cervicomental angle. Chin augmentation usually is performed at this point if indicated.

Once the adjunct procedures are completed, attention is then directed toward performing the rhytidectomy. Starting with a 2–3-cm incision in the anterior temporal hair tuft (Figs. 28.6 and 28.7), the incision is slightly curved posteriorly to meet the root of the helix. The temporal hairline incision should never be at the junction of the nonhair-bearing region as it has a high chance of being visible even with meticulous closure. From the root of the helix, the incision will continue along the preauricular contour down to the tragus inferiorly. The incision is then created in the retrotragal region in women, before following the natural crease just anterior to the lobule and then posteriorly onto the postauricular conchal bowl. In men, a pretragal incision is created to avoid placing the sideburn hair inside the ear. The postauricular incision is continued about 3 mm onto the conchal bowl to the junction of the helix and the occipital hair tuft before continuing into the occipital hair tuft for an additional 3 cm. The occipital incision is at a 45° angle and does not follow the hairline because of increased visibility.

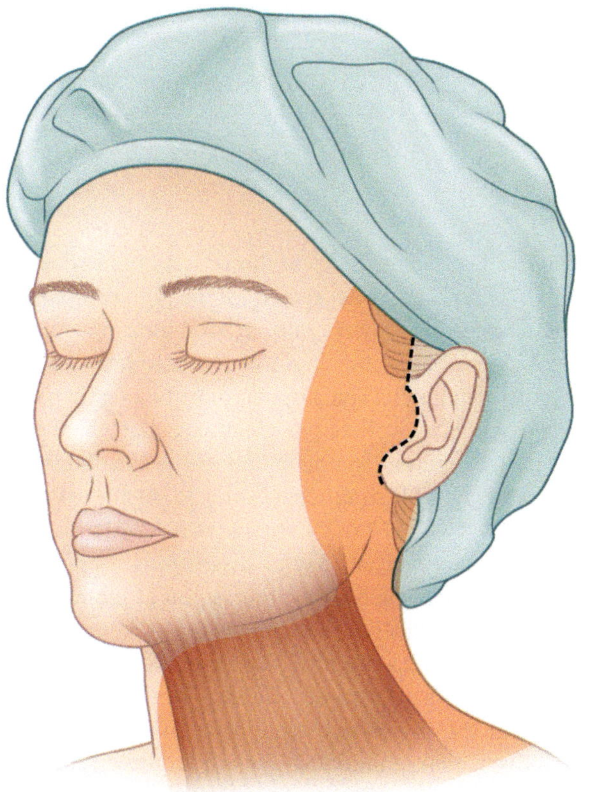

Fig. 28.6 The incision and area of dissection in short-flap rhytidectomy. The temporal and occipital incisions are limited. A retrotragal route is utilized. The facial region is dissected for 4–5 cm. The neck is widely dissected to the submental region

The postauricular incision is generally well camouflaged because of the inconspicuous location and heals unnoticeably. Occasionally, a short-scar facelift using a limited postauricular incision can be performed in a select number of patients.

A Brown Adson and No. 15 scalpel are used to begin the flap elevation in the subcutaneous plane at the temporal hair tuft and midface region (Fig. 28.8). Once the plane is identified, double prong skin hooks or 4-prong cat-paws are placed to aid the remainder of the undermining performed with Metzenbaum scissors. During the subcutaneous elevation, countertraction of the skin on the opposite side of the flap by the assistant is critical to preserve the appropriate plane of dissection. Of note, a thick skin flap is dissected at the level of the tragus, just above the perichondrium measuring approximately 8–10 mm. The facial skin is significantly thicker than the native tragal skin and obliteration of the pretragal notch is a telltale sign of facelift procedures. Aggressive thinning of the skin at the end of the procedure significantly limits postoperative tragal fullness, leading to a more appealing esthetic result.

The extent of facial skin undermining is minimal in the SFR. Skin elevation is performed for only 4–5 cm in the facial region. This limited skin dissection is the most important variation of the SFR as compared to other SMAS facelift procedure. Note that the most inferior aspect of the facial dissection at the angle of the mandible is not performed until the posterior neck elevation is completed. The temporal and zygomatic arch regions need to be dissected with extreme care in the subcutaneous plane, as it is very easy to dive down to a deeper plane where the frontal branch can be easily injured (Fig. 28.9).

Once the facial skin elevation is completed, the postauricular and cervical dissection is initiated. The posterior occipital area is elevated initially with a No. 10 or 15 blade (Fig. 28.10). This dissection is more fibrous and difficult than the anterior dissection. The subcutaneous plane is more

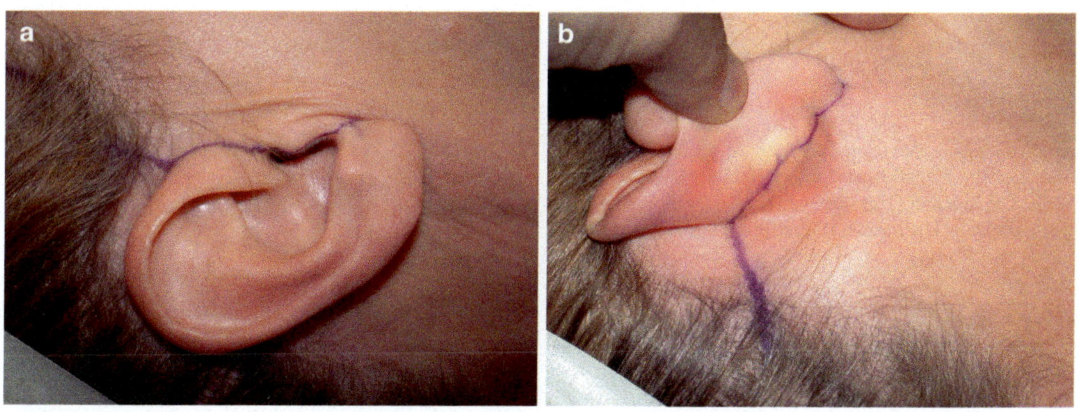

Fig. 28.7 Intraoperative markings for incisions. Preauricular incision (**a**). Postauricular incision (**b**)

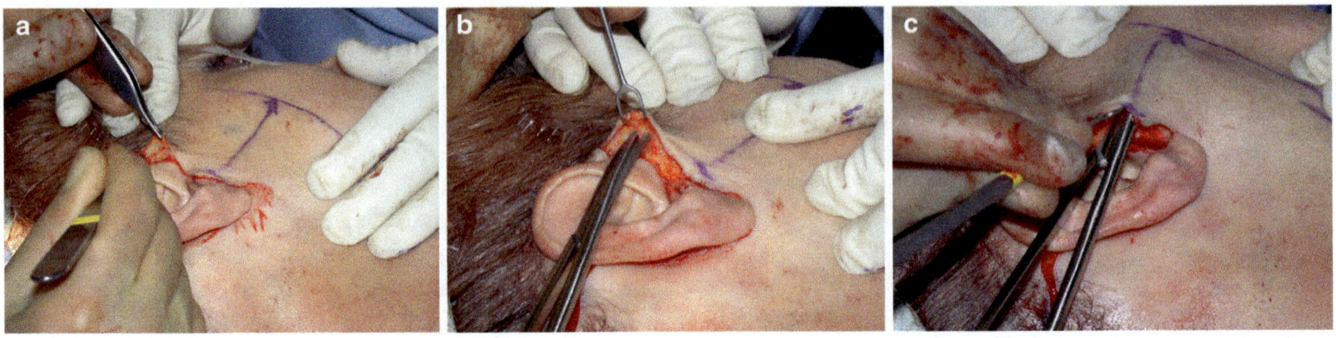

Fig. 28.8 Facial subcutaneous dissection. The flap elevation starts at the temporal hair (**a**). Brown Adson and 15 blade are utilized to start the dissection. Double hook is utilized with Metzenbaum scissors for the majority of the undermining (**b**, **c**). The assistant retracts the facial skin centrally

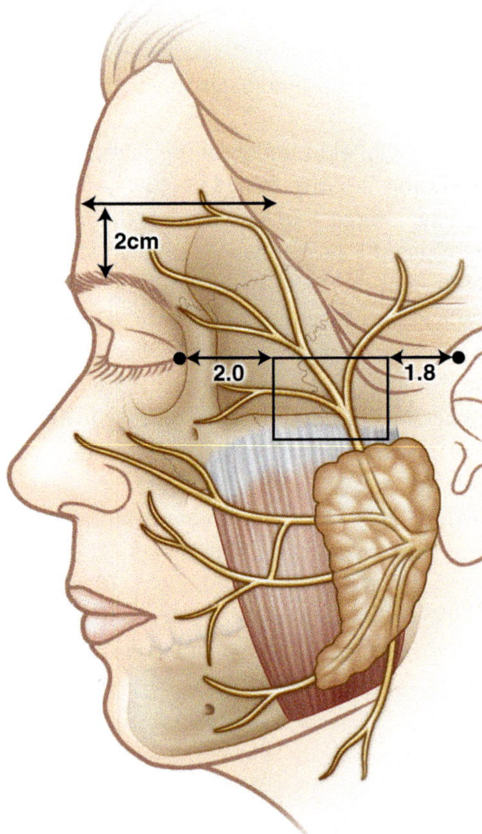

Fig. 28.9 Danger zone for the frontal branch of the facial nerve. Typically, four rami of the frontal branch of the facial nerve pass over the zygomatic arch. The most anterior rami runs about 2 cm posterior to the anterior zygomatic arch. The branch is almost always anterior to the superficial temporal vessels

difficult to ascertain. Supercut facelift scissors are utilized to complete the cervical dissection. Extensive cervical dissection may be necessary for individuals with significant neck skin laxity. The lateral cervical dissection is united with the central dissection that was created for the platysmaplasty and suction-assisted lipectomy. The inferior limit of the dissection is 4–5 cm below the angle of the mandible and at the level of thyroid notch. The surgeon must be cognizant of the external jugular as well as the great auricular nerve as they can be easily injured. Complete cervical dissection is necessary in patients with significant laxity to obtain exceptional results.

Once the cervical and facial dissections are completed independently, the interconnection region at the level of the angle of the mandible is elevated in a subcutaneous plane while the other areas are retracted (Fig. 28.11). Skin hooks are used in the facial and cervical regions to retract the ear and skin in the opposite direction to ensure a continuous level of dissection in the same plane. Furthermore, this technique allows increased protection of the marginal mandibular nerve. The anterior limit of this dissection is approximately 4–5 cm to preserve the continuity of the skin and SMAS layer as a functional unit as previously discussed. Facial liposuction is not recommended because of unpredictability of results.

Following complete elevation of the subcutaneous tissue in the facial and postauricular regions, the SMAS just anterior to the preauricular incision is grasped using a Brown Adson and excised using facelift scissors (Figs. 28.12 and 28.13). The SMAS is removed from the level of the root of the helix extending inferiorly to the infraauricular platysma. The SMAS could be safely undermined to the level of the anterior border of the parotid. For patients with significant facial laxity, the sub-SMAS dissection can be carried out bluntly past the anterior border of the parotid. This should be done with extreme caution. The edges of the SMAS are then imbricated with multiple buried 3–0 PDS sutures to suspend the continuous skin and SMAS layer in a posterosuperior direction

(Fig. 28.14). The direction of the SMAS suspension will depend on the patient's level of laxity and must be customized for each individual.

At this point, the excess skin is then redraped and excised to complete the rhytidectomy. The goal of skin redraping is to minimize tension in the facial region, while distributing any potential tension in the postauricular region of the occipital hair tuft. This portion of the procedure is critical for the outcome. A Brown Adson forcep is used to aid in the calculation of excess skin excision followed by placement of multiple anchor points to reapproximate the skin in the facial region (Fig. 28.15). Any intervening excess skin is then removed. The skin is then closed in two layers, with the helical root serving as the first major anchor point (AP1). Once AP1 has been determined and set using a 3–0 PDS suture, any excess temporal hair tuft superior to this point is excised using a No. 15 scalpel. The hair bearing temporal region is then closed using staples in a superior to inferior fashion to prevent potential "dog ear" deformity. Because the temporal incision is limited, no significant alteration in hairline positioning is experienced.

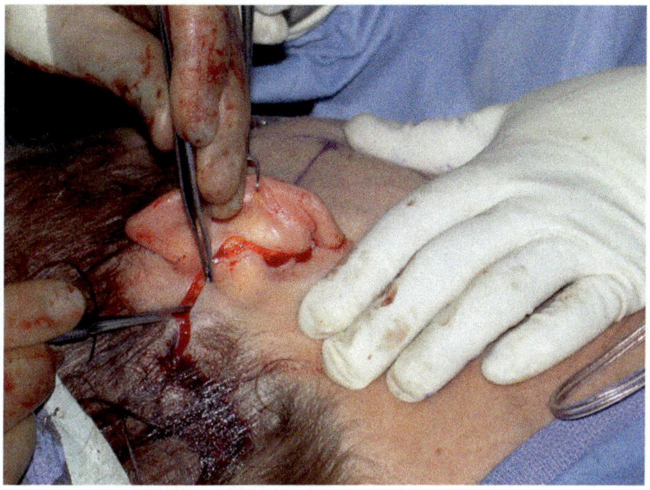

Fig. 28.10 Postauricular skin flap elevation. This posterior dissection is more fibrous and difficult than the anterior dissection. Facelift scissors and double-pronged hooks are utilized to complete the cervical dissection. The inferior limit of this dissection is 4–5 cm below the angle of the mandible. An extensive cervical elevation is performed in order to join the submental dissection

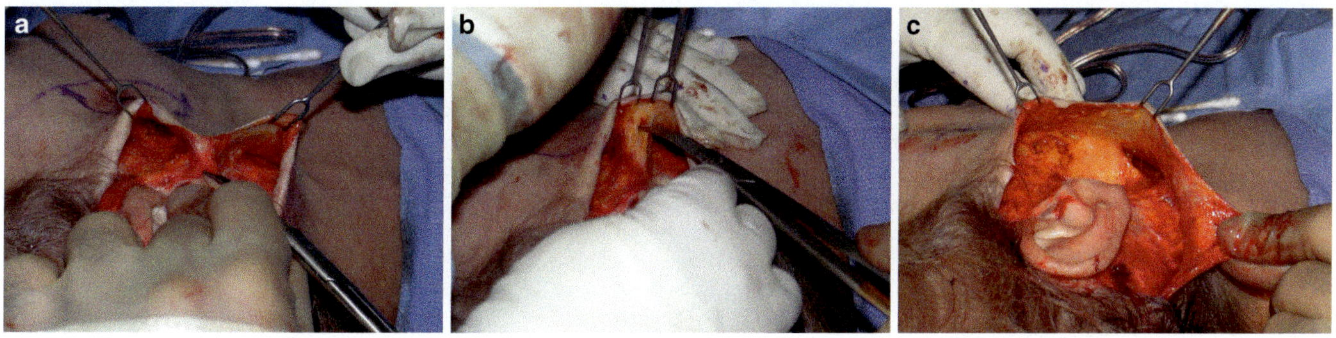

Fig. 28.11 The upper facial dissection and cervical dissection are joined. Once the cervical and superior facial dissections are completed, the lower facial subcutaneous elevation at the level of the angle of the mandible is performed (**a**). Hooks are placed on the facial and cervical regions as the ear and facial skin are retracted in opposite direction (**b**). The dissection is usually carried out for 4–5 cm (**c**).

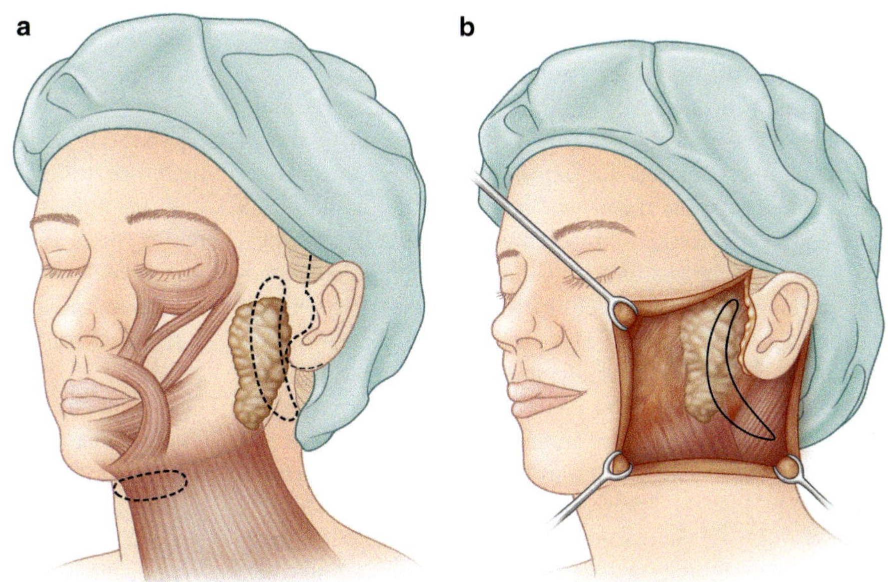

Fig. 28.12 Outline of the SMAS excision. A segment of SMAS is excised 1–2 cm anterior to the preauricular incision at the level of the root of the helix and extends inferiorly down to the infraauricular platysma (**a**, **b**)

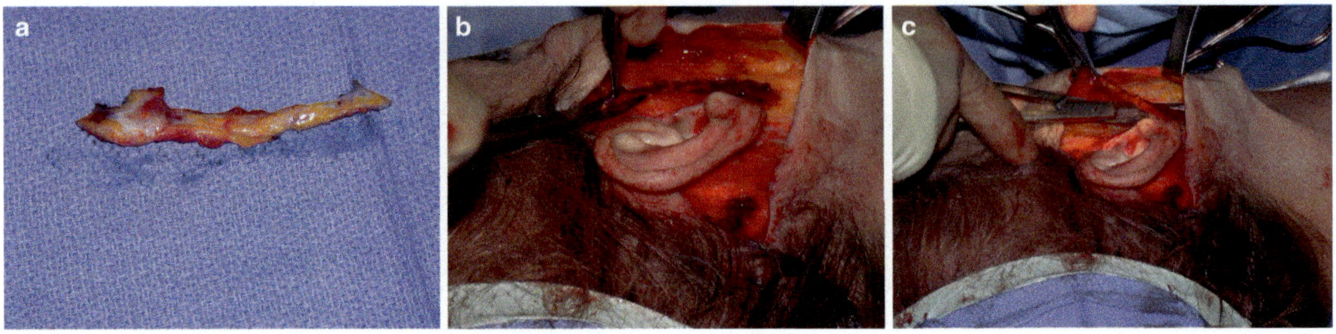

Fig. 28.13 Intraoperative excision of SMAS. A segment of SMAS is excised using Brown Adson and facelift scissors (**a**). The excision starts 1–2 cm anterior to the preauricular incision at the level of the root of the helix and extends inferiorly down to the infraauricular platysma (**b**, **c**)

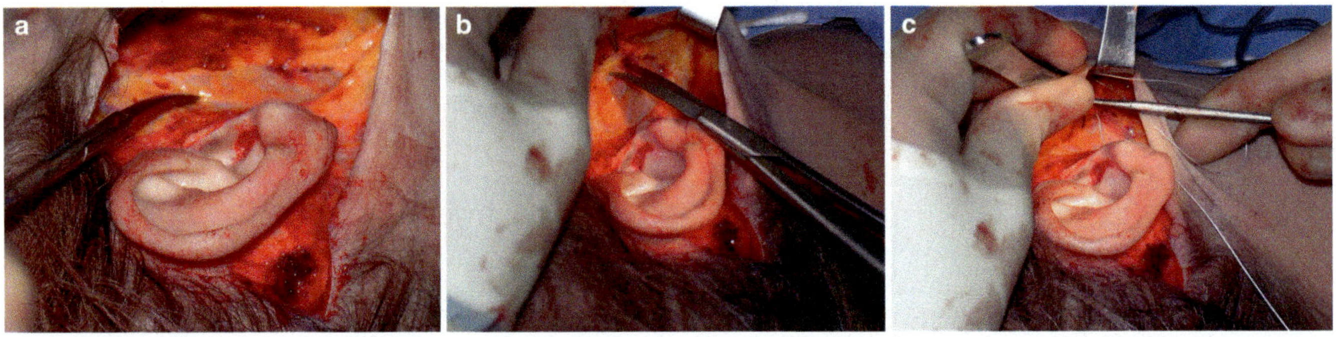

Fig. 28.14 SMAS imbrication. The anterior segment of the SMAS is elevated up to the anterior border of the parotid gland (**a**, **b**). The SMAS is imbricated with buried 3–0 Mersilene sutures (**c**). Multiple buried horizontal mattress sutures are placed. A posterosuperior vector is used for the SMAS imbrication.

The level of the antitragus serves as the second anchor point (AP2). Once AP2 has been placed, the intervening skin between AP1 and AP2 is judiciously excised to avoid over-excision of the skin, which can lead to a widened scar and displacement of the tragus anteriorly. A natural pretragal cleat should be surgically fashioned to conceal the facelift incision. This is easily completed by using facelift scissors and curved iris scissors to thin the newly positioned facial skin draped over the tragus. A buried, interrupted 4–0 PDS suture is then placed into the dermis of the skin flap to artificially recreate the anatomic tragal notch and to prevent inadvertent anterior displacement of the tragus during healing. The third anchor point (AP3) is placed toward the apex of the postauricular region. A single hook is then placed at the distal edge of the occipital incision to allow realignment of the skin and allows identification of the excess occipital skin that needs to be excised. Following excision, the occipital hairline is loosely approximated using deep dissolvable sutures followed by placement of staples to close the hair-bearing occipital hair tuft. The tissue between AP2 and AP3 is draped over the ear lobule to assess the amount of skin to excise. Facelift scissors are then used to carefully incise the postauricular excess skin, as the apex will become the anchor point of the lobule attachment (AP4). The excess skin between AP-2 and AP-4 is excised using a No. 15 scalpel to score the skin followed by excision using tenotomy scissors. Aggressive skin removal will lead to pixie ear deformity; therefore limited tension at AP4 is critical.

Prior to closure of the epidermal layer in the preauricular region, there should be a lack of tension following closure of the dermal layer. Should any tension be noted, additional subdermal absorbable sutures should be placed. Medium-sized Jackson-Pratt drains are placed prior to closure. Alternatively, Tisseel Fibrin Sealant (Baxter, Mississauga, ON, Canada) can be used to eliminate the need for drains. The preauricular incision is closed using a running locking 6–0 Nylon or Prolene suture between AP1 and AP4. In the postauricular region, a 4–0 plain gut suture is used to close the skin. The submental incision is closed with a 6–0 Nylon suture. Ice, placed in sterile gloves, is used throughout the

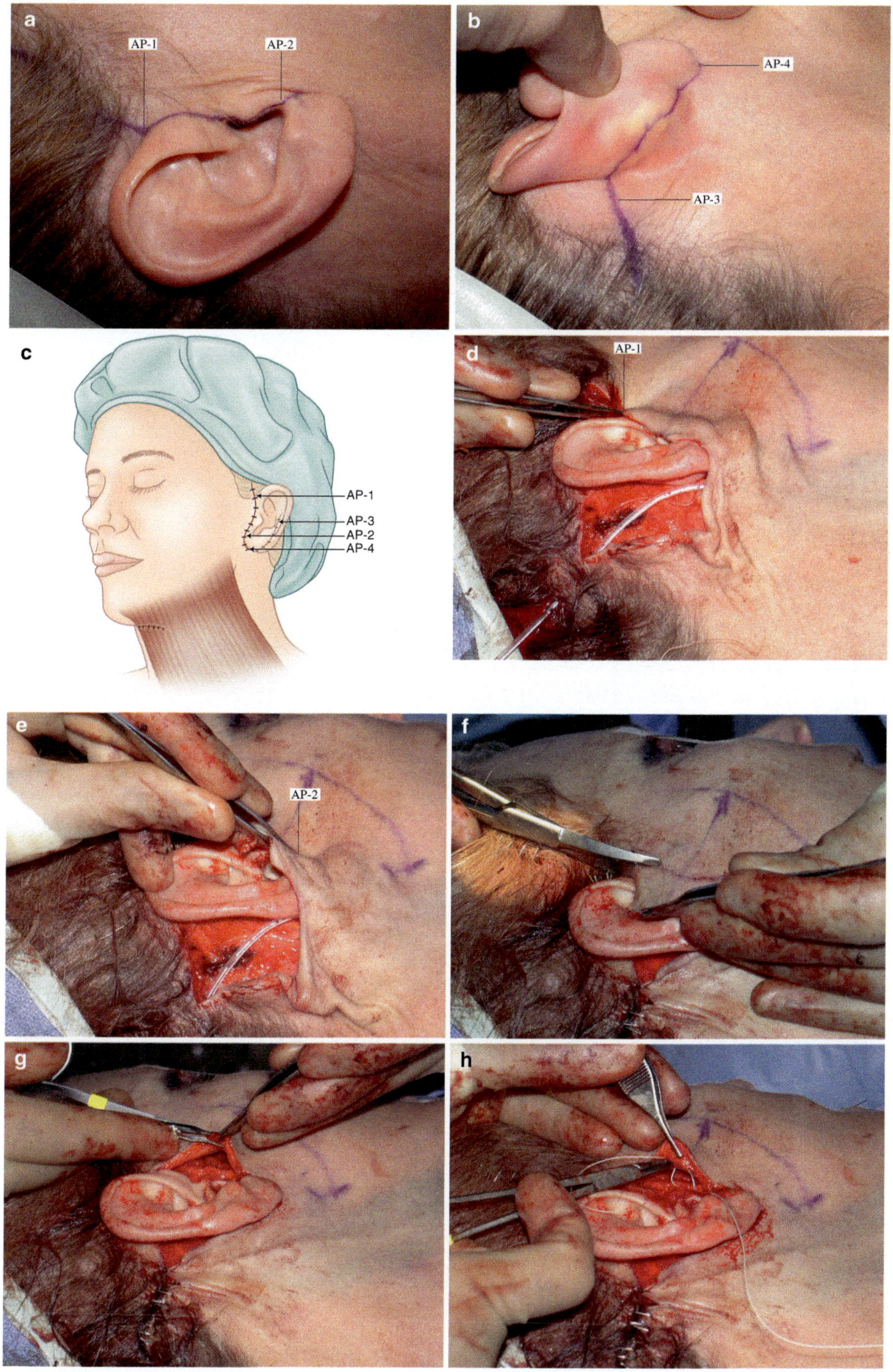

Fig. 28.15 Skin tailoring. Several anchor points are utilized for tailoring the skin (**a–c**). The root of the helix (AP-1) serves as the first anchor point (**d**). Once this location has been set, excess temporal hair tuft superior to AP-1 is excised and staples are used for closure. The second anchor point (AP-2) is at the level of the antitragus (**e**). The intervening skin between the first and second anchor point is removed

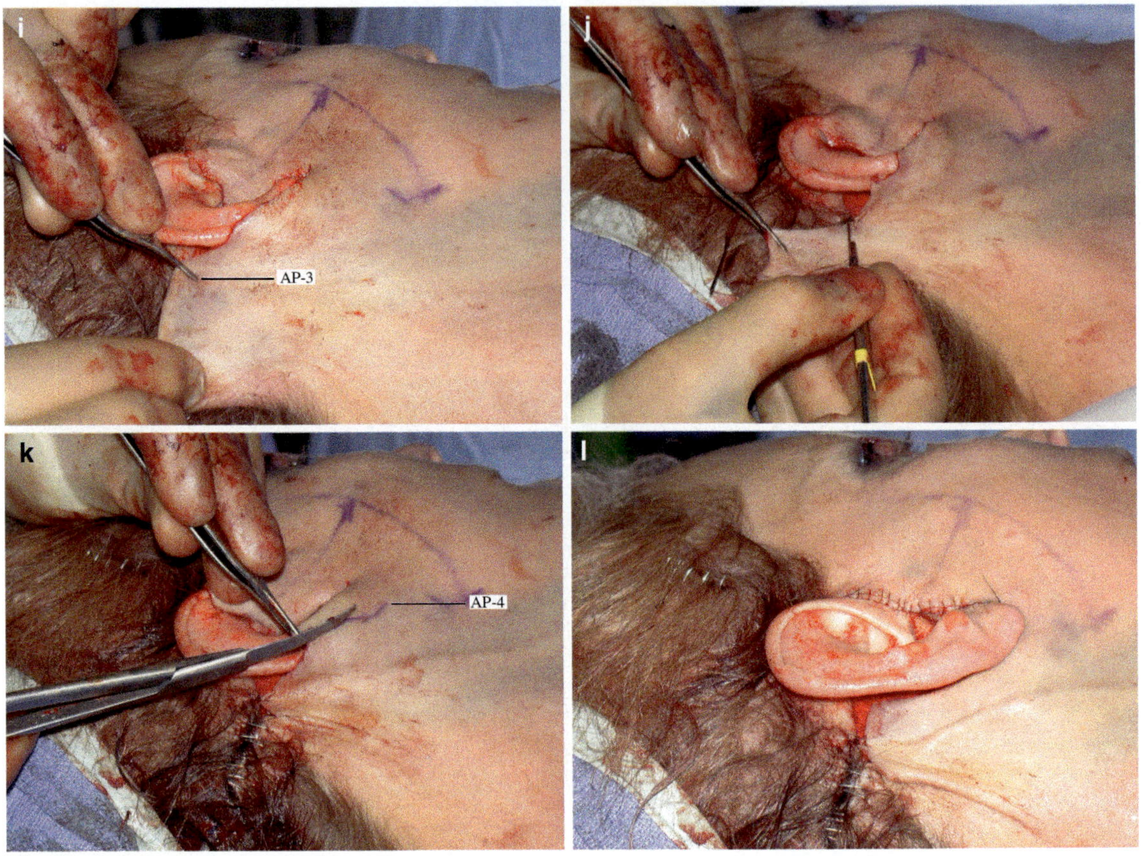

Fig. 28.15 (continued) (**f**) using curved iris scissors. The newly positioned facial skin over the tragus is aggressively thinned (**g**). A Vicryl suture is used to create a pretragal cleat; it penetrates the dermis of the facial skin and secured to the pretragal tissue (**h**). The third anchor point (AP-3) is the apex of postauricular incision (**i**). Excess occipital skin is excised with the help of a hook (**j**). The occipital hairline is aligned with deep dissolvable sutures. The intervening tissue between AP-2 and AP-3 is draped over the ear lobule (**k**). The inferior border of the lobule is then used to make a split into this intervening skin. The apex of this incision becomes the anchor point of lobule attachment (AP-4). The excess skin between AP2 and AP-4 is excised. In the postauricular area, the skin between AP-3 and AP-4 is also trimmed conservatively. The preauricular incision is closed with a 6–0 Nylon in a running locking manner (**l**)

procedure to promote vasoconstriction and limit perioperative ecchymoses. As discussed in earlier sections, volume restoration is a key component of facial rejuvenation and most patients at this point will undergo multilevel fat grafting, most commonly in the midface and prejowl sulcus regions. At the conclusion of all the procedures, a circumferential pressure dressing is placed and the patient is transported to the recovery room.

28.7 Postoperative Care

It is recommended that patients stay in an after-care facility for 24–48 hours where registered nurses can provide personal postoperative care, although patients can choose to recover at home if assistance is available. Patients are encouraged to elevate their heads and use cool compresses for the first 72 hours to minimize perioperative ecchymoses. Antibiotics, analgesics, sleep, and anti-nausea medications are prescribed for the recovery period.

Patients are seen on postoperative day No. 1 for dressing and drain removal as well as wound inspection. Hydrogen peroxide and antibiotic ointment are generously and continuously applied to keep the wounds clean and moist for the first 5 days. A Velcro head wrap is used continuously while the patient is at home during the first postoperative week. Patients are allowed to take light showers starting on the postoperative day No. 2. The preauricular sutures and all staples are removed on the seventh postoperative day and Steri-strips (3M, St. Paul, MN) are applied. The patients return around the fourth postoperative week for follow-up. At this follow-up visit, if indicated, dermal fillers, volumizers, and neuromodulators are used to address the midface as well as any perioral and periorbital rhytids (Figs. 28.16–28.18).

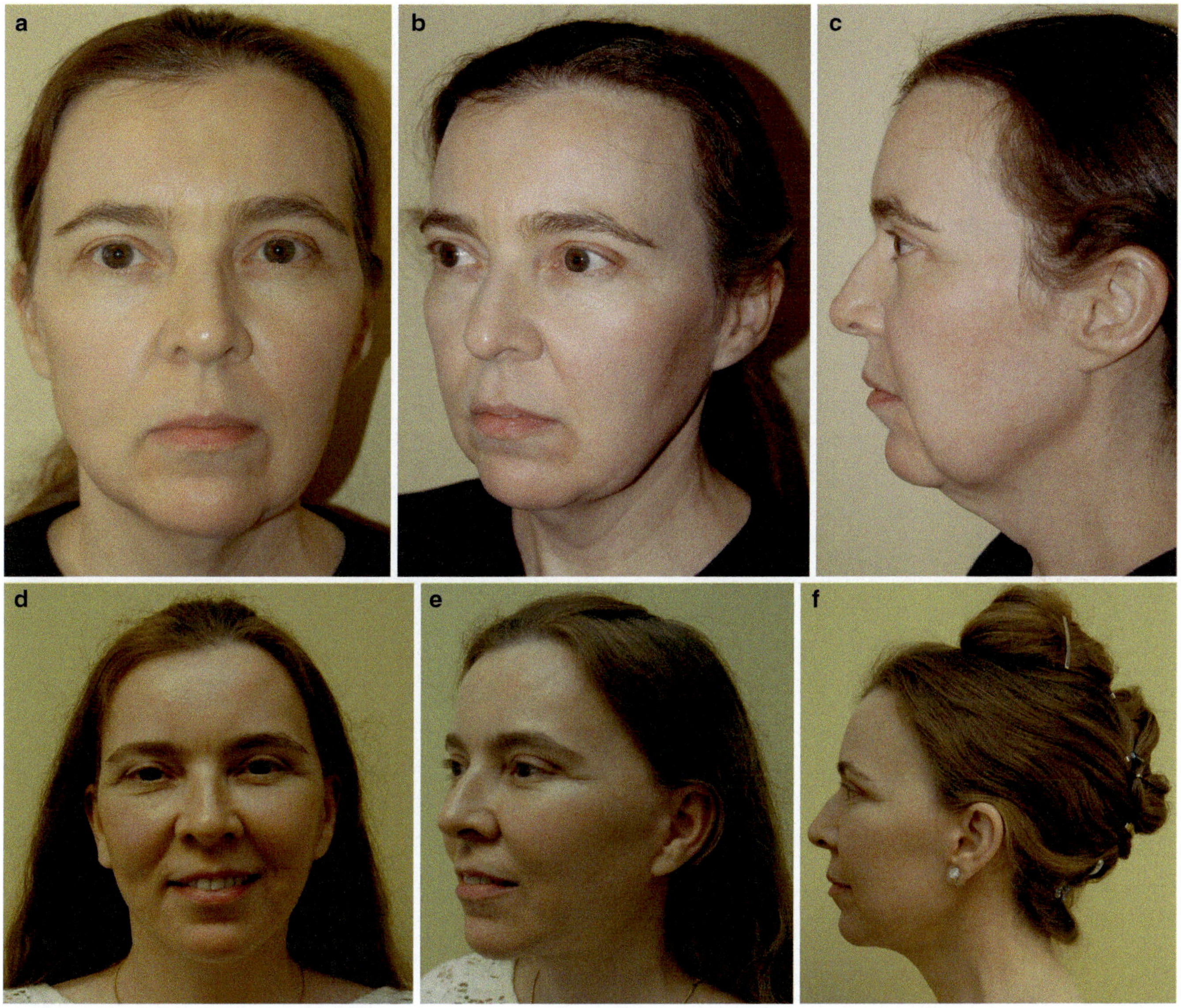

Fig. 28.16 Preoperative (**a–c**) and postoperative (**d–f**) photos of a patient who underwent short-flap SMAS rhytidectomy, upper blepharoplasty, and multilevel fat grafting.

Table 28.4 Potential complications

Cervicofacial hematoma
Alopecia
Poor scarring
Contour irregularities
Skin slough
Infection
Numbness
Need for revision surgery
Facial nerve injury

28.8 Potential Complications

Potential complications associated with the SFR are listed in Table 28.4. While the rate of cervical hematoma, postauricular skin necrosis, alopecia, and numbness is tantamount to other facelift techniques, our experience has shown that the SFR has a lower risk of facial hematoma, flap necrosis, and facial nerve palsy. The rate of revisional surgery has been observed to be similar to other SFR techniques.

28.9 Future Considerations

With the advent of less invasive facial rejuvenation options, patients' demand for minimally invasive procedures have skyrocketed over the past decade. This trend is expected to continue into the twenty-first century. The future of facial rejuvenation will likely depend on a combination of surgical and nonsurgical modalities to yield ideal results. While the advent of longer lasting fillers, volumizers, and noninvasive

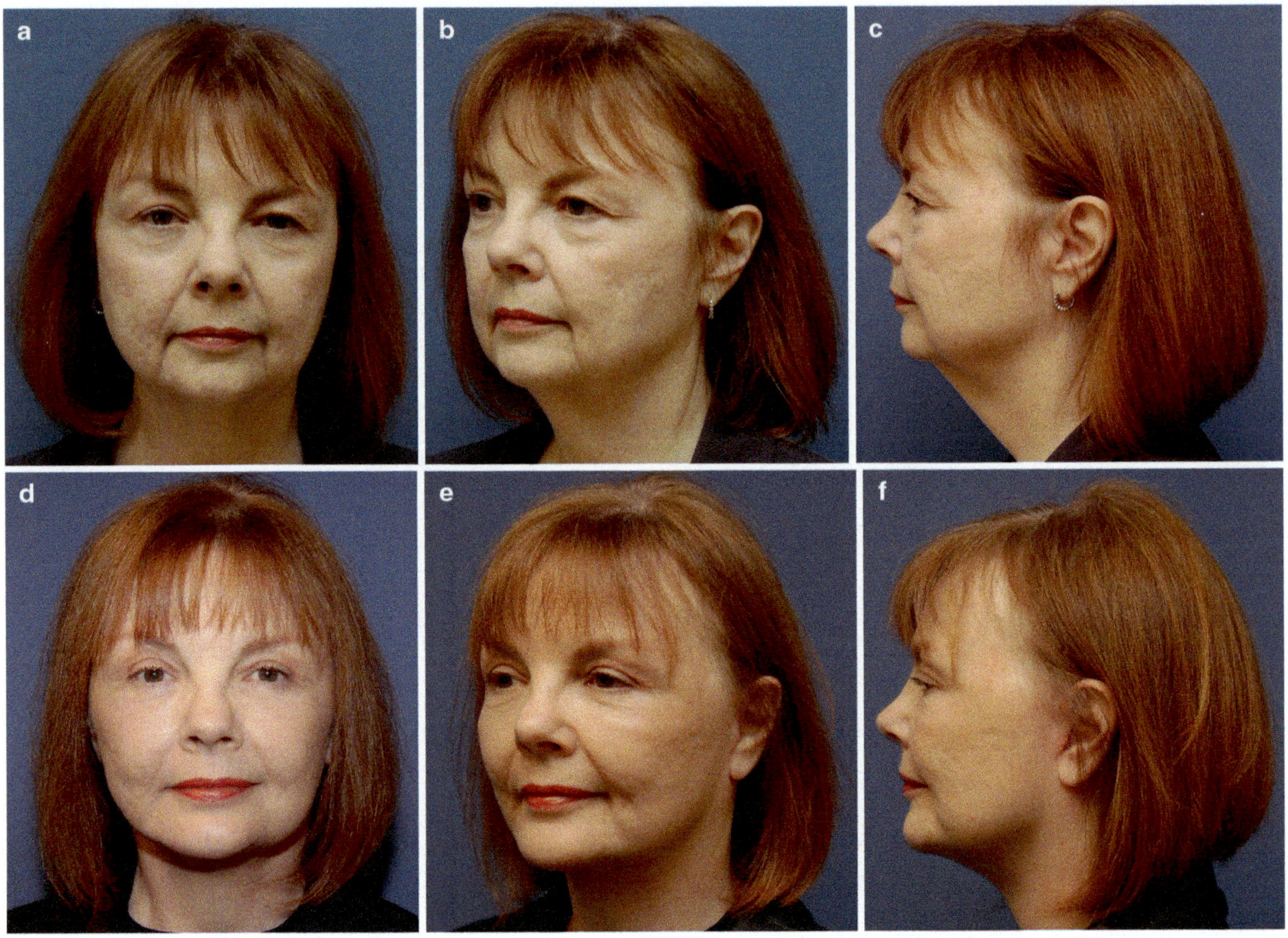

Fig. 28.17 Preoperative (**a–c**) and postoperative (**d–f**) photos of middle-aged female with aging face who underwent short-flap SMAS rhytidectomy, multilevel fat grafting, and blepharoplasty

tightening technology may diminish those interested in receiving surgery, time-tested surgical procedures, such as facelifts, blepharoplasty, fat grafting and brow lifts, will continue to be critical methods for maximizing facial rejuvenation results.

References

1. Bettman A. Plastic and cosmetic surgery of the face. Northwest Med. 1920;19:205.
2. Bourget J. La disparition chiurgicale des rides et plis du visage. Bull Acad Med (Paris). 1919;82:183.
3. Aufricht G. Surgery for excessive skin of the face. In: Transactions of the second international congress of plastic surgery. Edinburgh: Livingstone; 1960. p. 495.
4. Guerrero-Santos J, Espaillat L, Morales F. Muscular lift in cervical rhytidoplasty. Plast Reconstr Surg. 1974;54:127.
5. Webster RC, Smith RC, Papsidero MJ, et al. Comparison of SMAS plication with SMAS imbrication in face lifting. Laryngoscope. 1982;92:901.
6. Skoog T. Plastic surgery: new methods and refinements. Saunders: Philadelphia; 1974.
7. Mitz V, Peyronie M. The superficial musculoaponeurotic system (SMAS) in the parotid and cheek area. Plast Reconstr Surg. 1976;58:80.
8. Owsley Jr JO. SMAS-platysma face lift. Plast Reconstr Surg. 1983;71(4):573.
9. Fodor PB. Platysma-SMAS rhytidectomy – a personal modification. Aesthet Plast Surg. 1982;6(3):173.
10. Jost G, Lamouche G. SMAS in rhytidectomy. Aesthet Plast Surg. 1982;6(2):69.
11. Kamer FM, Halsey W. The two-layer rhytidectomy. Arch Otolaryngol. 1981;107(7):450.
12. Adamson JE, Todsu AE. Progress in rhytidectomy by platysma-SMAS rotation and elevation. Plast Reconstr Surg. 1981; 68(1):23.
13. Rees TD, Aston SJ. A clinical evaluation of the results of submusculo-aponeurotic dissection and fixation in face lifts. Plast Reconstr Surg. 1977;60(6):851.
14. Baker DC. Lateral SMASectomy. Plast Reconstr Surg. 1997;100(2): 509.
15. Hamra ST. The deep plane rhytidectomy. Plast Reconstr Surg. 1990;86(1):53–61; discussion 62.

16. Hamra ST. Composite rhytidectomy. Plast Reconstr Surg. 1992;90(1):1.
17. Kamer FM. One hundred consecutive deep plane face lifts. Arch Otolaryngol Head Neck Surg. 1996;122:17.
18. Godin MS, Johnson CM. Deep plane/composite rhytidectomy. Facial Plast Surg. 1996;12(3):231.
19. Alsarraf R, Johnson CM. The aging face: a systematic approach. WB Saunders: Philadelphia; 2002.
20. Baker SR. Triplane rhytidectomy. Combining the best of all worlds. Arch Otolaryngol Head Neck Surg. 1997;123:1167.
21. Tessier P. Lifting facial sous-perioste. Ann Chir Plast Esthét. 1989;34:193.
22. Psillakis JM, Rumley TO, Carmargos A. Subperiosteal approach as an improved concept for correction of the aging face. Plast Reconstr Surg. 1988;82:383.
23. Ramirez OM. The subperiosteal approach for the correction of the deep nasolabial fold and the central third of the face. Clin Plast Surg. 1995;22(2):341.
24. Ramirez OM, Maillard GF, Musolas A. The extended subperiosteal facelift: a definitive soft tissue remodeling for facial rejuvenation. Plast Reconstr Surg. 1991;88:227.
25. Ramirez OM. Endoscopic full facelift. Aesthet Plast Surg. 1994;18:363.
26. Ramirez OM. Three-dimensional endoscopic midface enhancement: a personal quest for the ideal cheek rejuvenation. Plast Reconstr Surg. 2002;109(1):329–40; discussion 341.
27. Quatela VC, Choe KS. Endobrow-midface lift. Facial Plast Surg. 2004;20(3):199.
28. Williams III EF, Vargas H, Dahiya R, et al. Midfacial rejuvenation via a minimal-incision brow-lift approach: critical evaluation of a 5-year experience. Arch Facial Plast Surg. 2003;5(6):470.
29. Quatela VC, Jacono AA. The extended centrolateral endoscopic midface lift. Facial Plast Surg. 2003;19(2):199.
30. Isse NG. Endoscopic facial rejuvenation: endoforehead, the functional lift. Aesthet Plast Surg. 1994;18:21.
31. Webster RC, Davidson TM, White MF, et al. Conservative face lift surgery. Arch Otolaryngol. 1976;102(11):657.
32. Webster RC, Smith RC, Smith KF. Face lift. Part I: extent of undermining of skin flaps. Head Neck Surg. 1983;5:525.
33. Webster RC. Facelifts: conservative vs. radical. In: Ward P, Berman W, editors. Plastic and reconstructive surgery of the head and neck. CV Mosby Co: St. Louis; 1984. p. 363–82.
34. Webster RC, Hamdan U, Fuleihan N, et al. The considered and considerate facelift. Am J Cosmet Surg. 1985;2:1.
35. Burgess LP, Casler JD, Kryzer TC. Wound tension in rhytidectomy: effects of skin flap underminig and superficial musculoaponeurotic system suspension. Arch Otolaryngol Head Neck Surg. 1993; 119(2):173.
36. McCollough EG, Perkins SW, Langsdon PR. SASMAS suspension rhytidectomy. Arch Otolaryngol Head Neck Surg. 1989;115:228.
37. Rees TD, Liverett DM, Guy CL. The effect of cigarette smoking on skin flap survival in the face lift patient. Plast Reconstr Surg. 1984;73:911.
38. Adamson PA, Moran ML. Complications of cervicofacial rhytidectomy. Facial Plast Surg Clin North Am. 1993;1(2):257.
39. Rohrich RJ, Pessa JE. The fat compartments of the face: anatomy and clinical implications. Plast Reconstr Surg. 2007;119(7):2219–27.
40. Lambros V. Fat injection for aesthetic facial rejuvenation. Aesthet Surg J. 1997;17(3):190–1.
41. Glasgold M, Lam SM, Glasgold R. Autologous fat grafting for cosmetic enhancement of the perioral region. Facial Plast Surg Clin North Am. 2007;15(4):461–70.
42. Coleman SR. Structural fat grafting: more than a permanent filler. Plast Reconstr Surg. 2006;118(3 Suppl):108S–20.
43. Furnas DW. The retaining ligaments of the cheek. Plast Reconstr Surg. 1989;83(1):11.
44. Stuzin JM, Baker TJ, Gordon HL. The relationship of the superficial and deep facial fascias: relevance to rhytidectomy and aging. Plast Reconstr Surg. 1992;89(3):441.
45. Hoefflin SM. The extended supraplatysmal plane (ESP) face lift. Plast Reconstr Surg. 1998;101(2):494.
46. Mendelson BC. SMAS fixation to the facial skeleton: Rationale and results. Plast Reconstr Surg. 1997;100(7):1834–42.
47. Ozdemir R, Kilinc H, Unlu RE, et al. Anatohistologic study of the retaining ligaments of the face and use in face lift: retaining ligament correction and SMAS placation. Plast Reconstr Surg. 2002;110(4):1134.
48. Mendelson BC, Muzaffar AR, Adams WP. Surgical anatomy of the midcheek and malar mounds. Plast Reconstr Surg. 2002;110:885.
49. Muzzaffar AR, Mendelson BC, Adams WP. Surgical anatomy of the ligamentous attachments of the lower lid and lateral canthus. Plast Reconstr Surg. 2002;110:873.
50. Seckel BR. Facial danger zones: avoiding nerve injury in facial plastic surgery. St. Louis: Quality Medical; 1994.
51. Owsley JQ. Rejuvenation of the midface. Plast Reconstr Surg. 2001;108(1):262.
52. Owsley JQ, Zweifler M. Midface lift of the malar fat pad: technical advances. Plast Reconstr Surg. 2002;110(2):674.
53. Owsley JQ. Face lifting: problems, solutions, and an outcome study. Plast Reconstr Surg. 2000;105(1):302.
54. Owsley JQ, Fiala TG. Update: lifting the malar fat pad for correction of prominent nasolabial folds. Plast Reconstr Surg. 1997;100(3):715.
55. Becker FF, Bassichis BA. Deep-plane vs. superficial musculoaponeurotic system placation face-lift. Arch Facial Plast Surg. 2004;6:8.
56. Ivy EJ, Lorenc ZP, Aston SJ. Is there a difference? A prospective study comparing lateral and standard SMAS face lifts with extended SMAS and composite rhytidectomies. Plast Reconstr Surg. 1996; 98(7):1135.
57. Binder WJ. Submalar augmentation: a procedure to enhance rhytidectomy. Ann Plast Surg. 1990;24(3):200.
58. Anderson JR. The tuck-up operation, a new technique of secondary rhytidectomy. Arch Otolaryngol. 1975;101(12):739.
59. Kamer FM, Parkes ML. Sequential rhytidectomy. Laryngoscope. 1978;88(7 Pt 1):1196.
60. Kamer FM. Sequential rhytidectomy and the two stage concept. Otolaryngol Clin North Am. 1980;13(2):305.
61. Rees TD, Aston SJ. Complications of rhytidectomy. Clin Plast Surg. 1978;5:109.
62. Baker DC. Complications of cervicofacial rhytidectomy. Clin Plast Surg. 1983;10(3):543.
63. Dedo DD. "How I do it" – plastic surgery. Practical suggestions on facial plastic surgery. A pre-operative classification of the neck for cervicofacial rhytidectomy. Laryngoscope. 1980; 90(II Pt I):1894.

Index

G.G. Massry et al. (eds.), *Master Techniques in Blepharoplasty and Periorbital Rejuvenation*,
DOI 10.1007/978-1-4614-0067-7, © Springer Science+Business Media, LLC 2011

C

G

H

Q

R

S